FAMILY PSYCHOPATHOLOGY

Family Psychopathology

The Relational Roots of Dysfunctional Behavior

Edited by

LUCIANO L'ABATE

THE GUILFORD PRESS
New York   London

© 1998 The Guilford Press
A Division of Guilford Publications, Inc.
72 Spring Street, New York, NY 10012
http://www.guilford.com

Printed in the United States of America

This book is printed on acid-free paper.

Last digit is print number: 9 8 7 6 5 4 3 2

Library of Congress Cataloging-in-Publication Data

Family psychopathology: the relational roots of dysfunctional
  behavior / Luciano L'Abate, editor.
      p. cm.
  Includes bibliographical references and index.
  ISBN 1-57230-369-7
  1. Family—Mental health. 2. Family psychotherapy. I. L'Abate,
Luciano, 1928- .
RC455.4.F3H354 1998
616.89′156—DC21   98-13462
                                                       CIP

*To the memory of Michael J. Goldstein, PhD, who
devoted most of his academic career
to the study of family psychopathology—as
a rigorous teacher, first-class researcher,
and unequaled gentleman.*

Contributors

Steven R. H. Beach, PhD, Department of Psychology, University of Georgia, Athens, Georgia

Thomas N. Bradbury, PhD, Department of Psychology, University of California, Los Angeles, Los Angeles, California

Ewald Johannes Brunner, MD, Institut für Erziehungswissenschaften, Lehrstuhl für Pedagogische Psychologie, Universität Jena, Jena, Germany

Victor G. Cicirelli, PhD, Department of Psychological Sciences, Purdue University, West Lafayette, Indiana

Manfred Cierpka, MD, Abteilung für Psychosomatische Kooperationsforschung und Familien Therapie, Universität Heidelberg, Heidelberg, Germany

Vittorio Cigoli, PhD, Centro Studi di Ricerche sulla Famiglia, Dipartimento di Psicologia, Universita' Cattolica del Sacro Cuore, Milan, Italy

Mario Cusinato, PhD, Centro Interdipartimentale di Ricerca sulla Famiglia, Dipartimento di Psicologia Generale, Universita' degli Studi, Padua, Italy

Mary E. Dankoski, PhD, Family Studies Center, Purdue University, Calumet, Hammond, Indiana

Joanne Davila, PhD, Department of Psychology, University of California, Los Angeles, Los Angeles, California

Frank D. Fincham, PhD, School of Psychology, University of Wales, Cardiff, Wales, United Kingdom

Hiram E. Fitzgerald, PhD, Department of Psychology, Michigan State University, East Lansing, Michigan

Ana G. Gardano, PhD, Department of Professional Psychology, George Washington University, Washington, D.C.; private practice, Chevy Chase, Maryland

Jan R. M. Gerris, PhD, Institute of Family Studies, University of Nijmegen, Nijmegen, The Netherlands

Deborah Gorman-Smith, PhD, Institute for Juvenile Research, University of Illinois, Chicago, Chicago, Illinois

Robert W. Heffer, PhD, Department of Psychology, Texas A&M University, College Station, Texas

Jan M. A. M. Janssens, PhD, Institute of Family Studies, University of Nijmegen, Nijmegen, The Netherlands

Gregory J. Jurkovic, PhD, Department of Psychology, Georgia State University, Atlanta, Georgia

Achim Kraul, PhD, Schwerpunkt Familientherapie, Georg-August-Universität, Göttingen, Germany

Luciano L'Abate, PhD, Department of Psychology, Georgia State University, Atlanta, Georgia; Institute for Life Empowerment, Atlanta, Georgia

Alexandra Loukas, PhD, Program for Prevention Research, Arizona State University, Tempe, Arizona

Ian R. Nicholson, PhD, London Health Sciences Centre, London, Ontario, Canada; Department of Psychiatry, University of Western Ontario, London, Ontario, Canada

Matthias Petzold, PhD, Department of Psychology, Universities of Dusselfdorf and Cologne, Germany

Lisa A. Piejak, PhD, Department of Psychology, Michigan State University, East Lansing, Michigan

Elena Quintana, PhD, Institute for Juvenile Research, University of Illinois, Chicago, Chicago, Illinois

Günter Reich, PhD, Schwerpunkt Familientherapie, Georg-August-Universität, Göttingen, Germany

Karen H. Rosen, EdD, Department of Human Development, Virginia Tech, Falls Church, Virginia

Matthew R. Sanders, PhD, Parenting and Family Support Centre, School of Psychology, University of Queensland, Brisbane, Queensland, Australia

Eugenia Scabini, PhD, Centro Studi di Ricerche sulla Famiglia, Universita' Cattolica del Sacro Cuore, Milan, Italy

Douglas K. Snyder, PhD, Department of Psychology, Texas A&M University, College Station, Texas

Patrick H. Tolan, PhD, Institute for Juvenile Research, University of Illinois, Chicago, Chicago, Illinois

Terry S. Trepper, PhD, Family Studies Center, Purdue University, Calumet, Hammond, Indiana

Wolfgang Tschacher, PhD, Universitare Psychiatrische Dienste, Universität Bern, Bern, Switzerland

Geoffrey R. Twitchell, MA, Department of Psychology, Michigan State University, East Lansing, Michigan

Nicole M. C. Van As, MA, Institute of Family Studies, University of Nijmegen, Nijmegen, The Netherlands

Paul M. A. Wels, PhD, Institute of Family Studies, University of Nijmegen, Nijmegen, The Netherlands

Robert A. Zucker, PhD, Departments of Psychiatry and Psychology, and University of Michigan Alcohol Research Center, University of Michigan, Ann Arbor, Michigan

Contents

FAMILY PSYCHOPATHOLOGY

Introduction

LUCIANO L'ABATE

PURPOSE OF THIS BOOK

The purpose of this book is to bring together diverse sources that cover the broad spectrum of family psychopathology not only from a research viewpoint, but also from theoretical, preventive, and therapeutic perspectives (Goldstein, 1988). The influence of the family on individual functional or dysfunctional behavior is still a matter of controversy and debate (Rowe, 1994). However, thus far no one has disputed or disproved the overall conclusion that functional individuals generally grow up in functional families and that dysfunctional individuals generally grow up in dysfunctional ones. To dispute or disprove this conclusion, one would need to demonstrate that dysfunctional individuals grow up in functional families and that functional individuals grow up in dysfunctional families. This argument, of course, depends on what is meant by "functional" and "dysfunctional." The controversy about this issue is still very much alive, as seen in Bergner's (1997) provocative paper and all the replies to it in the same journal issue (a list too long to include here). I hope that this book will be able to clarify the meanings of both attributes. If not, it will add fuel to the same fire.

Most of the mounting literature in psychological journals of all types, not just those in the area of family therapy, suggests that links between family and individual behavior are real, strong, and influential (Erel & Burman, 1995). Although the research literature is replete with studies that link individual with family behavior (Auhagen & Hinde, 1997), to date there is no encyclopedic treatise that covers all the literature in this area. One attempt at such a treatise in Great Britain (Frude, 1991) has not received the attention it deserves in the United States. A more recent

1

contextual and relational theory of personality socialization in the family and other settings makes the family the most important influence in the development of both functional and dysfunctional behavior (L'Abate, 1994a; L'Abate & Baggett, 1997, 1998).

Most textbooks and handbooks of abnormal psychology or psychopathology do mention (often in passing) the family as being one of the many causes or antecedents of psychopathology. However, this mention is more like lip service, because the orientation of most traditional textbooks in this area remains individually monadic at best or intrapsychic at worst; it is rarely contextual and certainly not relational (Mischel & Shoda, 1998). The "bad seed" theory of psychopathology is still rampant in the field of psychology and psychopathology, as indicated by emphases on psychopathology's neurological and physiological causations or concomitants (Heynes, 1992). In contrast to this viewpoint, supported mainly by geneticists and summarized fairly recently by Rowe (1994), there is the opposing viewpoint that most psychopathology, *in the absence of gross physical or physiological evidence,* is due to faulty or incomplete socialization (Frude, 1991; Helmersen, 1983; L'Abate, 1994a, 1994b; L'Abate & Baggett, 1997; White, 1991). Hence, the present volume gathers most of the evidence available to date in order to assess whether the family is indeed the major influence in the development of individual and family psychopathology. As indicated in Chapter 5, culture does have a distinct role in fostering psychopathological outcomes as well, but cultural influences (Cooper & Denner, 1998) are filtered through the family (in addition to occurring in such settings as work and leisure-time activities, as suggested in the past by Murphy, 1947).

Contributors, nominated by consensus from a distinguished panel of advisors, were requested to consider critically the evidence gathered to date in support of or in opposition to a socialization viewpoint. Only studies of individual functional, dysfunctional, or psychopathological behavior linked to family variables were considered. In contrast to previous treatises of psychopathology, where little if any consideration has been given to contextual studies of psychopathology, contributors were asked to stress instead those very studies that do evaluate the individual–family link. Is this link real or wishful thinking? Is this link a substantive one or just a figment of family therapists' imagination?

There is no doubt in my mind that a treatise of this kind is needed to summarize the status of this field. It is inevitable that this work will be needed by professionals, researchers, teachers, and students in the area of abnormal psychology, whether they are members of the disciplines of psychology, social work, family studies, family therapy, nursing, and psychiatry. Whether this book will eventually replace existing textbooks or other works in abnormal psychology remains to be seen. Nothing old is usually replaced with the new in the mental health literature; it is just added to existing knowledge.

The closest publication to this topic is the work of Jacob (1987), which was a very important and excellent contribution. However, by now it may be considered dated, since so much research has been done since its publication. Furthermore, Jacob's text was concerned with many methodological issues that, although relevant to the general topic of family psychopathology, may have detracted from the overall coverage of psychopathology. For instance, only 5 of the 17 chapters were dedicated to psychopathological topics (schizophrenia, depression, alcoholism, childhood psychopathology, and psychopathology from a genetic perspective). As the table of contents of the present work indicates, there is more to family psychopathology than these topics. This work is an attempt to make sure that the field is covered thoroughly and well.

The more recent *Handbook of Developmental Family Psychology and Psychopathology* (L'Abate, 1994b) may invite further comparison. At first blush, there may be a great deal of overlap between that book and the present work. In the 1994 handbook, however, 7 out of 20 chapters were devoted to dysfunctionalities from the viewpoint of the individual, marital, and family life cycles (marital conflict and divorce; mental illness and the family; chronic illness; and physical, sexual, psychological, and substance abuse). The present book, on the other hand, does not have as much of a developmental slant as the previous one. Of course, development is included, since this is not a topic that can be ignored (as many chapters attest). Most of the chapters in the 1994 book referred to the major antecedents or "roots" of psychopathology—mainly of physical, sexual, and emotional abuse—rather than to nosological psychiatric syndromes. The present book is more specific in that regard. It focuses on a more comprehensive, yet traditional, psychiatric classification of disorders. Whereas the 1994 book contained just one chapter on the implications of a developmental and contextual viewpoint for clinical practice, the present book includes one chapter on preventive approaches, one on parental training programs, and one on family therapy.

An even more important, very comprehensive contribution to the field of family psychopathology has been published under the editorship of Florence W. Kaslow (1996). Both the 1994 and the 1996 books are the forerunners and predecessors of the present one. I hope, however, that this book covers a much broader and much more differentiated domain than was possible earlier—that is, the family *qua* family. This book expands on and covers in greater specificity and detail whatever might have been covered previously. By now there is much more research on family psychopathology than was available just a few years ago, as indicated by the recent paper by Shealy (1995) on parental correlates of offspring psychopathology, and by a special issue of the *Clinical Psychology Review* entirely devoted to "The Impact of the Family on Child Adjustment and Psychopathology" (Faust, Bellack, & Hersen, 1995).

The contextual and relational family-oriented paradigm can be considered a part of the ecological perspective (Tudge, Gray, & Hogan, 1997). Tudge et al., in contrasting ecological perspectives with the traditional intrapsychic, nonrelational, and acontextual views, stated:

> These perspectives have never been at the forefront of psychology, particularly as practiced in the United States, where it has been and continues to be dominated by an experimental and reductionistic model adopted from the physical sciences, rather than an ecological perspective derived from biology. Although some psychologists have argued for a more holistic approach (considering the interrelatedness of individual, physical, sociohistorical, and cultural aspects of development), the discipline has been dominated by those who have taken a dichotomous stance on the relation between the individual and the environment. (p. 75)

In contrast to an internal, acontextual, nonrelational, physiological perspective, the ecological, family-oriented perspective has been strengthened by the arguments of Harrop, Trower, and Mitchell's (1996) review. Harrop et al. argued, as has been argued elsewhere (L'Abate & Baggett, 1997), that genetics and physiology (and, by extension, nature) may not in fact determine the most damaging of all psychopathologies (i.e., schizophrenia); instead, physiological differences may be produced by factors in socialization (nurture). That is, instead of internal factors' determining the course of this condition, external factors may produce as well as maintain this condition, and may even produce and maintain internal physiological and metabolic processes.

Harrop et al.'s review, however, falls short of explaining *how* symptoms of schizophrenia (or any other clinical condition, for that matter) are produced. If they are not produced internally, what kind of external context produces them? Hence, the present volume takes over where previous authors have feared to tread—that is, arguing that the most powerful determinant of individual psychopathology is the family. This statement does not mean that other settings, such as school/work and leisure-time activities, may not be just as powerful at different stages in the life cycle (L'Abate, in press-a, in press-b). Moreover, there may be predisposing conditions, either physiological, characterological, or both (i.e., temperament). However, thus far the search for a specific pathogenic gene for any genetic or physiological condition, aside from demonstrable brain damage, has been questionable if not unsuccessful.

Strong support for the socialization of functional and dysfunctional behavior, rather than for its origins in internal, acontextual factors, comes from at least six independent lines of research. Additional sources have been reviewed elsewhere (L'Abate & Baggett, 1997). The present discussion of these research lines is limited by my own knowledge. There may be additional sources of evidence unknown to me, as well as research that refutes this conclusion.

The first line of research consists of Gottman, Katz, and Hooven's (1996) work on metaemotions, thinking about emotions, and ways emotions are expressed within the family. These investigators found that "parental meta-emotion philosophy [relates] to parenting, *to child regulatory physiology*, to emotion regulation abilities in the child, and to child outcomes in middle childhood" (p. 243; emphasis added). Hence, what seemed a far-fetched hypothesis from past, internally oriented, acontextual viewpoints may indeed become an established position once contextual variables are considered.

The second line of research only adds evidence along the same lines. In a review of the role of expressed emotion (EE) in affective disorders—in addition to their role in the maintenance, if not the origins, of schizophrenia—Coiro and Gottesman (1996) found that "depressed patients with a high-EE relative are 13 times more likely to relapse than those with a low-EE relative" (p. 310). More often than not, the high-EE relative was a parent or a sibling.

The third line of research (Free, Alechina, & Zahn-Waxler, 1996) found that untreated depressed mothers may pass on to their children an inclination to distort and confuse such emotions as anger, sadness, contempt, disgust, and fear. These are the very same emotions found by Gottman et al. (1996) to be relevant to self-regulation in children. Especially in adults (Gottman, 1994), the emotions of contempt and disgust predispose adults to higher risk for divorce.

The fourth line of research consists of the work of Kiecolt-Glaser et al. (1996). Blood samples were taken from 90 newlywed couples at several points during a discussion that in some cases turned into an argument. In the latter case, women showed a significant increase in stress hormones (epinephrine, cortisol, and norepinephrine) and a consequent decrease in certain aspects of immune functions. The men did not show any relationship between conflict episodes and the release of stress hormones.

In the fifth line of research, Zajonc and Mullally (1997) demonstrated that birth order as an independent variable in intellectual test scores:

> The correspondence between the test trends and family trends is remarkable. Regression equations showed that the aggregate birth order was by far the major source of variation in test scores, for it alone accounted for as much as 81% of variance in SATs, 86% in the A-levels, and 89% in the Iowa scores. (p. 685) ... The trends and changes in scores ... are a clear reflection of family patterns, confirming the important role of environmental factors, and especially family and peer influences, which have been repeatedly downsized and outsourced in favor of genetic hypotheses. (p. 698)

The sixth line of research consists of the work of Reiss et al. (1995), who "sought to determine the relationship between differences in parenting styles and depressive symptoms and antisocial behavior in adolescence, and to compare the influence of these nonshared experiences with genetic influences" (p. 925). Parenting styles in 708 families were assessed via questionnaires and via video recordings of interactions between parents and adolescents. Reiss et al.'s findings were as follows:

> Almost 60% of variance in adolescent antisocial behavior and 37% of variance in depressive symptoms could be accounted for by conflictual and negative parental behavior directed specifically at the adolescent. In contrast, when a parent directed harsh, aggressive, explosive, and incon- sistent parenting toward the sibling [of the adolescent], we found less psychopathological outcome in the adolescent. (p. 925)

An additional line of research is found in the work of Dietz (1996). He and his collaborators discovered the negative effects that "inactivity" produces on the body. In addition, he and his collaborators followed up 854 boys and girls born in the late 1960s through young adulthood. These researchers found that among children younger than 10, having an over- weight parent roughly doubles the risk of a child becoming a heavy adult, even if the youngster is still of normal size. This is the first study to document the influence of parents' sizes on their children at very early ages.

This area requires further study, of course. However, it is most interesting that researchers are now finding evidence suggesting that physi- cal factors such as body weight, as well as emotional and personality factors, may be transmitted from one generation to the next via family influence rather than simply inheritance.

PLAN OF THE BOOK

The sections of this book follow a straightforward sequence, from general and abstract to more specific and concrete. The first section explores the overall foundations of this field. The first chapter, by, Eugenia Scabini and Vittorio Cigoli, reviews the role of theory in the study of family psychopa- thology. Without theory to give direction, it would be conceptually and practically impossible to understand the individual–family link. For Chapter 2, Alexandra Loukas, Geoffrey R. Twitchell, Lisa A. Piejak, Hiram E. Fitzgerald, and Robert A. Zucker take their title from the title of a paper originally given by sociologist E. W. Burgess in 1926. They explore changes in the structure and function of the family in today's American society. In Chapter 3, Matthias Petzold focuses on the concept of "the family" in family psychology; he notes that unless family psychology takes into account the broad diversity of living patterns in today's society, its useful- ness will be limited.

Historically, most theories of the family *qua* family have been either sociological or therapeutic, without much attention to the individual–family link. It is high time for family psychologists to become involved in looking at this link in its functional and dysfunctional implications. This is the very link covered in Chapter 4 by Ewald Johannes Brunner. Family therapy may have been the forerunner in stressing the importance of this link. On the other hand, it is just as important to establish empirical bases for clinical practices. These practices were originally dominated by vague and grandly (if not grandiosely) encompassing but unverifiable metaphors generated by general systems theory. Finally, just as the individual does not grow up in a relational vacuum, the family does not exist in a cultural vacuum. That is, a family's structure and functioning cannot be separated from its culture. Consequently, in Chapter 5, Ana C. Gardano shows how cultural differences contribute even greater variability and complexity to the individual–family–culture link. How is one to separate one element in this link from the others?

These discussions at abstract and general levels in the introductory section are followed by greater specificity and concreteness in Section II, "Dimensions of Family Structure." In Chapter 6, Joanne Davila and Thomas N. Bradbury consider the marital dyad: How do personal adjustment factors in partners as individuals affect their long-term adjustment as individuals and as a couple? This individual–couple link is probably the most important factor in determining the outcome of the offspring, because it produces the very family climate that may lead either to functionality or to dysfunctionality. In Chapter 7, Mario Cusinato expands on the link between parental styles and family psychopathology. Again, is this link a real one, based on reliably and validly established evidence, or has it been created by common sense and public opinion?

In Chapter 8, Victor G. Cicirelli examines the effects of multigenerational relationships and the extended family. It is often said that it takes three generations to develop dysfunctionality in one offspring. How many generations are needed to develop functionality? How much does "modernity" contribute to the development of functional or dysfunctional patterns? In Chapter 9, Robert W. Heffer and Douglas K. Snyder cover the topic of family assessment, evaluation, and diagnosis. How do we distinguish a functional from a dysfunctional family? If this differentiation cannot be made even empirically, how can it be reached impressionistically and subjectively (i.e., clinically)? Unfortunately, single and normative reliance on the interview, as practiced by most couple and family therapists, is insufficient to establish a meaningful and reliable differentiation between functional and dysfunctional families. There are probably more books published about family evaluation than there are therapists actually practicing it with a variety of instruments, in addition to the interview.

The third section, "Varieties of Individual and Family Psychopathology," is where the real substance of this book lies. What family patterns lead to what kinds of individual, marital, and family psychopathology? In Chapter 10, Gregory J. Jurkovic reviews the evidence concerning one of the most pernicious, yet difficult-to-measure, pathogenic processes: that of parentification, whereby the oldest child is given parental responsibilities over the younger siblings. If we could link data from this chapter to the individual, marital, and relational characteristics of couples as partners and couples as parents (reviewed in Chapters 6 and 7, respectively), it may become possible to predict which families will tend to use this pattern and which will not. In Chapter 11, Steven R. H. Beach and Frank D. Fincham cover one of the major but still often unreported and undetected determinants of family psychopathology—depression in either partner or in both. To add to the list of determinants, Ian R. Nicholson, in Chapter 12, summarizes the kind of family patterns that seem to predict and produce schizophrenia. Expressed emotions (EE) and communication deviance, two abusive patterns that thus far are well verified, may be the very determinants that will allow us to predict this extreme condition better than any physiological or genetic linkage can.

In Chapter 13, Manfred Cierpka, Günter Reich, and Achim Kraul not only review the evidence for psychosomatic illness, but raise extremely relevant questions about the issue of specificity: Which family patterns will predict externalization and which will predict internalization, and, in its extreme form in the latter case, psychosomatic illness? In Chapter 14, Karen H. Rosen reviews the role of the family in the production and maintenance of aggression and violence. This is another of the many battlegrounds over the role of nature versus nurture. Thus far, socialization patterns seem to predict externalization as well as, and internalization patterns as well as or better than, internal factors do. These patterns may turn out to be produced by the family context or nurture, rather than by heredity or nature. Is the jury in or out in this regard? In Chapter 15, Terry S. Trepper and Mary E. Dankoski review the relationship between family psychopathology and substance abuse and dependence within the context of systemic vulnerabilities to substance misuse. What kind of metabolic and physiological changes do substance abuse and dependence produce in individuals? Is this another area where nurture supersedes nature?

Section IV is titled "Helping Families at Risk, in Need, and in Crisis." In Chapter 16, Patrick H. Tolan, Elena Quintana, and Deborah Gorman-Smith review prevention approaches for families in need of targeted social skill training programs; in Chapter 17, Jan R. M. Gerris, Nicole M. C. Van As, Paul M. A. Wels, and Jan M. A. M. Janssens review various parenting programs for families at risk of possible breakdown in the future. In Chapter 18, Matthew R. Sanders reviews the empirical status of psychological interventions with families of children and adolescents, including crisis intervention as well as psychotherapy. Although originally many family therapists, flush with their success, took (at times smugly and even arrogantly) a decidedly antiempirical stance, it has dawned on many that without an empirical basis for clinical practice, the field would not survive under the onslaught of managed care constraints.

In Chapter 19, which constitutes the book's fifth and final section, Wolfgang Tschacher reviews some of the methodological problems in studying family psychopathology. Ideally, knowledge of these problems will help researchers and clinicians alike to improve their research and to link it more specifically with clinical practices (L'Abate, in press-a, in press-b).

REFERENCES

Auhagen, A. E., & Hinde, R. A. (1997). Individual characteristics and personal relationships. *Personal Relationships, 4,* 63–84.

Bergner, R. M. (1997). What is psychopathology? And so what? *Clinical Psychology: Science and Practice, 4,* 235–248.

Coiro, M. J., & Gottesman, I. I. (1996). The diathesis and/or stressor role of expressed emotion in affective illness. *Clinical Psychology: Science and Practice, 3,* 310–322.

Cooper, C. R., & Denner, J. (1998). Theories linking culture and psychology: Universal and community-specific processes. *Annual Review of Psychology, 49,* 559–584.

Dietz, W. H. (1996). The role of lifestyle in health: The epidemiology and consequences of inactivity. *Proceedings of the Nutrition Society, 55,* 829–840.

Erel, O., & Burman, B. (1995). Interrelatedness of marital relations and parent–child relations: A meta-analytic review. *Psychological Bulletin, 118,* 109–132.

Faust, J., Bellack, A. S., & Hersen, M. (Eds.). (1995). Special issue: The impact of the family on child adjustment and psychopathology. *Clinical Psychology Review, 15*(5), 371–474.

Free, K., Alechina, I., & Zahn-Waxler, C. (1996). Affective language between depressed mothers and their children: The potential impact of psychotherapy. *Journal of the American Academy of Child and Adolescent Psychiatry, 35,* 783–790.

Frude, N. (1991). *Understanding family problems: A psychological approach.* Chichester, UK. Wiley.

Goldstein, M. J. (1988). The family and psychopathology. *Annual Review of Psychology, 39,* 283–299.

Gottman, J. M. (1994). *What predicts divorce?: The relationship between marital processes and marital outcomes.* Hillsdale, NJ: Erlbaum.

Gottman, J. M., Katz, L. F., & Hooven, C. (1996). Parental meta-emotion philosophy and the emotional life of families: Theoretical models and preliminary data. *Journal of Family Psychology, 10,* 243–268.

Harrop, C. E., Trower, P., & Mitchell, I. J. (1996). Does the biology go around the symptoms?: A Copernican shift in schizophrenia paradigms. *Clinical Psychology Review, 16,* 641–654.

Helmersen, P. (1983). *Family interaction and communication psychopathology: An evaluation of recent perspectives.* London: Academic Press.

Heynes, S. N. (1992). *Models of causality in psychopathology: Toward dynamic, synthetic and nonlinear models of behavior disorders.* New York: Macmillan.

Jacob, T. (Ed.). (1987). *Family interaction and psychopathology: Theories, methods, and findings.* New York: Plenum Press.

Kaslow, F. W. (Ed.). (1996). *Handbook of relational diagnosis and dysfunctional family patterns.* New York: Wiley.

Kiecolt-Glaser, J. K., Newton, T., Cacioppo, J. T., MacCullum, R. C., Glaser, R. C., & Malarkey, W. B. (1996). Marital conflict and endocrine function: Are men really more physiologically more affected than women? *Journal of Consulting and Clinical Psychology, 61,* 324–342.

L'Abate, L. (1994a). *A theory of personality development.* New York: Wiley.

L'Abate, L. (Ed.). (1994b). *Handbook of developmental family psychology and psychopathology.* New York: Wiley.

L'Abate, L. (in press-a). How should a theory of personality socialization in the family be evaluated?: Strategies of theory testing. *Famiglia Interdisplinarita Ricerca.*

L'Abate, L. (in press-b). The discovery of the family: From the inside to the outside. *American Journal of Family Therapy.*

L'Abate, L., & Baggett, M. S. (1997). *The self in the family: Classification of personality, criminality, and psychopathology.* New York: Wiley.

L'Abate, L., & Baggett, M. S. (1998). *Personality socialization in the family and other settings.* Manuscript in preparation.

Mischel, W., & Shoda, Y. (1998). Reconciling processing dynamics and personality dispositions. *Annual Review of Psychology, 49,* 229–258.

Murphy, G. (1947). *Personality: A biosocial approach to origins and stucture.* New York: Harper.

Reiss, D., Howe, G. W., Simmens, S. J., Russell, D. A., Hetherington, E. M., Henderson, S. H., O'Connor, T. J., Law, T., Plomin, R., & Anderson, E. R. (1995). Genetic questions for environmental studies: Differential parenting and psychopathology in adolescents. *Archives of General Psychiatry, 52,* 925–936.

Rowe, D. C. (1994). *The limits of family influence: Genes, experience, and behavior.* New York: Guilford Press.

Shealy, C. N. (1995). From *Boys Town* to *Oliver Twist*: Separating fact from fiction in welfare reform and out-of-home placement in children an youth. *American Psychologist, 50,* 565–580.

Tudge, J., Gray, J. T., & Hogan, D. M. (1997). Ecological perspectives in human development: A comparison of Gibson and Bronfenbrenner. In J. Tudge, M. J. Shanahan, & J. Valsiner (Eds.), *Comparison in human development: Understanding time and context* (pp. 72–105). New York: Cambridge University Press.

White, J. M. (1991). *Dynamics of family development: A theoretical perspective.* New York: Guilford Press.

Zajonc, R. B., & Mullally, P. R. (1997). Birth order: Reconciling conflicting effects. *American Psychologist, 52,* 685–699.

SECTION I

—◆—

FOUNDATIONS

CHAPTER 1

The Role of Theory in the Study of Family Psychopathology

EUGENIA SCABINI
VITTORIO CIGOLI

The aim of this chapter is to highlight the theoretical aspects of the study of family psychopathology. As we will see, the role of theory in this area has changed as much for clinicians as for academic researchers. We first focus on the debate in the family field about normality versus pathology. We distinguish three phases of this debate. In the first phase, "strong" theories (psychoanalytic and systemic) were all the rage. However, psychoanalytic approaches were too individual-oriented to be adapted to family functioning, and systemic approaches did not actually focus on specifically distinguishing normal from pathological families; normality was seen merely as an absence of symptoms. This was followed by a phase in which normality came to be defined in terms of ideal functioning, and research and therapeutic models proliferated. Currently, theory-prone approaches are on the decline, as is beginning to be the case with the postpositivistic view, while more object-oriented approaches are gaining favor. We believe, though that theory must be given its due. In fact, giving up any thought of identifying psychological constructs able to "explain" the workings of the family obliges us either to accept a weak theoretical stance, which can only be basically self-referential and contextual, or to look elsewhere for a foundation—more often than not, in biology.

Second, we outline our own model. We stress both the specific identity of our object of study (family relationships), and three levels of family reality with specific constructs associated with them: the interactive, the relational, and the symbolic levels. Each of these has its own identity in space and time, and can provide plenty of information on the family. We believe that the theoretical model we present provides a suitable framework for both psychosocial and clinical research (Cigoli, 1993/1995; Scabini, 1995).

Finally, we focus on family psychopathology, comparing our relational (transgenerational, symbolic) approach with the psychoeducational and attachment approaches, and identifying similarities as well as differences among these viewpoints.

THE NORMALITY–PATHOLOGY DEBATE:
A BRIEF SURVEY

It is a generally acknowledged fact that the psychological approach to family studies has been affected by psychiatry. Links between forms of individual psychopathology (particularly, schizophrenia) and family relationships were intuited back in the 1950s and 1960s jointly and "across the board," as has been highlighted by all major historical accounts to date (Broderick & Schrader, 1991). In those years, investigations of these links followed one of two main approaches: the psychoanalytic approach (Ackerman and the Philadelphia school) or the systemic one (the Palo Alto school). However, the former was more clinical than theoretical. It geared the investigation toward identifying the mechanisms (basically defenses) underlying evolution or involution (regression), its attempt being to adapt a psychological theory centered on the individual to fit a strategy that had a group as its target (Ackerman, 1958). The systemic perspective generated a more lively and far-reaching theoretical debate, its attempt being to put forward a psychological theory accounting for normal as well as pathological family behavior. Actually, its pragmatic slant was more conducive to a strategy thriving on a closer link between theoretical and empirical research, which was indeed innovative. By actually monitoring families, sticklers for the systemic approach expected to gain better understanding of the rules underlying family behavior, whether such behavior was disturbed or not.

We can distinguish three phases of the evolution of the concepts of normality and pathology.

Phase 1: Observations of Pathological
versus Normal Families

As Haley (1972) stated, in the 1960s and 1970s the key questions raised by therapists and researchers alike could be summarized as follows:

1. Are families with an abnormal member different from families whose members are all "normal"?

2. Is a family with a member showing a given type of pathology (e.g., schizophrenia) different from a family with a member showing another type of pathology (e.g., delinquency)?

With a view to answering these questions, Haley thought it essential to back up the work of researchers with that of therapists. In fact, therapists resorted to research just to verify the theoretical diversity of pathology as opposed to normality, which was basically taken for granted in their everyday activity. Actually, the theoretical strategic/systemic view did not envisage *any* difference between normality and pathology. The symptoms of individual disturbance were nothing but failed attempts to solve an evolutionary crisis, and those very attempts were just part and parcel of the problem. This was a fine example, indeed, of a theoretical assumption that was not made explicit, but that nevertheless affected research. The data were there to prove what was actually the basic assumption. Consequently, systemic researchers and therapists just did their best to spot specific features pertaining to different types of families, which were distinguished according to their respective symptoms (the "anorexic" family, the "schizophrenic" family, etc.), with the "normal" family acting as control group (Ferreira & Winter, 1968). The normal family was viewed as such simply because of its lack of symptoms (Offer & Sabshin, 1974).

The most substantial body of research was thus devoted to the study of interaction (excellent reviews can be found in Jacob, 1975, and Doane, 1978). To researchers and therapists of all stripes, this approach did seem the safest ground on which to make substantial cognitive progress. However, as Eisler, Dare, and Szmuckler (1988) showed, such an approach proved unproductive. On the one hand, the needs of researchers were far too different from those of therapists; on the other hand, the experimental methodology adhered to was quite unsuitable for understanding the family as a whole.

Phase 2: Normal versus Pathological Functioning— From Mere Observation to the Building of Models

In the 1980s, the contrast between family normality and pathology took on newer and more critical overtones. To start with, it was no longer expected that the specific features of the various types of pathological families should surface vis-à-vis those of normal families. Rather, it became increasingly apparent that therapeutic practice in regard to pathological functioning was actually guided by the very concept of normal functioning. In Offer and Sabshin's (1974) words, there was a shift from normality viewed as the lack of symptoms typified by the control group to normality viewed as ideal functioning.

Thus therapists and researchers alike built their frames of reference into models. As we use the term, a "model" represents a construct halfway between theory and clinical practice. It actually identifies a number of variables within family functioning that prove useful to researchers and therapists alike. Klein and White (1996) maintain that "another kind of idea that must be distinguished from a theory is a model. A model is a representation of how something works. Models are usually scaled-down or simplified versions of complex relationships between phenomena. . . . Some scientific models are simplified versions of theories" (pp. 6–7).

The framing of theories contrasting normal with pathological functioning was the eventual result of models of intervention as they gradually developed out of actual clinical action. Thus, Broderick and Schrader (1991), in drawing up their history of family and couple therapy, provided contributors with a grid submitting questions such as these: "What does normal family functioning consist in? What does pathological functioning consist in?" In her important work, Froma Walsh (1982) formulated her hypothesis of normal versus disturbed functioning, and her related view of therapeutic goals, with reference to the chief models of family therapy (strategic, structural, psychodynamic, behavioral). The result, again, was a shift from a concept of normality viewed basically in a negative sense (lack of symptoms) to a concept of normality viewed in a positive sense (functioning). This brought about much stimulating debate and a wealth of models in the field of research proper (Olson, 1986; Hampson, Beavers, & Hulgus, 1988).

On the other hand, the new definition of normality also gave way to a different concept of pathology—this time not just defined in terms of sheer lack of something, but related to the actual resources available. In other words, therapists were asked to take into due account the actual resources of families when it came to planning treatment. Thus the new standpoint stressed not only the prerequisites of pathology, but also the prerequisites of health. By the way, this helped researchers and therapists to understand, for example, how high-risk children of seriously disturbed parents could manage to be "invulnerable" and avoid developing disturbed behavior (Wynne, Jones, & Al-Khayyal, 1982).

In a nutshell, the 1980s were the years of the proliferation of therapy and family functioning models. True enough, the theoretical energies that went into this proliferation spread themselves a bit too thin. However, contributors to the field also tried to build integrated models incapsulating within themselves all the key variables common to the various stances (Walsh, 1982).

Phase 3: The Decline of Theories as a Driving Force

However, in the late 1980s and 1990s, the effort to build models and to formalize the characteristics of both normal and pathological functioning appear to be on the decline, for a number of reasons:

1. From the point of view of therapy, theoretical aspects have actually been losing ground, since stances that used to be far apart have been gradually drawing closer together.
2. From the point of view of research, the "normal" family has proved to be less compact and uniform than expected when it has been examined more closely.
3. Radically new family forms have come to the fore of society, as a result of widely different cultural and ethnic realities.
4. Last, but not least, the theory–praxis relationship has undergone substantial change because of the shift in the conceptual framework.

In particular, the surge of the postpositivistic view of science has weakened the role of theory. In fact, in light of this new approach, any theory cannot help being self-referential and contextual, since each theory is restrained by and reflects the historical context in which it is generated (Boss, Doherty, La Rossa, Schumm, & Steinmetz, 1993). Standards for evaluating families keep cropping up, and all of them, especially in the social sciences, are clearly implicit in the respective theories. Thus, in the second edition of *Normal Family Processes*, Froma Walsh (1993) stresses the merely descriptive role of the expression "dysfunctional family," which must therefore be used with caution. Walsh now warns us against the danger of overpathologizing families: She maintains we must bear in mind that "individual problems are not invariably caused by family pathology" (p. 9).

Moreover, constructivist and social-constructivist positions, which are quite typical of the postpositivistic view and are all the rage now in other sectors of psychology, have basically changed the framework of the strategic and systemic approaches, at least according to some authors. Typical examples are supplied by Hoffman (1990), Goolishian and Anderson (1992), and White and Epston (1990). Such positions, if assumed radically, are actually conducive to theoretical–practical relativism and to a technique deprived of theory. The holders of these views have given up explaining family pathology. Instead, they are interested in defining the role of the therapist in new, more socially correct (less hierarchical) terms. The therapist is cocreator, together with the family, of new histories, which are being offered to the family members so that they can rely on a wider semantic scope of suggestions in order to better define the events they are involved in.

By attributing a limited role (if any) to theory, this approach strengthens the drive—always present in psychology—toward a reduction of psychic facts to mere biology. If therapists and researchers give up all efforts at finding out invariants (the categories underlying facts), they risk ousting psychology from the scientific field altogether by undervaluing the effort to identify regularities and make predictions. The universal features remaining are none other than the biological substratum of human nature (Donley,

1993). Thus, psychopathological symptoms and dysfunctions are often explained in terms of genetics of behavioral incompatibility, as is the case in the increasingly successful psychoeducational approach. Many commentators are actually trying to bypass this difficulty by smoothing the most radical stances. Thus, Boss et al. (1993), who in the early 1990s sided with the new trends in the family field (i.e., the trends toward greater professional inclusiveness, more theoretical and methodological diversity, more concern with language, more constructivist and contextual approaches, etc.), have more recently made a list of pitfalls and paradoxes these new trends give way to. In particular, they maintain that a radical constructivist position denying the power of reality is best avoided, and that standards for evaluating family theories must be firmly established.

We too believe that it is imperative for theory to be given its due, and, consequently, that epistemological aspects must be given due attention. By "epistemology" we mean the search for the foundations of any scientific approach to a given object of investigation. In actual fact, no one can possibly tackle the complexities of an object in constant flux (such as the family) by dreaming up a comprehensive theory, but one does have to make one's viewpoint and the constructs going with it quite explicit.

It is therefore possible to identify various levels of explanation, each autonomous in its own right and with its own method, and to show their articulation. Distinguishing different levels is not tantamount to actually integrating all of them into a whole. Each level has its own method and its own specificity. This strategy enables us to view things from a metatheoretical vantage point, and thus to detect points of convergence or divergence in the diverse levels. Identifying levels of analysis is a way of theorizing, and also of classifying and comparing different theoretical approaches. A number of authors, primarily in the sociological sector, have chosen to investigate the family by means of levels of analysis (Turner, 1991; Klein & White, 1996). The interpretative pattern we wish to put forward here tries to distinguish the main levels of the psychological analysis of the family.

LEVELS OF ANALYSIS OF FAMILY ORGANIZATION

Before we can point out the various levels though which we wish to investigate the family, it is imperative for us first of all to define the characteristics of this peculiar social group—in other words, to pinpoint, as it were, its very identity.

The family is not at all a simple object of study—far from it. Each culture is inclined to believe that the form of family most widespread in that specific culture and period is the only possible one. In fact, as Laslett and Wall (1972) duly showed in their investigation of the development of families in Europe, over the course of centuries a number of different types of families have evolved (nuclear, enlarged, multiple, etc.—now including broken families, stepfamilies, et al.). However, in order to investigate an object scientifically, we have to identify its basic traits (invariants), which remain such despite the different forms the family may have meanwhile taken on (and may still keep taking on). As a result, we need to define the very identity of the family in its structural and symbolic referents.

The family is a specific social form of human relationship with the features of a cultural universal (Lévi-Strauss, 1956; Héritier, 1996). In line with the organizational/relationship perspective of Sroufe and Fleeson (1988), we can say that the specific and universal aspect identifying the family is an organization of parental relationships based on a difference in gender (marital relationship) and a difference in generation (parental relationship). "Cultural and subcultural variations (extended families . . .) add complexities but typically do not alter these organizational features, and the common pattern well serves the central family features (i.e. the rearing of children and the meeting of adult intimacy support need)" (Sroufe & Fleeson, 1988, p. 42). If a family is in a position to fulfill its basic functions, it can reproduce itself through its children: "They internalize and take forward into adulthood both the capacity and inclination to nurture children and the meeting of adult intimacy support needs" (p. 43). However, if generational boundaries collapse—as is the case when children are pressed into the service of adult intimacy needs, or when gender-related expressions of intimacy are lacking—the family degenerates and shows symptoms of distress and pathology.

The exchanges between sexes and generations, which make up the specific aspects of family organization, can be conceptualized at three levels: interactive, relational and symbolic. Let us now consider these three levels separately.

The Interactive Level

When one is meeting a family for research or treatment, the level of exchange coming into play is interactive—literally, the "acting between" persons. True enough, the notion of interaction has now found pride of place in a number of diverse disciplines; yet, no precise definition of it has actually been supplied to date, given its complexity. In a nutshell, "interaction" can be defined as two or more phenomena affecting one another. In the social sciences, it is indeed defined as "the mutual influence the agents exert over their respective actions whenever they find themselves physically together. In this perspective, their action is de facto a joint action" (Trognon, 1991, p. 12; our translation). Be that as it may, from the very beginning of family studies interaction has proved to be the foundation of treatment. Research on family interaction can be traced back to the 1960s, when it was conducted very much in line with research on the social psychology of small groups. In this early phase, all those interested in the family—researchers and therapists alike—viewed this new and exciting psychosocial object of investigation as a system characterized by the interaction of one member with the other(s) as well as with the environment. Monitoring interaction is thus the major instrument to which both family research and therapy can resort.

This new approach has been fostered by two related factors. First, the gap between research and therapy has been getting smaller, and as a result, the respective objects of study and treatment have ended up sharing the same vision; second, greater scientific rigor is attained, thanks to the fact that the processes under scrutiny can now be duly quantified. More specifically, family researchers are now only too willing to buttress their pioneer studies with more established methods. For instance, they have borrowed a paradigm from social psychology in which interaction is somehow connected with the concept of the group, which in turn is viewed as a container or a background against which interactions can be investigated in their own right (Bales, 1950; Argyle, 1952; Hare, Borgatta, & Bales, 1955).

It is here that research on family interaction has its roots. Such research became full-fledged in the 1960s and the 1970s. As Eisler et al. (1988) pointed out, the chance to measure and classify interaction seemed to help researchers and therapists out of the quagmire they were bogged down in. As a matter of fact, their ventures were deemed to be not quite scientific, since they were simply untestable. However, as Eisler et al. duly noted, the greater the efforts to develop precise and viable measures of interaction became, the farther away the target of identifying psychological categories suitable for understanding the family as a group—as an organized whole—also became.

By the 1980s, researchers and therapists were well on the way to overcoming these difficulties. In point of fact, they managed to pinpoint the key dimensions of family interaction: cohesion, flexibility, intimacy, agreement–disagreement, support–aggression, communication, emotions, coalitions, power, and so on. In short, family research boils down to detecting transactive regularities in the here and now. It is thus possible to detect familial styles (formulated, as we have seen, in models), as well as functional and dysfunctional styles of marital interaction (Markman, 1981; Gottman & Levenson, 1992).

When it comes to treatment, the authors who have founded their approaches on problem solving (therapeuthic, structural, strategic, and behavioral models) are those who resort to interaction as the instrument for understanding the dysfunctional roles of the family system and stepping in. As is well known, the strategic model in particular has undergone transformations. To sum it all up in a few words, we can say that in the early phase the therapist, who viewed himself and herself as an observer outside the family, monitored the interactions between the family members with a view only to detecting the very rules and redundancies conducive to symptoms, in the attempt to prescribe behavior suitable for change. The approach was strictly behavioral, with the subjective aspects of the family members (meanings, motivations, expectations, and intentions) put aside, and the therapist's mind being just a "black box."

With the advent of second-order cybernetics (Von Foester, Prigogine, Haken, Varela, etc.), and the relationship of the system being watched and the system doing the watching changed radically. The therapist was no longer viewed as someone outside the family system, but as a member of the system itself. This way attention could be given to each individual as such, since each person is in a position to activate strategies, as well as to relational games geared to unveiling pathologies (Selvini Palazzoli, 1988). Morphogenetic aspects (positive feedback) and morphostatic mechanisms were also highlighted. In fact, the systemic model, which used to be typically behavioral in its setup, has undergone a thorough revision in cognitive and constructivist terms (Keeney, 1979; Keeney & Ross, 1984). Thus interaction proves to be made up not only of behavioral aspects but also of semantic and narrative components. Monitoring family members and getting them to interact through word and behavior are of paramount importance, both in research and in therapy. All clinical schools—although to different degrees—take this level into due account.

In short, the interactional level of analysis draws attention to the communication being exchanged in the here and now between family members (and/or the researcher/therapist). Reference is therefore made specifically to what happens and is being communicated between the participants, who here and now start and get interaction going. The spatial dimension centers on "here," whereas the temporal dimension centers on "now" (as well as on the sequence). As a rule, interaction comes into being through the constructs of distance–vicinity (cohesion) and of boundary (between family members and the social environment). Critical transitions in the life cycle and problem solving are investigated in terms of the flexibility (vs. rigidity) and abundance (vs. scarcity) of the strategies adopted. In turn, time is operationalized through the constructs of sequence (sequential process).

The Relational Level

Whether characterized by regularities or not, repeated interactions or sequences of interactive events do not encompass all that actually takes place in the exchange between persons. In fact, interaction casts into the shade what binds the subjects together: their sense of belonging. No one can possibly explain how an exchange can come about without hinting at what actually binds people together. What binds the members of a family together is the family history they share, and this cannot be reduced to the mere sum of the interactions hitherto performed. Any family history reflects a long-lasting tie or bind that is being continuously renewed and that is more than the sum of all exchanges between family members. This bind represents the relational level.

Too often, the relational level is used as a synonym for the interactional level. Its specificity is rarely taken into account. Instead, it precedes interaction (though not necessarily in a chronological sense) (Hinde, 1995). Interaction entails relationship, and vice versa, since interaction "fills up" relationship and lays the groundwork for it. And, in turn, relationship is the background against which interaction comes into its own. With reference to family vicissitudes, the unit of meaning is to be found at the relational level, where one can indeed read significance into interdependence/connection (and not just monitor sequences) and see the links among past, present, and future. Research on interaction focuses on the constructive level (what is actually being built jointly),whereas research on relationship focuses on the binding level (what is at once being structured and structuring), which "defines" and confines the subjects of the action. Relationship is the sediment that has meanwhile been sinking to the bottom. It is made up of norms, values, rites, models of behavior, and so on, but because of it, we perceive individuals as members of a family. Relationship therefore entails characteristics that pertain both to binding and to meaning. The etymology of "relationship" goes back to the Latin *re-fero* (which implies the meaning of "reference"), as well as to the Latin *re-ligo* (which conveys the meaning of "tie, bind").

Persons interacting and building a situation they share are not in a position actually to master the entire process. Partly, at least, the bind does have an impact on interaction. Sometimes those involved are not even aware of it; it is beyond their grasp. This goes without saying. Just think of how previous generations exert their influence over the family. The present members are subject to their generational history—after all, that is just what being a member of a family is all about. The specific aspect of relationship lies, then, in the processes of intergenerational transmission (Lieberman, 1979; Stierlin, 1972). Some events (e.g., death in the family, other losses) are indeed crucial to the intergenerational transmission (Walsh & McGoldrick, 1991). Relationship, which is by itself "vertical" (Carter & McGoldrick, 1980), is bound to affect interaction, which is by definition "horizontal." A member of a family is born into an order of action that is to a great extent quite unknown. Yet each person is called in to plan and build his or her relationship with the world—to come to grips with a story largely written by others. In fact, the parental systems with their transgenerational lines are what make up the generative devices, the cultural matrix of the individual life of each family member. And this is "the whole" that comes before and is actually more than the sum of its parts.

On the other hand, the intergenerational tie, binding though it might be, does not determine the action of the new generation. The latter is in fact called upon to bring to life a new family action/narration. In other words, each member of a single generation is personally responsible, although there is actually a more general responsibility pertaining to the generational line as a whole. Exchanges between generations can be more or less positive, and this is a key element of the bind/resource. Thus, a certain generation or a certain person in that generation, after interiorizing a positive quality drawn out of the intergenerational exchange, will find it easier to rewrite family or social history in a creative way, whereas another generation or person, burdened with some unhealthy experience, will not be quite up to the task and will be severely hampered. The latter's degrees of liberty are minimal (Framo, 1992). Nevertheless, these are degrees of actual liberty, which make the actions and decisions of the latest generation somewhat unpredictable.

Research has dealt with the relational aspect in a number of ways. Just think of the studies linking family psychology to the personality structure (L'Abate, 1994), the studies on the concept of family paradigm (Reiss, 1981), and the research on attachment theory (Main, Kaplan, & Cassidy, 1985; Doane & Diamond, 1994).

Therapy has generally stressed the psychodynamic intergenerational approach (Framo, 1992; Boszormenyi-Nagy & Spark, 1973; Paul, 1980; Williamson, 1981). However, in the past few years relational intergenerational aspects have been gaining ground. The Milan-based group of Nuovo Centro per lo Studio della Famiglia, for example, which started out from a rigidly interactive behavioral position, gradually got closer to the relational intergenerational stance, of which they are now among the leading representatives.

In order to gain insight into the family setup, one of the chief aims is to "dovetail" the interactive level with the relational level (and the other way round). Some researchers have actually done very well in this field. For instance, attachment researchers first stressed the interactive viewpoint (tackled through the "Strange Situation"), and complemented this later with the relational viewpoint (tackled through the Adult Attachment Interview). As for therapy, clinics espousing the psychodynamic intergenerational approach do get family members to interact, but on the whole, they basically focus on relational aspects viewed as "underground currents" (Framo, 1992) linking adult children to their parents. That is why particular attention is given to relational history and the modes of remembrance/memory.

Another important goal in therapy is inside the relational level itself: It consists of "dovetailing" the various types of relationship within the family. In particular, the relationship with the family of origin dovetails with the marital relationship. However, both theory and research have so far neglected to pursue this goal. Attachment researchers and therapists espousing the intergenerational approach (Donley, 1993) alike just "skip" the level of the couple.

We think it important, instead, to assign theoretical importance both to the intergenerational and to the marital relationships. We view the marital couple, for all its different degrees of liberty, as a living device geared to intergenerational transmission. It is a specific subsystem of generational exchange. The two partners represent the meeting point where the different family histories dovetail. As is the case with any encounter, there is a certain degree of unpredictability and emergency. It is, to a certain extent, "chancy." True enough, each of the two partners draws shortcomings and resources from his or her family of origin. Yet the couple's new bind does not quite amount to the sum of the partners' respective shortcomings and resources. This theoretical assumption can be backed up by empirical data. For instance, research contrasting "healthy" families with families with a young drug addict (Cigoli, 1994) showed that negative intergenerational transmission does not necessarily follow from a "critical" family history and frequent negative events, such as death in the family or parental neglect. "Healthy" families have also gone through painful experiences and have come to grips with no fewer drawbacks. What makes the difference seems to be the fact that there are families who can and families who cannot "manage" difficulties and generational strains as a couple. Some parents turn against their children just because they have themselves experienced situations of exploitation; other parents are capable of forgiveness, and thus redress the wrongs past generations have inflicted on them. In other words, the new couple may or may not be in a position to "work out" and "manage" the shortcomings of one or both partners. Doing this entails a specific type of interpersonal competence that comes in handy whenever the couple has, for instance, to manage conflict or to express affection.

Consequently, the major dimensions to be found in the relational level are temporality, the quality of ties, and the overall meaning each relationship takes on. Temporality can be investigated by monitoring the means by which families link past, present, and future. Ties can be investigated by evaluating the quality of the relationships between spouses, between parents and children, and between the partners and their families of origin. Meaning can be investigated by detecting the presence of values—spiritual, ethic, vital, cognitive, and material. On the whole, we can say that family health is related to the presence of a set of values.

The Symbolic Level

In addition, family relationships have a peculiar symbolic structure, epiphanized by language and a set of rituals. By "symbolic," we do not just refer to something standing for something else. We refer to the etymology of the term itself (symballein), meaning "bringing together"—linking items that otherwise would stand apart. In this case, it is imperative to find out what actually brings together the partners in the marital relationship, as well as those in the generational relationship.

A striking feature of this level is that its structure is latent and invariant. It cuts across and "trespasses on" the further two levels of family organization. We think that the symbolic reference family relationships have is species-specific. Let us now examine the symbolic aspects of both the marital and the intergenerational relationships.

The symbolic aspect of the marital relationship consists of unity–reciprocity. Human beings exist and have always existed in female and male forms. No single man or woman can actually represent the whole of humankind. We can speak of humankind just because the two modes of being, originally diverse, can be brought together. As the etymology of the term "symbolic" suggests (see above), they are but two sides of the same coin. Each side perceives within his or her innermost self that there is something lacking, and thus that there is a need to connect with the other side. The need for intimacy can be fulfilled by a mutual effort. The marital relationship is just the milieu where the two genders can strike an intimate and lasting binding deal. The marital relationship is supposed to take care of the respective differences, with this spouse looking after the difference of his or her partner. Thus reciprocity means facing up to the other's difference—in this case, to the spouse's different history and personality. At the same time, though, reciprocity also means acknowledging that the other is one's equal, and that one needs the other in order to be oneself. It is worth noting that the term "identity" has two linked senses: It relates at once to the Latin *idem* (the state of being exactly the same) and to the Latin *ipse* (being oneself, being specific). The identity of the couple comes into its own through reciprocity. Achieving reciprocity as a couple is a difficult task, since it means being up to an ideal relationship. No wonder, then, that the attempt is often bound to fail. Different cultures have also kept dealing with the theme of reciprocity. For example, Western culture has lately focused on reciprocity as equality of decision making within the couple.

The symbolic aspect of the intergenerational relationship consists, instead, of the exercise of maternal and paternal functions (tasks). The maternal functions are those of giving life, of containing anguish (the psychological equivalent of death), and of fostering hope and trust in human relationships. Maternity (motherhood) is connected to matrimony (marriage) and derives from the Latin *matri-munus*. It is parallel to patrimony, which derives from the Latin *patri-munus*. *Munus* pertains to a series of relational concepts. It is basically a gift that carries with it the onus of an exchange (Benveniste, 1969). The maternal function, on the psychological level, finds expression in the affective code of basic trust (in Erickson's sense). The hope–despair polarity represents the realization and the degeneration of the maternal function.

The paternal function, as noted above, refers to patrimony—to the transmission of material goods and moral lores. It gives a sense of belonging and acknowledgment. Belonging and inheritance are regulated by norms (each culture has its own, but no culture is without norms regulating property and its transmission). On the psychological level, the paternal function finds expression in the ethical codes of fairness and order.

As has been pointed out, invisible loyalties bind together the members of the various family generations. If the rules of fairness and order are not complied with, as is the case with the various forms of abuse or when one delegates one's duties, family pathology sets in (Boszormenyi-Nagy & Spark, 1973; Boszormenyi-Nagy, 1987). The ethical aspect (fairness included) does not quite fit into a double-entry logic of costs and benefits (Godbout, 1992), rather, far from it. In fact, pathology sets in just when such a logic becomes dominant. The symbolic intergenerational exchange is, by its very nature, asymmetrical and hierarchical. Its reciprocity is a long-term one, since the persons involved do not perform the same functions. The child who was given life and patrimony is in turn ready to give all this back in terms of loyalty to family values (e.g., loving care for an elderly parent). The child is also looking forward to taking on parental responsibilities, thus giving life and patrimony to the next generation. As anthropologist Marshall Sahlin (1976) stressed with the concept of "generalized reciprocity," sooner or later each member is called upon to give a "risky" gift, but he or she is confident the other will in turn reciprocate (with some relational goods or some symbolic token). If the rules of fairness are not complied with, a repetitive destructive cycle (of violence, for instance) may set in. Therapeutic treatment can help a family member who has suffered an injustice recognize it but break the cycle and press ahead notwithstanding (Doherty, 1995). As a matter of fact, through basic trust and forgiveness (exoneration, in Boszormenyi-Nagy's jargon), the chain of injustice can be broken and the order of fairness and loyalty can be restored. The maternal code (trust) and the paternal code (justice)—different though they are—are complementary, and each member must contribute to the system as a whole. The symbolic matrices of the ties between genders and generations are universal and invariant, but the ways they are embodied vary from one family to the other, and from one culture to the other, from one generation to the next.

Culture does influence the symbolic structures in quantitative terms. For example, it can highlight one element of a symbolic dyad and upstage the other. It cannot possibly rule out either, though. As we have pointed out, the symbolic register is, in fact, species-specific. Thus, for instance, from the Roman family (which was patrilinear—i.e., patrimony was of the utmost significance), we have passed on to the present-day family, which is matrifocal. In fact, the family is now characterized either by the centrality of the mother figure in family exchanges (as a number of studies have shown) or by greater emphasis on the themes of affect (support, care, empathy, good communication, etc.), all of which are included in *matrimunus* from the symbolic viewpoint.

We have thus far focused on the three levels of analysis under scrutiny (interactive, relational, and symbolic) and have duly underlined their specificity and articulation. We can now venture to state that interaction is placed on the level of verbal and nonverbal exchanges of those contents and observable processes. It highlights the "here" and reduces temporality to coexistence and sequence (the "now"). However, in order to gain an overall view of the family, it is imperative for us also to gain insight into the relational dimension—in other words, for us to pay attention to historical events (i.e., what has actually happened in the generational exchange). Also, some of the therapists who used to give more relevance to the exchange in the "here and now" and to resort to paradoxes and counterparadoxes or brilliant rituals (Selvini Palazzoli, Boscolo, Cecchin, & Prata, 1975) have now come to realize the need to investigate the exchange between generations with a view to better understanding of certain types of mental disorders (anorexia nervosa, schizophrenia, drug addiction, etc.). In this light, generational ties, their interiorizations, and their innermost meaning—not just their immediate significance—are indeed crucial when it comes to provoking some change conducive to treatment. Unlike significance, meaning rolls the whole register of values into one (expectations, ideals, et al.). As we have already stressed, the symbolic level cuts across both the interactive and the relational levels. It is, in other words, the invariant transcending all cultural variations. At this level, any generation must deal with universal issues and confront basic needs. The symbolic level, "deep-seated" as it is, is not detectable in itself as such. It must be tracked down on the other levels, in particular along with linguistic and cultural exchanges. When we mention the organizational identity of the family, we are simply referring to the structure resulting from the different levels' dovetailing together. In particular, the very term "organization" comes to signify the specific articulation of these levels within each cultural context and within each family's life.

THEORY AND FAMILY PATHOLOGY

The present chapter is intended to underline the importance of theory when it comes to tackling the "family issue." In particular, we want to stress the need for a specific theory that describes family relationships as clearly distinct from relationships in other social groups. We also maintain that culture and society are confronting issues that have their roots in "the family"; it should suffice to mention reciprocity (with reference to the marital couple) and fairness (with reference to the generational exchange).

The family dimension is likely to be given short shrift by research, which generally focuses either on the individual or on social issues at large. Instead, the family dimension must be recognized as a relational organization with a specific nature of its own, which is crucial to the formation and development of the individual's identity and sense of belonging in the social community. As we have specified, this identity comes from the fact that the family is an organization of parental relationships centered on the generative act, but one that is constantly confronting the issues of gender and generational differences. Thus, not all relationships, including the couple's, belong to the "family issue." There must be some kind of generational exchange, perhaps by way of biology, adoption, or guardianship.

Our use of the term "generational" stresses the difference between humans and other species. Humankind, in fact, is meant not just to reproduce itself or adjust to the environment, but rather to foster persons. This means that humankind activates mental devices capable of producing transformations through the ties binding parent and child. The family is up to its task if it can manage to enable its members to take an active and competent part in social life. "Competence" in this sense, as L'Abate (1986, 1994) has shown, pertains to the areas of being, doing/acting, and having/possessing; it finds expression in the fields of affect and work, as Freud pointed out long ago. The family is not up to its task whenever it fails to convey hope and fairness from one generation to the next, either because the spouses' reciprocity does not surface or because one spouse cripples the other. By the way, it is probably worth noting that the goals described above are not just ideals to be pursued, but actual "musts" if relationships between sexes and generations are to work properly.

Moreover, when we consider the links with anthropological and historical views of relationships, we feel that theory does require a model or idea of action. We wish to stress that both terms ("interaction" and "relationship") entail and express the idea of action; in this light, no family theory can do without a concept of action. In the tradition of Aristotle, we view "action" as the development of the plot, as drama (*mythos*). The drama in question is acted out by persons whom parental ties bind together. In addition, this very drama is something in its own right; that is to say, it transcends the actions performed by the individual family members, although it actually works through them. It can be traced back to the "principle of nonadditivity" espoused in philosophy by Husserl and Whitehead and in psychology by the Gestalt theorists and by Lewin. It is when drama turns into tragedy that we have psychopathology. Among tragedies, let us recall those pertaining to order (murders, vendettas, blind allegiance to ideas and norms), to passion (family feuds, fratricidal struggles, violent rebellions, wild love affairs), or to isolation (ban, excommunication, abandonment). One tragic form is likely to lead to another one. Unless the cycle is broken, pathology is bound to become chronic. Relational transformation can only be brought about by a turnabout, and this is signaled by the presence of "gestures" such as listening to the reasons of the other, reflecting on events and on self, redemption, forgiveness, and reconciliation. These are the actions that can alter the relational exchange.

Consequently, family pathology is not just supposed to result from shortcomings, lack of parental loving care, death in the family, or other critical events (e.g., emigration, sudden unexpected illnesses). All these are just part and parcel of everyday life. Family pathology results from generative failure: The latest generation turns out to be quite incapable of, or severely limited in, its mental and social competence. In this light, the severest forms of personality disorders are viewed as significantly related to particular forms of generational strains that have had little or no chance of being worked out in the generational exchange (Pontalti, 1996). For further discussion of this matter, see Morton Schatzman (1973) on the case of President Schreber, and Helm Stierlin (1972) on Adolf Hitler's family history.

More recently, a number of researchers and therapists—mainly Italian—have devoted their energies to investigating the link between severe personality troubles and the family matrix (Selvini Palazzoli, 1988; Pontalti & Menarini, 1985, 1994; Andolfi, 1994; Andolfi, & Angelo, 1987; Cirillo, Berrini, Cambiaso, & Mazza, 1996; Cigoli, 1994, 1997). Within a trans-generational perspective, they try to detect patterns and relational links conducive to severe forms of mental dysfunction (anorexia nervosa, psychosis, drug addiction, schizophrenia, etc.) or specific personality troubles—in other words, psychological structures of self that show limits and/or restrictions in cognitive, affective, or relational areas. This research does not rule out biological factors in pathology; neither does it underestimate sociocultural factors. However, relational factors are actually given top priority. The process of psychic degeneration is due to the unconscious transmission from one generation to the next of relational strains that were not properly dealt with. It goes without saying that a key role is played by the parental couple (whether one spouse's role dovetail with the other's). It takes more than a single critical family history to bring about pathology. In fact, it takes an unfortunate encounter of different family histories (Cigoli, 1994). Instead of acknowledging the respective shortcomings and managing or curing them, the unfortunate encounter magnifies the drawbacks and spreads them far and wide in the generations to come. The result is that the family group is doomed to sorrow, even if it is just one member who actually bears the stigmata. On the other hand, according to our clinical experience, as soon as therapy begins to tackle what the family fears most (be it a psychotic crisis, a depressive crisis, or the severe somatization of a family member), the mental strains of all come to the surface.

In order to clarify our stance further, this may now be the point at which to comment on the contrast between a theory (i.e., psychoeducational theory) that is definitely distant from our viewpoint, and one (i.e., attachment theory) that is certainly close to it. Let us start with the psychoeducational approach to pathology. In this approach, particularly as far as schizophrenia is concerned, the biological datum (i.e., the genetic transmission of the disease) comes right to the fore. As we have noted earlier, once the psychological/anthropological aspect is cut down to size and we come to the crunch, it is biology that reigns supreme. As a matter of fact, according to the psychoeducational approach, it is the very onset of the disease that triggers negative exchanges between family members, who thus give vent to dysfunction reactions, such as hyperinvolvement (symmetry of anxiety and protection between identified patient and family) and attack–counterattack (complementarity of conflictual relationships, which can even explode into violence). No wonder, then, that this approach gives short shrift to the relational aspect (Leff, Kuipers, Berkovitz, & Sturgeon, 1985; Miklowitz, Goldstein, Falloon, & Doane, 1984) while insisting on the interactive level (the transactive patterns between patient and family members). What is indeed striking is that the evidence presented in support of the biology deficit is dealt with as if it were a certainty, and that the experimental method is looked upon as the very paradigm of research, while no mention is made of the methodological debate the "theory of complexity" has stirred up in the past few years. When dealing with human relationships, one must take into due consideration not only the history of such relationships, but also the unconscious components of action, as well as their transmission between one generation and the next (Scabini & Donati, 1995). The "social advantage" of this approach is the fact that themes of family guilt and shame related to the mental disease of a member are simply removed, root and branch. On the other hand, though, out with the bathwater goes the baby of constructive responsibility and the chance to restore hope and fairness in the generational exchange.

Let us now turn to the attachment approach to pathology. The recent work by Doane and Diamond (1994), with its different types of families and specific models of treatment for each of them, provides a good example. Priority is given to each parent's attachment to the patient, on the one hand, and to each parent's attachment to his or her family of origin, on the other hand. As a result, the authors sketch out a number of different types of families: There are "disconnected" families, high-intensity families, and low-intensity families. Each of these presents a pathogenic "hard core." In particular, the authors stress the fact that the attachment between parents and children (and between family members) can be jeopardized by interiorized binds handed down from one generation to the next.

The major difference between Doane and Diamond's theory and our own lies in the value we assign to histories dovetailing through the marital couple. As we have amply stressed, the symbolic theme of reciprocity typical of conjugality dovetails with the distribution of gifts/tasks (hope and fairness) typical of the generational exchange. This dovetailing is indeed decisive in being conducive either to health or to disease. Incidentally, that is why the generational exchange itself is so very unpredictable. A couple can manage interiorized binds presenting particular difficulties and strains, but, in so doing, this very couple may hand a pathogenic malignant bind down to the next generation.

Those who endorse a relational (transgenerational, symbolic) theory are bound to take into account the interactive modes frequently associated with sorrow-inducing relationships. Hence, attention is given to the attribution of guilt, the threat of abandonment, emotional blackmail, escape into one's role, thought reading, standoffishness or communicative indifference, and spiteful communication. All of these reflect the difficulty (even impossibility) of the "me–other" relationship (between parents, or between one parent and his or her child). However, when considering crises related to binds, one must distinguish between defensive and chronic situations. In the latter case, it is the very bind that fails (i.e., is not up to its task), or is distorted or perverted out of all recognition. Here one can talk of family pathology proper. Hence, taking into account the relational level is a must. In turn, this means taking into account the history of relationships, as well as the ethical–affective symbolization (fairness and hope) that goes with it.

The task of therapy is to quench a pathology (if any), which arises out of the past but lives in the present of the relationship, by fostering hope and fairness in the generational exchange. To do so, a relational therapist must of necessity involve the parental couple: It is the dovetailing of painful generational histories within the couple that constitutes the major source of pathology. On the other hand, it is the couple itself that a therapist must look to when trying to find the resources needed to tackle a problem—in particular, a problem that affects one of its members.

REFERENCES

Ackerman, N. W. (1958). *The psychodynamics of family life.* New York: Basic Books.

Andolfi, M. (1994). *Il colloquio relazionale [The relational interview].* Rome: Accademia di Psicoterapia Familiare.

Andolfi, M., & Angelo, C. (1987). *Tempo e mito nella psicoterapia familiare [Time and myth in family psychotherapy].* Turin: Boringhieri.

Argyle, M. (1952). Methods of studying social groups. *British Journal of Psychology, 43,* 269–279.

Bales, R. F. (1950). *Interaction process analysis: A method for study of small groups.* Chicago: University of Chicago Press.

Benveniste, E. (1969). *Vocabulaire des institutions Indo-européennes [The vocabulary of Indo-European institutions].* Paris: Editions de Minuit.

Boss, G., Doherty, S., La Rossa, R., Schumm, W. R., & Steinmetz, S. K. (1993). *Sourcebook of family theories and methods: A contextual approach.* New York: Plenum Press.

Boszormenyi-Nagy, I. (1987). *Foundations of contextual family therapy.* New York: Brunner/Mazel.

Boszormenyi-Nagy, I., & Spark, G. (1973). *Invisible loyalties.* New York: Harper & Row.

Broderick, C. B., & Schrader, S. S. (1991). The history of professional marriage and family therapy. In A. S. Gurman & D. P. Kniskern (Eds.), *Handbook of family therapy* (pp. 5–35). New York: Brunner/Mazel.

Carter, E. A., & McGoldrick, M. (1980). *The family life cycle: A framework for family therapy.* New York: Gardner Press.

Cigoli, V. (Ed.). (1994). *Tossicomania: Passaggi generazionali e intervento di rete*

[*Drug abuse: Generational transitions and network intervention*]. Milan: Franco Angeli.

Cigoli, V. (1995). Il famigliare: Complessità delle forme o riconoscimento del legame? [The "familial": Complexity of forms or recognition of bonds?] In F. Walsh (Ed.), *Ciclo vitale e dinamiche familiari* [*Normal family processes*] (2nd ed., pp. 7–34). Milan: Franco Angeli. (Original work published 1993)

Cigoli, V. (1997). *Intrecci familiari: Realtà interiore e scenario relazionale* [*Family plots: Inner reality and relational scenery*]. Milan: Raffaello Cortina.

Cirillo, S., Berrini, R., Cambiaso, G., & Mazza, R. (1996). *La famiglia del tossicodipendente* [*The family of the drug abuser*]. Milan: Raffaello Cortina.

Doane, J. A. (1978). Family interaction and communication deviance in disturbed and normal families. *Family Process, 17,* 357–375.

Doane, J. A., & Diamond, D. (1994). *Affect and attachment in the family.* New York: Basic Books.

Doherty, W. J. (1995). *Soul searching: Why psychotherapy must promote moral responsibility.* New York: Basic Books.

Donley, M. (1993). Attachment and the emotional unit. *Family Process, 32,* 3–20.

Eisler, I., Dare, C., & Szmuckler, G. I. (1988). What's happened to family interaction research?: An historical account and a family systems viewpoint. *Journal of Marital and Family Therapy, 14,* 45–65.

Ferreira, A. J., & Winter, W. D. (1968). Decision-making in normal and abnormal two-child families. *Family Process, 7,* 17–36.

Framo, J. L. (1992). *Family of origin therapy.* New York: Brunner/Mazel.

Godbout, J. T. (1992). *L'ésprit du don* [*The spirit of the gift*]. Paris: La Découverte.

Goolishian, H. A., & Anderson, H. (1992). Some afterthoughts on reading Duncan and Held. *Journal of Marital and Family Therapy, 18,* 35–37.

Gottman, J., & Levenson, R. (1992). Marital processes predictive of later dissolution: Behavior, physiology, and health. *Journal of Personality and Social Psychology, 63,* 221–233.

Haley, J. (1972). Critical overview of present status of family interaction research. In J. L. Framo (Ed.), *Family interaction: A dialogue between family researchers and family therapists* (pp. 13–40). New York: Springer.

Hare, A. P., Borgatta, E. F., & Bales, R. F. (1955). *Small groups: Studies in social interaction.* New York: Knopf.

Hampson, R. B., Beavers, W. R., & Hulgus, Y. S. (1988). Comparing the Beavers and circumplex models of family functioning. *Family Process, 27*(1), 85–92.

Héritier, F. (1996). *Masculin, féminin: La pensée de la différence* [*Masculine, feminine: The thought of difference*]. Paris: O. Jacob.

Hinde, R. A. (1995). A suggested structure for a science of relationship. *Personal Relationships, 2,* 1–15.

Hoffman, L. W. (1990). Constructing realities: An art of lenses. *Family Process, 29,* 1–12.

Jacob, T. (1975). Family interaction in disturbed and normal families: A methodological and substantive review. *Psychological Bulletin, 82,* 133–165.

Keeney, B. (1979). Ecosystemic epistemology: An alternative paradigm for diagnosis. *Family Process, 18*(2), 117–129.

Keeney, B., & Ross, J. M. (1984). *Mind in therapy.* New York: Praeger.

Klein, D. M., & White, J. M. (1996). *Family theories: An introduction.* Thousand Oaks, CA: Sage.

L'Abate, L. (1986). *Systemic family therapy.* New York: Brunner/Mazel.

L'Abate, L. (1994). *A theory of personality development.* New York: Wiley.

Laslett, P., & Wall, R. (1972). *Household and family in past time.* Cambridge, England: Cambridge University Press.

Leff, J. P., Kuipers, L., Berkovitz, R., & Sturgeon, D. (1995). A controlled trial of social intervention in the families of schizophrenic patients: Two-year follow-up. *British Journal of Psychiatry, 146,* 594–600.

Lévi-Strauss, C. (1956). The family. In H. L. Shapiro (Ed.), *Man, culture, and society.* Oxford: Oxford University Press.

Lieberman, S. (1979). A transgenerational theory. *Journal of Family Therapy, 4,* 347–360.

Main, M., Kaplan, N., & Cassidy, J. (1985). Security in infancy, childhood, and adulthood: A move to the level of representation. In I. Bretherton & E. Waters (Eds.), *Growing points of attachment theory and research. Monographs of the Society for Research in Child Development, 50*(1–2 Serial No. 209), 66–104.

Markman, H. (1981). Predictions of marital distress: A 5-year follow-up. *Journal of Consulting and Clinical Psychology, 49,* 760–762.

Miklowitz, D. J., Goldstein, M. J., Falloon, I. R. H., & Doane, J. A. (1984). Interactional correlates of expressed emotion in the families of schizophrenics. *British Journal of Psychiatry, 144,* 482–487.

Offer, D., & Sabshin, M. (1974). *Normality: Theoretical and clinical concepts of mental health* (2nd ed.). New York: Basic Books.

Olson, D. H. (1986). Circumplex model VII: Validation studies and FACES III. *Family Process, 25,* 337–351.

Paul, N. L. (1980). Now and the past: Transgenerational analysis. *International Journal of Family Psychiatry, 1,* 235–248.

Pontalti, C. (1996). Epistemologia familiare e disturbi di identità. [Family Epistemology and Identity Disorders]. *Terapia Familiare, 52,* 33–44.

Pontalti, C., & Menarini, R. (1985). Le matrici gruppali in psicoterapia familiare. [Group Matrixes in Family Psychotherapy]. *Terapia Familiare, 19,* 55–64.

Pontalti, C., & Menarini, R. (1994). I disturbi di personalità: Dalla psicopatologia al progetto terapeutico [Personality disorders: From psychopathology to therapeutic project]. In G. Di Marco (Ed.), *A che punto è la psichiatria?* [*How far has psychiatry come?*] (pp. 53–68). Padua: Upsel-Domenghini.

Reiss, D. (1981). *The family construction of reality.* Cambridge, MA: Harvard University Press

Sahlin, M. (1976). *Âge de pierre, âge d'abundance: l'Économie des sociétés primitives.* Paris: Gallimard.

Scabini, E. (1995). *Psicologia sociale della famiglia* [*Social psychology of the family*]. Turin: Bollati Boringhieri.

Scabini, E., & Donati, P. (1995). *Nuovo lessico familiare* [*The new family lexicon*]. Milan: Vita e Pensiero.

Schatzman, M. (1973). *Soul murder: Persecution in the family.* New York: Random House.

Selvini Palazzoli, M. (1988). *I giochi psicotici della famiglia* [*Psychotic games in the family*]. Milan: Cortina.

Selvini Palazzoli, M., Boscolo, L., Cecchin, G., & Prata, G. (1975). *Paradosso e controparadosso* [*Paradox and counterparadox*]. Milan: Feltrinelli.

Sroufe, L., & Fleeson, J. (1988). The coherence of family relationship. In R. Hinde

& J. Stevenson-Hinde (Eds.), *Relationships within families: Mutual influences* (pp. 27–47). Oxford: Clarendon Press.

Stierlin, H. (1972). *Separating parents and adolescents.* New York: Quadrangle Press.

Trognon, A. (1991). L'interaction en général: Sujets, groupes, cognitions, représentations sociales. [Interaction in general: Subjects, groups, cognitions, social representations]. *Connexions, 57,* 9–25.

Turner, J. (1991). *The structure of sociological theory* (5th ed.). Belmont, CA: Wadsworth.

Walsh, F. (1982). Conceptualizations of normal family functioning. In F. Walsh (Ed.), *Normal family processes* (pp. 3–42). New York: Guilford Press.

Walsh, F. (Ed.). (1993). *Normal family processes* (2nd ed.). New York: Guilford Press.

Walsh, F., & McGoldrick, M. (1991). *Living beyond loss: Death in the family.* New York: Norton.

Williamson, D. S. (1981). Personal authority in family experience via termination of the intergenerational hierarchical boundary: Part II. The consultation process and the therapeutic method. *Journal of Marital and Family Therapy, 8,* 13–37.

White, M., & Epston, D. (1990). *Narrative means to therapeutic ends.* New York: Norton.

Wynne, L. C., Jones, J. E., & Al-Khayyal, M. (1982). Healthy family communication patterns: Observation in families "at risk" for psychopathology. In F. Walsh (Ed.), *Normal family processes* (pp. 142–164). New York: Guilford Press.

———⟫◆⟪———

CHAPTER 2

The Family as a Unity of Interacting Personalities

ALEXANDRA LOUKAS
GEOFFREY R. TWITCHELL
LISA A. PIEJAK
HIRAM E. FITZGERALD
ROBERT A. ZUCKER

> By a unity of interacting personalities is meant a living,
> changing, growing thing. . . . The actual unity of family life
> has its existence not in any legal conception, nor in any
> formal contract, but in the interaction of its members. For
> the family does not depend for its survival on the
> harmonious relations of its members, nor does it necessarily
> disintegrate as a result of conflicts between its members.
> The family lives as long as interaction is taking place and
> dies only when it ceases.
> —BURGESS (1926/1972, pp. 6–7)

Anticipating contemporary models of individual and family functioning,
Ernest Burgess (1926/1972) portrayed the early 20th-century family as a
dynamic interactional system—a mosaic of interacting personalities that
generates a "superpersonality," a family identity. Burgess commented on
the drastic changes taking place in the American family of the 1920s:
Family size was decreasing, roles of family members were changing, and
the "wild and reckless behavior . . . of youth in revolt" (p. 8) was of
concern. Historically, researchers and social critics alike have acknowledged
the importance of conceptualizing the family as a unity of interacting
personalities. Nevertheless, during the first half of the 20th century, the
dominant theories guiding the study of human development tended to focus
on intraindividual determinants of personality, or at best the dyadic

(mother–child) interactions underlying socialization of the child. Comparatively little attention was given to such issues as intergenerational family
structure, family composition, family rules and codes, neighborhoods, peer
influences on family functioning, and various ecological influences on
family structure and functioning. Moreover, the presumption was that the
normative setting for individual development and child socialization was
that provided by the nuclear family.

Today, as in 1926, family size is decreasing, roles of family members
are changing, and the wild and reckless behavior of youth is of societal
concern. Perhaps the diversity that is characteristic of the contemporary
American family is the natural outcome of cultural transitions begun over
70 years ago. Because of this diversity, today's challenge is to reach for an
inclusive definition of family—one that can incorporate "nontraditional"
families, such as those with single parents, cohabiting heterosexual couples,
cohabiting homosexual couples, blended families, extended families, and
an increasing number of interracial families (Melton & Wilcox, 1989).
Study of the family is affected by changes in sociocultural mores, as well
as by the paradigmatic models advanced to explain family dynamics. At
the same time that society struggles to frame a more inclusive definition of
the family, social and behavioral scientists struggle to reshape theoretical
and methodological approaches that will enhance understanding of family
dynamics. In the present chapter, the family is conceptualized as a unity or
system of interacting personalities, consistent with Burgess's analysis, but
cast in the framework of contemporary systems theory (Fitzgerald, Zucker,
& Yang, 1995; Ford & Lerner, 1992; Sameroff, 1995).

Systems theory (von Bertalanffy, 1968) is particularly well suited for
the study of the family as a unity of interacting personalities. From this
perspective, individuals are seen as embedded within families, families
within neighborhoods, neighborhoods within communities, and communities within an ever-expanding geopolitical macrospace (Bronfenbrenner,
1979). Bronfenbrenner proposed the "macrosystem" as the overarching
environment that includes the social, political, and cultural systems within
which the individual (family) develops. Although the political system is not
part of a child's proximal environment, political decisions and public policy
can have profound implications for child development and family life. For
example, individual family members are affected by policy decisions requiring welfare mothers to work, reducing funding for public day care programs, restricting advertising of cigarettes, and curtailing individual choice
on such issues as abortion and euthanasia. All of these policy issues have
an impact on family functioning and the nature of interpersonal interactions
among family members. For example, requiring welfare mothers to work
may negatively affect the quality of the mother–infant attachment relationship, or, for older children, may provide increased opportunities to be home
alone. On the other hand, the welfare-to-work policy could lead to
enhanced family resources, improved child care alternatives, and enriched

family relationships. In either case, the relationships among family members would be changed as a result of sociopolitical forces external to the family system.

In this chapter, we present a heuristic model for study of the family system that takes into account the various internal and external forces affecting both its structure and its function. Our reference to the broader literatures in the various fields that we touch upon is necessarily selective and limited, because our purpose is to whet the appetite for innovative thinking rather than to force dessert on an already sated palate.

CHILDREN'S CONCEPT OF FAMILY

Extensive work has focused on the development of the concept of family in children and adolescents (e.g., Borduin, Mann, Cone, & Borduin, 1990; Newman, Roberts, & Syre, 1993). Findings from such studies indicate that although affective ties (i.e., love) constitute the most commonly used basis for classifying a group of individuals as a family (Newman et al., 1993), as children grow older their concept of the family becomes increasingly abstract. For instance, first-grade children often use common residence to classify a family, whereas older elementary-school-age children use more abstract criteria (e.g., biological relatedness) in addition to common residence to classify a group of individuals as a family (Borduin et al., 1990). Furthermore, early elementary-school-age children often view the removal of an individual from the residence as permanent; thus, an individual who leaves the home is no longer part of the family. Older children, on the other hand, apply biological relatedness as a criterion for family membership; therefore, they are able to understand that cohabitation does not define family membership. Finally, older children are more likely than younger children to view nonrelative cohabiting individuals as part of the family unit. For example, among many urban, poor, single-parent families, social fathers are more likely to share or have greater family presence than are biological fathers.

Researchers have also been interested in assessing the concept of family in children of divorced parents (e.g., Kurdek, 1986; Newman et al., 1993). These studies report that children from intact homes are more likely to mention affective ties than are children from divorced homes (Newman et al., 1993). In general, more children are able to accept configurations of individuals in which some biological component is present (with or without coresidence). Fewer children, however, accept groupings united only by legal ties or only by coresidence. The fact that younger children have more trouble classifying nontraditional units as families may be due to the fact that the prototypical family or the family to which they are comparing these groups is the nuclear family (Pederson & Gilby, 1986). Societal processes play an important role in how children and adults view families. Thus, even today, the societal standard for the prototypical family is presumed to be one in which the biological mother, the biological father, and at least one child share a common residence. Considering the proportion of divorced and remarried couples and the high percentage of single-parent families in contemporary American society, the biological nuclear family seems more a cultural myth than a prototypical standard against which all family structures are to be compared. Burgess (1926/1972), in fact, suggested an alternative: conceptualizing the family in terms of a unity (system) of interacting personalities, rather than as a delimited unit of biologically related individuals.

SYSTEMS THEORY

A "system" can be defined as a set of interrelated units constituting a whole that is different from the sum of its constituent parts. A family is a system that is more than the sum of its members, although its dynamic characteristics are derived in large measure from its members. Systems are emergent, epigenetic, organizing, constructive, hierarchically integrated (Ford & Lerner, 1992; Gottlieb, 1991; Miller, 1978; Sameroff, 1995), and potentially chaotic (Levine & Fitzgerald, 1992). To the *developmental* systems theorist, the study of the family includes examination of the qualities of each individual member, the transactions among family members within the multiple contexts of development, and the transitions that occur over the life course. From this perspective, the individual is always embedded within a context that provides definition or boundaries to the system. Most systems are open and allow for rich intersystem commerce; that is, their boundaries are permeable, and transitions between systems are relatively easy to negotiate. Other systems are relatively closed, with rigid boundaries that pose barriers to transition, and therefore are especially vulnerable to chaotic, disruptive forces.

Developmental systems theory is an apt perspective for examining the dynamic nature of the family as a unity of interacting personalities. When change occurs within the family system, not only are individual family members affected, but the quality of their relationships and the family system itself change as well. Systemic change is regulated by transactional processes, which in turn are regulated by feedback mechanisms. Negative feedback dampens forces promoting change and helps to sustain continuity over the life course. Change, therefore, is gradual and viewed within the framework of normative developmental process, or in the framework of isolating the family from exogenous influences. Conversely, positive feedback overloads the system, stimulates change and systemic reorganization, and gives rise to discontinuities over the life course. Life course transitions provide the best examples of system reorganizations. The biobehavioral shift that occurs over the first 3 months after birth, and includes the emergence of the social smile, generally has a profound impact on the quality of parent–child relationships (Emde, Gaensbauer, & Harmon, 1976). When infants begin to produce social smiles, parents report for the first time that the infants are "really human." Increased parental efforts to engage an infant provide the context for the infant to produce more smiles, and a cyclic pattern of parent–infant engagement is repeatedly strengthened through reciprocal action. The onset of walking marks another transition that fundamentally changes the parent–child relationship, as does the transition to school, the accompanying set of systemic changes in child behavior that White (1965) labeled the "5-to-7 shift," the marriage of a child, or the death of a family member.

Many perturbations in system functioning occasioned by life course transitions are resolved by using resources internal to the family. In other instances, families draw upon external systems for emotional support, assistance with problem solving, help with child care, or spiritual guidance. In one example of an exosystem study, Muller, Fitzgerald, Sullivan, and Zucker (1994) examined the influence of maternal social support and stress on child behavior problems in a sample of alcoholic families. The researchers found that lack of parental social support was related to increased levels of parental daily stress, which in turn made child maltreatment more likely. Although parental social support is external to a child's immediate environment, it can have a direct impact on the mother–child relationship and thereby play a role in child adjustment.

Although social support may dampen the impact of family crisis on child behavior, individual child characteristics also influence the context in which change is occurring (Ge et al., 1996). Temperament provides an example of a factor that exerts its influence on individual–environment transactions (Lerner & Lerner, 1983). Children approach situations with distinct styles or ways of acting; however, such factors as the attitudes and values of parents, teachers, and peers can influence how children express their styles (Lerner, 1993). Thus, children vary greatly in their ability to adapt to contextual changes, such as parental divorce, death, or the birth of a sibling. Moreover, children vary greatly in their ability to negotiate boundaries and to make successful transitions across intrafamilial and interfamilial boundaries.

THE FAMILY AS A CONTEXT FOR DEVELOPMENT

Regardless of whether an investigator is interested in microsystem or macrosystem variables (Bronfenbrenner, 1979), the way the investigator approaches the analysis of a system is fundamentally the same. Figure 2.1 depicts a primary family system consisting of a mother, a father, and their children. The arrows indicate all possible transactional linkages among family members. An exemplar adjunctive system, exogenous to the primary

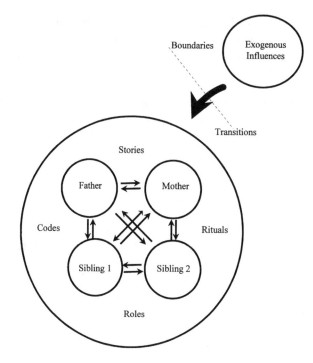

FIGURE 2.1. Possible transactional linkages in a primary family system consisting of a mother, a father, and their children.

system, illustrates that boundaries defining a system can create barriers to intersystem commerce (Fitzgerald et al., 1995). Keep in mind that barriers can also interfere with interpersonal relationships between and among family members, and that to the extent that such barriers involve pathology, transitions may require professional assistance.

From a developmental perspective, the effects of adjunctive systems on members of the family are most likely moderated by parents when children are young. For example, a change from employment to unemployment may exacerbate parental violence, which in turn may enhance risk for spouse or child abuse. When children are older, peers become more influential moderators of child behavior. Thus, the reciprocal interactions that take place between a child's peers and his or her family influence child development. Examples of such reciprocal interactions are provided by Gerald Patterson and his colleagues (Patterson, 1996; Patterson, DeBaryshe, & Ramsey, 1989), who examine the influence of peers and the family in the development of antisocial behavior. Results from Patterson's laboratory indicate that the development of antisocial behavior in a child occurs through a series of interactions with parents who display poor parental monitoring skills and coercive behaviors. From these interactions the child learns to display coercive and antisocial behavior, not only in the home environment but in other contexts, such as the school. The antisocial child enters school, performs poorly, and is rejected by normal peers; therefore, he or she socializes with delinquent peers who further reinforce the antisocial behavior and possibly model other problem behaviors as well. This process becomes cyclical and still further reinforces the child's antisocial behavior. However, the antisocial behavior is not confined to the home and school contexts, but spills over to other adjunctive systems, including the workplace and the courts. Thus, transactions between the family and peer network are not limited to these two contextual settings, but can embrace other adjunctive systems as well.

Systemic analysis of the family as a unity of interacting personalities requires one first to assess the presenting state characteristics of each member of the primary system (adaptive functioning, psychopathology, and family history). Then one would proceed to assess aspects of interindividual relationships, family structure and functioning, and influences from adjunctive systems, with the analysis usually guided by a theory-driven model of relationships predictive of an expected outcome. Presenting state characteristics change as a function of individual and family development and of the dynamic interplay of endogenous and exogenous influences on the primary system, so models predicting long-term outcomes must be able to deal with discontinuities as well as continuities over the life course. The challenge for behavioral science is to develop nonlinear models of development, which can capture change processes in ways that can only be inferred from linear models.

Sameroff's (1995) theory examines the individual in transaction with multiple levels of the environment, and emphasizes that development occurs within a regulated context to produce adaptive or maladaptive outcomes. Just as the genotype regulates the development of biological systems, Sameroff suggests that the "environtype" (external experience) regulates individual behavior; in particular, he draws attention to the "family code," which functions to organize individual members of the family system and to give members a sense of family boundaries. Four specific aspects of the family code serve as organizers or regulators of individual behavior. Sameroff (1995) refers to these as family "rituals," "stories," "myths," and "paradigms." The family code ensures that participating members carry out their roles and participate fully within the system. Through the use of rituals, stories, and roles, individuals are taught how to act within the system and in the larger society. Family rituals can offer options for making transitions between the family system and exogenous systems, or they can assist in isolating the family from such influences. For example, attendance at religious services and religious outreach projects can bring family members into direct contact with various adjunctive systems and can provide a means to practice social and interpersonal skills as well as experience diversity of life conditions. Family stories provide a means of transmitting family history and of connecting families intergenerationally, in addition to providing experience in conversational turn taking. Such stories sometimes feed family myths, which Sameroff points out may persist regardless of their basis in reality. Finally, paradigms are the core assumptions or basic beliefs that the family unit constructs about its experiential world.

"Cultural codes" represent the regulation of individuals within a society. These codes ensure that individuals fit into the society. Cultural codes consist of societal mores, norms, and fads, all of which can bring adjunctive systems into potential conflict with the family (Caspi, Elder, & Herbener, 1990). Finally, the "individual code" represents the independent contribution of each parent to the family. The cultural codes presented to children are in part the perceptions of their parents. Parents interpret culture and family codes, and present what they wish in the manner they wish to their children. Therefore, the individual characteristics of the parents will influence the children. However, Sameroff's (1995) analysis of individual, familial, and cultural regulation is deeply grounded in systems theory, so it demands recognition that parental behavior is always embedded within a context greater than that provided by the family and its interacting personalities.

INTERACTIONAL STYLE AND FAMILY DEVELOPMENT

The types and patterns of interaction styles used by individual family members may have important implications for the functioning of the family as a whole, in addition to influencing individual family members. However, few researchers have conceptualized the family unit as a whole; more often interactions in dyadic and triadic subsystems are examined. Interaction styles have most often been studied in terms of quality of the marital relationship and its influences on family functioning, influences of different parenting styles on child development, and interactions of dyads and triads within the family unit.

Impact of Marital Distress on Interacting Personalities in Families

The quality of the parental relationship is an important influence on many interactions within the family. Within a systems theory framework, marital interaction and parent–child interaction are viewed as reciprocally influencing each other (see Figure 2.1). The quality of the parental relationship clearly affects behaviors in the parent–parent dyad, but it also affects behaviors in the parent–child dyad, behaviors between siblings, and the various triadic combinations of parents and children (Wagner & Reiss, 1995). For example, parental expressed anger causes emotional reactions in children, who in turn are likely to strike out against others, including their siblings. Clearly there is a strong link between interdependency in sibling relationships and marital quality. Parent–child interactions are also linked to the quality of the marital relationship. Mothers in distressed marriages are found to be more actively responsive in interactions with their children by using more questions, positive feedback, informational feedback, and verbal task management (Brody, Pillegrini, & Sigel, 1986). Apparently mothers in unsatisfying marital relationships compensate by investing time in their children.

Marital conflict also predicts negative outcomes for children, including the incidence of both internalizing and externalizing problems (Harold, Fincham, Osborne, & Conger, 1997). The quality of the parental relationship, both before marriage and after the birth of a child, has been found to be associated with child functioning (Howes & Markman, 1989). For mothers, high satisfaction, low conflict, and high communication quality are related to security of attachment and to dependency in children, whereas for fathers, high levels of premarital conflict and low communication quality are positively related to child dependency. Gottman and Katz (1989) reported that marital discord was associated with poor health and poor peer relations in young children. In addition, the ways in which couples engage in conflict may have differential effects on child behavior. Specifically, patterns of conflict in which each spouse directly attacks the other's fundamental beliefs, feelings, and character are predictive of externalizing behavior problems in children, whereas patterns of conflict in which the husband exhibits stonewalling and anger are predictive of internalizing behavior problems in children (Katz & Gottman, 1993). The quality of the parents' relationship continues to have an impact on their children over the life span.

The mechanisms by which interparental conflict influences child outcome are less well understood, but the way in which such conflict is expressed may have important implications. Even young children respond with distress when exposed to angry adult interactions, and such exposure results in subsequent increased aggressive responses toward peers (Cummings, Iannotti, & Zahn-Waxler, 1985). As children get older, they perceive resolved anger as less negative and unresolved anger as more negative. Although children between the ages of 5 and 19 were found to respond negatively to unresolved anger, younger children were more likely to show fear responses, whereas younger girls and older boys were more likely to respond with sadness (Cummings, Ballard, El-Sheikh, & Lake, 1991). It has also been suggested that the links between marital relationships and child outcomes should be examined from the child's perspective (Grych & Fincham, 1993), thus focusing on the child's interpretation of interparental conflict.

The occurrence of marital conflict may be exacerbated when one parent in a marriage experiences problems with alcohol. Empirical findings suggest that alcoholic couples experience more marital complaints and expressed hostility, are less able to work cooperatively toward a mutual goal, and more actively avoid communication than do nonalcoholic couples (McCrady & Epstein, 1995).

Influences of Parenting Styles on Interacting Personalities in Families

Baumrind's (1989) seminal work has established the importance of parenting styles as influences on child development. Using a two-dimensional approach, Baumrind has identified styles of parenting that vary in levels of responsiveness and demandingness. Parents high on both responsiveness and demandingness are "authoritative"; those low on both responsiveness and demandingness are "neglectful"; those high on responsiveness and low on demandingness are "indulgent"; and those low on responsiveness and high on demandingness are "authoritarian."

Different parenting styles have been found to be associated with different outcomes for children, with the best outcomes associated with authoritative parenting. Boys of authoritative parents are friendly and cooperative, and girls of authoritative parents are purposive, dominant, and achievement-oriented (Baumrind, 1989). Parenting practices make a difference even after a child reaches high school (Dornbusch, Ritter, Leiderman, Roberts, & Fraleigh, 1987). There are clear advantages for adolescents raised in authoritative homes with respect to psychosocial development, school achievement, internalized distress, and problem behavior, and clear disadvantages for adolescents raised in neglectful homes; adolescents from authoritarian and indulgent households show more mixed outcomes (Lamborn, Mounts, Steinberg, & Dornbusch, 1991). Over time, the deleterious consequences for adolescents raised in homes characterized by neglectful parents continue to accumulate. However, the deleterious consequences of authoritarian parenting may not be as severe among youth from minority groups (Steinberg, Lamborn, Darling, Mounts, & Dornbusch, 1994). As Baumrind (1995) notes, child rearing occurs in a larger societal context; there is a paucity of research on how parenting objectives vary among cultures, and on how various parenting styles that produce negative child outcomes in some contexts may actually be adaptive in other contexts.

Rather than merely focusing on parental styles, some research has focused on general family styles of responsiveness (acceptance) and demandingness (control). Both of these dimensions have been linked to the adjustment of young adolescents, and each of these dimensions contributes independently to adolescent adjustment (Kurdek & Fine, 1994). Effects of parenting styles have also been investigated in stepfamilies. Despite family disruption, a caring and empathetic parenting style appears to be the main determinant of both family functioning and the well-being of adolescents (McFarlane, Bellissimo, & Norman, 1995). However, a word of caution is in order. Although the authoritative parenting pattern is associated with child competence and positive child outcomes in most samples, it is not yet clear how individual child characteristics or personality styles interact with particular parental styles, or why certain children are influenced by one parenting style more than another. This is an issue of "goodness of fit" that is also addressed in the temperament literature.

Family Interactions in Dyads and Triads

Family interactions are often studied via dyadic and triadic interactions within the larger family system (Wagner & Reiss, 1995). This work suggests that mothers interact differently with children than fathers do, and that dyadic parent–child interactions are different from triadic interactions in which both parents are involved with a child. Each parent's rate of engagement with the child decreases when the other parent is present (Lamb, 1976). For adolescents, however, father presence seems to enhance the quality of mother–son interactions, whereas the presence of the mother reduces the quality of father–son interactions (Gjerde, 1986).

Results of observations of mother–child, father–child, and mother–father–child groups suggest that mother–child interactions are qualitatively different from interactions in the other two groups. Although there are many similarities in mother–child and father–child interaction patterns, children are more likely to direct vocalizations to their mothers (Liddell, Henzi, & Drew, 1987) and to engage in rough-and-tumble play with their fathers. It seems evident, therefore, that mother–child dyads, father–child dyads, and mother–father–child triads should be simultaneously analyzed if one wishes to fully understand the family as a unity of interacting personalities.

Family interaction patterns also predict behavior problems among young children. Pettit and Bates (1989) found that the absence of behavior problems was predicted by affectively positive, educative interactions in the mother–child dyad, and that the absence of such exchanges predicted the development of behavior problems. Coercive family interactions were also predictive of behavior problem ratings. Similarly, interactions in families with a hyperactive son are characterized by a higher degree of coercion (Buhrmester, Camparo, Christensen, Gonzalez, & Hinshaw, 1992). This type of interaction is marked in mother–son dyads, in which mothers are more likely to make demands and express emotions, and in which sons are more likely to behave negatively.

Family interactions also vary when a parent experiences psychopathology. Among children of depressed mothers, girls were more caring toward their mothers whether they were depressed or not, and boys became more caring only when their mothers were severely depressed (Radke-Yarrow, Zahn-Waxler, Richardson, Susman, & Martinez, 1994). The constellation that produced the highest frequency of prosocial behaviors by children included severe maternal depression, secure attachment between mother and child, and child problems of affect regulation or impulse control. Families with an alcoholic father are also characterized by impaired parent–child interactions (Whipple, Fitzgerald, & Zucker, 1991). Parents in the alcoholic families were less able to engage their children during directed play in situations where a child was asked to operate in a more restrictive rule structure; they also showed lower positive affect during the latter situation.

Intergenerational Relationships

The multigenerational family is of increasing interest to developmentalists, especially as the study of cultural diversity in family life intensifies. Multigenerational family forms include grandparents residing in the home of a nuclear family, or grandparents raising grandchildren when parents are absent from the home (Uzoka, 1979). Multigenerational family structures are more common among African American, Asian American, and Hispanic families than they currently are among European American families in the United States (Carrasquillo, 1991; Fong & Browne, in press; Rueschenberg & Buriel, 1995). Nevertheless, there is as much diversity within a particular ethnic group as there is between groups (Min, 1995). Tolson and Wilson (1990) report that among African American families, different family structures are associated with different family climates. For example, three-generational families perceive less emphasis on organization, presumably because the presence of the grandmother allows for greater sharing of caregiving and nurturance. Whenever a second caregiver is present in a home, there is greater assistance with caregiving and more social support for the mother.

Grandparents play many roles in the family. One role involves teaching their daughters about child development (Stevens, 1984), thus providing an intergenerational link to family codes and family traditions. Family functioning may therefore be adversely affected when a grandparent is not present; for example, Fong and Browne (in press) note that U.S. immigration policy has had a negative impact on traditional Chinese family values, which include grandparents as members of the primary family system. Key determinants of shared roles involve the age and health of the grandparent, the developmental levels of the grandchildren, and the marital situation of the family (McGreal, 1994). Although grandfathers and grandmothers may see their grandchildren equally often, grandmothers interact more with their grandchildren during visits than do grandfathers (Eisenberg, 1988). Whereas grandmothers are more likely to engage in caregiving behaviors, grandfathers are more likely to engage in rough-and-tumble play behaviors (Russell, 1986), mirroring the caregiving behaviors of mothers and fathers. During interactions with infants, grandparents are likely to be gentler with babies than parents are (Tinsley & Parke, 1987). With older grandchildren, grandparent–grandchild interactions are likely to be characterized by companionship and discussions of personal issues (McGreal, 1994). Grandchildren are more likely to have closer relationships with grandparents when they perceive themselves to be similar to grandparents, when they perceive their grandparent to show special interest in them, and when they feel a sense of admiration for their grandparent (Kennedy, 1991).

Divorce and Child Outcomes

The nuclear family continues to be the "gold standard" for American family composition, despite the facts that nearly half of all marriages in the United States end in divorce, and that nearly 30% of all children under 6 years of age live in such single-parent homes. Parental divorce or separation is a transition that affects all members of the family. Divorce or separation is stressful for adults as well as children, and affects parenting attitudes as well as family interactions (Webster-Stratton, 1990). Immediately following a divorce or separation, parents are more punitive, more irritable, and less affectionate with their children. Furthermore, within 2 years of the divorce or separation, both parents and children exhibit increased emotional, physical, and behavioral problems (Hetherington, 1989).

Divorce does not result in increased problems or negative outcomes for all families. Rather, various factors influence the extent to which divorce or separation has negative effects on parents and children. For instance, the amount of time that has passed since the divorce or separation is an important predictor of child and adult outcomes. According to Hetherington (1989), the majority of families recover and are functioning well 2 or 3 years after the divorce. Thus, the effects of divorce on parents and children are highest immediately after the event as the family adjusts to the absence of one parent. In addition, the negative effects tend to be more evident in boys than in girls, especially with respect to externalizing behavior problems (Hetherington, 1989).

Finally, the amount of conflict parents experience both prior to and following the divorce is an important predictor of child outcomes (Emery, 1982; Hetherington, 1989; Shaw, Emery, & Tuer, 1993). Children are often aware of parental conflict, especially if the conflict is openly hostile rather than encapsulated. Such conflict can lead to increased levels of child stress and in turn to child behavior problems. Thus, several researchers have speculated that parental conflict, rather than divorce or separation per se, is at the root of increased child behavior problems. Shaw et al. (1993) found that the family environments of boys in to-be-divorced families were characterized by more rejection, more economic stress, and less parental concern than were the family environments of boys in intact homes, and that these factors were associated with an increase in behavioral problems following the divorce. Others have also reported that many of the negative child outcomes that are reported to follow a divorce or separation can be predicted by predivorce family conditions (Cherlin et al., 1991).

Although researchers have focused almost exclusively on the influence of the event of divorce or separation, few researchers have examined the influence of factors that accompany such family transitions. For instance, divorce or separation is often preceded by marital conflict (as noted above) and instability, both of which play important roles in child outcomes (Cherlin et al., 1991). Furthermore, many children experience a decrease in family income and an increase in economic insecurity after a divorce or separation, especially if they are living in a mother-headed household.

Divorce or separation changes the primary system by physically moving one parent outside the existing boundaries (see Figure 2.2). If the mother recouples, a new caregiver enters the primary system, but usually occupies psychological space somewhere on the perimeter of this system.

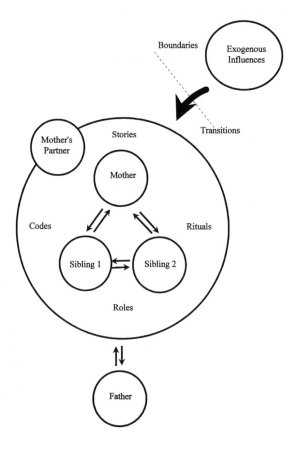

FIGURE 2.2. Possible transactional linkages in a primary family system in which the parents have divorced and the mother has recoupled.

The new member of the primary system brings new adjunctive systems, stories, rituals, codes, and roles to the primary system, and generates a new set of interpersonal relationships. In time, this individual may move more toward the core of the primary system and achieve a level of integration that may in fact exceed the biological parent's. If the new stepparent or partner is accompanied by children from a past relationship as well, the heuristic in Figure 2.2 becomes that much more complex.

When one is examining the influence of divorce or separation on children, it is important to remember that events both precede and follow the occurrence of the marital separation. These events may in some cases be as important as or even more important than the divorce itself. In addition, these events may predict changes in the child's behavior that are wrongly attributed to divorce. Therefore, investigators should take advantage of existing prospective longitudinal studies to assess the family situation prior to the occurrence of divorce, and to track family members for several years after the divorce to determine its long-term impact on family relationships. Future studies should also examine factors that predict positive outcomes, rather than just negative outcomes for divorced parents and their children.

FAMILY STRUCTURE
AND INDIVIDUAL DEVELOPMENT

Family research is struggling to keep up with the ever-changing and expanding landscape of family structure. Today's families reach far beyond the traditional two-parent nuclear family, on which so much early research was based. Current U.S. demographics have shown that families are taking on a variety of diverse structures (Flaks, Ficher, Masterpasqua, & Joseph, 1995). These include (but are not limited to) single-parent families, extended families, gay- and lesbian-parented families, and families with members of various races and ethnicities.

The social and legal implications surrounding nontraditional families have proven to be the main impetus for the current research on these families. As these new family entities are identified and become more visible, issues regarding the desirability of these families have moved from the social into the legal arena. Nontraditional families have been researched primarily within a deficit model and have had to exist within the context of legal and social systems that are frequently hostile. For example, child custody cases have often reflected questions concerning the ability of these families to raise healthy children. Increasing divorce rates have spurred research aimed at determining the deleterious effects of single parenthood on children. Similarly, much research on African American families has sought to examine the presumed negative impact of absent fathers, and has neglected the positive influence of extended family and community support.

More recently, the impact of cultural sanctions against homosexuality has resulted in a large number of homosexual parents' losing custody of their children because of their sexual orientation.

Single-Parent Families

The large majority of non-nuclear families are single-parent families. Given that women are granted custody of their children in the majority of cases, research on single-parent families has centered on female-headed households. Research on the single-parent family has been characterized by its comparisons of the traditional two-parent family with those families where a father is absent and either a single or a divorced woman is the head of the household.

Research on these families has frequently utilized the family deficit model. This model hypothesizes that families with an absent father will have poorer outcomes than families with two parents will (Partridge & Kotler, 1987). Research that has looked at associations between the developmental outcome of children and adolescents and these structural differences has generally reported that families with an absent father are plagued by poorer outcomes, including increased delinquency, greater rates of alcohol and drug use, and lower self-esteem. One study reported that youth in mother-only households were perceived as more likely to make decisions without parental input, and as more likely to exhibit deviant behavior (Dornbusch et al., 1987). Interestingly, these findings emerge even after family income and parental education are controlled for. Notably, most of this research has been done with middle-class European American families, and the few studies on African American families have shown equivocal results (Zimmerman, Salem, & Maton, 1995).

Another study examined the long term effects of single-parent and stepparent family structures on family solidarity (White, 1994). The findings suggested that divorced single-parent families were associated with reduced family solidarity in adulthood. Results also suggested that a custodial parent's remarriage positively affected parent–child solidarity in mother–stepfather families, but negatively affected solidarity in father–stepmother families. White suggested that this might be related to traditional gender roles of males being less engaged, as well as to children's normal resentment of a newcomer.

Ethnic Family Structures

The tradition of treating families as though they all involve a two-parent nuclear structure (see Figure 2.1) (Hill, 1980) has masked the true heterogeneity of the American family structure (Allen, 1978; Hill, 1972; Nobles, 1978; Uzoka, 1979). The adherence to this model in studying African American families has been especially inappropriate, due to the large numbers of African American families who live in nontraditional family structures (Glick, 1981; Reid, 1982). Tolson and Wilson (1990) reported 1985 findings from the U.S. Bureau of the Census showing that in 1984, 31% of African American children lived in an extended family with either one or both parents. This was contrasted with the appreciably smaller proportion of children from other ethnic groups who lived in nontraditional families (19.8%). In addition, these authors pointed out that greater numbers of African American children than children from other ethnic groups lived in single-parent families (53% vs. 17.1%). Notably, in a recent study of African American family structure, the only differences found were that those youth living in a single-mother household reported receiving more parental support than other youth (Zimmerman et al., 1995). This study also found that adolescent males living in single-mother households did not differ from other family structures in relation to alcohol and other substance use, school dropout, delinquency, or psychological distress.

Although the role of the African American extended family has been considered over the years, few research groups have empirically studied this aspect of African American life. Tolson and Wilson (1990) argue that because such studies typically have gathered data from only one or two family members, the full complexity of the interactions within the family system has not been assessed. They suggest that to better understand the family climate in African American families, researchers need to take issues of family structure into account at all stages of study (McAdoo, in press). Then relationships between family members and the systems they are involved in can be studied in a comprehensive, ecologically valid fashion.

Asian American family structures have been described as being traditionally extended in composition (Fong & Browne, in press). Although these families have also been described as patriarchal, achievement-oriented, and highly encouraging of independence, the effects of these dynamics on the individual and the family system are not yet fully understood. Hispanic families have similarly been characterized as patriarchal in nature, family-centered, and highly cohesive (Carrasquillo, 1991). Future research on these families may warrant the examination of relationships between family members and how family cohesion affects individual development.

African American individuals have had to deal explicitly with racism and prejudice. African American families have helped their children survive in this hostile environment by teaching coping skills through racial socialization. The effect of minority status on the individual and the family in African American culture is an area that is in need of further research. In addition, some researchers have pointed out that the traditional between-group design used to explore differences between African American and European American samples is flawed, because European Americans may not be similar to African Americans on several dimensions (Zimmerman et al., 1995). Therefore, examining differences within groups of African Americans, instead of comparing African Americans to European American mainstream culture, may provide a more accurate, fuller, and more ecologically valid understanding of these families. The same reasoning applies to other ethnic groups within the United States.

Gay and Lesbian Families

Lesbian women and gay men have always been involved in parenting. However, research has typically emphasized a conceptualization of gay and lesbian people as individuals, rather than as family members or parents (Allen & Demo, 1995). Laird (1993) has suggested that this limited and inaccurate perception is related to heterosexist assumptions reflecting society's belief that gayness and family are mutually exclusive concepts. Laird has stated that this belief continues because "the same-sex family, more than any other form, challenges fundamental patriarchal notions of family and gender relationships" (Laird, 1993, p. 259). Thus, experience outside the confines of the more narrow and traditional definition of family are not identified, remain nameless, and are largely ignored in the realm of family research (Allen & Demo, 1995). In a review of the three leading family journals between 1980 and 1993, Allen and Demo (1995) discovered that of the 2,598 articles published, only 12 articles focused on families of lesbians and gays.

Although lesbian women and gay men have achieved heightened visibility, basic demographic information regarding the size of the lesbian and gay populations has remained difficult to obtain. Current estimates of gay and lesbian parents in the United States have been reported to range between 2 and 8 million, while estimates of children of lesbian and gay parents range from 4 to 14 million (Patterson, 1995). Current estimates suggest that there are between 1.5 and 5 million lesbian mothers who live with their children in the United States (Falk, 1989; Turner, Scadden, & Harris, 1990). Many of these women had children within a heterosexual marriage and then divorced, came out as lesbian, and continued raising their children with a same-sex partner or alone. Currently there are many "out" lesbian women who are choosing to have families through donor insemination, adoption, or foster care (Flaks et al., 1995). It has also been estimated that there are between 1 and 3 million gay men who are natural fathers of children (Bozett, 1987). Moreover, at least 6 million children under the age of 18 have been estimated to have gay or lesbian parents (Schulenberg, 1985). Whatever the exact numbers, the prevalence of lesbian and gay families alone justifies further research on the interactions among its family members. Figure 2.3 illustrates a conceptual model of a lesbian family with a known biological father who is not part of the primary system. The boundaries constructed between the biological father and members of the primary system will depend in large measure on the

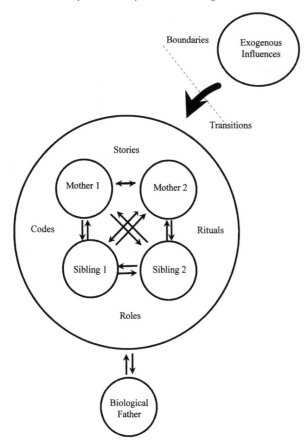

FIGURE 2.3. Possible transactional linkages in a primary family system headed by two lesbian women with a known biological father who is not part of the system.

parenting partners and the extent to which they or the biological father want him to participate in a caregiving role. Key adjunctive systems may play a major role in structuring the boundaries that surround the primary system.

Current research on lesbian and gay families has been spurred by the legal system's attempts to grapple with issues surrounding child custody. As the prevalence of gay and lesbian families receives more widespread attention, gay and lesbian parents' desirability as parents has been questioned. Concern is centered around the possible negative developmental effects of gay and lesbian parenting and the possibility that exposure to gay or lesbian parents may result in gay or lesbian offspring (Bailey, Bobrow, Wolfe, & Mikach, 1995). Reviews of gender identity, gender role behavior, sexual orientation, psychological well-being, and social relationships have failed to find any greater risk for difficulty in children of gay or lesbian parents (Patterson, 1992).

The lack of research on these families may be related to the treatment of gay and lesbian households as a "social address" (Allen & Demo, 1995). The "social address" has been described by Bronfenbrenner and Crouter (1983) as an "environmental label—with no attention to what the environment is like, what people are living there, what they are doing, or how the activities taking place could affect the child" (pp. 361–362). What is needed, in addition to the study of family structure in gay- and lesbian-headed families, is more attention to family interactions and processes. Similar to the study of ethnic minority families, the impact of sexual minority membership on the family members and the family unit is an area of needed research. Lastly, research must sample the diversity of gay and lesbian families (Allen & Demo, 1995; Gartrell et al., 1996). Most studies of gay and lesbian families to date have sampled a unique subset of families that are predominantly European American, middle-class, urban, highly educated, and strongly identified with their lesbian and gay identities (Laird, 1993; Patterson, 1992).

CONCLUSION

A more dynamic and pluralistic definition of family is necessary to guide the study of contemporary family systems. The diversity of the American family of the 21st century requires equally diverse and innovative research methodologies to capture the essence and subtlety of the family and the interacting personalities that define it. High priority should be given to study of culturally diverse families, in order to heighten societal understanding of the rich cultural and family codes that help shape individual differences in a pluralistic society. Equally high priority should be given to understanding the impact of nontraditional parenting structures on child behavior and development. As the numbers of families headed by single fathers, homosexual partners, and multiracial couples continue to increase, study of the transactions among family members and the ways that families deal with exogenous forces will provide deeper insight into the policies and societal resources necessary to assure optimal rearing environments and the integrity of family life for future generations.

ACKNOWLEDGMENT

Preparation of this chapter was supported in part by Grant No. AA07065 from the National Institute on Alcohol Abuse and Alcoholism to Robert A. Zucker and Hiram E. Fitzgerald.

REFERENCES

Allen, K. R., & Demo, D. H. (1995). The families of lesbians and gay men: A new frontier in family research. *Journal of Marriage and the Family, 57,* 111–127.

Allen, W. R. (1978). The search for applicable theories of black family life. *Journal of Marriage and the Family, 40,* 117–129.

Bailey, J. M., Bobrow, D., Wolfe, M., & Mikach, S. (1995). Sexual orientation of adult sons of gay fathers. *Developmental Psychology, 31,* 124–129.

Baumrind, D. (1989). Rearing competent children. In W. Damon (Ed.), *Child development today and tomorrow* (pp. 349–378). San Francisco: Jossey-Bass.

Baumrind, D. (1995). *Child maltreatment and optimal caregiving in social contexts.* New York: Garland Press.

Borduin, C. M., Mann, B. J., Cone, L., & Borduin, B. J. (1990). Development of the concept of family in elementary school children. *Journal of Genetic Psychology, 15,* 33–43.

Bozett, F. W. (1987). Children of gay fathers. In F. W. Bozett (Ed.), *Gay and lesbian parents* (pp. 39–57). New York: Praeger.

Brody, G. H., Pillegrini, A. D., & Sigel, I. E. (1986). Marital quality and mother–child and father–child interactions with school-aged children. *Developmental Psychology, 22,* 291–296.

Bronfenbrenner, U. (1979). *The ecology of human development: Experiments by nature and design.* Cambridge, MA: Harvard University Press.

Bronfenbrenner, U., & Crouter, A. C. (1983). The evolution of environmental models in developmental research. In P. H. Mussen (Series Ed.) & W. Kessen (Vol. Ed.), *Handbook of child psychology: Vol. 1. History, theory, and methods* (4th ed., pp. 357–414). New York: Wiley.

Buhrmester, D., Camparo, L., Christensen, A., Gonzalez, L. S., & Hinshaw, S. P. (1992). Mothers and fathers interacting in dyads and triads with normal and hyperactive sons. *Developmental Psychology, 28,* 500–509.

Burgess, E. W. (1972). The family as a unity of interacting personalities. In G. D. Erikson & T. P. Hogan (Eds.), *Family therapy: An introduction to theory and technique* (pp. 4–15). Monterey, CA: Brooks/Cole. (Original work published 1926)

Carrasquillo, A. L. (1991). *Hispanic children and youth in the United States.* New York: Garland Press.

Caspi, A., Elder, G. H., Jr., & Herbener, E. S. (1990). Childhood personality and the prediction of life-course patterns. In L. Robins & M. Rutter (Eds.), *Straight and devious pathways from childhood to adulthood* (pp. 13–35). New York: Cambridge University Press.

Cherlin, A. J., Furstenberg, F. F., Jr., Chase-Lansdale, P. L., Kiernan, K. E., Robins, P. K., Morrison, D. R., & Teitler, J. O. (1991). Longitudinal studies of effects of divorce on children in Great Britain and the United States. *Science, 252,* 1386–1389.

Cummings, E. M., Ballard, M., El-Sheikh, M., & Lake, M. (1991). Resolution and children's responses to interadult anger. *Developmental Psychology, 27,* 462–470.

Cummings, E. M., Iannotti, R. J., & Zahn-Waxler, C. (1985). Influence of conflict between adults on the emotions and aggression of young children. *Developmental Psychology, 21,* 495–507.

Dornbusch, S. M., Ritter, P. L., Leiderman, P. H., Roberts, D. F., & Fraleigh, M. J. (1987). The relationship of parenting style to adolescent school performance. *Child Development, 58,* 1244–1257.

Eisenberg, A. R. (1988). Grandchildren's perspectives on relationships with grandparents: The influence of gender across generations. *Sex Roles: A Journal of Research, 19,* 205–217.

Emde, R. N., Gaensbauer, T. J., & Harmon, R. J. (1976). Emotional expression in infancy: A biobehavioral shift. *Psychological Issues, 10*(1, Whole No. 37).

Emery, R. E. (1982). Interparental conflict and the children of discord and divorce. *Psychological Bulletin, 92,* 310–330.

Falk, P. (1989). Lesbian mothers: Psychosocial assumptions in family law. *American Psychologist, 44,* 941–947.

Fitzgerald, H. E., Zucker, R. A., & Yang, H.-Y. (1995). Developmental systems theory and alcoholism: Analyzing patterns of variation in high-risk families. *Psychology of Addictive Behaviors, 9,* 8–22.

Flaks, D. K., Ficher, I., Masterpasqua, F., & Joseph, G. (1995). Lesbians choosing motherhood: A comparative study. *Developmental Psychology, 31,* 105–114.

Fong, R., & Browne, C. (in press). United States immigration policy and Chinese children and families. In H. E. Fitzgerald, B. M. Lester, & B. Zuckerman (Eds.), *Children of color: Research, health, and policy issues.* New York: Garland Press.

Ford, D. H., & Lerner, R. M. (1992). *Developmental systems theory: An integrative approach.* Newbury Park, CA: Sage.

Gartrell, N., Hamilton, J., Banks, A., Mosbacher, D., Reed, N., Sparks, C. H., & Bishop, H. (1996). The national lesbian family study: 1. Interviews with prospective mothers. *American Journal of Orthopsychiatry, 66,* 272–281.

Ge, X., Conger, R. D., Cadoret, R. J., Neiderhiser, J. M., Yates, W., Troughton, E., & Stewart, M. A. (1996). The development interface between nature and nurture: A mutual influence model of child antisocial behavior and parent behaviors. *Developmental Psychology, 32,* 574–589.

Gjerde, P. F. (1986). The interpersonal structure of family interaction settings: Parent–adolescent relations in dyads and triads. *Developmental Psychology, 22,* 297–304.

Glick, P. C. (1981). A demographic picture of black families. In H. P. McAdoo (Ed.), *Black families* (pp. 106–126). Beverly Hills, CA: Sage.

Gottlieb, G. (1991). Experiential canalization of behavioral development: Theory. *Developmental Psychology, 27,* 4–13.

Gottman, J. M., & Katz, L. F. (1989). Effects of marital discord on young children's peer interaction and health. *Developmental Psychology, 25,* 373–381.

Grych, J. H., & Fincham, F. D. (1993). Children's appraisals of interparental conflict: Initial investigations of the cognitive-contextual framework. *Child Development, 64,* 215–230.

Harold, G. T., Fincham, F. D., Osborne, L. N., & Conger, R. D. (1997). Mom and dad are at it again: Adolescent perceptions of marital conflict and adolescent distress. *Developmental Psychology, 33,* 333–350.

Hetherington, E. M. (1989). Coping with family transitions: Winners, losers and survivors. *Child Development, 60,* 1–14.

Hill, J. P. (1980). The family. In M. Johnson (Ed.), *Toward adolescence: The middle school years* (pp. 32–55). Chicago: University of Chicago Press.

Hill, R. (1972). *The strengths of black families.* New York: Emerson-Hall.

Howes, P., & Markman, H. J. (1989). Marital quality and child functioning: A longitudinal investigation. *Child Development, 60,* 1044–1051.

Katz, L. F., & Gottman, J. M. (1993). Patterns of marital conflict predict children's internalizing and externalizing behaviors. *Developmental Psychology, 29,* 940–950.

Kennedy, G. E. (1991). Grandchildren's reasons for closeness with grandparents. *Journal of Social Behavior and Personality, 12,* 435–443.

Kurdek, L. A. (1986). Children's reasoning about parental divorce. In R. D. Ashmore & D. M. Brodzinsky (Eds.), *Thinking about the family: Views of parents and children* (pp. 233–276). Hillsdale, NJ: Erlbaum.

Kurdek, L. A., & Fine, M. A. (1994). Family acceptance and family control as predictors of adjustment in young adolescents: Linear, curvilinear, or interactive effects? *Child Development, 65,* 1137–1146.

Laird, J. (1993). Lesbian and gay families. In F. Walsh (Ed.), *Normal family processes* (2nd ed., pp. 282–328). New York: Guilford Press.

Lamb, M. E. (1976). Effects of stress and cohort on mother- and father–infant interaction. *Developmental Psychology, 12,* 435–443.

Lamborn, S. D., Mounts, N. S., Steinberg, L., & Dornbusch, S. M. (1991). Patterns of competence and adjustment among adolescents from authoritative, authoritarian, indulgent, and neglectful families. *Child Development, 62,* 1049–1065.

Lerner, J. V. (1993). The influence of child temperamental characteristics on parent behaviors. In T. Luster & L. Okagaki (Eds.), *Parenting: An ecological perspective* (pp. 101–118). Hillsdale, NJ: Erlbaum.

Lerner, J. V., & Lerner, R. M. (1983). Temperament and adaptation across life: Theoretical and empirical issues. In P. B. Baltes & O. G. Brim, Jr. (Ed.), *Life-span development and behavior* (Vol. 5, pp. 197–230). New York: Academic Press.

Levine, R. L., & Fitzgerald, H. E. (Eds.). (1992). *Analysis of dynamic psychological systems: Vol. 1. Basic approaches to general systems, dynamic systems, and cybernetics.* New York: Plenum Press.

Liddell, C., Henzi, S. P., & Drew, M. (1987). Mothers, fathers, and children in an urban park playground: A comparison of dyads and triads. *Developmental Psychology, 23,* 262–266.

McAdoo, H. P. (in press). Diverse children of color: Research and policy implications. In H. E. Fitzgerald, B. M. Lester, & B. Zuckerman (Eds.), *Children of color: Research, health, and policy issues.* New York: Garland Press.

McCrady, B. S., & Epstein, E. E. (1995). Directions for research on alcoholic relationships: Marital- and individual-based model of heterogeneity. *Psychology of Addictive Behaviors, 9,* 157–166.

McFarlane, A. H., Bellissimo, A., & Norman, G. R. (1995). Family structure, family functioning and adolescent well-being: The transcendent influence of parental style. *Journal of Child Psychology and Psychiatry, 36,* 847–864.

McGreal, C. E. (1994). The family across generations: Grandparenthood. In L.

L'Abate (Ed.), *Handbook of developmental family psychology and psychopathology* (pp. 116–131). New York: Wiley.

Melton, G. B., & Wilcox, B. L. (1989). Changes in family law and family life: Challenges for psychology. *American Psychologist, 44,* 1213–1216.

Miller, J. G. (1978). *Living systems.* New York: McGraw-Hill.

Min, P. G. (1995). *Asian Americans: Contemporary trends and issues.* Thousand Oaks, CA: Sage.

Muller, R. T., Fitzgerald, H. E., Sullivan, L. A., & Zucker, R. A. (1994). Social support and stress factors in child maltreatment among alcoholic families. *Canadian Journal of Behavioural Science, 26,* 438–461.

Newman, J. L., Roberts, L. R., & Syre, C. R. (1993). Concepts of family among children and adolescents: Effect of cognitive level, gender, and family structure. *Developmental Psychology, 29,* 951–962.

Nobles, W. W. (1978). Toward an empirical and theoretical framework for defining black families. *Journal of Marriage and the Family, 40,* 679–688.

Partridge, S., & Kotler, T. (1987). Self-esteem and adjustment in adolescents from bereaved, divorced, and intact families: Family type versus family environment. *Australian Journal of Psychology, 8,* 427–432.

Patterson, C. J. (1992). Children of lesbian and gay parents. *Child Development, 63,* 1025–1042.

Patterson, C. J. (1995). Families of the lesbian baby boom: Parents' division of labor and children's adjustment. *Developmental Psychology, 31,* 115–123.

Patterson, G. R. (1996). Some characteristics of a developmental theory for early-onset delinquency. In M. F. Lenzenwenger & J. J. Haugaard (Eds.), *Frontiers of developmental psychopathology* (pp. 81–124). New York: Oxford University Press.

Patterson, G. R., DeBaryshe, B. D., & Ramsey, E. (1989). A developmental perspective on antisocial behavior. *American Psychologist, 44,* 329–335.

Pederson, D. R., & Gilby, R. L. (1986). Children's concepts of family. In R. D. Ashmore & D. M. Brodzinsky (Eds.), *Thinking about the family: Views of parents and children* (pp. 181–204). Hillsdale, NJ: Erlbaum.

Pettit, G. S., & Bates, J. E. (1989). Family interaction patterns and children's behavior problems from infancy to 4 years. *Developmental Psychology, 25,* 413–420.

Radke-Yarrow, M., Zahn-Waxler, C., Richardson, D. T., Susman, A., & Martinez, P. (1994). Caring behavior in children of clinically depressed and well mothers. *Child Development, 65,* 1405–1414.

Reid, J. (1982). Black America in the 1980's. *Population Bulletin, 37,* 1–37.

Rueschenberg, E. J., & Buriel, R. (1995). Mexican-American family functioning and acculturation: A family systems perspective. In A. M. Padilla (Ed.), *Hispanic psychology* (pp. 15–25). Thousand Oaks, CA: Sage.

Russell, G. (1986). Grandfathers: Making up for lost opportunities. In R. A. Lewis & R. E. Salt (Eds.), *Men in families* (pp. 233–259). Beverly Hills, CA: Sage.

Sameroff, A. J. (1995). General systems theories and developmental psychopathology. In D. Cicchetti & D. J. Cohen (Eds.), *Developmental psychopathology: Vol. 1. Theory and methods* (pp. 659–695). New York: Wiley.

Schulenberg, J. (1985). *Gay parenting.* New York: Doubleday.

Shaw, D. S., Emery, R. E., & Tuer, M. D. (1993). Parental functioning and children's adjustment in families of divorce: A prospective study. *Journal of Abnormal Child Psychology, 21,* 119–134.

Steinberg, L., Lamborn, S. D., Darling, N., Mounts, N. S., & Dornbusch, S. M. (1994). Over-time changes in adjustment and competence among adolescents from authoritative, authoritarian, indulgent, and neglectful families. *Child Development, 65,* 754–770.

Stevens, J. H. (1984). Black grandmothers' and black adolescent mothers' knowledge about parenting. *Developmental Psychology, 20,* 1017–1025.

Tinsley, B. J., & Parke, R. D. (1987). Grandparents as interactive and social support agents for families with young infants. *International Journal of Aging and Human Development, 25,* 259–277.

Tolson, T. F. J., & Wilson, M. N. (1990). The impact of two- and three-generational black family structure on perceived family climate. *Child Development, 61,* 416–428.

Turner, P. H., Scadden, L., & Harris, M. B. (1990). Parenting in gay and lesbian families. *Journal of Gay and Lesbian Psychotherapy, 1,* 55–66.

Uzoka, A. F. (1979). The myth of the nuclear family: Historical background and clinical implications. *American Psychologist, 34,* 1095–1106.

von Bertalanffy, L. (1968). *General systems theory.* New York: Braziller.

Wagner, B. M., & Reiss, D. (1995). Family systems and developmental psychopathology: Courtship, marriage, or divorce? In D. Cicchetti & D. J. Cohen (Eds.), *Developmental psychopathology: Vol. 1. Theory and methods* (pp. 696–730). New York: Wiley.

Webster-Stratton, C. (1990). Stress: A potential disrupter of parent perceptions and family interactions. *Journal of Clinical Child Psychology, 19,* 302–312.

Whipple, E. E., Fitzgerald, H. E., & Zucker, R. A. (1995). Parent–child interactions in alcoholic and non-alcoholic families. *American Journal of Orthopsychiatry, 65,* 153–159.

White, L. (1994). Growing up with single parents and stepparents: Long-term effects on family solidarity. *Journal of Marriage and the Family, 56,* 935–948.

White, S. H. (1965). Evidence for a hierarchical arrangement of learning processes. In L. P. Lipsitt & C. C. Spiker (Eds.), *Advances in child development and behavior* (Vol. 2, pp. 187–220). New York: Academic Press.

Zimmerman, M. A., Salem, D. A., & Maton, K. I. (1995). Family structure and psychosocial correlates among urban African-American adolescent males. *Child Development, 66,* 1598–1613.

CHAPTER 3

The Concept of
"the Family"
in Family Psychology

MATTHIAS PETZOLD

THE STATE OF THE MODERN FAMILY

Nearly every human being on earth has at least some family ties. Everyone is at least a member of a family of origin, and many people are also currently members of a primary living group. In this way, most of us have multiple family memberships. Therefore, "the family" is without question a very important concept for almost everybody.

The family must cope with heavy duties and social demands. Furthermore, the ideological biases concerning the family are rather strong too. It is assumed that the family gives its members the psychological support that they need in their lifelong development as human beings. Infants need shelter and warmth. Preschool children need guidance in acquiring basic cognitive and social competence. Older children will not be successful in school without social support from parents or caregivers (e.g., help with homework). Adolescents need room and support in developing their own identities. Most adults seek support for productivity at work, intimacy with spouses or partners, and nurturant relationships with children. And elderly people need physical and psychological support, especially if they are disabled in some way.

Individual life span development is thus marked by many tasks involving a need for general social support. These tasks are part of the basic social problems unique to humankind, and should thus be considered as public problems—problems requiring attention from the state. But instead of making efforts to solve these problems, most public officials consider them responsibilities of private families. Nowadays in most Western countries, giving support to individual development is not recognized as a public affair, but is delegated to the family. In order to avoid creating more public social support programs, many politicians call for a revival of "the family," which is supposed to give us all the support we need in our individual development.

Such public calls for strengthening "the family" have influenced traditional legal forms (e.g., in family laws, social welfare regulations, etc.). Politicians of all main parties around the globe rely on the family. However, they only give minor financial grants or tax breaks to families. Nevertheless, families do a lot of unpaid work in raising and socializing children. It has been estimated that in Western countries, raising one child from birth until the child leaves home or finishes his or her education costs as much as half a million U.S. dollars. This is calculated on the basis of the mother's not being paid at all or being paid at the level of an unskilled worker. On the basis of this calculation, by far the largest component of the gross national product is this work that is done free or nearly free of charge within families—by mothers, mainly. Keeping this huge labor force happy in continuing to work with little or no compensation is the main reason why all the politicians praise "the family." These ideological biases are still present in the mass media as well, but times are changing, and the family is changing even more.

Within the last 200 years, there have been major revolutions in history and society that have shaped the family. The shift from an agrarian to an industrial society started 200 years ago in England and is even now reshaping some former Third World countries. Within this industrial revolution a new urban family type developed, characterized by a clear distinction between work and family, and by the father as the breadwinner working somewhere in the industrial sector. For many years, this was the dominant form of families. But within the last few decades, this type has shown a sharply decreasing frequency. Dual-career families, one-parent families, and many other new forms have started flourishing within the last two decades. Hernandez (1993), analyzing the development of family forms in the United States, has shown that the typical family consisting of father as breadwinner, mother as caregiver and child(ren) has only marginal relevance today. Meanwhile, the old ideological biases have lost some of their basis because of these strong shifts within family development. The 21st century will not be characterized by the traditional nuclear family as the basic unit of Western society. Again, times are changing, and the family is changing. Indeed, who knows what new shapes the family will take in the future?

The debate on this development in the social sciences is already rather old, and some investigators have even discarded "the family" as a basic term for a social unit. However, in psychology, family research has become a newly fashionable area. Several psychological subdisciplines have been involved in research on family psychology from their respective viewpoints. Families' educational styles and similar questions have been studied in educational psychology for some time; developmental psychologists have shifted from descriptions of single family members toward descriptions of the family as a group; and social psychologists have examined familial interaction patterns and different types of family structures (Markman, 1992; Gable et al., 1992).

Despite all these research activities, not much has been done in constructing new theoretical perspectives, and only a few publications have focused on the theory of the family (e.g., Cheal, 1991; Fine, 1993). Family psychology still lacks sound theoretical work. This is especially true for the basic term itself: Although the concept of "the family" is widespread in psychological research and practice, a clear definition of what the term really means has not yet been established. Without a theoretical framework, a definition of the term can only be an operational definition within a particular investigation. Before outlining some ideas on how to define "the family" within an ecopsychological theory of family development, however, I want to show that in Western countries no single family form currently prevails. Rather, taking Germany and the United States as examples of modern Western nations, I show that "the family" consists not of one but of many different basic living forms.

Status of the Nuclear Family in Germany and the United States

To throw some light on the current situation in Germany and the United States, let us look at recent demographic data. The following statements are based on statistical data from the German Federal Bureau of Statistics (Statistisches Bundesamt) and the U.S. Bureau of the Census. One has to take into account that these institutions themselves are still clearly employing an operational definition of "the family" as a traditional nuclear family, or at least a parent–child unit. Statistisches Bundesamt (1995) uses this definition of families: "parental couples or single parents living with their unmarried children in a shared household" (p. 10; my translation). This restricted definition describes two important forms, but by no means the only forms, of primary living situations. I discuss alternative forms later after looking at some general demographic trends.

In 1992, the population of the reunited Germany consisted of 80.7 million people living in 35.6 million households. Only 13.3 million of these households were families with children. Of these 13.4 million, 6.8 million consisted of families with one child, 4.9 million had two children, 1.3 million had three children, and only 0.4 million had four or more children. The rest of the households consisted of persons living alone (12.0 million), couples without children (8.4 million), and a minority of other household forms (Statistisches Bundesamt, 1995).

Therefore, according to the household structures, the trend toward living alone or as part of a childless couple is striking. Moreover, although the family is still the dominant primary living form in Germany, this family is not the traditional father–mother–child triad. Although more than half of the Germans live in a kind of family, the number of single parents is rising (5.3% in 1992). This trend toward single-parent families is especially strong in ethnically diverse cultures, as indicated by a look at the state of the family in the United States (see Table 3.1). Most notably, in black U.S. culture the single-parent family is already the prevailing form.

Because of this trend, even in Germany less than half of the population (47.8%) lives in the traditional form of a nuclear family (two parents with at least one child). From an overview of the major household forms in Germany and the United States, it is obvious that the traditional family is only one of many living patterns (see Table 3.2). If one compares the different household forms, the picture is even more striking, because only 31.9% of German households and 25.8% of U.S. households exhibit the traditional father–mother–child(ren) family form. The predominant German household form consists of singles without children, and the predominant U.S. form consists of couples without children.

General Trends in Western Countries

Therefore, the full-fledged nuclear parental family is no longer the prevailing family form in the United States and Germany. There are several reasons for this situation: The marriage rate is declining, the number of divorces is increasing, the number of children per family is decreasing, and new primary living forms are emerging.

First, a striking event is occurring in all the modern industrialized countries: The birth rate and the death rate are both declining. This trend is continuous for Germany but similar in the United States, where the birth rate is lower but the death rate is higher (see Table 3.3). The German trend is typical for the West European nations, all of which are characterized by a growing proportion of elderly people. This trend is causing a change in the age structure of the population, with a growing number of old and a declining number of young people. This is exemplified in an evaluation made for the European Commission (see Table 3.4).

TABLE 3.1. U.S. Families with Children in 1994: Percentage of Different Forms by Ethnic Group

Family form	White	Black	Hispanic	Total
Two-parent	75.3	35.2	63.8	69.2
Single-mother	20.7	59.7	31.2	26.6
Single-father	4.0	5.1	5.0	4.2

Note. The data are from U.S. Bureau of the Census (1995).

TABLE 3.2. Major Household Forms in Germany (1992) and the United States (1994)

	Without children	With children
Germany		
Singles	33.6% (12.0 mil.)	5.3% (1.9 mil.)
Couples	23.5% (8.4 mil.)	31.9% (11.4 mil.)
Others	5.3% (1.9 mil.)	
United States		
Singles	24.3% (23.6 mil.)	11.7% (11.4 mil.)
Couples	29.0% (28.2 mil.)	25.8% (25.1 mil.)
Others	6.6% (6.4 mil.)	9.2% (8.9 mil.)

Note. The data are from Statistisches Bundesamt (1995) and U.S. Bureau of the Census (1995). Total household *n*'s are 35.6 million for Germany and 103.6 for the United States.

One reason for the decline of the birth rate in Germany, at least, might be the rise in the age at first marriage. Whereas in the 1950s the mean age at first marriage was 25 years for German women, nowadays German women first marry at a mean age of over 30 years (with husbands at a mean age of 32.8 years). Furthermore, the marriage rate is steadily declining in general. Young couples choose to live together and place a high emphasis on intimate relationship, but not necessarily on marriage. However, marriage usually takes place before or at childbirth, because unmarried parents in Germany receive fewer social benefits and experience legal restrictions in parental rights. These facts demonstrate that there is a slow but strongly continuing trend against marriage in Germany, mainly due to the tendency to postpone marriage to a later age. In particular, young people choose to

TABLE 3.3. Birth and Death Rates per 1,000 in Germany (1988–1995) and the United States (1994)

Year	Birth rate	Death rate
Germany		
1988	11.4	11.5
1989	11.2	11.5
1990	11.4	11.6
1991	10.4	11.4
1992	10.4	11.3
1993	9.8	11.1
1994	9.5	10.9
1995	9.4	10.8
United States		
1994	8.8	15.3

Note. The data are from Statistisches Bundesamt (1995) and U.S. Bureau of the Census (1995).

TABLE 3.4. Age Structure of the Population in Selected European Countries

	1900	1950	1980	2000 (est.)	2020 (est.)
Age 0–14					
France	—	26.1	22.7	22.3	19.2
Germany	34.8	23.5	18.2	15.5	13.4
Italy	—	34.4	26.4	22.0	17.1
Sweden	32.5	23.4	19.6	17.4	16.3
Age 15–64					
France	—	65.7	65.9	63.8	65.5
Germany	60.4	67.1	66.3	67.4	64.8
Italy	59.5	65.5	64.6	67.6	66.0
Sweden	59.1	66.3	64.1	66.0	62.9
Age 65+					
France	8.2	11.3	14.0	15.3	19.5
Germany	4.8	9.3	15.5	17.1	21.1
Italy	6.1	8.0	13.4	15.3	19.4
Sweden	8.4	10.2	16.3	16.6	20.8

Note. Data from European Centre (cited in Overtrup, 1991, p. 21).

live together for several years before marriage, and often marriage is considered only because of the increased social benefits that result after in-wedlock childbirth.

The currently widespread pattern of a long "trial period" of sharing a household before getting married does not prevent the breakup of marriages. Although many couples have a long period of living together before marriage, the number of divorces is rising steadily. Although many of the marriages break up in the early years, the mean time for most divorces is after 5 years of marriage. This means that in most cases of divorce, children are involved in this change of their family. The trend toward more and more divorces has been generally increasing since the end of the 1950s. This development means that only half of recent marriages will be terminated by the death of one of the partners, because every second marriage will end earlier—by divorce.

Alternative Forms of Modern Family Life

There is a strong trend toward newly emerging alternatives to the traditional family. Some selected alternative family forms are discussed in detail here:

- Singles
- Childless couples
- Homosexual couples
- Unmarried cohabitation
- Successive families

- "Living apart together"
- Care for the elderly

In Germany, where (as noted above) only half of the population now lives in a traditional nuclear family, many people have chosen to live in other basic household forms, which in most cases are also perceived subjectively as family forms. It is a complicated matter to show how important these alternative forms of family life really are, because it is very much a question of the subjective feelings of the persons involved. If one abandons the nomothetic tradition of defining the family according to legal norms or social stereotypes, one has to listen to the subjective under-standings of individuals. One implication of this is that statistical data for a general analysis cannot be gained any more, because the same form may be considered a family by one person but not by another. This can even be true for different people living in the same shared environment.

The basic living form of singles who decide to stay alone has become more and more attractive. In some big Western cities (e.g., San Francisco, Paris, or Munich), it has even been estimated that far more than half of the population consists of singles in one-person households. The number of singles has also gone up because of a large group of young adults who have not yet decided to enter into a couple relationship or marriage, but stay single for some time. Similarly, there is a slight tendency not to marry again after a divorce, especially for women. When one looks at all those different forms of singles, it is very hard to say whether some of the people living this way understand themselves as a family; some of them may, but most probably do not. Nevertheless, this form of basic living is becoming more and more important.

Childless couples are also more common; indeed, this is a newly strong trend. Here again, it is difficult to decide whether such couples form a type of family. At least by their own subjective understanding, many do. Even within the legal norms, a married couple without children is considered a family by the state for taxation and other purposes in Germany.

In recent years, homosexual couples have been "coming out" to the public, and many such couples have called for the right to marry. With some restrictions, such marriages were recently legalized in the Netherlands and Sweden. Some homosexual couples have even applied to adopt a child, or to care for one full-time at least. In these cases, the conflict between the nomothetical stereotype and a clear subjective understanding is evident: Whereas by law in most countries a married couple must be heterosexual to form a family, many homosexual couples are keen on marriage and on being recognized as families.

Living together without legal marriage is a very fashionable form for young couples nowadays. One can even say that it is a "must" for young people planning to start a family. Therefore, many of these young people marry after or shortly before the birth of a child. Some family sociologists believe this form only to be a kind of preparatory stage for traditional family life. However, a growing large number of young couples—even with children—refrain from marrying and stay unmarried, although clearly understanding themselves as families. Such couples represent a kind of traditional nuclear family without marriage.

Stepparentship is an old divergent form of the traditional family. With the rising number of divorces, however, a new form of "double stepparentship" has emerged: If a family breaks up and each parent separately forms a new family with a partner who has also come from a broken-up family, successive families come into being. Most remarkable is that within such a family a child has four parents and eight grandparents. Because of the trend for divorced partners to marry again, successive families have emerged as an important family form after childbirth. In discussions of matters of family law, it is nowadays often stressed that after divorce a couple is separated, but both partners still have to be responsible parents. In this respect one can argue that although divorced, a couple still forms a family because of the ex-partners' shared responsibility as parents. This is especially true if this couple really shares child care responsibilities (e.g., the children live for part of the week with the mother and for the rest of the time with the father). Although the couple is not characterized by intimacy, this can still be a kind of family.

The new term "living apart together" has been used to note a different type of family. This is a new trend that thus far has only been chosen by a few people. The partners are very often related to each other very strongly by intimacy and a shared perspective, but they still do not decide to share living quarters. (The philosophers Jean-Paul Sartre and Simone de Beauvoir were one of the most prominent couples of this kind.) Such a construction can even include shared responsibility for children. Most of these couples, if asked, would describe themselves as families.

On the one hand, the need for child care is slowly declining in Western countries. On the other hand, the need for care for the elderly is rapidly growing in our current society, with its rising number of old people. Part of this trend is that many persons in middle adulthood do not have any obligation to look after children, but they have the responsibility of caring for an elderly person from their family of origin. In many psychological aspects, such new living forms resemble the traditional parent–child family, and many people living this way feel the same.

APPROACHES TO DEFINING THE FAMILY

In short, during the last few decades social life has changed a great deal, especially with regard to the family. These changes have led many investigators to the conclusion that it is no longer possible to use the traditional concept of "the family" for scientific research. It has even been suggested that the term "family" should not be used anymore, because this type of primary living form has vanished in social reality. Therefore, a thorough discussion of the various approaches to defining the family seems to be necessary.

Traditional Definitions

Traditional definitions of the family stress various different characteristics:

- Law and legal restrictions link family and marriage.
- The genealogical approach to understanding the family refers to various types and degrees of ancestry and blood relationship.
- Indeed, sometimes the terms "family" and "relatives" are mixed up, and both are seen as referring to biological or blood ties.
- In modern government statistics, the unit of the family is often operationally defined in terms of a household shared with one's children, leaving aside the question of marriage of any kind.

Although the traditional nuclear family is a basic stereotype within society, and the various definitions listed above reflect very different orientations. General law regulations in most countries tie family and marriage together; nevertheless, a growing number of young people stay unmarried. Most important in any application for social benefits is the responsibility for other family members. According to the calculations of social benefits, not only married partners but also first-degree biological relatives are also seen as family members. In common public understanding, the concept of marriage is often seen as secondary to the family tradition of genealogical bonds through ancestry and blood relationship. Although this perspective might have been stronger in the last century, this is still an important view of what may be meant by "the family." Because of the growing diversity in real social life, the official statistics have not kept to the legal restrictions of linking family with marriage. Thus, for example, the Statistisches Bundesamt (1995) has stressed the variables of shared household and care for children as key variables for defining "the family," as noted earlier.

Older scientific approaches kept to the traditional understanding of the nuclear mother–father–child (Süssmuth, 1981). In family sociology, René König (1974) stressed the biosocial double nature of the family. In German family psychology, Schneewind (1987) refers to "intimacy" as the basic variable for defining a family; a colleague and I (Petzold & Nickel, 1989) base our definition on "intimacy and intergenerational relations."

Modern Sociological Approaches

In modern sociological surveys, an "ego-centered" approach to defining the family has been used. The main assumption of this approach is based on the statement that a "family" has to be defined according to the subjective understanding of those forming the family; this is called the "ego-centered" method of definition (see Nyer, Bien, Marbach, & Templeton, 1991). This approach is very close to a psychological understanding, because the definition of the term "family" is not developed out of political norms, but out of the subjective feelings of people who believe themselves to be members of a family. Researchers from the Deutsches Jugendinstitut (Nyer et al., 1991) asked their subjects several questions about those with whom they believed they had a kind of familial relationship. The classificatory analysis of these data yielded three bases for these beliefs:

- Blood relationship
- Shared household
- Shared functions

These groups overlapped, but each group represented a distinct family characteristic.

Such a sociological approach supports the idea that there is no one specific family form. Based on the subjective feelings of their subjects, Nyer et al. (1991) suggested defining "the family" therefore in terms of different kinds of perceived family forms. This approach is also very fruitful for a new psychological definition of the term.

Psychological Approaches

In recent years, Klaus A. Schneewind (1987, 1991) has opened this debate in Germany and has suggested using the principle of intimacy as the basic variable for defining a family. This means that couples without children are also acknowledged as families. This concept has been critiqued, but has generally been accepted as a fruitful approach (see Voss, 1989; Petzold & Nickel, 1989).

Within our theoretical framework of family psychology, a colleague and I have stressed that intergenerational relations—not just intimacy—have to be considered as part of the basis for a definition of the family (Petzold & Nickel, 1989; Petzold, 1992). Therefore, we define "the family" as "a special social group, characterized by intimacy and intergenerational relations" (Petzold, 1992, p. 42). Variables such as lifelong continuity, heterosexual relationship, sharing a household and so on are all *not* part of our definition.

THEORETICAL CORNERSTONES
FOR FAMILY PSYCHOLOGY

Family psychology is a new, emerging subdiscipline with roots from various sources. Thus, the task of constructing theoretical models and systems is still open. Theoretical work should start with a discussion of the subject as it is investigated in scientific analysis. The subject of this new subdiscipline, the family, is not a given subject with compact theory.

Family Psychology in the Context of Systems Theory

Family psychology can learn a lot from other disciplines and scientific orientations. In particular, systems theory has stimulated much research and therapeutic work. However, there are several systems orientations with very different backgrounds. At least three approaches in systems theory are of relevance for family psychology (see Herlth, Brunner, Tyrell, & Kriz, 1994):

- The sciences approach and cybernetics (see von Bertalanffy, 1968)
- The analytical approach (see Parsons & Shils, 1951)
- The constructivist approach (see Luhmann, 1988)

In a kind of eclecticism, one can pick several ideas from each of these approaches. The sciences/cybernetics approach has been useful in describing the many regulatory processes within the family in its ecological setting and in society. The analytic perspective, derived from traditional empirical sociology and psychology, has yielded many insights on intergenerational relations (especially parent–child interactions). Within the constructivist view, the family is not considered as a natural object but as an idea, a concept, or a mythology that people share and live.

These three approaches enable us to understand three different perspectives on the family as an institution. One perspective is a pure theoretical construct, which comes to life in any kind of ideological stereotype of "the family" as an ideal concept. Such a perspective refers to social constructs, not to real entities. Another perspective is a view based on legal or religious convictions, which assume marriage as the basis of the family. This is a perspective often found in law and social policy. A third perspective emerges out of the genealogical function of the family and refers to childbirth and parenthood. Such an approach is often used in pedagogic, educational, and psychological treatment of family matters. These perspectives shape people's views of the family; they are the bases for the development of all the different realized forms of primary living. As such, it is fruitful to use them for an understanding of the plurality of current family life. It is even more fascinating to combine these perspectives as suggested in Figure 3.1.

A systemic understanding of the perspectives needs an analysis of how these perspectives interact with one another. If one conceives each perspective as a subsystem, and if we concede that these subsystems overlap, our analysis results in seven different family forms:

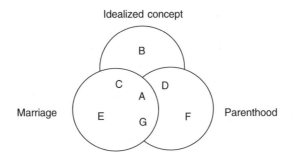

FIGURE 3.1. Three perspectives on the family as an institution: The family as an idealized concept (social construct), marriage, or parenthood. For definitions of family forms A–G, see text.

A. The traditional nuclear family (i.e., the traditional mother–father–child triad).

B. The family as a pure idealized concept or set of aspirations, such as that shared by family politicians and some family researchers.

C. The spousal relationship with an idealized family orientation, but no children (i.e., involuntarily childless couples).

D. Unmarried parenthood with an idealized family orientation, which is often the case in modern unmarried dual-career families and in some single-parent families.

E. Postmodern married couples without children and without an idealized family orientation (i.e., a job- and partner-oriented couple).

F. Alternative unmarried parenthood without an idealized family orientation (i.e., cohabitation with children, or alternative single parenthood).

G. Married couples with children but without an idealized family orientation (i.e., a new alternative family type).

The traditional nuclear family can be considered from each of these three perspectives, whereas the family forms B, E, and F can only be understood from one of the three perspectives. Therefore, it is necessary for a scientific approach to the definition of the family to take all three perspectives into account.

Although this analysis enables us to take a new look at the definition of the family, the setting of the family in social life needs further discussion. Following up the ecopsychological approach in developmental psychology, Bronfenbrenner (1986) has suggested some conclusions for family research.

An Ecopsychological Model of the Family

My ecopsychological approach (see Petzold, 1992) to defining the primary living group or the family takes into account that there is a broad range of different traditional and many new alternative forms of family living, and thus that any ideological biases should be avoided. As noted above, this model is based on intimacy and intergenerational relations. It incorporates external variables, characteristics of the spouses' or partners' relationship, and characteristics of the parent–child relationship; it also takes into account that other persons may be part of the family. Moreover, it incorporates the subsystems of Bronfenbrenner's (1986) human ecology: the macro-, exo-, meso-, and microsystems (see Figure 3.2).

In the ecopsychological model, within the general social setting (macrosystem), there are four variables influencing the family:

1. Legal marriage versus an extramarital arrangement
2. Lifelong versus time-limited or undefined arrangement
3. Shared versus separate income and revenues
4. Cohabitation versus living apart

Apart from general social settings, individuals belong to a special network (exosystem), which also shapes family life. This network can be constituted of the following:

5. Persons related by blood or marriage
6. Self-reliant or care-dependent persons
7. Economically independent or dependent persons
8. Persons who share the same culture or come from a different culture

In regard to children (mesosystem), three more variables influence the family:

9. Childlessness or child(ren)
10. Biological or adopted child(ren)
11. Parental or stepparental status of adults

Finally, aspects of the dyadic relationship of the partners themselves (microsystem) contribute to the family form:

12. Dual or single living style
13. Hetero- or homosexual relations
14. Egalitarian or dominant–subordinate roles

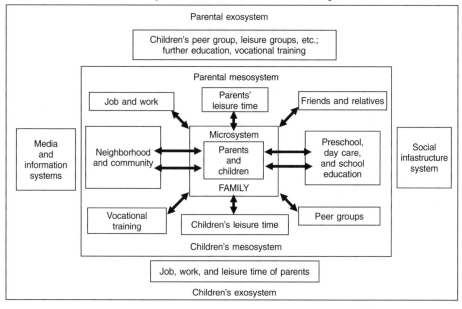

Macrosystem: Social, economic, and cultural settings

Parental exosystem

Children's peer group, leisure groups, etc.;
further education, vocational training

Parental mesosystem

Job and work

Parents'
leisure time

Friends and relatives

Media
and
information
systems

Neighborhood
and community

Microsystem

Parents
and
children

FAMILY

Preschool,
day care,
and school
education

Social
infastructure
system

Vocational
training

Children's leisure time

Peer groups

Children's mesosystem

Job, work, and leisure time of parents

Children's exosystem

FIGURE 3.2. Ecopsychological model of the family in the social setting. Adapted from Petzold (1992). Copyright 1992 by Matthias Petzold. Adapted by permission.

Any definition of the family needs to take into account this broad range of different variables, which contribute in different respects to the particular form of a specific family. In other words, there is no single form for families, but a pluralistic variety. If one accepts the suggested 14 variables, the possible number of different family forms (14 × 14) arising out of this schema comes to 196!

Family psychology has to take into account this broad diversity of different living patterns in today's society. Some members of the population do not live in any kind of family, although almost everybody is tied to a personal kind of family relationship. For those who do live in families, their particular positions on the broad spectrum of possible family patterns need to be understood. Moreover, each family member has a subjective image of the family's living pattern; therefore, it is even possible that people belonging to the same family have different psychological conceptions of the family they live in. For this reason, it is very useful to base a psychological analysis on a flexible model of the family that incorporates systemic approaches and individual constructs. In particular, when psychopathology is diagnosed, a knowledge of the individual's concept of family is necessary before any therapeutic intervention can start. Rather than attempting to reestablish the traditional concept of family, modern family psychology should help the individual to stabilize a healthy family concept compatible with his or her specific ecopsychological setting.

74 FOUNDATIONS

REFERENCES

Bronfenbrenner, U. (1986). Ecology of the family as a context for human development. *Developmental Psychology, 22,* 723–742.

Cheal, D. (1991). *Family and the state of theory.* New York: Harvester/Wheatsheaf.

Fine, M. A. (1993). Current approaches to understanding family diversity: An overview of the special issue. *Family Relations, 42,* 235–238.

Gable, S., Belsky, J., & Crnic, K. (1992). Marriage, parenting, and child development: Progress and prospects. *Journal of Family Psychology, 5,* 276–294.

Herlth, A., Brunner, E. J., Tyrell, H., & Kriz, J. (1994). *Abschied von der Normalfamilie?* Heidelberg: Springer-Verlag.

Hernandez, D. J. (1993). *America's children.* New York: Russell Sage Foundation.

König, R. (1974). *Die Familie der Gegenwart.* Munich: Beck.

Luhmann, N. (1988). Sozialsystem Familie. *System Familie, 1,* 75–91.

Markman, H. J. (1992). Marital and family psychology: Burning issues. *Journal of Family Psychology, 5,* 264–275.

Nyer, G., Bien, W., Marbach, J., & Templeton, R. (1991). Obtaining reliable data about family life: A methodological examination of egocentered networks in survey research. *Connections, 14,* 14–26.

Overtrup, J. (1991). *Childhood as a social phenomenon* (Eurosocial Report No. 36). Vienna: European Centre.

Parsons, T., & Shils, E. A. (1951). *Toward a general theory of action.* Cambridge, MA: Harvard University Press.

Petzold, M. (1992). *Familienentwicklungspsychologie.* Munich: Quintessenz.

Petzold, M., & Nickel, H. (1989). Grundlagen und Konzept einer entwicklungspsychologischen Familienforschung. *Psychologie in Erziehung und Unterricht, 36,* 241–257.

Schneewind, K. A. (1987). Familienpsychologie: Argumente für eine neue psychologische Disziplin. *Zeitschrift für Pädagogische Psychologie, 1,* 79–90.

Schneewind, K. A. (1991). *Familienpsychologie.* Stuttgart: Kohlhammer.

Statistisches Bundesamt. (1990). *Familien heute: Strukturen, Verläufe und Einstellungen (Ausgabe 1990).* Stuttgart: Metzler-Poeschel.

Statistisches Bundesamt. (1995). *Im Blickpunkt: Familien heute.* Stuttgart: Metzler-Poeschel.

Süssmuth, R. (1981). Familie. In H. Schiefele & A. Krapp (Eds.), *Handlexikon zur Pädagogischen Psychologie* (pp. 124–129). Munich: Ehrenwirth.

U.S. Bureau of the Census. (1995). Demographic data. Washington, DC: U.S. Government Printing Office.

von Bertalanffy, L. (1968). *General systems theory.* New York: Braziller.

Voss, H. G. (1989). Entwicklungspsychologische Familienforschung und Generationenfolge. In H. Keller (Ed.), *Handbuch der Kleinkindforschung* (pp. 207–228). Neuwied, Germany: Luchterhand.

CHAPTER 4

Family Interaction and Family Psychopathology

EWALD JOHANNES BRUNNER

THERAPIST: Can you imagine what it is your wife wants?
HE: No. She gets all she needs. I'm not stingy to her.
SHE: But that isn't what I mean!
HE: So what *do* you mean?
SHE: You'll never understand!

This short sequence from a session of couple therapy (Georgi, Levold, & Wedekind, 1990, p. 71; my translation) highlights what an important role dysfunctional communication can play in the development of psychopathology. We witness here a sequence or pattern of communication that has obviously taken place time and again. The pathologizing patterns of communication with which family therapists are often confronted have been characterized by Haley (1978) in the following way: "It is the rigid, repetitive sequence of a narrow range that defines pathology" (p. 105). These continually recurring sequences and patterns are referred to in the family therapy literature as "games" (Selvini Palazzoli, Boscolo, Cecchin, & Prata, 1975/1978). What in the world makes the members of a family play these eternal, complex games? It is hard to understand why people who are so familiar to one another, and so dependent on one another in their need for protection and support, should create a form of interaction that causes them real distress and brings on further suffering (e.g., in the form of illnesses).

The most spectacular new development in the clinical-psychological field since Sigmund Freud—the invention of family therapy—took these games themselves as its point of reference (leaving the question of why they are played open). Whereas in the past the focus had been on deficits in the individual, the emphasis now shifted to interaction sequences between members of the communication system (the family) and to the web of moves and countermoves and the apparent chaos of their sequence; to communication barriers and traps; and to the regulation of distance and closeness by verbal and nonverbal communication. Family therapists began to ask about the function of the games for the psychological "health" of the family system. Where family therapy broke new ground was in recognizing the importance of communication/interaction for psychopathology.

Interactions, as they take place and can be observed between members of a family, came to be seen as the keys that could open the system. Corresponding to the observable patterns of communication, specific structures are formed in self-organizing processes in the course of the family's life, and these break out dangerously in moments of family stress. Family therapists have spoken here of the occurrence of specific interaction and communication patterns.

We have to thank the pioneers of family therapy for seeing a link between the development of schizophrenic phenomena and the communication style of the family members. According to this perception, the so-called "double-bind" communication, as described by the members of the Palo Alto school, can induce schizophrenia (Bateson, Jackson, Haley, & Weakland, 1956; see below).

THE APPROACH TO FAMILY PSYCHOPATHOLOGY VIA FAMILY INTERACTION: THEORETICAL FOUNDATIONS

To regard a psychosocial problem not as the problem of an individual but as one of communication made the traditional pathologizing concept superfluous (as I have suggested in the preceding paragraph), in that it debunked the notion of the "psychologically sick" patient or the "social misfit." Beyond that, communication semantics with its focus on configuration patterns (e.g., on "games") liberated the patient from the weight of earlier, more traditional attempts to solve his or her problems in psychotherapy. Neither the psychoanalytical search for buried traumas in the individual's psyche (or in the collective psyche) nor the behaviorist researches into the patient's reinforcement history were any longer in demand. It was now only a question of analyzing communication in the here and now—apparently without any need of prerequisites.

Up to the present, this refraining from any concentration on "previous history" has been experienced in the psychotherapeutic field as liberating. The only problem is that in a scientific discussion of communication, we are reduced to a purely formal "accounting": Communications are analyzed in their sequence, and patterns are registered. This mode of operating, with its formalistic character, leaves the content open to interpretation in practice as in theory.

Correspondingly, various approaches have been explored in the history of family therapy. In the first phase, many different constructs were tested with the new paradigms; when disturbances occurred in families, the degree of organization–disorganization in the family was seen as responsible for these (Brown, 1972, p. 970). At first, from time to time, the psychoanalytical concept of ego development was forced into service (Brown, 1972, p. 971). Lidz, however, introduced another approach, in which the "intrafamily schisms" in disturbed families were described in the following terms: "In such families there is a chronic failure over many years to achieve appropriate complementary roles in the marriage" (quoted by Brown, 1972, p. 979). Lidz in this way filled, as it were, the construct of "communication" with the concept of "roles." What is interesting here is the way in which Lidz conceived of a distortion of the roles in concrete terms. For instance, a mother is discounted and grossly devalued by the father; the daughter forms a coalition with the father, because she cannot identify with her mother; and so on.

In the formalistic approach to psychopathology via family interaction, the differences between the sexes and the generations have also been brought into play. Differentiation according to sex and generation played a role in at an early stage in the formation of a theory of family therapy. As an example, I have chosen Fleck's (1972) characterization in the *Manual of Child Psychopathology* (p. 190):

> Before family functions can be outlined as a preliminary to considering pathology, two important and basic divisions that govern family structure and dynamics must be understood. These can be viewed as the two axes of family life. One is the generation boundary. . . . The other division is that between the two sexes.

Indeed, dysfunctional communication in the family can occasionally (under certain conditions) be described in terms of the difference between the sexes or the generations, as seen in some recent studies (see below).

A further approach to characterizing the nature of communication or interaction patterns is expressed in terms of conflict theory. Two partners in an interaction can easily find themselves in the dilemma that either one partner wins and the other loses, or the relationship breaks up. In these circumstances, more possible solutions can be found if a third party is drawn in. The partner who is manifestly in the weaker position can compensate for his or her defeat via a secret bond with a third party, and can thus restore balance to the relationship within the dyad. Furthermore, conflict can be avoided if the third party (usually a child) provides a common problem or has this role delegated to him or her (Simon & Stierlin, 1984, p. 366).

In other words, we are confronted with an extension of a conflict-laden partnership to include a third party, who covers up or neutralizes the conflict. This is a phenomenon often observed in the practice of family therapy and known as "triangulation." It is no coincidence that in Simon and Stierlin's definition, this type of conflict is often a conflict between husband and wife—a conflict that can be avoided or neutralized (in the sense of triangulation) by involving a child of the couple in question.

Family therapist Virginia Satir has used the following formula to describe the theoretical basis of this observation: The husband-and-wife relationship is the axis around which all other family relations are formed. The spouses are the "architects" of the family (Satir, 1973, p. 13). The fact that parents use their child to redirect or avoid their marital conflict (Minuchin, 1974, p. 130) accentuates the specific character of the parental/marital subsystem, as it shows itself in Satir's formula. Whereas the psychoanalytical tradition's starting point was a disturbed and eventually pathological relationship between parent and child, in family therapy the point of departure is a disturbed relation between the parents, which may be mirrored in disturbances in the child.

According to Minuchin, the marital subsystem has vital functions for the family—simply because the parents, after all, started the family in the first place. The interaction patterns between the partners ought, to a large extent, to be complementary, so that both partners can "give in" without the feeling of having 'given themselves up' (Minuchin, 1974, p. 76). The boundaries between the couple and other members of the family have to be particularly clearly marked, as husband and wife require a refuge from the many and various demands made on them by life. James G. Miller's (1978) systems conception shows the parental subsystem acquiring the function of the "decider" (one of the Miller subsystems). As long as the children are very small, the functions of feeding and protecting are predominant. Later, control and guidance become more important (Minuchin, 1974, p. 78).

As Minuchin sees it, insistence on overly rigid boundaries is pathologizing, but transgression or violation of boundaries can be even more so. Above all, transgressing the boundaries between the generations can have a pathological effect. Examples of this include grandparents' interfering with the raising of the children (and parents' not sufficiently defending their boundaries); a parent's delegating parenting tasks to a child subsystem; and a parent's forming an alliance with a child across the generational borders against his or her partner. All of these examples violate boundaries in Minuchin's sense, with consequences that are sometimes devastating.

Up to this point, I have been discussing the grounding for a theory of family psychopathology in some concepts from communication theory. Here metatheoretical considerations are as interesting as the theoretical. Students of the semantics of communication were able to borrow from the following metatheoretical concepts:

- General systems theory, following von Bertalanffy (1969)
- The autopoesis theory, following Maturana and Varela (1987)
- Systems theory, in Luhmann's sense (1984)
- Chaos and self-organization theory (cf. Tschacher, Schiepek, & Brunner, 1992)

As a result of these borrowings, communications semantics became "communication systems semantics": The communications that were observed were interpreted systemically—according to the systems theory orientation of the author(s) in question—and thus supplemented with metaphors from systems theory. A number of theoretical outlines for "communication and systems-based family therapy" followed as a result (for summaries, see Kriz, 1985, Part IV, and Hoffman, 1982; on the question of the theoretical foundations of communications and systems-oriented family therapy, see Brunner, 1986). Although these deliberations play a central role in the current debate among family therapists on constructivism (see Dell, 1982, and those in his wake), they will not be discussed further in this chapter.

At this point, it is also appropriate to quote Kantor and Lehr (1975) on the question of a possible systems theory categorization of psychopathological phenomena in the family. For example, these authors define the members of the family not only as system elements, but as subsystems of the complete family system. Indeed, they postulate three different system categories: "The family system is composed of three subsystems that interact with each other as well as with the world outside: these are the family-unit subsystem, the interpersonal subsystem, and the personal subsystem" (Kantor & Lehr, 1975, p. 23).

THE PROBLEM OF THE EMPIRICAL BASIS OF ASSUMPTIONS ABOUT PSYCHOPATHOLOGY AND FAMILY INTERACTION

In family therapy, relationships between individual behavior (respective individual dysfunctions) and the family group are analyzed within the conceptual framework derived from communication theory and systems theory. However, not enough empirical investigations have been carried out to provide genuine empirical support for these theoretical assumptions. Studies on a link between specific structures and modes of communication within families and particular problems of the identified patient (e.g., anorexia nervosa) are still in their initial stages. Altogether, we can look back on a rich history of clinical knowledge and anecdotal reports, but the field of family interaction research is still at an early stage in its development. Undoubtedly this has a lot to do with the development of family therapy in general, where, by and large, clinicians pay no attention to research evidence (Wynne, McDaniel, & Weber, 1987). While acknowledging the obvious and visible success of family therapy in practice, Wynne (1988) conceded, "with dismay, that research on family therapy was strikingly limited in quantity and quality, that it was piecemeal and not keeping pace with clinical practice" (p. 5).

There are a number of reasons why research in this field is not in the best shape. The study of family interaction sets researchers delicate and tricky tasks, of which only a few are mentioned here (see also Tschacher, Chapter 19, this volume):

• Family interaction is a complex object to examine. Research into dyadic communication has already produced unexpected difficulties, as work in the field of social psychology has shown. Studies of communication that attempt to include more than two people at a time in their analyses require the surmounting of even higher methodological hurdles. For the assessment of family interaction, there are relatively few standardized tests or procedures to draw on.

• "Family interaction" refers not only to the verbal and nonverbal exchange of communication between the separate members of the family, but also to mutual influence on several system levels (in the sense suggested in the quotation above from Kantor & Lehr, 1975). All levels of the family system are potentially important for the researcher's and clinician's "need to know" about specific phenomena within or across subsytem levels.

• What this implies is that in order to register family interaction fully and accurately, multiple descriptions are required. Bateson (1979) argued that multiple descriptions, rather than singular descriptions, enable one to construct a satisfactory view of human relationships and interaction (Keeney and Siegel, 1986, p. 69). For comprehensive analyses of this kind, relatively few standardized tests or procedures exist. Also, family interaction studies can obviously soon become unwieldy and uneconomical.

• Yet another methodological hurdle causes difficulties: A systemic mode of viewing phenomena requires the analysis of processes of recursive causality. For example, we know about the impact of family interaction on somatic health outcome, but simultaneously we know about the influence of somatic health on family functioning. Even if we had sufficient information on family interaction, we would still know little about the complex transactions between family interaction and outcome variables of whatever kind—somatic, psychological, and/or social.

FUNCTIONAL FAMILY COMMUNICATION

"Communication is a basic requirement for the development and maintenance of any interpersonal relationship" (L'Abate, 1986, p. 166). The importance of family interaction for the socialization process, and in particular for the development of self-worth, is unquestioned. Everywhere in the world, the family is the primary social authority responsible for looking after the biological needs of children and steering their development, so that they can turn into integrated persons capable of living in society and of preserving and handing on its culture (Lidz, 1971, p. 3). The acculturation of the individual is the result of a myriad of family interaction processes.

If we turn our attention to disturbed processes of socialization (with their corresponding somatic, psychological, and/or social consequences), we become aware that they can be seen in direct relation to dysfunctional family interaction. In order to understand family psychopathology, we can therefore take a very specific route: The effects of dysfunctional family interaction should show up clearly against the contrasting background of functional family interaction.

Frude (1991, pp. 46–47) draws the following portrait of the optimal family and of functional family communication:

> In healthy families, members have warm and close relationships with one another. . . . The internal structure is clear and boundaries (for example, between the parental subsystem and the child subsystem) are adequately maintained. Power is distributed relatively equally within generations, and not between generations. . . . Roles are clearly differentiated and are complementary. . . . There are clear rules that are understood and supported by all members. . . .
>
> Healthy families engage in open and effective communication. The meaning of messages is clear and it is always apparent to whom the message is addressed. Questions are clearly asked and plainly answered, and all transactions have a clear ending. The way in which a message is expressed is almost congruent with the verbal content.

Compared with such optimal family interaction, dysfunctional communication in families provides a contrasting picture of corresponding deficits. This way of seeing communication goes back to the formulation of the double-bind theory by Bateson et al. (1956). Haley (1959) described how a schizophrenic's communication is marked by the way the schizophrenic denies that he or she is defining the relationship to the other person in a communication situation. The schizophrenic remains unclear or produces discrepant utterances as regards his or her role as the transmitter of the message, the receiver, the content, and/or the context.

The double-bind theory is the prototype of a theory of family psychopathology built on assumptions about communication. The research questions linked with these assumptions lead directly to an assumption of specificity—the assumption of a relationship between a specific family interaction and a defined clinical picture of a family member. The simple monocausal relationship that is assumed here does not, however, seem to be confirmed by the results of research into schizophrenia (Goldstein & Rodnick, 1975; Hahlweg, 1986). Steinhauer, Santa Barbara, and Skinner

(1984) use a considerably more complex model ("a process model of family functioning"), which assumes that mental diseases occur when particular individual, psychodynamic, and/or genetic components and particular family interaction patterns all influence one another (Cierpka, 1989). Signs of disturbance are thus always the systems product of all the contributing subsystems. When, in what follows, I talk of an influence of dysfunctional family interaction on the genesis and/or maintenance of a social or psychological disturbance, it must be kept in mind that a field of mutually interacting factors is responsible for the emergence of the disturbance—as the findings will show in each particular case.

The following classification attempts to link disturbed family interactions with particular outcome variables. In the spirit of the specificity hypothesis, interrelations between particular interaction behaviors and specific effects are described, provided that evidence can be shown for them in empirical findings.

DYSFUNCTIONAL FAMILY COMMUNICATION

Dysfunctional family communication in general and conflictual communication between parents in particular can have a marked effect on the general state of mind of all family members, especially children. For example, aggressive behavior in children can be linked directly with disturbed patterns of parental communication, especially if the conflict between parents occurs in front of a child or incorporates the child (Forehand, 1993, p. 81). Overt parental conflict seems to be the strongest predictor of children's problems. In the following, I focus first on parental communication in conflict situations, and then on the consequences of interparental conflict for children and adolescents in the family.

Marital/Parental Communication in Conflict Situations

Many studies (cf. Halford & Markman, 1997) show that interparental conflict has an immediate effect on the behavior and subjective experience of the partners. In this, the manner in which the conflict is dealt with plays a decisive role. Burman, John, and Margolin (1992) showed that conflictual couples, compared to nondistressed couples, exhibited rigid, contingent behavioral sequences, in addition to a greater amount of negative behavior and a lesser amount of positive behavior (see also Fitzpatrick, Fey, Segrin, & Schiff, 1993).

Gottman (1991) found that "some patterns of marital conflict were beneficial to the marriage in the long run even if they were upsetting at the time. In contrast when wives were only agreeable and compliant the marriage would deteriorate over time" (p. 4). The corresponding destructive pattern of husbands in this research was, according to Gottman, their withdrawal as listeners ("stonewalling"). Dysfunctional marital interaction varies in form, therefore, in a way linked to the sex of each partner. What the two styles have in common is that neither husband nor wife is able or willing to deal with differences in a positive manner. According to these observations, the decisive role is played by the destructive forms of conflict management. "A major determinant of future outcomes for a relationship may be the extent to which wives can bring up negative feelings constructively and the extent to which husbands can respond . . . constructively" (Markman, 1991, p. 91).

Akister, Meekings, and Stevenson-Hinde (1993) have examined the various possibilities of more or less constructive–destructive marital interaction with the help of sophisticated assessment methods. Their Couple Interaction Categories cover the following classifications: Adaptive, Stable, Cooperative, Disengaged/Anxious, Parallel, or Failing. For example, Disengaged/Anxious couples "are more disruptive and attention-seeking than [those] in other groups. . . . The Disengaged/Anxious pattern as well as the Failing pattern may be indicators of risk of marital and/or family difficulties" (Akister et al., 1993, p. 19).

Sex-related differences in dealing with marital conflicts have come to the fore in two further studies. In the first of these, Haefner, Notarius, and Pelegrini (1991) examined how marital satisfaction was affected if the partners were drawn into a problem-solving discussion. The authors were able to show that the determinants of discussion satisfaction differed for husbands and wives. The discussion satisfaction of the husbands depended in an *additive* fashion on their own marital satisfaction and their wives' interactional behavior; by contrast, this additive way of experiencing discussion satisfaction played hardly any role for the wives, whose discussion satisfaction depended *interactionally* on both their own level of marital satisfaction and their husbands' interactional behavior. "Specifically, maritally satisfied wives whose husbands engaged in behaviors that inhibited problem-solving experienced these discussions as dissatisfying" (Haefner et al., 1991, p. 67).

In the second study, Wichstrom and Holte (1991) pursued the question of whether there were any connections between maturity of personality (measured by the Consensus Couples Rorschach) and marital communication (assessed via a coding system in an observation setting). In these settings, too, situations of conflict were engineered. The results pointed to an association of a low level of maturity with egocentric and self-disqualifying communication. And here, too, the sexes showed different patterns: "In mature couples the wife tended to be more dominant—and the husband more submissive—than in immature couples" (Wichstrom & Holte, 1991, p. 381).

What all these studies show, therefore, is that parental communication patterns can lead to considerable family distress, which may also have a tremendous effect on the entire family's life.

Effects of Parental Communication Deviance on Offspring

Since the work of Wynne and Singer (1963), it has been assumed that continued exposure to disturbed communication in the day-to-day environment can contribute to the development of schizophrenia in children and adolescents. High levels of communication deviance are considered characteristic of the parents of schizophrenics. However, it has not been possible in all studies to differentiate between parents of schizophrenics and parents of "normal" or nonpsychotic patients in regard to communication deviance (Doane, 1978; Liem, 1980; Helmersen, 1983; Miklowitz et al., 1991). In a survey, Miklowitz (1994) noted that at least 12 published studies have found higher levels of overall communication deviance in parents of schizophrenics; still, it was not clear "whether high levels of communication deviance are specific to families of schizophrenia patients or whether levels of communication deviance are simply correlated with illness severity in the offspring" (p. 138). Rund, Oie, Borchgrevink, and Fjell (1995) conjecture that uncertainty is aroused in a child when a parent's communication is extremely egocentric.

> In egocentric communication, the sender and the receiver do not speak and listen according to each other's premises. They do not take each other's perspective—a phenomenon characterized by monologues, lack of reaction to feedback, and use of words or expressions lacking agreed-on referents. (Rund et al., 1995, p. 224)

Miklowitz (1994, p. 138) sketches communication deviance as a measure of unclear, amorphous, disruptive, or fragmented communication. Velligan, Funderberg, Giesecke, and Miller (1995, p. 6) say that "communication deviance" refers to instances in which speakers leave ideas incomplete, use language in an odd manner, use unclear referents, contradict previously made statements with little explanation, or make unintelligible or tangential statements. As all of these authors point out, researchers into family structure are confronted by the task of defining what exactly communication deviance is; one conjecture might be that communication deviance is a indirect measure of the distress a parent might experience from interaction with a disturbed child at risk for schizophrenia (Miklowitz, 1994, p. 143 ff.). Here this question—touched on in the section above on problems of methodology—is posed: What models of causality are to be the basis of our understanding?

In an effort to answer this methodological question, Velligan et al. (1995) carried out a longitudinal analysis of communication deviance in families with a schizophrenic patient. With the data they collected these authors were not able to prove a monocausal explanation for the direct influence of dysfunctional parental speech on the development of schizophrenia. On the basis of their concept of communication deviance as a *transactional* process between speaker and listener, the authors nevertheless came to the conclusion that interactional communication deviance—that is, communication deviance expressed in the context of family problem-solving discussions—is a stable attribute within schizophrenic patients over time (Velligan et al., 1995, p. 15).

THE EFFECTS OF FAMILY DYSFUNCTION ON CHILD DEVELOPMENT
Psychosomatic Symptom Patterns

Child development and child welfare are closely related to family function and dysfunction. Numerous studies agree on this point. The connections between family dysfunction and children's state have been demonstrated in the psychosomatic family model. According to Kog, Vandereycken, and Vertommen (1989, p. 81), this model claims that a typical family organization, together with a special physiological vulnerability of the child, is the chief underlying factor in the occurrence of a psychosomatic symptom in the child. What is typical here is the involvement of the child in parental conflicts, either as an avoider or as a coalition partner. The psychosomatic symptom in the child is, according to this view, accentuated by the child's involvement in the parental conflict.

Classic examples of symptom patterns that exhibit this link are anorexia nervosa, bulimia nervosa, and similar disorders. Families with an anorexic patient appear to be characterized most significantly by this psychosomatic family organization. Minuchin and his colleagues (Minuchin, 1974; Minuchin, Rosman, & Baker, 1978) discovered four characteristics of families that may exacerbate, or even produce, anorexic symptom patterns in a child: enmeshment, overprotectiveness, rigidity, and an absence of conflict resolution (Hurtig, 1994, p. 268). These assumptions were at least partially reinforced by a recent investigation: Blair, Freeman, and Cull (1995, p. 985) reported that in families with anorexia nervosa, "Over-involvement correlated with illness severity. More households in the anorexia group were enmeshed, over-protective and poor at problem solving" when compared to the control groups. In the case of diabetes, Mengel et al. (1992) found relationships between several dysfunctional family dynamics (particularly family disengagement) on the one hand, and poor diabetic control and adolescent physiological hyporesponsiveness on the other. (See also Minuchin et al.'s [1978] study of the effect of family enmeshment on diabetic control.)

On no account, however, should the family interaction variables be overrated or viewed as the sole factors causing these disorders. Hurtig (1994) points to the fact that for psychosomatic phenomena, organic, psychological, and cultural factors all play a role alongside social factors. Moreover, careful, detailed studies of the specific family dysfunction are needed. Kern and Hastings (1995) were able to show in a study of the family environment of bulimics that bulimics reported less cohesive, more conflictual, less independent, more achievement-oriented, and more controlling family environments than did normal eaters. The significance of these findings was altered, however, when the variable of childhood sexual abuse was taken into consideration. The authors noted: "When eating behavior and abuse status were analyzed concurrently, significant differences between bulimics and normal eaters failed to emerge. Abnormal family environment was associated more closely with childhood sexual abuse than with bulimia" (Kern & Hastings, 1995, p. 499). That is, according to these researchers, childhood sexual abuse is the major factor in bulimia; the family communication pattern functions merely as a moderator variable. Obviously, further researches are required here.

Eme and Danielak (1995) showed that daughters with maladaptive eating attitudes, compared with daughters without such attitudes, "reported problems with their fathers on communication, problem solving, autonomy issues and expression of warmth, while reporting problems in communication and expression of warmth with their mothers" (p. 40). The parents themselves did not report any differences in either group; however, correlational data indicated that "parents of daughters who reported more maladaptive eating disorders were more likely to report family structural problems involving triangulation" (Eme & Danielak, 1995, p. 40). What family therapists have sensed and supposed—namely, that eating problems are connected with family problems—is supported by this study, as well as by case studies. For instance, Merl (1989) described family therapy in the case of a 15-year-old boy with anorexia nervosa; the function of the boy's illness within the family system was emphasized. A 7-year follow-up documented the effectiveness of the systems-oriented approach in this case.

Behavior Disorders

Dysfunctional family interaction may produce not only psychosomatic symptoms, but also significant behavioral problems. The child's difficulties are then thought of as reflections of troubled interactions in the family. For example, parents who are unhappy with each other and engage in chronic bickering may aggravate the symptoms of attention-deficit/hyperactivity disorder (Bruno, 1992, p. 119). Whether the assumption of specificity in this particular case can be regarded as more generally valid is a question that further research must answer.

Research on behavior disorders in families is dependent to a great extent on conceptual and methodological prerequisites, as will be shown in two examples—a case study of an adolescent with suicidal tendencies, and an observational study of mother–son interactions showing varying degrees of aggression in both mothers' and sons' reactions to family discussions, in induced situations.

Koopmans (1995) based his case study on an initial hypothesis that suicidal behavior in adolescence is related to dysfunctional family processes. In this study the author investigated this relationship, focusing on the concepts of boundary transgression, double-bind interactions, and the demarcation of kinship roles in the family. Koopmans discussed the possibility that suicidal behavior in adolescence is a double-bind response to contradictions in the way roles and responsibilities are distributed in the family.

In contrast to a methodological concept of research into behavior disorders that one could call "soft," the second study followed a more experimental approach. O'Brien, Margolin, John, and Krueger (1991) examined cognitive and emotional reactions to family discussions as experienced by mothers and sons from homes with physically aggressive, verbally aggressive, and low-conflict marital relationships. Significant differences in the experience of the simulated situation appeared: Sons of parents who showed physically aggressive behavior "demonstrated more self-interference, self-distraction and arousal and less criticism than did other sons in reaction to simulated parental conflict," whereas sons of low-conflict parents "were more optimistic about family conflict and articulated more ideas concerning family structure and how conflict 'should' proceed than did other sons" (O'Brien et al., 1991, p. 692). It can therefore be assumed that chronic stress factors, such as parent and family conflict, may influence family interactions.

Over and above these indicators, there are numerous powerful signs that parental aggression has an effect on children's behavior. For instance, research on physical abuse during childhood and young adulthood shows the far-reaching consequences of violence in families:

> The most striking finding by intrafamily violence researchers is the relative stability or consistency in the occurrence of physical abuse across the life cycle. Children who are abused or who witness spouse abuse in their families of origin are at risk for physically abusing a child or spouse in their family of procreation. In turn, their abused or witnessing children are at risk for growing up to abuse their own. (Arias & Pape, 1994, p. 301)

In an examination of Family Environment Scale profiles, Glaser, Sayger, and Horne (1993) showed that three types of scale profiles emerged: profiles from abusive, distressed (clinic-referred for child behavior problems), and functional families.

The fact that the behavior of parents has an effect on their children is borne out indirectly by comparative studies of social behavior in differing cultures. Kornadt (1991), in a longitudinal study of the ways German and Japanese mothers raised their children, was able to show that Japanese mothers demonstrated far more patience and wisdom in day-to-day stressful situations with children than the German mothers did. A parallel

88

FOUNDATIONS

observation is that there is strikingly less aggressive behavior in Japan than in the Western world. This points to the effects of aggressive parental behavior on the behavior of children.

IMPROVING FAMILY COMMUNICATION

If one is to do full justice to the role of family communication in the development of children and adolescents, it is highly appropriate to foster good family communication in the spirit of prevention. Both in dysfunctional and in "normal" families, all family members gain in competence and self-assurance when communication skills are improved. This is particularly the case when one member of a family has a physical disability or a chronic illness. In families containing a disabled or chronically ill person, the communication structure is affected. One observation is that families with an epileptic child have different interaction patterns from those of families without such a child. For example, the mothers of these families seem to have a "take-charge attitude," and the parents seem to experience significant marital distress (Dakof, 1987, p. 137).

The atypically developing child plays a focal role in the family system. McGillicuddy-DeLisi (1993) points to the changes in family interaction that arise. This author examined 44 children who had been diagnosed as communication-handicapped and their parents. Because of such a child's position "as the special child in the family, his or her competency level becomes an object of attention and concern, with the result that interaction patterns are regulated to a greater degree by that individual than by the others, such as the sibling, in the family" (McGillicuddy-DeLisi, 1993, p. 231). For this sample of handicapped children, the author was able to determine that the pattern of distancing behavior obtained for fathers was similar to that for mothers. In the case where a member of the family suffers from hearing loss, family interaction can be shown to be severely affected (Clymer, 1993). The role of supportive family interaction is obvious in such a case.

Gotcher (1993) examined the effects of family communication on the psychosocial adjustment of cancer patients, who were interviewed on the subject of their families. The author found that interactions with immediate family members were important in determining effective adjustment. What emerged as most vital was emotional support; communication satisfaction, frequency of communication, and honesty had a limited effect on adjustment.

According to a study by Miller et al. (1992) of depressive patients from dysfunctional families, the course of the depression took a significantly more negative turn in these patients than it did in a sample of patients from functional families. In a 12-month follow-up investigation, the depressives from dysfunctional families manifested higher levels of depression and lower levels of overall adjustment. The authors concluded that "impaired family functioning appears to be an important prognostic factor in major depression" (Miller et al., 1992, p. 637).

Breitenstein, Flor, and Birbaumer (1994) compared chronic back pain patients and their partners to a parallel sample of healthy couples. Patient couples (particularly the significant others of the patients) showed more positive and accepting utterances during an induced conflict dialogue than did the healthy couples. However, when negative escalations occurred, the patients were more likely to respond with criticism and disagreement; the altercations also lasted longer and suggested an inflexible problem-solving style. We might question what these findings indicate. Were the significant others becoming overresponsible and the patients more rigid? Or was the overall communication pattern in these couples different from that in "normal" couples? Were the "sick" couples communicatively sick? Given the model of circular causality, we might conclude well that both the dysfunctional communicative pattern and the dysfunctional communicative styles of the individual partners were probably responsible for the phenomena of distress.

The implications of successful and unsuccessful patterns of communication in the family can also be seen in studies of addictive behaviors. Several studies have shown that children or young adults from homes in which the parents abuse or are dependent on alcohol or other drugs are at risk for a wide range of developmental problems (see, e.g., Buelow, 1995). But here too, as I have emphasized repeatedly above, it is problematic to assume a simple monocausal chain of cause and effect. Blackson (1995) examined sons of substance-abusing fathers and was able to confirm empirically that sons' positive affective temperament and intellectual ability mediated the effects of paternal substance abuse (the dependent variable was the reading achievement score). This study did not concern itself with the softening effects of family communication on addictive behavior and its consequences, but it could nevertheless be regarded as a prototype in this field.

Research on families with a disabled, chronically ill, or disturbed member is a many-faceted field, and there is much in the findings to make us appreciate the striking advantages of functional family communication. In fact, I feel that introducing families to the practice of functional communication is a goal of great importance (cf. Ginsberg, 1997). The effect of communication training on parents and young adolescents has been proven in several studies; I will only mention that of Riesch et al. (1993).

Andrews and Andrews (1993) describe the use of family-centered early intervention services to empower families in which a member has a communication disorder. The following are two of the strategies seen as creating an empowering environment: the encouragement of all family members to participate, and the practice of listening to all family members.

Similarly, Clymer (1993) calls for support for family members affected by the illness or disability of one member of the family, in the form of training in communicating inside the family. When family members are given the opportunity to express frustration while showing acceptance, the result is a strong, mutually beneficial family relationship.

REFERENCES

Akister, J., Meekings, E., & Stevenson-Hinde, J. (1993). The spouse subsystem in the family context: Couple interaction categories. *Journal of Family Therapy, 15*, 1–21.

Andrews, M. A., & Andrews, J. R. (1993). Family-centered techniques: Integrating enablement into the IFSP process. *Journal of Childhood Communication Disorders, 15*, 41–46.

Arias, I., & Pape, K. T. (1994). Physical abuse. In L. L'Abate (Ed.), *Handbook of developmental family psychology and psychopathology* (pp. 284–308). New York: Wiley.

Bateson, G. (1979). *Mind and nature: A necessary unity.* New York: Dutton.

Bateson, G., Jackson, D. D., Haley, J., & Weakland, J. (1956). Towards a theory of schizophrenia. *Behavioral Science, 1*, 251–264.

Blackson, T. C. (1995). Temperament and IQ mediate the effect of family history of substance abuse and family dysfunction on academic achievement. *Journal of Clinical Psychology, 51*, 113–122.

Blair, C., Freeman, C., & Cull, A. (1995). The families of anorexia nervosa and cystic fibrosis patients. *Psychological Medicine, 25*, 985–993.

Breitenstein, C., Flor, H., & Birbaumer, N. (1994). Kommunikations und Problemlöseverhalten von chronischen Schmerzpatienten und ihren Partnern [Communication and problem solving of chronic pain patients and their partners]. *Zeitschrift für Klinische Psychologie, 23*, 105–116.

Brown, S. L. (1972). Family group therapy. In B. B. Wolman (Ed.), *Manual of child psychopathology* (pp. 969–1009). New York: McGraw-Hill.

Brunner, E. J. (1986). *Grundfragen der Familientherapie: Systemische Theorie und Methodologie [Basic questions of family therapy: Systemic theory and methodology].* Berlin: Springer-Verlag.

Bruno, F. J. (1992). *The family encyclopedia of child psychology and development.* New York: Wiley.

Buelow, G. (1995). Comparing students from substance abusing and dysfunctional families: Implications for counseling. *Journal of Counseling and Development, 73*, 327–330.

Burman, B., John, R. S., & Margolin, G. (1992). Observed patterns of conflict in violent, nonviolent, and nondistressed couples. *Behavioral Assessment, 14*, 15–37.

Cierpka, M. (1989). Das Problem der Spezifität in der Familientheorie [The problem of specifity in family theory]. *System Familie, 2*, 197–216.

Clymer, E. C. (1993). The practitioner's challenge: The family system and hearing loss. *Family Therapy, 20*, 217–223.

Dakof, G. A. (1987). At the starting gate: Research and theory on families and somatic health. *Journal of Family Psychology, 1*, 135–141.

Dell, P. F. (1982). In search of truth: On the way to clinical epistemology. *Family Process, 21*, 21–41.

Doane, J. A. (1978). Family interaction and communication deviance in disturbed and normal families: A review of research. *Family Process, 17*, 357–375.

Eme, R. F., & Danielak, M. H. (1995). Comparison of fathers of daughters with and without maladaptive eating attitudes. *Journal of Emotional and Behavioral Disorders, 3*, 40–45.

Fitzpatrick, M. A., Fey, J., Segrin, C., & Schiff, J. L. (1993). Internal working models of relationships and marital communication. *Journal of Language and Social Psychology, 12*, 103–131.

Fleck, S. (1972). Some basic aspects of family pathology. In B. B. Wolman (Ed.), *Manual of child psychopathology* (pp. 189–204). New York: McGraw-Hill.

Forehand, R. (1993). Family psychopathology and child functioning. *Journal of Child and Family Studies, 2*, 79–85.

Frude, N. (1991). *Understanding family problems: A psychological approach.* Chichester, England: Wiley.

Georgi, H., Levold, T., & Wedekind, E. (1990). *Familientherapie: Was sie kann, wie sie wirkt und wem sie hilft.* Mannheim, Germany: PAL Verlagsgesellschaft.

Ginsberg, B. G. (1997). *Relationship enhancement family therapy.* Chichester, England: Wiley.

Glaser, B. A., Sayger, T. V., & Horne, A. M. (1993). Three types of Family Environment Scale profiles: Functional, distressed, and abusive families. *Journal of Family Violence, 8*, 303–311.

Goldstein, M. J., & Rodnick, E. H. (1975). The family's contribution to the etiology of schizophrenia: Current status. *Schizophrenia Bulletin, 14*, 48–63.

Gotcher, J. M. (1993). The effects of family communication on psychosocial adjustment of cancer patients. *Journal of Applied Communication Research, 21*, 176–188.

Gottman, J. M. (1991). Predicting the longitudinal course of marriages. *Journal of Marital and Family Therapy 17*, 3–7.

Haefner, P. T., Notarius, C. I., & Pelegrini, D. S. (1991). Determinants of satisfaction with marital discussions: An exploration of husband–wife differences. *Behavioral Assessment, 13*, 67–82.

Hahlweg, K. (1986). Einfluss der Familieninteraktion auf Entsehung, Verlauf und Therapie schizophrener Störungen [Effects of family interactions on onset, process, and therapy of schizophrenia]. In E. Nordmann & M. Cierpka (Eds.), *Familienforschung in Psychiatrie und Psychotherapie* [*Family research in psychiatry and psychotherapy*]. Berlin: Springer-Verlag.

Haley, J. (1959). An interactional description of schizophrenia. *Psychiatry, 22*, 321–332.

Haley, J. (1976). *Problem-solving therapy.* New York: Harper & Row.

Halford, W. K., & Markman, H. J. (Eds.). (1997). *Clinical handbook of marriage and couple intervention.* Chichester, England: Wiley.

Helmerson, P. (1983). *Family interaction and communication in psychopathology: An evaluation of recent perspectives.* London: Academic Press.

Hoffman, L. (1982). *Grundlagen der Familientherapie: Konzepte für die Entwicklung von Systemen* [*Foundations of family therapy: A conceptual framework for systems change*]. Hamburg: Isko-Press.

Hurtig, A. L. (1994). Chronic illness and developmental family psychology. In L.

L'Abate (Ed.), *Handbook of developmental family psychology and psychopathology* (pp. 265–283). New York: Wiley.

Kantor, D., & Lehr, W. (1975). *Inside the family: Toward a theory of family process.* San Francisco: Jossey-Bass.

Keeney, B. P., & Siegel, S. (1986). The use of multiple communication in systemic couples therapy. *American Journal of Family Therapy, 14,* 69–79.

Kern, J. M., & Hastings, T. (1995). Differential family environments of bulimics and victims of childhood sexual abuse: Achievement orientation. *Journal of Clinical Psychology, 51,* 499–506.

Kog, E., Vandereycken, W., & Vertommen, H. (1989). Multimethod investigation of eating disorder families. In W. Vandereycken, E. Kog, & J. Vanderlinden (Eds.), *The family approach to eating disorders: Assessment and treatment of anorexia nervosa and bulimia* (pp. 81–106). New York: PMA.

Koopmans, M. (1995). A case of family dysfunction and teenage suicide attempt: Applicability of a family systems paradigm. *Adolescence, 30,* 87–94.

Kornadt, H.-J. (1991). Aggression motive and its development conditions in eastern and western cultures. In N. Bleichrodt & P. J. D. Drenth (Eds.), *Contemporary issues in cross-cultural psychology* (pp. 155–167). Amsterdam: Swets & Schwarzenberg.

Kriz, J. (1985). *Grundkonzepte der Psychotherapie [Basic concepts of psychotherapy].* Munich: Urban & Schwarzenberg.

L'Abate, L. L. (1986). *Systematic family therapy.* New York: Brunner/Mazel.

Lidz, T. (1971). *Familie und psychosoziale Entwicklung [The family and human adaptation].* Frankfurt: S. Fischer.

Liem, J. H. (1980). Family studies of schizophrenia: An update and commentary. *Schizophrenia Bulletin, 6,* 429–455.

Luhmann, N. (1984). *Soziale systeme [Social systems].* Frankfurt: Suhrkamp.

Markman, H. J. (1991). Constructive marital conflict is NOT an oxymoron. *Behavioral Assessment, 13,* 83–96.

Maturana, H. R., & Varela, F. J. (1987). *The tree of knowledge.* Boston: New Science Library.

McGillicuddy-DeLisi, A. V. (1992). Correlates of parental teaching strategies in families of children evidencing normal and atypical development. *Journal of Applied Developmental Psychology, 13,* 215–234.

Mengel, M. B., Blackett, P. R., Lawler, M. K., Volk, R. J., Viviani, N. J., Stamps, G. S., Dees, M. S., Davis, A. B., & Lovallo, W. R. (1992). Cardiovascular and neuroendocrine responsiveness in diabetic adolescents within a family context: Association with poor diabetic control and dysfunctional family dynamics. *Family Systems Medicine, 10,* 5–33.

Merl, H. (1989). Systemische Familientherapie bei einem Fall von Anorexia nervosa bei einem Knaben: Eine Falldarstellung im Spiegel der Schlussinterventionen [Systemic family therapy in the case of an anorexic boy as reflected by interventions at the end of sessions]. *Psychotherapie, Psychosomatik, Medizinische Psychologie, 39,* 444–451.

Miklowitz, D. J. (1994). Family risk indicators in schizophrenia. *Schizophrenia Bulletin, 20,* 137–149.

Miklowitz, D. J., Velligan, D. I., Goldstein, M. J., Nuechterlein, K. H., Gitlin, M. J., Ranlett, G., & Doane, J. A. (1991). Communication deviance in families of schizophrenic and manic patients. *Journal of Abnormal Psychology, 100,* 163–173.

Miller, I. W., Keitner, G. I., Wishman, M. A., Ryan, C. E., Epstein, N. B., & Bishop, D. S. (1992). Depressed patients with dysfunctional families: Description and course of illness. *Journal of Abnormal Psychology, 101,* 637–646.

Miller, J. G. (1978). *Living systems.* New York: McGraw-Hill.

Minuchin, S. (1974). *Families and family therapy.* Cambridge, MA: Harvard University Press.

Minuchin, S., Rosman, G. L., & Baker, L. (1978). *Psychosomatic families: Anorexia nervosa in context.* Cambridge, MA: Harvard University Press.

O'Brien, M., Margolin, G., John, R. S., & Krueger, L. (1991). Mothers' and sons' cognitive and emotional reactions to simulated marital and family conflict. *Journal of Consulting and Clinical Psychology, 59,* 692–703.

Riesch, S. K., Tosi, C. B., Thurston, C. A., Forsyth, D. M., et al. (1993). Effects of communication training on parents and young adolescents. *Nursing Research, 42,* 10–16.

Rund, B. R., Oie, M., Borchgrevink, T. S., & Fjell, A. (1995). Expressed emotion, communication deviance and schizophrenia. *Psychopathology, 28,* 220–228.

Satir, V. (1973). *Familienbehandlung. Kommunikation und Beziehung in Theorie, Erleben und Therapie [Conjoint family therapy].* Freiburg, Germany: Lambertus.

Selvini Palazzoli, M., Boscolo, L., Cecchin, G., & Prata, G. (1978). *Paradoxon und Gegenparadoxon: Ein neues Therapiemodell für die Familie mit schizophrener Störung.* Stuttgart: Klett-Cotta. (Original work published 1975)

Simon, F. B., & Stierlin, H. (1984). *Die Sprache der Familientherapie: Ein Vokabular. Überblick, Kritik und Integration systemtherapeutischer Begriffe, Konzepte und Methoden [The language of family therapy: A systematic vocabulary and source book].* Stuttgart: Klett-Cotta.

Steinhauer, P. D., Santa Barbara, J., & Skinner, H. A. (1984). The process model of family functioning. *Canadian Journal of Psychiatry, 29,* 77–88.

Tschacher, W., Schiepek, G., & Brunner, E. J. (Eds.). (1992). *Self-organization and clinical psychology.* Berlin: Springer-Verlag.

Velligan, D. I., Funderburg, L. G., Giesecke, S. L., & Miller, A. L. (1995). Longitudinal analysis of communication deviance in the families of schizophrenic patients. *Psychiatry, 58,* 6–19.

von Bertalanffy, L. (1969). General systems theory and psychiatry: An overview. In W. Gray, F. J. Duhl, & N. D. Rizzo (Eds.), *General systems theory and psychiatry* (pp. 33–50). Boston: Little, Brown.

Wichstrom, L., & Holte, A. (1991). Maturity of personality and family communication. *Scandinavian Journal of Psychology, 32,* 372–383.

Wynne, L. C. (1988). Zum Stand der Forschung in der Familientherapie: Probleme und Trends [The state of the art in family therapy: Problems and trends]. *System Familie: Forschung und Therapie, 1,* 4–22.

Wynne, L. C., McDaniel, S. H., & Weber, T. T. (1987). Professional politics and the concepts of family therapy, family consultation, and systems consultation. *Family Process, 26,* 153–166.

Wynne, L. C., & Singer, M. T. (1963). Thought disorder and family relations of schizophrenics: A research strategy. *Archives of General Psychiatry, 9,* 191–198.

CHAPTER 5

Risk and Resiliency
Factors among Culturally
Diverse Families:
Implications for
Family Psychopathology

ANA C. GARDANO

This chapter examines how current cross-cultural research, combined with a family systems framework, can serve as a way to conceptualize and understand families within their cultural contexts, specifically with regard to family dysfunction and resiliency. The theme of mental health problems among ethnic groups is best addressed by examining the types of factors that either promote or detract from a successful adjustment to a new lifestyle and the development of effective family relations. Although there is a substantial body of cross-cultural research literature and theories, few of these have addressed the issue of cultural diversity from the perspective of family relationships, ethnic/racial identity, and discrimination.

It is essential that clinicians, researchers, supervisors, and those in training become aware of cultures other than their own. As Pedersen (1994, p. 18) stated, "it is rare for any human being . . . ever to behave without responding to some aspect of culture." In addition, no society or culture has remained static, without any influences from other cultures, over either short or extended periods of time in world history. As we approach the 21st century, most societies will continue to experience an influx of culturally diverse people due to economic and political pressures. In this chapter, the term "culturally diverse people or families" refers to those of different races or cultures/ethnicities residing as minorities in a host culture. The process of inclusion or exclusion of a variety of racial and ethnic groups will necessitate the redefinition of nations as culturally pluralistic or multicultural. The United States may be a natural testing ground for building societies of the future, because of its origins and legacy as a nation founded by immigrants and refugees. The United States has also experienced relatively extreme conditions in dealing with ethnic and racial groups, such as the enslavement of Africans and the displacement of Native Americans and Mexicans. In 1964, the Civil Rights Act abolished segregation by race or ethnicity. These experiences of the past continue to have long-term effects on the values of U.S. culture, families, and individuals.

More recently, the impact of culturally diverse people on the U.S. majority culture has become a topic of concern in all fields, including psychology. Perhaps this is due to the shifts in population that are projected to occur in the next century. The U.S. Bureau of the Census (1996) estimates that by the year 2050, the fastest-growing ethnic group in the United States will be Hispanics, followed by Asians and African American/Blacks, while European American/Whites[1] will remain the largest group. The number of Hispanics will quadruple by then, from 27.8 million to 96.5 million, and will be the largest minority group; the number of Asians will more than triple, from 9.0 million to 32.4 million; and the number of African American/Blacks will almost double, from 31.8 million to 53.6 million. The number of European American/White is expected to increase by about 5%, from 194.1 million to 207.9 million.

Given the projected increase of culturally diverse groups in the United States, most of this chapter concentrates on research studies conducted with these populations, but any international research or small studies that address the topics of this chapter are also included. Most of the research studies selected were conducted over the last 10–15 years, included a substantial number of subjects (about 100 subjects or more), and involved a variety of measures and analyses.

Some of the concepts presented in this chapter have received consid-

---

[1]In this chapter, the term "White" refers to people belonging to the mainstream culture in the United States. "White" implies a racial identity and a set of values that represent the majority culture. Most recently, the term "European American" is being used in the literature to represent the White majority. However, oftentimes, Hispanics, Middle Easterners, or others may identify themselves as "White" in research instruments because there may not be a specific category for "White Hispanic, Black Hispanic," and there is hardly ever a category for Middle Eastern, mixed race, or biracial. Similarly, the term "Black" may represent those belonging to this racial group, whether they are born in the United States, other countries, or are of Hispanic origin. In addition, the cultural origin of the "White" subjects (e.g., German, English, Eastern European) or "Black" (e.g., African, West Indian, or North American) is hardly ever specified in the research literature. In this chapter, the term "European American/White" and "African American/Black" refers to the definition of "White" or "Black" aforementioned, unless otherwise stated.

erable attention in the cross-cultural research literature in terms of comparing and contrasting *individuals* in different cultures. Few studies, however, have concentrated on the relevance of these concepts to the study of culturally diverse *families*. Current concepts that support both cross-cultural and family systems theories are discussed, in order to provide a framework for the interpretation of the research findings. Cross-cultural research emphasizes the concepts of individualism and collectivism (Berry, Poortinga, Segall, & Dasen, 1992; Triandis, 1995; Schwartz, 1994). Most cultures of the world are primarily based on the natural support systems of the family; thus, family systems concepts are highly relevant ways of understanding any culture. The integration of cross-cultural and family systems theories is an original concept, which I have termed the "culturally integrated family systems model" (Gardano, 1996, in press). This global approach should prove helpful to both clinicians and researchers who wish to understand families of any culture, while at the same time it provides a basis for working with one cultural group in depth.

Next, a review is presented of current cross-cultural research studies that focus on identifying the risk and resiliency factors for culturally diverse families within the cultural constructs of individualism–collectivism and family systems. One way to study risk and resiliency factors for culturally diverse families is to address the incidence of mental health problems across cultures. Most studies with culturally diverse groups, however, focus on socialization factors, ethnic/racial identity, family functioning, acculturation, biculturation, intergenerational conflicts, and gender issues. In terms of methodology, the studies reviewed here demonstrate that research with culturally diverse families is complex. Cross-cultural studies require special attention to defining the hypotheses, samples, instruments, and conclusions within a context relevant to the sociocultural, developmental, linguistic, and family structure of the populations being studied. Additional issues related to research methodology and the assessment of psychopathology with different cultural groups are found in Sartorius and Janca (1996); Dana (1996); Verhulst and Achenbach (1995); and Canino and Bravo (1994); for issues related to alcohol use see Gureje, Mavreas, Vazquez-Barquero, and Janca (1997); and for research with children see Canino, Bird, and Canino (1997) and Foster and Martinez (1995).

THEORETICAL CONSTRUCTS
ABOUT CULTURE AND FAMILIES

This section focuses on providing a framework of basic definitions and theoretical concepts to facilitate the understanding of culturally diverse families, especially those in the process of adapting from one culture to another. First, key terms in the cultural diversity literature are defined, as well as concepts related to ethnic and racial identity development. The next subsections define and describe the relationship between basic theories about individualism and collectivism from the cross-cultural literature and family systems concepts. The integration of these concepts is the basis for my culturally integrated family systems model.

Culture and Racial Identity

It is no easy task to find definitions and theoretical constructs about culture that are adequate and applicable to culturally diverse families. "Race," as opposed to culture, is an attribute that individuals inherit and are born with, such as skin color. "Culture," on the other hand, consists of values that are learned after birth (Gardano, Davis, & Jones, 1994; Pedersen, 1994). Definitions of culture include sharing similar norms and values, speaking a particular language, and living in the same geographic location. Definitions of culture also include categorizing experiences in the same way—for example, how families are defined and how families transmit cultural values from one generation to the next. Thus, any group that meets this criteria can be considered a culture. Social organizations, such as government institutions, schools, and family units facilitate the transmission of cultural values within a society or community. This process, also termed "enculturation" (Berry et al., 1992), includes the many ways that families transmit their own cultural values and organizational patterns from one generation to the next. Whereas one culture may emphasize the importance of the nuclear family, another will emphasize the influence of the extended family. In any attempt to further understand families of different cultures, one should look at the similarities and differences in terms of family structure, values, and norms of each culture (Gardano, 1996; Gardano et al., 1994). However, focusing only on similarities may ignore differences, while focusing only on differences may result in stereotyping (Pedersen, 1994). Some publications are useful references that describe specific family characteristics of various ethnic groups (McGoldrick, Pearce, & Giordano, 1996) or focus on one group, such as African American/Black families (Boyd-Franklin, 1989), or a specific issue, such as the parenting values of minority families (Forehand & Kotchick, 1996).

Other important terms (Berry et al., 1992) that relate to culture are "acculturation," "assimilation," "biculturation," "marginalization," and "acculturative stress." "Acculturation" refers to the process of adaptation that individuals and families undergo while living in a culture different from the culture of origin. "Biculturation" refers to the development of adaptive skills to cope with two cultures. Typically, families that experience living in a new culture are in the minority, compared to those already of the new culture, who may be described as the "majority," "mainstream," or "dominant" culture. Individuals and families in a new culture "assimilate," or adopt, some of its values, while others are rejected. When values from the new culture and the culture of origin merge, families have integrated values from both cultures. Families that consolidate values tend to experience more successful adaptation than those that either totally adopt the new culture's values or exclusively maintain those of the culture of origin. However, each family member may experience this process in a different way and at a different rate. Individuals who totally reject the new culture or experience themselves as excluded or discriminated against within the new culture are described as "marginalized." The differences between the acculturation processes of different family members are more clearly seen when examining the acculturation rates of family members in each generation. The many ways in which individuals adjust to a new culture are termed "acculturation strategies." The conflicts, identity confusion, and emotional symptoms that individuals and families exhibit during the acculturation process is termed *acculturative stress*. These processes are much more evident in immigrant families because of the drastic changes that these families undergo, such as language, geographic location, socioeconomic status, and often family structure. However, even ethnic groups whose members have been born in the United States, such as African American/Blacks, experience stress related to discrimination and lack of acceptance by the majority culture.

Another important concept to take into account in the evaluation of culturally diverse families is the process of ethnic and racial identity development (Gardano, 1996; Helms, 1995; Spencer & Markstrom-Adams, 1990; Sue & Sue, 1990). Basically, this process is part of the development of autonomous behaviors and self-identity that everyone experiences, regardless of culture or race. The process of identity development is the major task during the stage of adolescence in any culture. Adolescents usually explore alternatives that shape the way to self-identity through discussion of ideas, experimentation with different behaviors and ways of dressing, and challenges to parental rules and expectations. A community that supports a wide range of opportunities for adolescents to pursue these goals (e.g., recreational activities) also contributes to adolescents' identity formation. Racial and cultural identity is part of this process. When adolescents are raised within the confines of conflicting cultural values, lack of opportunities, or discrimination within one society, problems in achieving identity formation will arise. Most often, minorities feel disempowered by the majority culture. This power inequity has a negative impact on positive self-esteem, which is further intensified through the expected conflicts between parents and adolescents.

The process of cultural and racial identity development parallels the acculturation process. Some of the most recent and comprehensive concepts in this area have been proposed by Helms (1995). She has suggested two sets of stages, or statuses, of racial identity development—one for "Whites" and one for other racial groups. She defines the term "White" as the mainstream group in U.S. society that has the most privileges, as opposed to "Caucasian" (or the newer term "European American/White"), which defines a race. Each of the stages includes moral dilemmas, such as conflicts of loyalties between the culture of origin and the mainstream for both

Whites and other racial groups. For the most part, the stages involve various degrees of either identification or rejection of one's own culture and the mainstream. She proposes that it is much more adaptive to integrate aspects of both cultures, and emphasizes that racial identity development is also predicated on social power inequities. For example, in any culture parents and children have unequal power relationships. Similarly, men and women have unequal power relationships in most cultures. Members of minority groups experience a low status in society, compared to the majority or dominant culture. Gushue and Sciarra (1995) suggest a model of examining family interactions in terms of the racial identity development of each family member.

Racial and cultural identity issues are in the initial stages of development in the fields of research, child development, and diagnosis. Diagnostic classifications are the most controversial. Some of the literature suggests that definitions of psychopathology tend to exclude cultural considerations and to represent primarily the views of the dominant culture in the United States (e.g., Sue & Sue, 1990). Definitions found in diagnostic manuals may not correspond to definitions of psychopathology in some cultures. For example, the definition of problem drinking (e.g., usage rates) may vary considerably by culture and by region (Gureje et al., 1997). At a national conference regarding the publication of the fourth edition of the *Diagnostic and Statistical Manual of Mental Disorders* (DSM-IV; American Psychiatric Association, 1994), Good (1996) and other participants acknowledged so many diagnostic dilemmas that the development of case illustrations (termed "minority casebook") was suggested. DSM-IV and the "Guidelines for Providers of Psychological Services to Ethnic, Linguistic, and Culturally Diverse Populations" (American Psychological Association, 1993) mark the first efforts to address these problems.

Individualism and Collectivism

Cross-cultural research by Berry et al. (1992), Triandis (1995), and Schwartz (1994) is particularly relevant and useful in understanding cultures and families. Most cross-cultural theorists and researchers subscribe to the notions of "individualism" and "collectivism." As the words imply, individualism emphasizes individual goals and competition, whereas collectivism emphasizes collaborative efforts to achieve goals. At the root of these concepts is extensive cross-cultural research. Berry et al. (1992) conceptualize the collectivistic trends in a culture as a result of the need to develop strategies to maintain a continuous food supply throughout evolution. In agricultural or herding societies, loyalty, compliance, and cooperation among family groups protected their territories and ensured their survival. In societies where food was scarce, daily hunting was needed to preserve the family groups, so more individualistic forms of behavior were promoted. In addition, the roles of males and females are conceptualized as largely dependent on biological correlates. Thus, males tend to be more dominant and achievement-oriented (individualistic) than females because of their greater physical strength. Females bear and socialize children, and thus tend to be more socially responsive (collectivistic) than males. Berry et al. (1992) also suggest that there are no societies in which males have full child-rearing roles.

Tannen (1990) has also concluded from her psycholinguistic research that males and females have different ways of communicating, because of their biologically based roles throughout evolution. Therefore, males tend to use more words and strategies related to action, and females use more words and strategies related to cooperation and socialization, in communication patterns. In his work on individualism and collectivism, Triandis (1995) observes that in most societies women are responsible for the educational level of the family, especially when they have a considerable role in providing economic resources for the family. Currently, the growing scarcity of economic and food resources in the world has propelled women into the work force; it has also caused many cultural groups to seek economic resources outside their own culture. Therefore, economic need may override biological and evolutionary dispositions. These concepts signal that the availability of economic resources in a culture or society may shape cultural, family, and gender values. It also signals a shift in the power balance between different groups in society.

Schwartz's (1994) innovative research reveals that cultures cannot be neatly categorized as individualistic or collectivistic. Rather, these concepts coexist in every culture as a bipolar dimension. In each culture the dimension that is emphasized, either individualism or collectivism, depends on what a culture values more highly. Some cultures, such as Iran's current culture and most other cultures of the world, emphasize collectivism and downplay individualism. Others, such as U.S. culture, emphasize individualism and downplay collectivism. In every culture, there is a need for communities to function within a hierarchy with the collaboration of all institutions, for the collective good of the society. There is also a need for individual achievement and pursuit of individual talents, such as scientific discoveries, that contribute to the society as a whole.

How are these concepts relevant to family systems? In every family, there is a need for family members to have distinct roles and to communicate and interact for the collective good of the family. There is also a need for each individual family member to express opinions and talents and to develop as a distinct human being. In every family, an individual functions simultaneously in relation to his or her own interests and within the context of the group and its culture. The concept of viewing individuals within their family and environmental contexts has been expanded by the theories of Bronfenbrenner (1979) and Szapocznik and Kurtines (1993). They support the ecosystemic approach in understanding cultures, which emphasizes contextualism. Specifically, Szapocznik and Kurtines (1993) define "contextualism" as placing individuals and their families within the context of their *current* sociocultural environment, rather than a historical or idealized concept of culture. In addition, their research lends further support to the notion that the individual needs to be understood not only within his or her culture, but also within the culture of his or her family (microcontext) and the environment (macrocontext) as one entity or system. Szapocznik and his colleagues have discovered in their research with Cuban families in Miami, Florida, that the problematic behaviors of adolescents have a direct link to cultural conflicts between the collectivistic views of the less acculturated parents and the individualistic views of their highly acculturated adolescent children. Such parent–child acculturative stress can be redefined from a systemic point of view, as a power struggle between the authority of the parental subsystem and the child subsystem. Thus, another way to define cultural differences is to examine differences between the structure and role expectancies of family members within their current environment, and to show how these differences affect the psychological well-being of its members.

Structural Family Systems Theory in the Context of Culture

In the next few subsections, differences between the family structures of culturally diverse families and mainstream families are described. Specifically, general differences in the distribution of authority in the family, communication patterns, and gender roles are suggested. Issues of inequities in social power and conflicts are highlighted in terms of the process of adjustment for culturally diverse families. These ideas further expand the culturally integrated family systems model.

Basic Concepts

Together with many others in the field (Minuchin, 1974; Minuchin & Fishman, 1981), I consider structural family therapy quite relevant to the assessment of family functioning. Minuchin's theory suggests that the family is organized into various subsystems. Within the nuclear family, there are the parental, spousal, and child subsystems. A family system can also include the extended family, schoolteachers, neighbors, and anyone else who is influential in the functioning of a family. Structural theory emphasizes the identification of roles of authority, or power, and communication patterns within the family. The way family members communicate and interact can promote either an "enmeshed" or "closed" family system, where members depend greatly on each other to make decisions, or a "disengaged" system, where family members do not communicate much and generally make decisions on their own. Individual family members can also become enmeshed with other family members or can disengage from the family system. Family members do not always function as either enmeshed or disengaged, but these patterns can sometimes either intensify or modify at a time of crisis and can promote dysfunction within the family, especially during abrupt changes in sociocultural and economic status. For example, a teenage Hispanic boy may experience ambivalence between taking care of his own needs and the needs of his family. He may feel more compelled to accompany a non-English-speaking grandparent to medical appointments than to go to school. His loyalty to the family may overpower him to the extent that when there is a financial crisis in the family, he develops panic anxiety and school refusal. Families also experience healthy enmeshment or disengagement. For example, some degree of enmeshment is expected between infants and their mothers for a period of time. Adolescents are expected to experience disengagement from their parents. The enmeshment–disengagement dimension parallels the collectivist–individualistic dimension as envisioned by Schwartz (1994). He emphasizes that both collective and individual characteristics coexist within a culture as a bipolar dimension. The bipolarity inherent in these dimensions is also evident in family functioning. A well-balanced family system enables the family to make decisions as a group and still supports each family member's opinions. A family psychologist also stands inside the family system by collectively joining it and stands outside the family system by individually assessing and designing strategies for change.

Family theories are useful in identifying patterns of risk and resiliency for culturally diverse families, because of the value placed on the family and its interactions within its sociocultural environment. To seek help within the natural support systems of the family is consistent with the world view of any family, but it is especially relevant for culturally diverse families (Gardano et al., 1994; Ho, 1987; Sue & Sue, 1990).

Common Patterns in Family Structures

Culturally Diverse Families. The trends described in this and the next subsection should be regarded as general guidelines rather than stereotypical; these patterns may vary from one family to another. Common patterns in the family structure (Boyd-Franklin, 1989; Gardano et al., 1994; Gardano, 1996; Ho, 1987; Sue & Sue, 1990) of culturally diverse families are as follows: (1) an emphasis on collectivism, harmony with nature, and spirituality, which highlights the welfare of the group; (2) hierarchical relationships between societal systems and within the family; and (3) hierarchical and sharp distinctions between the roles of males and females (except for African American/Black families, where egalitarianism is prevalent). Nuclear families rely greatly on the extended family and kinship ties for support and guidance, especially during family stress, and for help with the socialization of children. In addition, religious affiliation plays a major role in supporting the values of culturally diverse families.

Among culturally diverse families, marriages are generally perceived as the union of two families in a long-term relationship. There is also a strong emphasis on a highly delineated relationship between husband and wife, as well as between parents and children. Husbands are expected to be the main economic providers and to make most of the decisions in the family, whereas wives are expected to socialize and care for the children. Accordingly, male children are allowed much more freedom than females, especially during adolescence. Generally, parents adopt an authoritarian style toward the children, who are not expected to question the authority of the parents. There is thus an underlying need for dominant and submissive qualities between these subsystems in culturally diverse families. Family conflicts are usually resolved within the confines of the family context, and professional help is rarely sought.

U.S. Mainstream Families. Family values of culturally diverse families often clash or are in direct contrast to the family values of mainstream families in the United States. In most mainstream families, there is a great emphasis on the nuclear family and individual achievement is encouraged. Marriage is seen as a joining together of two individuals, rather than two families. Each nuclear family is generally expected to resolve problems on its own or to seek professional help, rather than help from its extended family (McGill & Pearce, 1982). Although gender role differences do exist—for example, women are still generally dependent on their husbands, who are the main breadwinners—this trend has changed considerably since the 1960s as women have joined the work force in great numbers. The greater economic power of women has shifted the traditional roles of husband and wife. The wife's role has changed from dependent housewife to sharing the status of breadwinner in the family. This shift in power has also resulted in greater demands for men to take on more child-rearing roles. Triandis (1995) suggests that bilateral (egalitarian) child rearing promotes individualism, because the child has to decide on his or her own which values to integrate from both mother and father.

Family Systems Issues and Conflicts in the Acculturation Process: Social Power Inequities

Despite these general trends for culturally diverse families and mainstream families in the United States, all families and their cultures are always in transition. Culture is not static; it is in a constant process of redefining itself. Families go through a constant process of adaptation and negotiation that reshapes the family subsystems and communication each time there is a transaction with other systems. U.S. society is currently undergoing slow but definite changes with the increase of culturally diverse families. Culturally diverse families, especially immigrants, experience high degrees of acute stress and conflict in the process of adapting from the original culture to the mainstream culture, or acculturation (Gushue & Sciarra, 1995; Szapocznik et al., 1986).

The process of acculturation for culturally diverse families largely involves sudden shifts from a primarily collectivistic society to a primarily individualistic society. Abrupt changes such as these may bring about a change in social power, as Helms (1995), Pinderhughes (1989), and Sue and Sue (1990) have pointed out. Very often, immigrant families experience a loss of status and economic stability, a disruption of family ties, and discrimination. It is important to assess how families are negotiating with the systems in their new environment, how they are establishing their role in the community, and how fully they are being accepted by the majority culture, in order to determine the families' level of adaptation to the new culture. These are also factors for African American/Black families as they move out of their neighborhood culture into the mainstream community.

Within any family, there are also differences of power within the spousal subsystem and between the parental and child subsystems. As culturally diverse women work and become economically viable, their role is strengthened and they gain authority over decisions in the family. As the traditional roles of men and women in culturally diverse families are challenged, major marital conflicts may arise. In addition, as children (including African American/Blacks) become more acculturated to U.S. mainstream values, they begin to challenge their parents, and frequently intergenerational conflicts emerge. Some adolescents experience extreme biculturation conflicts and become dysfunctional, sometimes choosing self-destructive actions. Others are able to integrate aspects of both cultures successfully, with parental support (Gardano, 1996; Ho, 1987).

Other investigators and I have speculated (Gardano, 1996; Ho, 1987; Pinderhughes, 1989) that the transactions and shifts of power between family members are also relevant to any culture or society. As wives gain economic power, husbands may lose authority in the home. However, both gain economic power for their families. Mainstream U.S. families may experience a loss of power as more and more culturally diverse groups attempt to integrate. Immigrant families also experience great losses from their culture of origin. On the other hand, the contribution of diverse cultures can also provide further dynamic power to Americans as a world culture.

The ideas presented in the previous sections demonstrate that the culturally integrated family systems model is primarily based on factors that are common to all societies and all families. Cross-cultural researchers suggest that cultures define themselves according to varied degrees of both individual and collective needs. I suggest that there is a reciprocal relationship between these cultural dimensions and the structure of families, in terms of the distribution of authority in a family and communication patterns both within and outside the family system. The role of gender differences is also an essential part of the model. From this starting point, the evaluation of other factors—such as specific characteristics of a family or cultural group, as well as the impact of acculturation and family crises—is facilitated.

REVIEW OF RESEARCH: RISK AND RESILIENCY FACTORS IN RELATION TO FAMILY PSYCHOPATHOLOGY

In this section, I discuss current cross-cultural research studies relevant to risk and resiliency factors in the mental health of culturally diverse families. In the first half of this section, the review of studies addresses common issues in cross-cultural research with families, such as the prevalence of mental health disorders and issues pertaining to child socialization, parenting styles, and family communication patterns. In the second half, the review addresses issues frequently found among culturally diverse families, especially families with adolescents. The discussion includes both the negative and positive impact of acculturation and biculturation relevant to racial and ethnic identity and their influence on family structure, communication, and gender roles. The review also includes interpretations relevant to the *culturally integrated family systems model.*

Prevalence of Mental Disorders among Ethnic Groups

A few studies reported in the literature since the 1970s attempted to investigate specific patterns of psychopathology among different ethnic groups. Reviews of studies on this topic have not identified any specific types of psychopathology common to various ethnic groups. The prevalence of certain disorders may be higher or lower in some cultures or ethnic groups than in others, which raises questions about diagnostic definitions. For example, studies reviewed by Ruiz (1985) suggested that Manic Depressive illness was three times higher for Hispanics, and four times higher for African American/Blacks, than national hospital admission rates. Similarly, symptoms of schizophrenia may differ among ethnic groups and between urban and rural groups, according to some studies reviewed by Ruiz. For example, African American/Black schizophrenics living in urban areas were found to display higher levels of anger, impulsiveness, and hallucinations than European American/Whites. African American/Blacks living in rural areas displayed more severe symptoms, such as affective lability, than those living in urban areas. Schizophrenia was found to have a more positive outcome in developing countries where socioeconomic status is higher, according to a review of the cross-cultural research literature in the 1990s (Davidson & McGlashan, 1997).

The prevalence of mental disorders may also differ between one group and another, depending on the context of sociocultural and environmental influences. Trevino and Bruhn (1977) surveyed Mexican Americans receiving services at a community mental health center in Laredo, a Texas town in the Mexican border. Adjustment disorders were the most common diagnoses, followed by alcoholism, drug dependence, and major affective and psychotic disorders. The frequency of these problems, especially adjustment disorders, was attributed to the transient nature of the area, which had approximately 11,000 migrants per year crossing the border.

One of the most comprehensive surveys to date about the prevalence of mental disorders among ethnic groups was conducted by Regier et al. (1993). The U.S. portion of this survey was undertaken during 1 month in five U.S. sites of the National Institute of Mental Health (NIMH) Epidemiologic Catchment Area program with more than 18,000 people, aged 18 to over 65; the survey also included an international study with more than 3,000 people in seven sites in Europe and Australia. The Diagnostic Interview Schedule (Robins, Helzer, Croughan, Williams & Spitzer, 1981), based on DSM-III (American Psychiatric Association, 1980), was used with the NIMH sample, and the Present State Examination of the World Health Organization, based on the ninth revision of the *International Classification of Diseases* (World Health Organization, 1977) was used for the international study. In the international study, all diagnostic categories were lumped into one large category that included any mental disorder. In the U.S. study, major diagnostic categories were surveyed, including schizophrenia; affective and anxiety disorders, such as dysthymia; obsessive–compulsive disorders; as well as antisocial personality and alcohol/drug abuse or dependence (also grouped as substance use disorder). The subject pool was categorized by race or ethnicity as follows: "Non-Black, non-Hispanic" (European American/White), "Black, non-Hispanic" (African American/Black) and "Hispanic."

The results of the U.S. study were given in two forms—percentages and odds ratios—that measured the strength of risk factors in proportion to a mental disorder. Sociodemographic risk factors were considered to be age, gender, marital status, socioeconomic status, and race or ethnicity. When the risk factors were controlled for, the odds that ethnicity would be statistically significant among any of the diagnostic categories were not borne out. However, there were some trends worth noting for specific diagnostic categories among the ethnic groups surveyed in the United States. Overall, the odds of European Americans/Whites having a substance use disorder were higher than for the other ethnic groups. Frequency rates, however, showed that Hispanics had slightly higher (nonsignificant) rates of substance use disorders (4.8%), as compared to African American/Blacks (4.5%) and European American/Whites (3.7%). Hispanics also had higher (nonsignificant) rates of antisocial personality disorder and affective disorders overall, including dysthymia. African American/Blacks had rates of anxiety disorders (11.5%), especially phobias that, though still not of statistical significance, were almost double those of the other groups (anxiety disorders: 6.9% Hispanics; 6.8% European American/White); they also had higher rates of schizophrenia and severe cognitive impairments. However, again, the odds ratio do not show any significant differences in these categories by ethnicity when all other sociodemographic risk factors were taken into consideration.

Socioeconomic status was the factor most strongly associated with high rates of most psychiatric disorders, according to Regier et al.'s (1993) U.S. study. Socioeconomic status was evaluated by a combined measure of occupation, education, and income. Individuals in the lowest socioeconomic group were 2.5 times more likely to have a psychiatric disorder than those in the highest socioeconomic group. For example, schizophrenia was eight times more prevalent in the lowest than in the highest socioeconomic group, regardless of ethnicity. The authors also cited earlier literature to support this conclusion and so did a later study (Verhulst & Achenbach, 1995). In addition, anxiety disorders, antisocial personality disorder, and severe cognitive impairment were higher in the lowest socioeconomic group.

In the international study by Regier et al. (1993), there was also a higher rate of any mental disorder among those in the lowest socioeconomic group. In Edinburgh, Athens, London, and Finland the rates for any mental illness were twice as high between the lowest and highest socioeconomic groups. Another study by Sundquist (1993) also showed that Latin American political refugees of low socioeconomic status in Sweden had a higher incidence of mental illness. In this case, situational stress may also have been a contributing factor.

Both the U.S. and international studies (Regier et al., 1993) also showed a difference in the prevalence of psychiatric problems due to marital status or gender. Single, separated, divorced, or widowed persons were 2.0 times more likely to have a psychiatric disorder than those who were married. There were also indications of a higher incidence of affective and anxiety disorders in women and a higher incidence of substance use disorders among men, especially those in the 18- to 24-year-old group.

Substance use disorders are among the most frequently studied disorders in the research literature on adolescents. The National Institute on Drug Abuse has conducted longitudinal surveys over the past 20 years with adolescents in U.S. high schools regarding the prevalence of substance use and misuse. Data collected between 1991 and 1994 (Johnston, O'Malley, & Bachman, 1995) showed that the substance use rate was lower for Hispanics and African American/Blacks than European American/Whites. Survey results indicated that among high school seniors (approximately 15,000 subjects), binge drinking was more common among European American/Whites (32%), especially males, than among Hispanics (24%) and African American/Blacks (14%). European American/White high school seniors also had higher rates of illicit drug use (e.g., use of marijuana,

LSD, barbiturates, and amphetamines). Overall, in 12th grade males had higher rates of heavy drinking and annual use of most illicit drugs (except stimulants) than females. Among 8th-graders, use of marijuana doubled, and it increased by up to 10% in other grades; cigarette use increased by 30% in 8th grade and by close to 5% in other grades. Use of specific drugs varied by ethnicity. For example, European American/White and Hispanic seniors showed the same rate of heroin use, whereas Hispanics showed a higher rate of cocaine use. However, Hispanics also showed the strongest decline in drug use of all ethnic groups between the 8th and 12th grades, although they also had the highest dropout rates from high school. African American/Black seniors had the lowest rates of alcohol and drug use, as well as daily cigarette use, of all three groups, but they also had the lowest rates of decline in substance use between the 8th and 12th grades. Nevertheless, ethnicity was not the primary factor associated with substance misuse in adolescence. There was also no difference in alcohol or drug usage rates related to socioeconomic status (based on parental education).

The studies reviewed here demonstrate that variations in symptoms of psychiatric disorders appear to be linked to socioeconomic, marital, gender, and situational factors rather than to ethnicity per se. Substance misuse is common among U.S. adolescents of various socioeconomic levels, but some differences by ethnicity and gender have been noted.

Socialization Issues within Cultural Contexts

Theories and research studies that focus on socialization patterns of children of different cultures reveal some important differences in parenting methods used. In particular, Zayas and Solaris (1994) have reviewed research studies on infant–mother attachment using the "Strange Situation" technique (Ainsworth, Blehar, Waters & Walls, 1978, as described in Zayas & Solaris, 1994, p. 201), which involves the study of infants' reactions after separation from their mothers. Studies using this technique with different cultural groups demonstrate that early experiences promote cultural values. A basic premise is that mothers generally expect to have a positive relationship with their infants. However, cultural values may influence the quality of the mother–infant relationship. In cultures where solidarity and interdependence among family members are promoted (collectivism), such as Japanese culture, infants are seldom separated from their mothers. In a Japanese study, infants experienced a great deal of anxiety when reunited with their mothers after a brief separation (Miyake, Chen, & Campos, 1985). In contrast, infants in a similar German study evidenced tendencies toward anxious avoidance, because the mothers frequently separated from the infants as a way to encourage independence (Grossman, Grossman, Spangler, Suess, & Unzner, 1985). European American/White infants tested in the Ainsworth et al. (1978) study spent a balanced amount of time away and with their mothers. These infants showed a desire to be comforted by their mothers after separation, which was a sign of secure attachment to the mothers. The results of these research studies can be interpreted from a family systems perspective. Whereas Japanese mothers can be characterized as enmeshed with their infants, German mothers can be characterized as disengaged.

An important influence in the socialization of culturally diverse children is the role of the extended family. The extended family acts simultaneously as a socializing agent for cultural values and as a cushion against traumatic changes and adaptations (Harrison, Wilson, Pine, Chan, & Buriel, 1990). In essence, the power or authority of the parents is shared with members of the extended family as socializing agents of the children. According to some surveys, approximately 53% of African American/Black households include an elderly extended family member (usually a grandparent), as compared to 40% of European American/White households (Beck & Beck, 1989). African American/Black families also often include persons other than blood relatives (Boyd-Franklin, 1989). The support of the extended family system among African American/Blacks continues throughout life. There was more family support, caregiving, and contact among relatives of elderly childless African American/Blacks, as compared to a comparison group of European American/Whites in a study by Johnson and Barer (1995). These patterns are also common in Hispanic and Asian families. Native Americans expect most of their tribal members to function as a collateral support group. The ongoing support of the extended family may be diminished when relatives are separated by a change of environment (Gardano, 1996; Ho, 1987; Sue & Sue, 1990). The reliance and value placed on connectedness among family members may be misinterpreted as dependency, rather than as a source of resiliency. The role of the extended family should be researched to aid in the diagnosis and treatment of culturally diverse families.

Other differences in socialization patterns deal with the values most emphasized by the parents, such as cognitive achievement, motivation, social skills, creativity, and problem solving. Studies reviewed by Zayas and Solaris (1994) on the parental beliefs of various groups, such as Asian and Mexican cultures, showed an emphasis on motivation and social skills related to cooperative behaviors, whereas European American/White parents emphasized cognitive achievement and competitiveness much more than the other skills (e.g., Okagaki & Sternberg, 1993). In terms of methods used to transmit the cultural values of collectivism among culturally diverse families, some studies show that conformity to authority is encouraged much more than autonomy. In order to socialize children into conformity, high levels of modeling and an authoritarian and punitive style of parenting are common among Hispanic, African American/Black, and Asian families, especially those undergoing adjustment and economic stress (Lamborn, Dornbusch, & Steinberg, 1996). The authoritarian style of parenting may be reinforced because the parents may be unavailable due to a loss of or increase in levels of employment. The authoritarian style, coupled with an emphasis on cooperation and social skills, fosters collectivism and a hierarchical family structure. Acculturated families may deviate from the authoritarian model because they may have adopted democratic decision-making and communication patterns between the parents and children.

Few studies exist that compare cultural differences in terms of parenting methods and their effectiveness. Most of the literature focusing on parenting methods (Lamborn et al., 1996) suggests that the democratic style promotes better adjustment and psychosocial outcomes for children and adolescents than does either the permissive or the authoritarian parenting style. The democratic style mainly features freedom within limits, whereas in the permissive style parents have abdicated their authority and have few rules, and children have considerable power. In the authoritarian style, the parents are the primary decision makers, have strictly delineated rules, and possess most of the power. Sue and Sue (1990) question whether studies of this nature are intended to support mainstream values.

One study that examined the effect of parenting styles on adolescent adjustment by ethnicity was conducted by Lamborn et al. (1996). Differences in family decision making and self-reliance were evaluated through the ratings of 3,597 adolescents in 9th to 11th grades in two California public school communities. By testing students from two different communities—a predominantly European American/White community (at least 75%) and a predominantly ethnically mixed community (at least 25% were ethnic families)—the study also compared whether environmental influences played an important role. Measures of family decision making and self-reliance, as well as a self-esteem inventory, were used. Results showed that patterns in parenting style and decision making were predictive of adolescent adjustment, but there was no significant relationship to ethnicity. Adolescents under the influence of a permissive parenting style, who were allowed ample freedom to make decisions (termed "unilateral adolescent decision making" by Lamborn et al., 1996, p. 284), exhibited lower academic functioning and poorer psychosocial functioning than those who made joint decisions with their parents. Adolescent maladjustment was high among Hispanic adolescents whose parents were permissive in their parenting style and lived in ethnically mixed communities. African American/Black families tended to use the authoritarian style and were more vulnerable in European American/White communities. It is possible that African American/Black parents feel their children are more vulnerable to the effects of discrimination, and thus feel more compelled to protect them.

Family communication is another area that is often addressed in the family systems literature (Gardano, 1996; Ho, 1987; Sue & Sue, 1990). Most ethnic cultures do not support open expression of feelings. Some cultures, such as Asian and Hispanic cultures, may interpret the expression of anger as a sign of disrespect or shame. Humor sometimes disguises annoyance and anger. Most often, feelings of anger may be expressed to an extended family member who will intervene in the nuclear family. Generally, women are expected not to disagree with men. Children are not expected to show open feelings of disagreement toward parents, because this would challenge their authority in the hierarchy. Signs of affection are often expressed more openly or through actively participating in family obligations or rituals, or doing special favors for family members. Differences in the communication styles of families were studied with respect to ethnicity by Hampson, Beavers, and Hulgus (1990). The study compared the responses to the Beavers Systems Model Scales among European American/White, African American/Black, and Mexican American parents who had a developmentally disabled child. Overall, the Beavers Scales primarily measure dimensions related to emotional closeness–distance, such as openness and receptivity to others' feelings, including both warm and angry feelings. These scales also include measures of power relationships and enmeshment–disengagement. Results indicated that there were no statistically significant differences between the three ethnic groups on global scale ratings of emotional closeness–distance, but subtle differences were found in the way feelings are expressed. For example, African American/Black families, especially those of lower socioeconomic status, were less likely to express thoughts and feelings directly and clearly. These results and other studies reviewed by Hampson et al. (1990) suggest that differences in communication styles between cultural groups do not necessarily have a negative impact on general family functioning.

The research described here shows that the patterns of socialization, motivation, parenting style, and expression of feelings in families with a collectivistic orientation, as compared to families with an individualistic orientation, do not evidence any risk factors for psychopathology. The reliance on the extended family by families from a collectivist orientation actually represents a unique source of resiliency. The findings reveal that an authoritarian parenting style may have a more positive outcome for some ethnic families than the democratic parenting style, because it lends support to collectivism and a hierarchical family structure. The authoritarian style may also serve as a protective factor for families that experience marginalization. Some of the research demonstrates that when culturally diverse families with adolescents adopt a permissive style of parenting characterized by blurred authority roles, and live in a predominantly European American/White community, they are at much greater risk for maladjustment. When parents of any culture abdicate authority, the family becomes disorganized, and adolescents for the most part are not prepared to take on responsibilities of adults.

Biculturation/Acculturation

Racial and Cultural Identity

Part of the process of adaptation to another culture, or acculturation, includes the acquisition and management of bicultural skills. One of the most important issues in differentiating the family functioning styles and socialization skills of minority, culturally diverse families in the United States (such as Hispanics, Asians, and African American/Blacks) from those of mainstream families is the development of adaptive skills to manage a bicultural environment. Minority children learn adaptive skills that will help them cope with more than one culture (also termed "bicultural skills") as well as with potential discrimination and alienation. Basically, minority children have to learn to live in a primarily collectivistic system at home and an individualistic system outside the home, including the latter system's institutions, such as schools (Triandis, 1995). The skills involved in teaching children how to perform well in more than one culture include role flexibility, such as loyalty to the culture of origin and adaptability to the host culture; cognitive flexibility, in terms of adapting to discontinuity between one culture and another; and the ability to infer multiple meanings if more than one language is spoken (Harrison et al., 1990). These can all be considered strengths or resiliency factors.

The adaptive skills of minority children have been interpreted both as resources and as liabilities (Gardano, 1996; Ho, 1987; Spencer & Markstrom-Adams, 1990; Sue & Sue, 1990). On the one hand, minority children are quite resilient because they learn a wide range of adaptive skills that can help them to thrive in a multicultural system. However, many develop a negative self-image and identity conflicts in adolescence, which can sometimes result in depression and anxiety, conduct problems, substance misuse, and severe conflicts with parents. The expected conflicts between parents and adolescents are assumed to be more acute among ethnic minority children, and consequently to have a more negative impact on family cohesiveness, than among mainstream children. For example, the discontinuity of roles in shifting from one culture to another was found to be detrimental to African American/Blacks in a study by Tanner (1992). The subjects consisted of 172 adolescents attending regular and alternative middle schools for at-risk students. Although results demonstrated that both African American/Black and European American/White at-risk students showed disengagement, higher rates were found among the African American/Black at-risk group. In this group, a higher rate of disengagement was associated with more interchangeability of family roles and leadership among family members.

The values of the majority culture may exert a strong influence on minority children because of a greater exposure to these values than to those of their own culture (Spencer & Markstrom-Adams, 1990). The values of the majority are often promoted through the school environment, peers and their families, neighbors, and the mass media. Thus, minority children may perceive the mainstream culture as more powerful than their own culture, which may lead to marginalization. During adolescence, individuals forge an identity through exploration and interactions with others in their environment. Negative influences and experiences can damage an adolescent's quest for a positive self-identity. Ambivalence about racial/ethnic identity in minority children may emerge because of conflicts in expectations between school (individualistic) and home (collectivistic); differences in language and economic power; and images of racial/ethnic groups as powerless and negative, such as those sometimes aired in the media. Continued marginalization and discrimination experienced by adults may also contribute to a disconnection with the culture of origin, according to a study with African American/Black and Hispanic mothers (Ruggiero, Taylor, & Lambert, 1996). The lack of positive identification with the culture of origin may thus be transmitted to subsequent generations.

The effects of biculturation conflicts on identity development also needs to be studied in depth by examining the identity development of children living with biracial and bicultural parents. The effect of biculturation was the focus of a study by Georgas and Kalantzi-Azizi (1992) with 326 adolescents of Greek or part-Greek origin who were living in either Greece, Germany, or The Netherlands. In Greece, there were two groups of 16- to 17-year-old high school students: one group with homoethnic parents (i.e., both parents in each family were Greek) and one group with biethnic parents (i.e., one parent in each family was Greek and the other was either Italian, German, or American). The groups outside of Greece consisted of 17-year-olds who were living with their homoethnic Greek immigrant parents in either Germany or The Netherlands. Results of this study revealed less adherence to traditional Greek family values for the groups outside of Greece. The adolescents living in Greece with biethnic parents tended to identify with and be influenced by both parental cultures (biculturalism), suggesting that the cultural identity of individual family members is also a function of the cultural membership of the family as a whole.

Intergenerational Differences

Other studies, which focus on the influence of acculturation, shed further light on the question of racial and bicultural identity development in families. Acculturation can also be defined as a transformation process between individualism and collectivism (Triandis, 1995) within a family. Thus, a family that has primarily collectivistic values may shift its emphasis to more individualistic values, or vice versa. These shifts involve the development of bicultural skills to create a consolidated cultural point of view, coping mechanisms, and strategies for survival. However, not all family members acculturate at the same rate; this is especially true of parents from a collectivistic culture and highly assimilated adolescents.

The majority of research studies concerning culturally diverse families focus on the intergenerational differences between the values of immigrant parents and their adolescents. Szapocznik and colleagues (Szapocznik et al., 1986; Szapocznik & Kurtines, 1993; Kurtines & Szapocznik, 1996) developed theories and research based on ecosystemic and structural family therapy methods in their work with Cuban immigrant families in Miami, Florida. The results of most of these investigators' studies indicated that parents, especially mothers, who adhered to traditional values tended to have highly assimilated adolescents who exhibited higher risks for conduct problems and substance use. The combination of the individualistic value system of U.S. mainstream culture; the lack of positive role models and reinforcement for ethnic minority values; and parents who are traditionally collectivistic often results in what may be best described as an ethnic war between parents and their offspring. When parents of any culture demand rigid adherence to clear lines of authority, family obligations, closeness, and conformity, adolescents are more likely to rebel, because at this stage of development they need to be able to challenge family authority and rules in order to promote their autonomy and self-identity. In Szapocznik and colleagues' studies, parents and their adolescent children who successfully integrated values from both the Cuban culture and the U.S. mainstream cultures were functioning better than those whose values were entrenched in either culture.

Conflicts and risks for emotional difficulties arise within the realm of the parent–child relationship in culturally diverse families. Research demonstrates that there are few, if any, differences between mainstream adolescents and those of other cultures in terms of adherence to mainstream cultural values. For example, a study in Hawaii with 121 Japanese American and 126 European American/White middle-class adolescents aged 13 to 20 showed no differences in their attitudes about family values (McDermott, Char, et al., 1984). The adolescents and their parents rated agreement or disagreement about the expression of thoughts and feelings in various situations. There were significant differences between all of the parents and all of the adolescents, but not by ethnicity. For example, most adolescents preferred to keep their thoughts and feelings private, whereas parents of both groups wanted them shared with the family. However, affective and parenting styles varied by ethnicity, although the differences were not statistically significant. Japanese parents considered open displays of feelings as a sign of disrespect, whereas European American/White parents promoted open expression of feelings and the right to privacy. Japanese parents also showed a preference to make important decisions within the family in a hierarchical manner, whereas European American/White parents were more flexible about making decisions as a group.

Another study with young adult college students found that it is important to distinguish between first- and second-generation ethnic youth (Heras & Revilla, 1994). There was no significant relationship between family cohesiveness scores and either low or high acculturation scores among 61 Filipino American college students. However, second-generation Filipino Americans reported lower self-esteem and self-concept than first-generation subjects did. By the second generation, the bonds and identification with the culture of origin, including language, are not as strong as in first-generation offspring.

Two studies with Chinese immigrant families in the United States and Australia examined in depth the impact of acculturation and intergenerational differences (Chiu, Feldman, & Rosenthal, 1992; Feldman, Mont-Reynaud, & Rosenthal, 1992). These studies evaluated adolescents aged 15 to 18 in three different cultural environments: the United States (San Francisco), Australia, and Hong Kong. In each location, there were 100 adolescent subjects in each of the ethnic groups. In both studies, the adolescent samples included Chinese from Hong Kong or Canton who had emigrated 3 years before the study (first generation); Chinese Americans and Chinese Australians, born in the United States or Australia (second generation); and Americans and Australians of West European descent. In addition, there was a control group of about 100 Chinese adolescents in Hong Kong in each of the studies. Chiu et al. (1992) examined whether the impact of immigration and acculturation had any effect on the level of emotional distress in adolescence (in terms of anxiety, depression, self-esteem, and psychosomatic symptoms) or on the quality of parenting behaviors related to control, monitoring, and emotional support by parents (termed "warmth," p. 213). Feldman et al. (1992) focused on the impact of acculturation on Chinese family values, such as self-control, politeness, and outward success. A measure of individualism and collectivism (Triandis et al., 1986, as cited in Feldman et al., 1992) was also included to compare collectivistic values (e.g., having unmarried children and elderly parents living at home—termed "family as a residential unit," p. 155) with individualistic values (e.g., self-reliance).

The impact of acculturation on emotional distress in adolescence and parenting behaviors was analyzed by comparing all of the adolescent adjustment measures with all of the parenting behavior measures (Chiu et al., 1992). The results showed no differences in degrees of emotional distress between all of the Chinese samples and samples of Americans and Australians of Western European descent. However, there was a difference in the type of emotional problem reported by Chinese immigrants by generation: First-generation Chinese adolescents, especially in the United States, reported more psychosomatic complaints, depression, and anxiety than those in the second generation. The results also showed that some parental behaviors and expectations were related to acculturation. Second-generation Chinese adolescents reported more rule setting and monitoring by their parents than first-generation adolescents did; they also indicated that the parent–adolescent relationship was not as positive. Chinese adolescents and adolescents of Western European descent gave their parents higher parental control ratings in terms of rule setting and decision making than the Chinese adolescents in Hong Kong did. The high ratings of parental monitoring and control by adolescents with Chinese mothers and fathers in the United States and especially in Australia was attributed to a protective parental strategy. The families were living in relatively unfamiliar cultures, both parents were working full-time, and there was possibly a lack of proximity to the extended family. In addition, it was surmised that the adolescents' lack of strong identification with the culture of origin may be predictive of intergenerational conflicts. Other parenting behaviors did not show differences by ethnicity. In both the Chinese group and the group of Western European descent, less parental warmth was associated with more emotional distress (e.g., depression and psychosomatic symptoms).

The impact of acculturation on Chinese family values showed that all Chinese groups valued individualism, especially in the United States (Feldman et al., 1992). Chinese adolescents in the United States and Australia placed more emphasis on success and individualism than on living with the family, compared to those in Hong Kong. However, the concept of living with the family in the same residential unit seemed resistant to acculturation, since it was still relatively valued by immigrant first- and second-generation Chinese adolescents, compared to the groups of Western European descent.

Gender Issues

Only a few of the studies reviewed for this chapter evaluated gender differences. Findings suggest that gender differences may sometimes override cultural differences, in terms of parenting styles and expected roles of family members. Most of the cross-cultural literature (Berry et al., 1992; Triandis, 1995) indicates that generally males are more oriented to achievement and leadership, whereas females are more oriented toward cooperation and egalitarianism, child rearing, and socialization of family members. These assumptions are based on biological factors, methods of gathering resources for the family, and socialization patterns that have developed through evolution. Furthermore, gender roles may be highly interdependent in hierarchical, male-dominated societies because the distribution of power and role expectations are clearly delineated by gender. In societies like the United States, gender roles are influenced by egalitarianism, which promotes a struggle for power and dominance between men and women (Wagner, Kirchler, Clack, Tekarslan, & Verma, 1990).

The results of various studies provide significant evidence that gender differences may be stronger than cultural differences in terms of family functioning. Findings from the study by McDermott, Robillard, et al. (1984) in Hawaii revealed that there were differences in the responses of male and female adolescents belonging to two cultural groups. Both European American/White and Japanese American girls tended to seek emotional closeness within the family, whereas the boys in both groups tended to seek more individual achievement and privacy. In another study with adolescents from various cultures (Hungary, Italy, Sweden, India, and Yemen), girls reported interpersonal-based strategies and boys reported problem-solving strategies as ways to cope with anxiety-provoking situations (Olah, 1995). These results suggest more universal assumptions along gender lines, such as the collectivistic and individualistic orientations for females and males, respectively. These studies also suggest that risks for emotional distress in adolescence may also be gender-based: Boys may be at risk when there are extreme levels of interdependence (enmeshment), and girls may be at risk when there are extreme levels of independence (disengagement), in family interactions. These trends suggest that there is a balance between females' need for interdependence and males' need for independence that fosters family functioning.

However, gender patterns are not static and do not always fit into stereotypes. Attitudes toward gender roles, such as those pertaining to decision making, household tasks, and child care, were researched in a study with 100 adult married Mexican American men and women in California (Ybarra, 1982). It was found that the wife's employment situation had the most impact on gender roles. When both spouses worked, the relationship was more egalitarian. For example, husbands were more likely to help with household chores and child rearing if their wives worked, whereas husbands helped minimally on these tasks if their wives stayed at home. Berry et al. (1992) also suggest that in cultures or families where the roles of spouses are clearly delineated, the role of women is diminished. However, in cultures or families where women make a contribution of resources to the family, their role and the educational level of the family are both enhanced. Some immigrant families may indeed benefit from individualism and egalitarianism, whereas others may experience significant spousal conflicts. Men and women may experience role conflict stress because of shifts in the expected distribution of authority in the family from a hierarchical to a more egalitarian system. Men may feel diminished in their role as head of the household, while women may be ambivalent about their increased power (Gardano, 1996).

The effects of gender on emotional distress in adolescence, parenting behaviors, cultural values, and perceptions of individualism–collectivism were studied with samples of adolescents of Chinese and Western European origin in the United States and Australia in two studies cited earlier (Chiu et al., 1992; Feldman et al., 1992). Significant gender-linked differences were found. Results of both of these studies showed that most males reported a preference for individualistic values (e.g., achievement) and females for collectivistic values (e.g., family security). Most female adolescents in all of the U.S. and Australian groups reported higher parental monitoring of their activities and higher levels of emotional and psychosomatic distress than male adolescents did. Chinese American females reported less family cohesiveness, more parental monitoring, and more emphasis on rule setting than males did. In view of the results on gender and intergenerational factors in these studies, the researchers suggest that for immigrant families there are stronger role expectations for females in order to maintain family cohesiveness. In this sense, acculturation does account for relative variations in gender roles.

It is suggested that any future research concerned with the individualism–collectivism paradigm in relation to families will need to consider gender as a factor because of its association with family roles. Specifically, the roles of spouses and parents, and the socialization of children by gender, need to be examined. In addition, family members may experience significant conflicts when gender roles shift or are modified as a result of acculturation.

RECOMMENDATIONS FOR FURTHER RESEARCH

Cross-cultural studies support findings that cultures throughout the ages developed either primarily collectivistic or individualistic values, due to the economic resources and survival of families within a community. This, in turn, shaped differences in cultural values, gender roles, and family structures. As nations forge new identities because of the influx of immigrant families from a variety of mostly collectivistic cultures, it is important for clinicians and researchers alike to become familiar with cultural constructs that integrate both the individualism–collectivism paradigm and family systems theories, such as the culturally integrated family systems model suggested in this chapter.

The prevalence studies reviewed here demonstrate that although symptoms vary, the same types of mental health problems exist across cultures at approximately the same rates. Some of the variables that most strongly differentiate higher from lower levels of mental disorders are low socioeconomic status, marital status, and gender. Other studies reviewed here have compared and contrasted the impact of collectivistic family values with that of individualistic values in terms of socialization patterns, family structure, biculturation, and acculturation. Differences in parenting methods, community influences, and gender appear to be much stronger determinants of emotional distress than cultural differences related to socialization patterns or affective styles. The socialization of children by gender may be an extremely powerful variable that deserves further study within different cultural contexts.

Studies with adolescents reveal that although collectivistic values are reinforced in culturally diverse families, adolescents do tend to become independent and achievement-oriented, especially when they live in an individualistic society such as the United States. Research with various ethnic groups has revealed significant differences between the values of adolescents and their parents in terms of individualism–collectivism. Since there are no significant differences between mainstream and culturally diverse adolescents in terms of individualistic values, intergenerational differences seem largely related to developmental issues.

However, most research has also found that adolescents tend to acculturate to the host culture at a faster rate than their parents. Differences in acculturation rates may account for most psychopathology within culturally diverse families. Studies show that those who experience the most significant emotional problems are highly acculturated adolescents who are extremely disengaged from parents who strongly adhere to the culture of origin. Second-generation adolescents may be at higher risks for intergenerational and identity conflicts because of proportionately more contact with the mainstream culture and less contact with the culture of origin. The literature reviewed here also suggests that emotional distress in adolescence is related to a redefinition of cultural identity. Living and coping within a bicultural environment, and often doing so in two languages, may indeed be a source of resiliency and progressive development for culturally diverse families. However, racial/ethnic identity may suffer in the process of adjusting to the majority culture, because of inequities in social power between the majority and minority cultures and discrimination against the minority. These factors certainly need further investigation.

Parents of various cultures share the same goals—to foster family cohesiveness, as well as their children's independence and self-identity—but the family values and methods are varied. Finally, it is important to recognize that the losses and gains experienced by culturally diverse families and families in the host culture are inevitable; this interaction often promotes dynamic societies. No culture ever remains static—not even the culture of origin.

The results of acculturation studies challenge researchers and clinicians to address the following questions/issues: How do variations in the acculturation levels of different family members affect the structure, interaction, communication patterns, and cultural identification of the family? What is the cultural orientation of the family in transition from a collectivistic to an individualistic mode? What is the impact of the loss or presence of the extended family? Are family roles primarily defined along gender lines? Is this true for any culture? Are bicultural adaptive skills and strategies the model for future culturally pluralistic societies?

CONCLUSIONS

The theoretical constructs about cultures and families developed in this chapter, and the supporting review of studies, identify risk and resiliency factors for families in transition from one culture to another. The results of these studies suggest that in order to investigate and treat family psychopathology adequately, it is essential to tease out such factors as development, gender, parenting methods, socioeconomic status, and environmental influences from such factors as stages of cultural and racial identity, biculturation, acculturation, and intergenerational conflicts. The interplay of these factors deserves further study within a framework that includes both cross-cultural and family theories, such as the culturally integrated family systems model.

This chapter is primarily based on the notion that most societies are and will be experiencing rapid changes in the composition of their familial and cultural identities. In the latter part of the 20th century, families have experienced marked redefinitions in the structure and the quality of family relationships. The concept of "family" in this century has been challenged by such changes as economic instability and increasing rates of divorce. The shift in gender roles in many societies has created new ways to manage a balance in the lines of authority in the family system. Many families find themselves in transition from one culture to another because of economic and political factors. For some culturally diverse families, these are additional stressors that pose significant risks for psychopathology. Others find strength and creative resources to cope with a bicultural environment that is often stressful and uninviting.

In the 21st century, families will be challenged more than ever to manage rapid changes that will continue to have an impact on the family system. The challenge to both researchers and clinicians is to shift the focus from psychopathology to the identification of family resources that strengthen and facilitate changes, while maintaining an adaptive balance in family life. The field of work with culturally diverse families is rich in such resources, which may provide fertile ground for innovative research and treatment methods that will benefit families of any culture.

REFERENCES

Ainsworth, M. D. S., Blehar, M. C., Waters, E., & Walls, S. (1978). *Patterns of attachment: A psychological study of the Strange Situation.* Hillsdale, NJ: Erlbaum.
American Psychiatric Association. (1980). *Diagnostic and statistical manual of mental disorders* (3rd ed.). Washington, DC: Author.
American Psychiatric Association. (1994). *Diagnostic and statistical manual of mental disorders* (4th ed.). Washington, DC: Author.
American Psychological Association. (1993). Guidelines for providers of psychological services to ethnic, linguistic, and culturally diverse populations. *American Psychologist, 48,* 45–48.
Beck, R. W., & Beck, S. H. (1989). The incidence of extended households among middle-aged black and white women. *Journal of Family Issues, 10,* 147–168.
Berry, J. W., Poortinga, Y. H., Segall, M. H., & Dasen, P. R. (1992). *Cross-cultural psychology: Research and applications.* New York: Cambridge University Press.

Boyd-Franklin, N. (1989). *Black families in therapy.* New York: Guilford Press.

Bronfenbrenner, U. (1979). *The ecology of human development: Experiments by nature and design.* Cambridge, MA: Harvard University Press.

Canino, G., Bird, H. R., & Canino, I. A. (1997). Methodological challenges in cross-cultural research of childhood psychopathology: Risk and protective factors. In C. T. Nixon & D. A. Northrup (Eds.), *Children's mental health services, 3: Evaluating mental health services: How do programs for children "work" in the real world?* (pp. 259–276). Thousand Oaks, CA: Sage.

Canino, G., & Bravo, M. (1994). The adaptation and testing of diagnostic and outcome measures for cross-cultural research. *International Review of Psychiatry, 6*(4), 281–286.

Chiu, M. L., Feldman, S. S., & Rosenthal, D. A. (1992). The influence of immigration on parental behavior and adolescent distress in Chinese families residing in two Western nations. *Journal of Research on Adolescence, 2*(3), 205–239.

Dana, R. (1996). Culturally competent assessment practice in the United States. *Journal of Personality Assessment, 66*(3), 472–487.

Davidson, L., & McGlashan, T. H. (1997). The varied outcomes of schizophrenia. *Canadian Journal of Psychiatry, 42*(1), 34–43.

Feldman, S. S., Mont-Reynaud, R., & Rosenthal, D. A. (1992). When East moves West: The acculturation of values of Chinese adolescents in the U.S. and Australia. *Journal of Research on Adolescence, 2*(2), 147–173.

Forehand, R., & Kotchick, B. A. (1996). Cultural diversity: A wake-up call for parent training. *Behavior Therapy, 27*(2), 187–206.

Foster, S. L., & Martinez, C. R. (1995). Ethnicity: Conceptual and methodological issues in child clinical research. Special issue: Methodological issues in clinical child psychology research. *Journal of Clinical Child Psychology, 24*(2), 214–226.

Gardano, A. C. (1996, August). *Individualism/collectivism, family structure, and communication: Practical knowledge and skills for work with culturally-diverse families.* Paper presented at the annual meeting of the American Psychological Association, Toronto.

Gardano, A. C. (in press). Assessment of culturally diverse families: Culturally integrated family systems model. *The Family Psychologist.*

Gardano, A. C., Davis, R. M., & Jones, E. (1994). Promoting receptivity to issues of cultural diversity in mental health services at health maintenance organizations. *The Family Psychologist, 10*(2), 15–18.

Georgas, J., & Kalantzi-Azizi, A. (1992). Value acculturation and response tendencies of biethnic adolescents. *Journal of Cross-Cultural Psychology, 23*(2), 228–239.

Good, B. J. (1996). Culture and DSM-IV: Diagnosis, knowledge and power. *Culture, Medicine and Psychiatry, 20*(2), 127–132.

Grossman, K., Grossman, K. E., Spangler, G., Suess, G., & Unzner, L. (1985). Maternal sensitivity and newborns' orientation responses as related to quality of attachment in northern Germany. In I. Bretherton & E. Waters (Eds.), Growing points of attachment theory and research. *Monographs of the Society for Research in Child Development, 50*(1–2, Serial No. 209), 233–255.

Gureje, O., Mavreas, V., Vazquez-Barquero, J. L., & Janca, A. (1997). Problems related to alcohol use: A cross-cultural perspective. *Culture, Medicine and Psychiatry, 21*(2), 199–211.

Gushue, G. V., & Sciarra, D. T. (1995). Culture and families: A multidimensional approach. In J. G. Ponterotto, J. M. Casas, L. A. Suzuki, & C. M. Alexander (Eds.), *Handbook of multicultural counseling* (pp. 586–606). Thousand Oaks, CA: Sage.

Hampson, R. B., Beavers, W. R., & Hulgus, Y. (1990). Cross-ethnic family differences: Interactional assessment of white, black, and Mexican-American families. *Journal of Marital and Family Therapy, 16*(3), 307–319.

Harrison, A. O., Wilson, M. N., Pine, C. J., Chan, S. Q., & Buriel, R. (1990). Family ecologies of ethnic minority children. *Child Development, 61,* 347–362.

Helms, J. E. (1995). An update of Helms's white and people of color racial identity models. In J. G. Ponterotto, J. M. Casas, L. A. Suzuki, & C. M. Alexander (Eds.), *Handbook of multicultural counseling* (pp. 181–198). Thousand Oaks, CA: Sage.

Heras, P., & Revilla, L. A. (1994). Acculturation, generational status, and family environment of Pilipino Americans: A study in cultural adaptation. *Family Therapy, 21*(2), 129–138.

Ho, M. K. (1987). *Family therapy with ethnic minorities.* Newbury Park, CA: Sage.

Johnson, C. L., & Barer, B. M. (1995). Childlessness and kinship organization: Comparisons of very old Whites and Blacks. *Journal of Cross-Cultural Gerontology, 10*(4), 289–306.

Johnston, L. D., O'Malley, P. M., & Bachman, J. G. (1995). *National survey results on drug use from the Monitoring the Future study, 1975–1994: Vol. 1. Secondary school students* (DHHS Publication No. 95-4026). Washington, DC: U.S. Government Printing Office.

Kurtines, W. M., & Szapocznik, J. (1996). Family interaction patterns: Structural family therapy in contexts of cultural diversity. In E. D. Hibbs & P. S. Jensen (Eds.), *Psychosocial treatments for child and adolescent disorders: Empirically based strategies for clinical practice* (pp. 671–697). Washington, DC: American Psychological Association.

Lamborn, S. D., Dornbusch, S. M., & Steinberg, L. (1996). Ethnicity and community context as moderators of the relations between family decision making and adolescent adjustment. *Child Development, 67,* 283–301.

McDermott, J. F., Jr., Char, W. F., Robillard, A. B., Hsu, J., Tseng, W., & Ashton, G. C. (1984). Cultural variations in family attitudes and their implication for therapy. *Annual Progress in Child Psychiatry and Child Development,* 145–154.

McDermott, J. F., Jr., Robillard, A. B., Char, W. F., Hsu, J., Tseng, W., & Ashton, G. C. (1984). Reexamining the concept of adolescence: Differences between adolescent boys and girls in the context of their families. *Annual Progress in Child Psychiatry and Child Development,* 155–165.

McGill, D., & Pearce, J. K. (1982). British families. In M. McGoldrick, J. K. Pearce, & J. Giordano (Eds.), *Ethnicity and family therapy* (pp. 457–479). New York: Guilford Press.

McGoldrick, M., Pearce, J. K., & Giordano, J. (Eds.). (1996). *Ethnicity and family therapy* (2nd ed.). New York: Guilford Press.

Minuchin, S. (1974). *Families and family therapy.* Cambridge, MA: Harvard University Press.

Minuchin, S., & Fishman, H. C. (1981). *Family therapy techniques*. Cambridge, MA: Harvard University Press.

Miyake, K., Chen, S. J., & Campos, J. J. (1985). Infant temperament, mother's mode of interaction, and infant attachment in Japan: An interim report. In I. Bretherton & E. Waters (Eds.), Growing points of attachment theory and research. *Monographs of the Society for Research in Child Development, 50*(1–2, Serial No. 209), 276–297.

Okagaki, L., & Sternberg, R. J. (1993). Parental beliefs and children's school performance. *Child Development, 64,* 36–56.

Olah, A. (1995). Coping strategies among adolescents: A cross-cultural study. Special Issue: Adolescent research: A European perspective. *Journal of Adolescence, 18*(4), 491–512.

Pedersen, P. (1994). *A handbook for developing multicultural awareness* (2nd ed.). Alexandria, VA: American Counseling Association.

Pinderhughes, E. (1989). *Understanding race, ethnicity and power.* New York: Free Press.

Regier, D. A., Farmer, M. E., Rae, D. S., Myers, J. K., Kramer, M., Robins, L. N., George, L. K., Karno, M., & Locke, B. Z. (1993). One-month prevalence of mental disorders in the United States and sociodemographic characteristics: The Epidemiologic Catchment Area study. *Acta Psychiatrica Scandinavica, 88,* 35–47.

Robins, L. N., Helzer, J. E., Croughan, J., Williams, J. W. B., & Spitzer, R. L. (1981). *NIMH Diagnostic Interview Schedule: Version III.* Rockville, MD: National Institute of Mental Health.

Ruggiero, K. M., Taylor, D. M., & Lambert, W. E. (1996). A model of heritage culture maintenance: The role of discrimination. *International Journal of Intercultural Relations, 20*(1), 47–67.

Ruiz, P. (1985). Clinical care update: The minority patient. *Community Mental Health Journal, 21*(3), 208–216.

Sartorius, N., & Janca, A. (1996). Psychiatric assessment instruments developed by the World Health Organization. *Social Psychiatry and Psychiatric Epidemiology, 31*(2), 55–69.

Schwartz, S. H. (1994). Beyond individualism/collectivism: New cultural dimensions of values. In U. Kim, H. C. Triandis, C. Kagitcibasi, S. Choi, & G. Yoon (Eds.), *Individualism and collectivism: Theory, method, and applications* (pp. 85–119). Thousand Oaks, CA: Sage.

Spencer, M. B., & Markstrom-Adams, C. (1990). Identity processes among racial and ethnic minority children in America. *Child Development, 61,* 290–310.

Szapocznik, J., & Kurtines, W. M. (1993). Family psychology and cultural diversity: Opportunities for theory, research and application. *American Psychologist, 48*(4), 400–407.

Szapocznik, J., Rio, A., Perez Vidal, A., Kurtines, W. M., Hervis, O., & Santisteban, D. (1986). Bicultural effectiveness training (BET): An intervention modality for families experiencing intergenerational/intercultural conflict. *Hispanic Journal of Behavioral Sciences, 8*(4), 303–330.

Sue, D. W., & Sue, D. (1990). *Counseling the culturally different: Theory and practice* (2nd ed.). New York: Wiley.

Sundquist, J. (1993). Ethnicity as a risk factor for mental illness: A population-based study of 338 Latin American refugees and 996 age, sex and education-matched Swedish controls. *Acta Psychiatrica Scandinavica, 87,* 208–212.

Tannen, D. (1990). *You just don't understand: Women and men in conversation.* New York: Ballantine Books.

Tanner, Z. (1992). School counselors and at-risk adolescents: Integrating family and subcultural perspectives. *Family Therapy, 19*(1), 33–42.

Trevino, F. M., & Bruhn, J. G. (1977). Incidence of mental illness in a Mexican-American community. *Psychiatric Annals, 7*(12), 33–51.

Triandis, H. C. (1995). *Individualism and collectivism.* Boulder, CO: Westview Press.

U.S. Bureau of the Census. (1996). *Resident population—estimates by age, sex, race, and Hispanic origin: Appendix A. Projections of the population by age, sex, race and Hispanic origin for the U.S.: 1995 to 2050.* Washington, DC: U.S. Government Printing Office.

Verhulst, F. C., & Achenbach, T. M. (1995). Empirically based assessment and taxonomy of psychopathology: Cross-cultural applications: A review. *European Child and Adolescent Psychiatry, 4*(2), 61–76.

Wagner, W., Kirchler, E., Clack, F., Tekarslan, E., & Verma, J. (1990). Male dominance, role segregation and spouses' interdependence in conflict: A cross-cultural study. *Journal of Cross-Cultural Psychology, 21*(1), 48–70.

World Health Organization. (1977). *International classification of diseases: Manual of the international statistical classification of diseases, injuries, and causes of death* (9th rev., Vol. 1). Geneva: Author.

Ybarra, L. (1982). When wives work: The impact on the Chicano family. *Journal of Marriage and the Family, 44*(1), 169–178.

Zayas, L. H., & Solaris, F. (1994). Early childhood socialization in Hispanic families: Context, culture, and practice implications. *Professional Psychology: Research and Practice, 25*(3), 200–206.

SECTION II

---◆---

DIMENSIONS OF FAMILY STRUCTURE

CHAPTER 6

Psychopathology and the Marital Dyad

JOANNE DAVILA
THOMAS N. BRADBURY

An association between marital functioning and psychopathology has been observed by numerous theorists, researchers, and clinicians. For example, evidence has shown that psychopathology is associated with divorce and other poor marital outcomes (e.g., Regier et al., 1993). This outcome is not surprising, given that skillful communication, adaptive emotion regulation, and the ability to be physically and emotionally available and supportive are important to good marital functioning, but are often impaired by various disorders. In line with this conclusion, forms of marital or couple therapy are now being considered to treat a number of individual disorders. For example, the *Clinical Handbook of Couple Therapy* (Jacobson & Gurman, 1995) includes chapters on couple therapy for depression, anxiety disorders, alcohol problems, eating disorders, sexual desire disorders, and personality disorders. This suggests that in addition to being aware of the association between marital functioning and psychopathology, researchers and clinicians also think that including the spouse in treatment might be beneficial for both the symptomatic partner and the marriage.

The goal of this chapter is to describe the status of current research on marital functioning and psychopathology. Attention is given to the nature of the association between marital functioning and psychopathology, the way this association develops, and the course it follows. A major focus is on whether and how psychopathology affects marital functioning, and, conversely, on whether and how marital functioning affects psychopathology. To set the stage for addressing these questions, we first identify those aspects of marital functioning that are typically considered important to good marital outcome, and those aspects of marital functioning that may be most likely to affect and be affected by psychopathology. These aspects of marriage are discussed next, followed by a discussion of different types of psychopathology. In these discussions, we have aimed for breadth over depth in our coverage, as our goal is to provide an illustrative rather than an exhaustive review.

FACTORS ASSOCIATED WITH MARITAL FUNCTIONING AND MARITAL OUTCOME

Many studies of marital functioning and marital outcome have employed a diverse set of predictor variables from the behavioral, intrapersonal, and cognitive traditions. Karney and Bradbury (1995) provide a coherent way to organize the numerous variables that are involved in producing variation in marital outcome, and we adopt their framework in our review. They suggest that marital satisfaction and, ultimately, marital stability are affected by the interplay of three broad factors: enduring vulnerabilities, adaptive processes, and stressful life events. These factors represent the two most common traditions in marital research, for which the greatest amount of empirical support exists—the intrapersonal tradition (via enduring vulnerabilities) and the behavioral tradition (via adaptive processes). Also included is the relatively understudied factor of life stressors. In our analysis, we identify which of these three factors may be implicated in the association between the various types of psychopathology and marital functioning. Specifically, we examine whether psychopathology may affect marital functioning through any of these factors, and whether any of these factors may put individuals at risk for continued psychopathology.

Enduring vulnerabilities in models of marital outcome reflect the intrapersonal tradition in marital research, which suggests that the qualities of each spouse are what affect marital functioning and marital outcome. Enduring vulnerabilities are thus the enduring characteristics (e.g., personality traits, family-of-origin experiences) that spouses would bring to any marriage, and that may put them at risk for marital dysfunction. One example of this approach is the application of attachment theory (Bowlby, 1969) to adult romantic relationships, which suggests that experiences in early attachment relationships (e.g., parent–child relationships) may be carried over into adult romantic relationships and affect the course of such relationships (e.g., Hazan & Shaver, 1987). Indeed, research suggests that an insecure attachment style in adulthood is associated with marital discord and with various aspects of marital functioning, such as poor problem solving and communication behaviors (e.g., Feeney, Noller, & Callan, 1994; Kobak & Hazan, 1991; Senchak & Leonard, 1992). Another example of the enduring vulnerabilities approach is that of trait theorists, and psychodynamic theorists who suggest that the personality characteristics of each spouse predict marital outcome. Empirical evidence exists for this hypothesis as well, and the personality traits with the most potent negative effects appear to be neuroticism and impulsivity (e.g., Karney & Bradbury, 1995; Kelly & Conley, 1987).

Of course, a history of or propensity for psychopathology can be considered an enduring vulnerability, and the hypothesis that psychopathology is associated with marital dysfunction is consistent with the enduring vulnerabilities approach. In addition, psychopathology may be associated with other types of enduring vulnerabilities, and as such may be part of a group of related vulnerability factors that interact to affect marital outcome. For example, to the extent that a disordered spouse manifests other enduring vulnerabilities, marital functioning may be impaired and dissatisfaction may result (e.g., Beach & Fincham, 1995; Davila, Christian-Herman, & Bradbury, 1996).

Adaptive processes refer to the manner in which spouses interact—in particular to how they negotiate disagreements, individual or marital difficulties, and transitions. Adaptive processes are necessarily interpersonal in nature and reflect the behavioral tradition in marital research, which has focused on predicting marital outcome from the behaviors exchanged by spouses. This approach suggests that the ways in which spouses treat and respond to each other, and their reactions to such responses, will influence satisfaction and the course of marriage. The particular processes that are likely to be most critical to marital outcomes may have to do with communication, support, and affect regulation skills. Spouses who cannot regulate their emotions, communicate appropriately and effectively, or provide and receive support and nurturance may be unlikely to negotiate important interpersonal interactions, resolve disagreements and difficulties, or weather stressful circumstances and transitions. Many studies in the behavioral tradition that have examined observable couple interaction behavior support these hypotheses (e.g., Pasch & Bradbury, 1998; see Weiss & Heyman, 1990).

As noted above, adaptive processes concern spouses' reactions to each other as well as their observable behaviors, and thus include the cognitive reactions and expectations that spouses generate when interacting (Bradbury, 1995; Karney & Bradbury, 1995). Such cognitions are thought to affect marital behavior further. For example, if a spouse believes that his or her partner is to blame for marital problems, or that the partner always causes problems, then the spouse may be likely to behave more negatively toward the partner when attempting to negotiate marital problems and to be less maritally satisfied. Research has supported this hypothesis (e.g., Bradbury & Fincham, 1992), thus offering further evidence of the critical role of adaptive processes in marital functioning.

In a discussion of adaptive processes and how they relate to psychopathology, it is useful to consider particular aspects of the marital relationship to which couples may need to adapt. Some marital situations may be more or less problematic for spouses dealing with psychopathology, because psychopathology may increase the likelihood that a particular aspect of the marital relationship may become a source of conflict. Thus, marital conflicts may be caused by psychopathology, and the couple may be less able to negotiate and adapt to these conflicts because of the psychopathology. One particular aspect of the marital relationship that may become a source of conflict for couples with psychopathology is the sexual relationship, because many disorders impair sexual functioning. Thus, impairment in this arena is a specific focus in our discussions of psychopathology.

Stressful life events are any events, within or outside of the marriage, that affect the couple or an individual spouse and to which the couple must adapt. Both types of stressors, when not handled effectively by the individual spouse or the couple, are likely to result in marital dysfunction. The occurrence of a stressful life event can have a number of negative effects on marital functioning. For example, the spouses may devote more time and energy to managing the stressor and neglect each other, or they may disagree about how to manage the stressful event. Moreover, managing a stressful event or ongoing stressful circumstances requires good individual and marital coping skills, including the skills identified above in regard to adaptive processes (e.g., conflict negotiation, affect regulation, support skills). If a couple can successfully manage a stressful event, the marriage may not suffer. Although the effects of stressors on the course of marriage has been a relatively neglected area of research, there is evidence that supports the role of stressors in the course of marital functioning. For example, stressful life events that occurred during a 2-year period subsequent to marital therapy were the best predictors of relapse (e.g., marital discord) among couples (Jacobson, 1989; Jacobson, Schmaling, & Holtzworth-Munroe, 1987). Moreover, this effect held even when marital events were excluded, suggesting that marital and external events can have significant negative impact on the marriage. Cohan and Bradbury (1997) have further shown that stressors interact with problem-solving behaviors to predict marital outcome. For example, among spouses with poor problem-solving skills, major life stressors predict marital discord and instability. Even daily work-related stressors can affect marital functioning, and spousal support in response to these stressors has important moderating effects on marital functioning (Repetti, 1989).

The three factors that we have just discussed are relevant to marital functioning once a couple is married or in the relationship. Another factor that may be important to future marital and individual functioning, but that has to do with how the couple gets involved in the relationship, is *mate selection*—that is, who people marry and why. It has been suggested that people marry others who are similar to them and that similarity has a positive effect on marriage, with the notion being that people who are similar will get along better and negotiate problems more easily. Research supports spousal assortment by similarity. Spouses tend to be initially similar on personality traits, attitudes, and levels of psychological distress and well-being (e.g., Caspi & Herbener, 1993; Du Fort, Kovess, & Boivin, 1994; Feng & Baker, 1994). In addition, initial similarity appears to be associated with greater marital stability (e.g., Bentler & Newcomb, 1978). Whereas this line of theorizing suggests that similarity has positive effects on marriage, it is also possible that similarity may have negative effects if spouses are similar on variables thought to be risk factors for marital discord. For example, the assortative mating approach to mate selection has suggested that people with psychopathology marry others with psychopathology (e.g., Hagnell & Kreitman, 1974). If this is true, then such a pairing may have significant negative implications for the future of the marriage and the future of each individual's psychological health. In support of this hypothesis, one study has shown that similarity on attachment insecurity has a negative effect on marital functioning: Couples in which both partners have insecure attachment styles show greater conflict when interacting than do other couples (Cohn, Silver, Cowan, Cowan, & Pearson, 1992). It has also been suggested that negative outcomes may occur if people marry specific types of spouses in order to satisfy unmet needs (e.g., Heavey, Parker, Vhat, Crisp, & Gower, 1989; Slipp, 1995). For example, a person who desires to satisfy unmet childhood needs for attention may marry someone who seems very attentive. If the partner cannot meet those needs, marital discord and poor individual functioning may result. Given the potential for marital dysfunction based on the nature of spousal pairing, we also examine the literature relevant to mate selection and spousal similarity.

PSYCHOLOGICAL DISORDERS AND THEIR ASSOCIATION WITH MARITAL FUNCTIONING AND OUTCOME

In the preceding section, we have identified four broadly defined factors—enduring vulnerabilities, adaptive processes, stressful life events, and mate selection—that have been shown to be important for marital functioning and that may therefore be implicated in the association between marital functioning and psychopathology. We now review research relevant to each of these factors for six types of disorders: depression, alcoholism, anxiety disorders, eating disorders, schizophrenia, and personality disorders. These six types were chosen because there is at least some empirical research relevant to marital functioning for each, and because some form of couple, marital, or family treatment has been designed for each.

Depression

Depression has been shown to be associated consistently with marital dysfunction. Of existing theory and research on marital functioning and psychopathology, theory and research on depression is by far the most extensive. We provide a brief review of this literature, following the guidelines we have set out for this chapter. For further details, the reader is referred to the chapter on marital processes and depression in this book (see Beach & Fincham, Chapter 11).

Direct Associations between Depression and Marital Outcomes

Depression has been shown to be related to marital dysfunction in a number of ways. First, depression is associated with marital dissatisfaction both concurrently and longitudinally. Regarding the longitudinal association, three findings are important: Depression predicts increases in dissatisfaction over time (e.g., Beach & O'Leary, 1993a); dissatisfaction predicts increases in depression over time (e.g., Beach & O'Leary, 1993b); and the concurrent association between depression and dissatisfaction increases over time (Beach & O'Leary, 1993b). Thus, depression and marital dissatisfaction follow a course in which each affects the other, and this pattern may become stronger as the marriage goes on.

Second, depression is associated with divorce. Epidemiological studies have shown that the odds of separated/divorced persons' having major depressive disorder are two to three times those of people with other marital statuses (see Smith & Weissman, 1992). Although this type of data does not address causality, divorce has been shown to put people at risk for depression (e.g., Bruce & Kim, 1992; Kendler et al., 1995), and depression may put people at risk for divorce through its effect on marital satisfaction. Thus, the effect may be bidirectional.

Associations with the Four Marital Factors

Depression is associated with a number of enduring vulnerabilities that may increase risk for marital dysfunction. For example, depression is associated with high levels of neuroticism (e.g., Saklofske, Kelly, & Janzen, 1995; Scott, Williams, Brittleband, & Ferrier, 1995), an insecure attachment style (e.g., Hammen et al., 1995; Carnelley, Pietromonaco, & Jaffe, 1994), low self-esteem (e.g., Roberts, Kassell, & Gotlib, 1995), and high levels of personality disturbance (e.g., Farmer & Nelson-Gray, 1990; Shea, Glass, Pilkonis, Watkins, & Docherty, 1987). Depressed people also tend to be interpersonally sensitive, as well as highly self-critical (see Beck, 1983; Blatt & Zuroff, 1992). All of these qualities may make depressed spouses more reactive to marital events and stressors, and/or lead them to misperceive interpersonal interactions. Depressed people also have a tendency to view themselves, the world, and the future negatively (Beck, 1967), and thus may be vulnerable to making dysfunctional marital attributions.

Depression is also associated with various adaptive processes. For example, depression is associated with a diminished capacity to provide support to and receive support from the spouse (Cutrona & Suhr, 1994; Davila, Bradbury, Cohan, & Tochluk, 1997). Spouses with depressive symptoms also expect their partners to be less supportive and that expectation leads them to provide and solicit support in a negative manner (Davila et al., 1997). Depression is associated with maladaptive behavior in problem-solving interactions. Depressed spouses exhibit high levels of conflict, tension, negativity, ambivalence, hostility, and criticism (e.g., Gotlib & Whiffen, 1989; see Gotlib & Beach, 1995, for a review). They also display certain "depressive behaviors" (e.g., Biglan et al., 1985), including depressed affect, self-degradation, and physical and psychological complaints. Depression is also associated with negative marital attributions (see Horneffer & Fincham, 1996), which have been shown to be associated with negative problem-solving behavior (see Bradbury, Beach, Fincham, & Nelson, 1996). The behaviors and attributions of the depressed person's partner affect marital functioning as well. For example, partners of depressed spouses behave more negatively during conflict resolution (e.g., Hautzinger, Linden, & Hoffman, 1982; see Gotlib & Beach, 1995, for a review). In addition, the partner's behavior can have significant effects on the depressed spouse's level of symptoms. Previously depressed spouses are more likely to relapse if their partners are critical of them and if their partners do not provide adequate support (e.g., Hooley & Teasdale, 1989; Jacobson, Fruzzetti, Dobson, Whisman, & Hops, 1993). Finally, depression is often accompanied by decreased sexual interest and may thus disrupt the sexual functioning of the couple, potentially leading to marital conflict and dissatisfaction.

In addition, depression is associated with stressful life events. Evidence suggests that stressful life events, particularly severe marital events, put people at risk for depression (e.g., Christian-Herman, O'Leary, & Avery-Leaf, in press; Kendler et al., 1995). Moreover, there is evidence that depression puts people at risk for increased stress in their lives. Hammen's (1991) stress generation model of depression suggests that depressed people may contribute to the occurrence of stressors in their lives, particularly interpersonal stressors. We (Davila et al., 1997) applied this model to marriage and suggested that the association between depressive symptoms and marital discord can be understood as a process of stress generation. We showed that for wives, depressive symptoms lead to increases in marital stress, which in turn lead to increases in depressive symptoms. Thus, depression and marital stress affect each other reciprocally, potentially creating a vicious cycle of marital dysfunction and depression.

Finally, regarding mate selection, there is some evidence that depressed people marry similar spouses. At least one study suggests that assortative mating occurs among patients with affective disorders. Merikangas and Spiker (1982) found that men and women with affective disorders tended to be married to spouses with psychiatric illnesses, especially affective disorders. In addition, couples in which both members had a psychiatric illness had significantly higher divorce rates than couples in which only one spouse had a psychiatric illness (Merikangas, 1984). However, other studies have not replicated the basic finding of assortative mating (e.g., Huen & Maier, 1993; Waters, Marchenko, Abrams, Smiley, & Kalin, 1983).

From this brief review, it is evident that depression is associated both with marital satisfaction directly and with factors that affect marital satisfaction. In addition to being an enduring vulnerability, depression is associated with other enduring vulnerabilities. Depression increases and is increased by stressful life events (particularly those within the marriage); it is also associated with important adaptive processes, such as problem-solving and social support behavior, as well as marital attributions. In addition, the behavior of the depressed spouse's partner has effects on whether the depressed spouse will experience symptoms in the future. Depressed people may also be more likely to marry spouses who are similar to them with regard to psychopathology. Thus, there is sufficient evidence showing that depression both affects and is affected by marital functioning, and there is evidence to suggest that this may be an ongoing process with great potential for negative marital and individual outcomes.

Alcoholism

Direct Associations between Alcoholism and Marital Outcomes

There is a growing body of literature that examines the association between alcoholism and marital functioning. Much work suggests that alcoholism can exert significant negative effects on marriage (e.g., Moos, Finney, & Gamble, 1982; Moos & Moos, 1984), and that marriages in which one spouse is alcoholic are comparable to distressed marriages in their level of marital satisfaction (e.g., Billings, Kessler, Gomberg, & Weiner, 1979; Jacob & Leonard, 1992; Leonard, 1990; O'Farrell & Birchler, 1987). However, it is also the case that many such marriages remain intact and stable. A number of theorists, primarily from the family systems perspective, have suggested that alcoholism may play various roles in a marriage (e.g., disrupting, stabilizing) and may lead to various outcomes (e.g., Steinglass, Bennett, Wolin, & Reiss, 1987). For example, drinking may be adaptive to the family by allowing for the expression of certain family behaviors and the accomplishment of family tasks that could not be done when the alcoholic is sober. Recent work has expanded on these ideas and has focused on different types of alcoholics and the effects they have on marital functioning (e.g., Leonard, 1990).

Associations with the Four Marital Factors

The bulk of the research on alcoholism and marital functioning focuses on the effect of alcoholism on adaptive processes. Early studies typically found that when discussing a marital problem, the alcoholic spouses (almost always the husband) tended to be more negative and hostile, and the nonalcoholic spouses (almost always the wife) tended to be more positive (e.g., Billings et al., 1979; Frankenstein, Hay, & Nathan, 1985; Jacob, Ritchey, Cvitkovic, & Blane, 1981). Within these studies, some showed that interactions were more negative when the spouse was drinking during experimental procedures (e.g., Jacob et al., 1981); some showed no differences (e.g., Billings et al., 1979); and some showed that interactions actually became more focused on problem solving (e.g., Frankenstein et al., 1985). These mixed results highlighted the notion that alcoholism is a heterogeneous disorder likely to affect a marriage in multiple ways.

Recent research has elaborated on this line of work by focusing on subtypes of alcoholics. One promising distinction appears to be between "steady drinkers," who drink about the same amount every day, and "episodic drinkers," who engage in binge drinking. Research has suggested that episodic drinking may have more negative effects on marriage, whereas steady drinking appears to have some positive effects under certain circumstances. For example, among steady alcoholics, higher alcohol consumption in the previous month is associated with higher marital satisfaction among wives (Jacob, Dunn, & Leonard, 1983). Thus, ironically, steady alcoholics' drinking may have a positive effect on their wives. Moreover, when actually drinking under experimental procedures, episodic alcoholic couples appear to engage in an interaction pattern suggestive of coercive control, whereas steady alcoholic couples appear to engage in an interaction pattern suggestive of high levels of problem solving (Jacob & Leonard, 1988; Leonard, 1990). As Jacob and Leonard (1988) describe, the episodic drinker may behave in a hostile manner in order to avoid dealing with conflictual issues while drinking. This pattern may discourage direct problem solving, while at the same time allowing the episodic drinker not to take responsibility for his behavior by blaming it on the alcohol. The pattern among steady alcoholic couples suggests that problem-solving activities may be energized when the husband has been drinking.

Although these patterns suggest that the episodic pattern may have negative long-term effects and the steady pattern may have positive long-term effects, these types of outcomes are presently unknown, and researchers caution that both patterns may have positive and negative effects. For example, the steady pattern may have positive consequences in that it may allow for successful management of family problems. However, it may also have negative consequences if periods of sobriety result in decreased problem solving (Jacob & Leonard, 1988). Moreover, there may be subtypes within the steady and episodic categories that have further differential effects. For example, among steady alcoholics, wives of those who primarily drank outside the home had lower levels of marital satisfaction than wives of those who primarily drank inside the home (Dunn, Jacob, Hummon, & Seilhammer, 1987). Researchers are now considering the possibility that "families in which the drinking style of the alcoholic and the family reaction to the drinking 'fit' are more likely to remain intact than families in which there is a lack of fit" (Leonard, 1990, p. 240).

Another aspect of adaptive functioning that may be impaired in alcoholic marriages is sexual functioning. A large body of evidence shows that compared to normal controls (i.e., individuals with no alcohol, medical, psychiatric, or marital problems), male alcoholics experience more sexual dysfunction, greater impotence, lower frequency of intercourse, and less sexual satisfaction (see O'Farrell, 1990). In addition to numerous physical and psychological causes for these problems, interpersonal factors play a role. In particular, male alcoholics' reports of sexual dysfunction and dissatisfaction are similar to those of nonalcoholic but maritally discordant males, suggesting that the marital discord that often characterizes marriages in which one partner is alcoholic contributes to sexual dysfunction (e.g., O'Farrell, Choquette, & Birchler, 1991).

A third important issue relevant to the adaptive processes of the couple is the role of alcoholism in marital violence. The prevalence of marital violence is becoming increasingly recognized, as are the serious effects of violence on individual and marital functioning (e.g., Leonard & Roberts, 1998; Straus & Gelles, 1990). Moreover, excessive alcohol use is associated with marital violence (e.g., Pan, Neidig, & O'Leary, 1994; see Leonard & Jacob, 1988, and Leonard, 1993, for reviews). This association is not accounted for by such factors as socioeconomic status or attitudes about violence, but it is moderated by a number of other demographic, person-ality, and cognitive variables (e.g., Kantor & Straus, 1987; Leonard & Blane, 1992). For example, "risky drinking" (e.g., high scores on alcohol use measures) is strongly associated with marital violence among men with high levels of hostility and negative affect (Leonard & Blane, 1992). In addition, male alcoholics who report an early onset of drinking, antisocial behavior, binge drinking, and out-of-home drinking are more maritally aggressive (Murphy & O'Farrell, 1994). Although this type of research is useful for identifying potential risk factors for marital violence among alcohol users, little is known about the proximal factors that affect the association between alcohol use and violence. For example, little is known about the nature of the interactions that lead to violence or about the role of alcohol in determining which interactions become violent. Given that marital violence may be one of the most damaging correlates of alcohol use, continued research that further specifies the role of alcohol in the development and course of marital violence is critical.

Although not as prominent as the research on adaptive qualities, a growing body of research suggests that alcoholism is associated with certain enduring vulnerabilities that may affect marital functioning. Some of these are noted above in the discussion of moderators of the alcohol–marital violence association, but independent of the literature on violence, research has shown that one particularly problematic enduring vulnerability is antisocial personality disorder (e.g., Hesselbrock, Hesselbrock, & Stabenau,

1985). Importantly, episodic alcoholics or binge drinkers, rather than steady drinkers, appear to be those who possess traits of antisocial personality disorder (e.g., hostility, impulsivity, and social disruptiveness; see Leonard, 1990). Episodic alcoholics may also have an early onset of problem drinking and a family history of alcoholism (see Leonard, 1990). Steady drinkers may be more likely to have passive, dependent personality traits, a later onset of alcohol problems, and fewer social and aggressive problems (Leonard, 1990). Thus, age at onset, family history, and antisocial personality traits may be particular vulnerabilities that moderate the impact of alcoholism on marital functioning.

Stressful life events may play a role in the association between alcoholism and marital functioning. Brown et al. (1990) found that acute, severe stressors and highly threatening chronic difficulties were associated with relapse among alcoholics. This finding raises the possibility that stress may affect marital discord through its effect on alcohol relapse. It is also possible that marital events themselves, if severe or threatening, may affect relapse. This is consistent with the finding that alcoholics tend to attribute their relapses to interpersonal factors involving their spouses (Maisto, O'Farrell, Connors, McKay, & Pelcovits, 1988), although the extent to which such self-reports correspond to actual marital events is unknown. However, alcoholic patients with spouses who are high on expressed emotion (EE) are more likely to relapse following treatment than are alcoholic patients with spouses who are low on EE (O'Farrell, Cutter, Hooley, & Fals-Stewart, 1996).

Regarding mate selection, early theories focused on the female's choice of an alcoholic male. It was suggested that women chose alcoholic men as a defense against conflicts regarding dependency or control, and that wives needed their husbands to continue drinking to avoid their own decompensation (e.g., Lewis, 1937). However, research has not supported this theory. Although wives of alcoholics may have elevated levels of symptomatology while their husbands are alcoholic, when alcoholics decrease their drinking or became abstinent, wives' symptom levels also decrease (e.g., Moos et al., 1982). The elevation of wives' symptoms is now seen as a reaction to the stress of the husbands' alcoholism. However, there is some evidence that nonalcoholic daughters of alcoholics are more likely to marry alcoholics than are nonalcoholic daughters of nonalcoholics (Schuckit, Tipp, & Kelner, 1994), suggesting that spousal selection factors may be at work in certain circumstances. Finally, although it was initially contended that there was a higher level of assortative mating among female alcoholics, there is some evidence that such rates are similar for males and females (Jacob & Bremer, 1986).

To summarize, alcoholism can lead to negative interactions between spouses, marital violence, and marital dissatisfaction. This appears to be the case particularly for episodic alcoholics, who possess a number of additional vulnerabilities—namely, an early onset of drinking and antisocial personality traits, including impulsivity. Alcoholism can also impair the sexual relations of couples, potentially leading to further marital discord, and marital discord may lead to further sexual impairment and dissatisfaction. Chronic marital discord or severe marital events may maintain or exacerbate alcoholism, as these sorts of stressors can lead to relapse among treated alcoholics. Thus, there is growing evidence that alcoholism both affects and is affected by marital functioning, although the exact nature of these associations is far from being fully understood.

Anxiety Disorders

Researchers have theorized that certain anxiety disorders may be associated with marital dysfunction. For example, it has been suggested that agoraphobia may manifest itself following marital conflict surrounding issues of autonomy–dependency (e.g., Goldstein & Chambless, 1978). However, very little empirical research on the association between anxiety disorders and marital functioning has been conducted. The anxiety disorders for which the most research exists are agoraphobia and obsessive–compulsive disorder (OCD).

Agoraphobia

Agoraphobia and Marital Outcomes. The results of research on agoraphobia with regard to marital functioning is mixed (see Emmelkamp & Gerlsma, 1994, and Steketee & Shapiro, 1995, for reviews). Some research suggests that a high proportion of agoraphobics are married women (e.g., Vose, 1981). On the other hand, Epidemiologic Catchment Area data have shown that there is an increased prevalence of agoraphobia among people who are separated or divorced (Boyd, 1985). These data also show that, compared with normal controls, people with panic disorder get along less well with their spouses and confide in their spouses less. Other studies show instead that agoraphobic wives (without comorbid depression) do not appear to be less maritally satisfied, on average, than wives without a psychiatric disorder (Arrindell & Emmelkamp, 1986; Buglass, Clarke, Henderson, Kreitman, & Presley, 1977). In one study, only 20% of agoraphobics were dissatisfied with their marriages (Arrindell, Emmelkamp, & Sanderman, 1986).

Associations with the Four Marital Factors. Although the magnitude of the association between marital dysfunction and agoraphobia is unclear, at least some proportion of agoraphobics have marital difficulties, and agoraphobia is associated with a number of factors that influence marriage. Regarding enduring vulnerabilities, agoraphobics tend to have dependent and avoidant personality characteristics (e.g., Barlow, 1988), which are often associated with interpersonal dysfunction. Severe agoraphobics also tend to be high on interpersonal sensitivity (Noyes et al., 1993), which may make them more sensitive to marital events or bias their interpretations of marital events. More generally, anxiety symptoms are also associated with insecure attachment (e.g., Fonagy et al., 1996; Hammen et al., 1995) and with neuroticism (e.g., Kenardy, Oei, & Evans, 1990). However, there is no research documenting how, or whether, these vulnerabilities specifically affect marital functioning in the context of agoraphobia or other anxiety disorders.

There are also no direct examinations of the association between agoraphobia and adaptive processes in marriage. One study relevant to adaptive marital processes found that better self-reported spousal communication predicted good response at follow-up after couple therapy for agoraphobia (Craske, Burton, & Barlow, 1989). Another related study examined EE in couples with an agoraphobic spouse and found that patients' high criticism and low warmth were associated with higher concurrent agoraphobic symptomatology, but, surprisingly, with greater reduction in symptomatology as well (Peter & Hand, 1988). Partners' high criticism was also significantly correlated with greater symptom reduction in their spouses. The contradictory nature of the results of these studies highlights the need for further understanding of communication and support among couples in which one spouse is agoraphobic. Finally, there is also some evidence that agoraphobia is associated with the sexual functioning of a couple. In one study, wives with agoraphobia reported a marked loss of sexual drive (Buglass et al., 1977). Similarly, among married agoraphobics, better initial sexual adjustment (pretreatment) was associated with greater improvement in symptoms 2 years following treatment (Monteiro, Marks, & Ramm, 1985).

There is evidence that the onset of anxiety disorders may be preceded by stressful life events (e.g., Pollard, Pollard, & Corn, 1990; see Barlow, 1988). Moreover, interpersonal stressors are particularly common precursors of anxiety disorders (Doctor, 1982). For example, separation from or loss of a spouse, and relationship problems, were reported as the most common antecedents of panic and agoraphobia.

Regarding mate selection, women who are vulnerable to agoraphobia and/or are highly dependent may marry men who want to protect and support them (see Hafner, 1986). This may set up a situation that can lead to anxiety on the part of the wife in response to conflicts about dependency–autonomy. Empirical evidence for this viewpoint is limited. Another study of assortative mating examined whether people with anxiety disorders tend to marry others with anxiety disorders, but there was no evidence to support this hypothesis (Columbo, Cox, & Dunner, 1990).

To summarize, the findings regarding agoraphobia and marital dysfunction are mixed, with some studies suggesting that associations exist and other studies showing relatively low rates of marital dissatisfaction among agoraphobics. There is, however, some evidence that certain types of marital events (e.g., conflict, separation) may be implicated in the onset of agoraphobia. There is also some evidence that certain important marital domains (e.g., sexual relations) may be disrupted by agoraphobia; there is indirect evidence that concurrent personality vulnerabilities may affect marital functioning, and that communication and support in marriage may be associated with agoraphobia. However, the lack of research in this area makes firm conclusions impossible.

Obsessive–Compulsive Disorder

Despite the fact that OCD is associated with disruptions in social functioning, very little attention has been paid to marital difficulties in particular. To date, there are just a few studies relevant to the association between OCD and marital dysfunction, and they suggest that OCD is associated with marital dissatisfaction. For example, among married people seeking treatment for OCD, approximately half are maritally distressed (Emmelkamp, Hann, & Hoogduin, 1990; Riggs, Hiss, & Foa, 1992). In addition, individual behavior therapy (i.e., exposure and response prevention) appears to increase marital satisfaction as well as to decrease OCD symptomatology in people who were initially maritally distressed (Cobb, McDonald, Marks, & Stern, 1980; Emmelkamp et al., 1990; Riggs et al., 1992; see Emmelkamp & De Lange, 1983, for an exception). This reduction in marital distress occurs independently of the reduction in depressive symptoms that also follows OCD treatment (Riggs et al., 1992). In addition to having a beneficial effect on marital satisfaction, OCD treatment has been shown in one study to reduce patients' levels of demandingness and dependency on their spouses, and to decrease frequency of arguments between spouses (Riggs et al., 1992). Finally, Steketee (1988, 1993) found that criticism and anger expressed by close family members (half of the sample were spouses) was associated with poorer outcome among OCD patients 9 months following treatment. Close family members' beliefs that OCD patients could control their symptoms were also associated with poorer long-term outcome. Thus, despite the limited research on this topic, it appears that OCD and marital dysfunction are associated, with some evidence that OCD may affect marital functioning and some evidence that marital functioning may affect OCD. Of course, this area of research is at a very early stage.

Other Anxiety Disorders

Even less research exists for other anxiety disorders than for OCD. However, one study has shown that generalized anxiety disorder (GAD)—in particular, early-onset GAD (i.e., GAD beginning in childhood or adolescence)—is associated with marital functioning. People with early-onset GAD reported more marital difficulties than people with later-onset GAD (Hoehn-Saric, Hazlett, & McLeod, 1990). In addition, people with early-onset GAD reported higher levels of neuroticism and greater interpersonal sensitivity, both of which may make them increasingly vulnerable to marital dysfunction. Social phobia is also associated with marital dysfunction. Schneier et al. (1994) found, using both self-report and clinician ratings, that social phobia patients were significantly more impaired in their marital functioning (and general romantic relationship functioning) than nonpsychiatric controls.

Eating Disorders

Many theories of eating disorders stress the importance of interpersonal factors, particularly family relations, in the development and course of these disorders. Such approaches suggest that families in which an eating disorder develops manifest communication problems and problems with interpersonal boundaries (e.g., Minuchin, Rosman, & Baker, 1978). These problems, according to family systems and psychodynamic theorists, often result in conflicts surrounding independence/autonomy and avoidance of intimacy for women with eating disorders. Because eating disorders have been conceptualized as disorders of adolescence, very little theory or research exists regarding the association between eating disorders and adult interpersonal relations, although evidence does suggest that eating-disordered women have impaired social functioning (e.g., Johnson & Berndt, 1983; Norman & Herzog, 1984). Some theorists have suggested that the developmental difficulties in the family of origin are carried over into the marital relationship and even drive the choice of partner (see Root, 1995). Given that many eating disordered women go on to marry, and that some women develop eating disorders in adulthood when married, investigation of the impact of eating disorders on marriage and of marriage on eating disorders seems warranted (see Vandereycken, 1995).

Direct Associations between Eating Disorders and Marital Satisfaction

In a sample of 246 anorexic women, Heavey et al. (1989) found that 21% were married. Of these married anorexics, 69% had a premarital onset of anorexia nervosa, and 30% had a postmarital onset. Estimates of marriage among bulimic women range from 7% to 33% (e.g., Garfinkel & Garner, 1982; Huon, 1985; Russell, 1979; Sykes, Leuser, Melia, & Gross, 1988). The few existing empirical studies of eating disorders and marital functioning suggest that bulimics, anorexics, and their husbands show levels of marital satisfaction comparable to those of maritally discordant couples and lower than those of controls (e.g., Van Buren & Williamson, 1988; Van den Broucke & Vandereycken, 1989a). In addition, husbands of anorexics and bulimics describe their marriages as severely maladjusted—even more so than their eating-disordered spouses do (Van den Broucke & Vandereycken, 1989a). Thus, eating disorders appear to be associated with dissatisfaction in marriage. Unfortunately, there is very little research that addresses the mechanisms of that association.

Associations with the Four Marital Factors

Regarding adaptive processes, there is only one study, and it examined self-reported conflict resolution styles among married bulimics. Bulimics reported poor conflict resolution abilities, in the form of high levels of conflict avoidance and low levels of problem-solving behaviors (Van Buren & Williamson, 1988). Their reports were significantly worse than those of normal controls, but the same as those of maritally discordant wives. Root, Fallon, and Friedrich (1986) have suggested that power is a significant issue in the relationships of eating-disordered women. Power struggles in relationships certainly may impede adaptive functioning, but empirical studies on this issue are lacking. One study failed to find support for power differentials in marriage (Van den Broucke & Vandereycken, 1989a).

Some research suggests that sexual functioning may be a source of conflict among couples with an eating-disordered spouse. During active phases of anorexia nervosa (i.e., at a low body weight), women may be uninterested in sexual activity (see Abraham & Llewellyn-Jones, 1995). Among anorexic patients who had inpatient treatment, many reported avoidance of sexual matters and behavior 4 years following treatment (Steinhausen & Seidel, 1992). Although bulimic women tend to have normal sexual desire and arousal, and may even be sexually assertive, they may withdraw from sexual activity during times when their weight is high (see Abraham, 1985; Abraham & Llewellyn-Jones, 1995). As regards marriage, Van den Broucke and Vandereycken (1989a) found that anorexics, bulimics, and their husbands all reported lower levels of sexual satisfaction than normal control couples did, although the eating-disordered couples' reports were similar to those of couples in which one partner was depressed or anxious.

One finding that may be relevant to the adaptive processes in the marital relationship comes from a study of EE in bulimic families. In this study, maternal criticism accounted for 28–34% of the variance in eating-disordered adolescents' symptom outcome (van Furth et al., 1996). EE in family members of adults with various forms of psychopathology has been found to predict relapse in these patients (e.g., Hooley & Teasdale, 1989). Thus, the examination of EE in the marital relationships of eating-disordered women may shed light on the adult course of eating disorders.

Studies of social support among eating-disordered women may also provide clues about how adaptive processes in marriage may be associated with eating disorders. Bulimics report significant social difficulties, a sense of social isolation (e.g., Silberstein, Striegel-Moore, & Rodin, 1987), and difficulty dealing with time alone (Cullari & Redmon, 1984). Thus, social support may be critical to bulimics' functioning. There is more direct evidence for the role of social support deficits in marriage among anorexic women. Anorexic women living without a partner or with an unsupportive partner (as rated by interviewers) reported more symptoms than women living with supportive partners did (Manz, Deter, & Herzog, 1992). Thus a supportive partner may protect against typical anorexic behavior.

Eating disorders may be associated with a number of enduring vulnerabilities that have the potential to affect marital functioning. For example, eating disorders are associated with attachment insecurity (see O'Kearney, 1996, for a review), neuroticism (see Vitousek & Manke, 1994), and impulsivity (for bulimics; e.g., Swift & Wonderlich, 1988). In addition, there is high comorbidity among eating disorders and various personality disorders, including obsessive–compulsive, avoidant, and dependent personality disorders for anorexics, and borderline and histrionic personality disorders for bulimics (see Vitousek & Manke, 1994; Wonderlich, 1995).

Regarding stressful life events, perceptions of stress are associated with worsening of eating disorders (Striegel-Moore, Silberstein, Frensch, & Rodin, 1989). The onset of bulimia nervosa is associated with stressful life events (Lacey, Coker, & Birtchnell, 1986; Strober, 1984)—especially interpersonal events, including loss, separation, and conflict (Lacey et al., 1986; Pyle, Mitchell, & Eckert, 1981). However, because all of the research is self-report, it is unclear whether bulimics simply experience events as more stressful. Still, these findings suggest that eating-disordered patients may be vulnerable to stressors, even if this association is mediated or moderated by their perceptions.

Regarding mate selection, some theorists have suggested that eating-disordered women may reenact unresolved family-of-origin conflicts in their marriages (e.g., Heavey et al., 1989), and even choose husbands with whom this reenactment will occur and/or with whom the eating-disordered behavior can recur (e.g., Dally, 1984; Root et al., 1986). Many have proposed psychological deficits in the husbands of eating-disordered women and have emphasized that certain men may have unresolved issues that attract them to eating-disordered women, again making the marriage a place where earlier conflicts get played out (e.g., Dally, 1984; Van den Broucke & Vandereycken, 1989b). There is a great lack of empirical work addressing these issues. One study did find that husbands of anorexic and bulimic women reported elevated levels of psychological symptomatology, compared to husbands of nondisordered women, but that they did not differ from husbands of depressed and anxious women (Van den Broucke & Vandereycken, 1989a). Whether this is evidence of assortative mating or evidence of a response to a stressful marital environment is unknown.

To summarize, despite the paucity of empirical research, the research that does exist indicates that eating disorders may affect marital satisfaction of both partners, may be associated with poor problem solving, and may result in poor sexual relations. Eating disorders are also associated with personality vulnerabilities that may affect marital functioning. In addition, eating disorder symptoms may be affected by levels of support and criticism in the marriage, and by stressful marital and nonmarital events.

Schizophrenia

There is a large literature highlighting the importance of the family environment for the course of schizophrenia (see Goldstein & Strachan, 1987) and demonstrating the success of family interventions as adjuncts to the treatment of schizophrenia (see Goldstein & Miklowitz, 1995; Penn & Mueser, 1996). By contrast, there is very little work specifically on marital functioning and schizophrenia, because schizophrenics tend not to marry. Those who do marry have typically had good premorbid functioning and a less severe type and course of illness (e.g., Gittelman-Klein & Klein, 1968; see Saugstad, 1989). One study suggests, however, that once schizophrenics are married, the type of symptoms that they experience, and the attributions that their spouses make for those symptoms, may be associated with marital satisfaction (Hooley, Richters, Weintraub, & Neale, 1987). Spouses' marital satisfaction was lower among couples in which the schizophrenic partner exhibited negative symptoms (e.g., depression, social isolation, lack of emotion) than among couples in which the partner exhibited positive symptoms (e.g., hallucinations, delusions, disorganization; Hooley et al., 1987). Hooley et al. (1987) theorized that a spouse may blame a partner for negative symptoms, but may blame the illness for positive symptoms. Such causal or controllability attributions should affect marital satisfaction. In particular, when a spouse believes that the partner is the cause of the symptoms, or that the symptoms are under the partner's control, then marital satisfaction should decline. Although some support for this attributional model exists for depressed patients (e.g., Bauserman, Arias, & Craighead, 1995), the model has not been tested in schizophrenic samples. Nevertheless, both the Hooley et al. (1987) study and findings that communication and criticism within families affect the course of schizophrenia (e.g., Vaughn & Leff, 1976) suggest that for those schizophrenics who are married, aspects of their marital interactions and the attributions their spouses make may affect the course of their marriages and the course of the illness.

Personality Disorders

There is a great deal of theory regarding borderline and narcissistic personality disorders in marital functioning; however, this literature focuses not on personality disorders as defined in the *Diagnostic and Statistical Manual of Mental Disorders,* but on self-psychological (e.g., Kohut, 1977) and object relations (e.g., Kernberg, 1975) conceptualizations of borderline and narcissistic personality organization. According to these approaches, the nature of each individual's personality pathology may result in a marital situation in which neither partner believes that his or her needs are being met, and in which neither partner can meet the needs of the other because both are attempting to get their earlier childhood needs met through the relationship. As a result, the marital relationship ends up as a replay of the childhood problematic relationships that probably led to the personality pathology in the first place. "Ultimately a to and fro dance ensues, with each partner attempting to manipulate, control, and punish the other into being the way he/she requires" (Slipp, 1995, p. 463). Inherent in these ideas is that the personality-disordered person selects a mate who also has a personality disorder. At present, support for this hypothesis comes only from clinical observation (see Slipp, 1995).

The meager empirical research that does exist on diagnosable personality disorders supports an association between marital functioning and personality disorders; given that personality disorders, by definition, should cause significant interpersonal impairment, it would be surprising if they were not associated. Reich, Yates, and Nduaguda (1989) found that more people with personality disorders reported marital difficulties than did people without personality disorders. Lavik (1982) reported a high proportion of nonmarried people among those diagnosed with personality disorders, especially among men. In the one study that directly addressed family and marital functioning, Hooley and Hoffman (1996) examined the role of EE in relapse among patients diagnosed with borderline personality disorder. They found, surprisingly, that patients whose family members expressed high levels of emotional overinvolvement were *less* likely to relapse than patients whose family members expressed low levels. Although only 16% of the family members assessed were spouses or partners of the borderline patients, this study does suggest that adaptive processes in the families, and possibly marriages, of borderline patients have a significant effect on the patients' future psychological functioning. In this case, the effect appears contrary to what might be expected. However, Hooley and Hoffman (1996) suggest that borderline patients, because of their specific personality dynamics and emotional needs, may experience emotional overinvolvement as a satisfying, validating form of attention that subsequently allows them to function better. This line of research is clearly in a very early stage, but it has the potential to shed light on important aspects of marital functioning among people with borderline personality disorder.

DISCUSSION AND DIRECTIONS FOR RESEARCH

The goal of this chapter has been to provide a broad review of the literature on the association between marital functioning and various types of psychopathology. In particular, our emphasis has been on clarifying the extent to which marital functioning and psychopathology affect each other and the mechanisms by which they do so. In summary, we can safely say that there is at least some evidence for an association between marital functioning and each type of disorder covered in this chapter. For some disorders, such as depression, entire theories have been devoted to describing and testing the nature of this association (e.g., Beach, Sandeen, & O'Leary, 1990), and research has provided insight into the direction and mechanisms of the association. For most other disorders (especially anxiety, personality, and eating disorders), programmatic research on marital functioning does not exist, and the little existing research has provided nothing more than suggestions or hints that an association exists. As such, an obvious conclusion of this chapter is that a great deal of research is needed to provide even a basic understanding of the association in question, especially if appropriate marital treatments are to be designed and implemented. We suggest that future research will benefit from (1) moving from an examination of associations between symptoms and marital satisfaction to an examination of the processes involved in the development and course of the association between marital dysfunction and psychopathology; (2) employing longitudinal research designs, although for many types of psychopathology, adequate cross-sectional research will be necessary first; and (3) examining the marital factors identified in this review.

We would like to describe this last point in more detail. We believe that having a coherent framework for identifying variables that are likely to be relevant to the marital functioning–psychopathology association is critical for the development of a comprehensive body of work in this area. Focusing on the marital factors identified here covers a broad range of relevant issues. For example, investigations of concomitant enduring vulnerabilities may help identify subtypes of individuals with each disorder who may be more or less at risk for marital discord. Also in the service of identifying at-risk individuals, investigations of mate selection processes (i.e., how people choose their spouses and the types of spouses they choose) may help identify early indicators of who will be at risk for marital dysfunction or instability. Investigations of similarity between spouses on identified risk factors may help identify couples at greater risk for marital discord or instability. Investigations of associations between psychopathology and stressful life events, particularly marital events, may help shed light on whether symptoms can both affect and be affected by stressors. Among the most important marital factors to examine are adaptive processes in marriage. Studying adaptive processes is valuable for two reasons. First, it requires researchers to examine mechanisms of the association between marital quality and psychopathology. As such, studies of adaptive processes may get at the heart of how and why marital quality and symptoms are related, rather than just finding or implying that they are associated. Second, it requires researchers to focus on the way in which spouses interact. Doing so retains the emphasis on the actual interpersonal context in which symptomatology occurs.

In addition, although we have described each marital factor in isolation, studies of the relationships among these factors (e.g., how psychopathology may affect adaptive functioning and marital satisfaction in the face of severe stress) would lead to further refinement of the specific processes that characterize the association between, and course of, psychopathology and marital dysfunction.

In addition to the research directions just identified, two additional issues deserve attention in future work. These issues have not been the focus of the present chapter, but they are issues that are relevant to understanding psychopathology and marital functioning. One issue regards the specificity of particular types of disorders to marital dysfunction. Two findings bear on this issue. First, there is significant evidence of comorbidity within Axis I disorders and across Axis I and Axis II disorders (e.g., Oldham et al., 1995; Sanderson, Beck, & Beck, 1990). Second, a number of associations involving interpersonal functioning that were thought to be specific to a particular disorder may actually be general to many forms of psychopathology (e.g., Gotlib, Lewinsohn, & Seeley, 1996; Hammen et al., 1995). This raises the question of whether theories and findings regarding specific disorders apply to all disorders.

The second issue regards the timing of marriage or age at which people marry. This is an important issue, because research indicates that marrying at a young age is itself a risk factor for marital discord and instability (see Karney & Bradbury, 1995). Thus, to the extent that people are more likely to marry early, they are at greater risk for negative marital outcomes. Recent research has shown that adolescents who experienced any form of psychopathology were more likely to marry early than adolescents without psychopathology were (Gotlib et al., 1996). Moreover, among those with early marriages, the people who experienced psychopathology in adolescence had significantly more marital discord than the people who did not experience psychopathology in adolescence. These data provide strong evidence for the idea that the association between psychopathology and interpersonal dysfunction begins early in life and has implications for subsequent marital functioning. Future research might thus be directed at further explorations of how psychopathology may set people on an unfortunate course of relationship dysfunction, and, ultimately, marital dysfunction.

REFERENCES

Abraham, S. F. (1985). The psychosexual histories of young women with bulimia. *Australian and New Zealand Journal of Psychiatry, 19,* 72–76.

Abraham, S. F., & Llewellyn-Jones, D. (1995). Sexual and reproductive function in eating disorders and obesity. In K. D. Brownell & C. G. Fairburn (Eds.), *Eating disorders and obesity: A comprehensive handbook* (pp. 281–288). New York: Guilford Press.

Arrindell, W. A., & Emmelkamp, P. M. (1986). Marital adjustment, intimacy, and needs in female agoraphobics and their partners: A controlled study. *British Journal of Psychiatry, 149*, 592–602.

Arrindell, W. A., Emmelkamp, P. M., & Sanderman, R. (1986). Marital quality and general life adjustment in relation to treatment outcome in agoraphobia. *Advances in Behaviour Research and Therapy, 8*, 139–185.

Barlow, D. H. (1988). *Anxiety and its disorders: The nature and treatment of anxiety and panic.* New York: Guilford Press.

Bauserman, S. K., Arias, I., & Craighead, W. E. (1995). Marital attributions in spouses of depressed patients. *Journal of Psychopathology and Behavioral Assessment, 17*, 231–249.

Beach, S. R. H., & Fincham, F. D. (1995). Toward an integrated model of negative affectivity in marriage. In S. M. Johnson & L. S. Greenberg (Eds.), *The heart of the matter: Perspectives on emotion in marital therapy* (pp. 227–255). New York: Brunner/Mazel.

Beach, S. R. H., & O'Leary, K. D. (1993a). Dysphoria and marital discord: Are dysphoric individuals at risk for marital maladjustment? *Journal of Marital and Family Therapy, 19*, 355–368.

Beach, S. R. H., & O'Leary, K. D. (1993b). Marital discord and dysphoria: For whom does the marital relationship predict depressive symptomatology? *Journal of Social and Personal Relationships, 10*, 405–420.

Beach, S. R. H., Sandeen, E. E., & O'Leary, K. D. (1990). *Depression in marriage: A model for etiology and treatment.* New York: Guilford Press.

Beck, A. T. (1967). *Depression: Causes and treatment.* Philadelphia: University of Pennsylvania Press.

Beck, A. T. (1983). Cognitive therapy of depression: New perspectives. In P. J. Clayton & J. E. Barrett (Eds.), *Treatment of depression: Old controversies and new approaches* (pp. 265–290). New York: Raven Press.

Bentler, P. M., & Newcomb, M. D. (1978). Longitudinal study of marital success and failure. *Journal of Consulting and Clinical Psychology, 46*, 1053–1070.

Biglan, A., Hops, H., Sherman, L., Friedman, L. S., Arthur, J., & Osteen, V. (1985). Problem solving interactions of depressed women and their spouses. *Behavior Therapy, 16*, 431–451.

Billings, A. G., Kessler, M., Gomberg, C. A., & Weiner, S. (1979). Marital conflict resolution of alcoholic and nonalcoholic couples during sobriety and experimental drinking. *Journal of Studies on Alcohol, 40*, 183–195.

Blatt, S. J., & Zuroff, D. C. (1992). Interpersonal relatedness and self-definition: Two prototypes for depression. *Clinical Psychology Review, 12*, 527–562.

Bowlby, J. (1969). *Attachment and loss: Vol. 1. Attachment.* New York: Basic Books.

Boyd, J. H. (1985). *Panic prevalence, risk factors, and treatment rates.* Paper presented at the annual meeting of the American Psychiatric Association, Dallas, TX.

Bradbury, T. N. (1995). Assessing the four fundamental domains of marriage. *Family Relations, 44*, 459–468.

Bradbury, T. N., Beach, S. R. H., Fincham, F. D., & Nelson, G. M. (1996).

Attributions and behavior in functional and dysfunctional marriages. *Journal of Consulting and Clinical Psychology, 64,* 569–576.

Bradbury, T. N., & Fincham, F. D. (1992). Attributions and behavior in marital interaction. *Journal of Personality and Social Psychology, 63,* 613–628.

Brown, S. A., Vik, P. W., McQuaid, J. R., Patterson, T. L., Irwin, M. R., & Grant, I. (1990). Severity of psychosocial stress and outcome of alcoholism treatment. *Journal of Abnormal Psychology, 99,* 344–348.

Bruce, M. L., & Kim, K. M. (1992). Differences in the effects of divorce on major depression in men and women. *American Journal of Psychiatry, 149,* 914–917.

Buglass, D., Clarke, J., Henderson, A. S., Kreitman, N., & Presley, A. S. (1977). A study of agoraphobic housewives. *Psychological Medicine, 7,* 73–86.

Carnelley, K. B., Pietromonaco, P. R., & Jaffe, K. (1994). Depression, working models of others, and relationship functioning. *Journal of Personality and Social Psychology, 66,* 127–140.

Caspi, A., & Herbener, E. S. (1993). Marital assortment and phenotypic convergence: Longitudinal evidence. *Social Biology, 40,* 48–60.

Christian-Herman, J., O'Leary, K. D., & Avery-Leaf, S. (in press). The impact of severe negative life events in marriage on depression. *Journal of Social and Clinical Psychology.*

Cobb, J. P., McDonald, R., Marks, I., & Stern, R. (1980). Marital versus exposure therapy: Psychological treatments of co-existing marital and phobic–obsessive problems. *Behavioural Analysis and Modification, 4,* 3–16.

Cohan, C. L., & Bradbury, T. N. (1997). Negative life events, marital interaction, and the longitudinal course of newlywed marriage. *Journal of Personality and Social Psychology, 73,* 114–128.

Cohn, D. A., Silver, D. H., Cowan, C. P., Cowan, P. A., & Pearson, J. (1992). Working models of childhood attachment and couple relationships. *Journal of Family Issues, 13,* 432–449.

Columbo, M., Cox, G., & Dunner, D. L. (1990). Assortative mating in affective and anxiety disorders: Preliminary findings. *Psychiatric Genetics, 1,* 35–44.

Craske, M. G., Burton, T., & Barlow, D. H. (1989). Relationships among measures of communication, marital satisfaction, and exposure during couples treatment of agoraphobia. *Behaviour Research and Therapy, 28,* 395–400.

Cullari, S., & Redmon, W. K. (1984). Questionnaire responses from self-identified binge-eaters and purgers. *Psychological Reports, 54,* 232–234.

Cutrona, C. E., & Suhr, J. A. (1994). Social support communication in the context of marriage: An analysis of couples' supportive interaction. In B. R. Burleson, T. L. Albrecht, & I. G. Sarason (Eds.), *Communication of social support: Messages, interactions, relationships, and community* (pp. 113–135). Thousand Oaks, CA: Sage.

Dally, P. (1984). Anorexia tardive: Late onset marital anorexia nervosa. *Journal of Psychosomatic Research, 18,* 423–428.

Davila, J., Bradbury, T. N., Cohan, C. L., & Tochluk, S. (1997). Marital functioning and depressive symptoms: Evidence for a stress generation model. *Journal of Personality and Social Psychology, 73,* 849–861.

Davila, J., Christian-Herman, J., & Bradbury, T. N. (1996). *Moderators of the depression and marital discord relation: Negative affectivity, personal history of affective disorder, and family psychopathology.* Unpublished manuscript, University of California, Los Angeles.

Doctor, R. M. (1982). Major results of a large-scale pretreatment survey of agoraphobics. In R. L. DuPont (Ed.), *Phobia: A comprehensive summary of modern treatments* (pp. 203–214). New York: Brunner/Mazel.

Du Fort, G. G., Kovess, V., & Boivin, J. F. (1994). Spouse similarity for psychological distress and well-being: A population study. *Psychological Medicine, 24,* 431–447.

Dunn, N., Jacob, T., Hummon, N., & Seilhammer, R. (1987). Marital stability in alcoholic–spouse relationships as a function of drinking pattern and location. *Journal of Abnormal Psychology, 96,* 99–107.

Emmelkamp, P. M., & De Lange, I. (1983). Spouse involvement in the treatment of obsessive–compulsive patients. *Behaviour Research and Therapy, 21,* 341–346.

Emmelkamp, P. M., & Gerlsma, C. (1994). Marital functioning and the anxiety disorders. *Behavior Therapy, 25,* 407–429.

Emmelkamp, P. M. G., de Hann, E., & Hoogduin, C. A. (1990). Marital adjustment and obsessive–compulsive disorder. *British Journal of Psychiatry, 156,* 55–60.

Farmer, R., & Nelson-Gray, R. (1990). Personality disorders and depression: Hypothetical relations, empirical findings, and methodological considerations. *Clinical Psychology Review, 10,* 453–476.

Feeney, J. A., Noller, P., & Callan, V. J. (1994). Attachment style, communication, and satisfaction in the early years of marriage. *Advances in Personal Relationships, 5,* 269–308.

Feng, D., & Baker, L. (1994). Spouse similarity in attitudes, personality, and psychological well-being. *Behavior Genetics, 24,* 357–364.

Fonagy, P., Leigh, T., Steele, M., Steele, H., Kennedy, R., Mattoon, G., Target, M., & Gerber, A. (1996). The relationship of attachment status, psychiatric classification, and response to psychotherapy. *Journal of Consulting and Clinical Psychology, 64,* 22–31.

Frankenstein, W., Hay, W. M., & Nathan, P. E. (1985). Effects of intoxication on alcoholics' marital communication and problem-solving. *Journal of Studies on Alcohol, 46,* 1–6.

Garfinkel, P. E., & Garner, D. M. (1982). *Anorexia nervosa: A multidimensional perspective.* New York: Brunner/Mazel.

Gittelman-Klein, R., & Klein, D. (1968). Marital status as a prognostic indicator in schizophrenia. *Journal of Nervous and Mental Disease, 147,* 289–296.

Goldstein, A. J., & Chambless, D. L. (1978). A reanalysis of agoraphobia. *Behavior Therapy, 9,* 47–59.

Goldstein, M. J., & Miklowitz, D. J. (1995). The effectiveness of psychoeducational family therapy in the treatment of schizophrenic disorders. *Journal of Marital and Family Therapy, 21,* 361–376.

Goldstein, M. J., & Strachan, A. M. (1987). The family and schizophrenia. In T. Jacob (Ed.), *Family interaction and psychopathology: Theories, methods, and findings* (pp. 481–508). New York: Plenum Press.

Gotlib, I. H., & Beach, S. R. H. (1995). A marital/family discord model of depression: Implications for therapeutic intervention. In N. S. Jacobson & A. S. Gurman (Eds.), *Clinical handbook of couple therapy* (pp. 411–436). New York: Guilford Press.

Gotlib, I. H., Lewinsohn, P. M., & Seeley, J. R. (1996). *Consequences of depression during adolescence: Marital status and marital functioning in early adulthood.*

Paper presented at the annual meeting of the Association for Advancement of Behavior Therapy, New York.

Gotlib, I. H., & Whiffen, V. E. (1989). Depression and marital functioning: An examination of specificity and gender differences. *Journal of Abnormal Psychology, 98,* 23–30.

Hafner, R. J. (1986). Marital therapy for agoraphobia. In N. S. Jacobson & A. S. Gurman (Eds.), *Clinical handbook of marital therapy* (pp. 471–494). New York: Guilford Press.

Hagnell, O., & Kreitman, N. (1974). Mental illness in married pairs in a total population. *British Journal of Psychiatry, 125,* 203–302.

Hammen, C. (1991). The generation of stress in the course of unipolar depression. *Journal of Abnormal Psychology, 100,* 555–561.

Hammen, C., Burge, D., Daley, S. E., Davila, J., Paley, B., & Rudolph, K. (1995). Interpersonal attachment cognitions and prediction of symptomatic responses to interpersonal stress. *Journal of Abnormal Psychology, 104,* 436–443.

Hautzinger, M., Linden, M., & Hoffman, N. (1982). Distressed couples with and without a depressed partner: An analysis of their verbal interaction. *Journal of Behavior Therapy and Experimental Psychology, 13,* 307–314.

Hazan, C., & Shaver, P. R. (1987). Romantic love conceptualized as an attachment process. *Journal of Personality and Social Psychology, 52,* 511–524.

Heavey, A., Parker, Y., Vhat, A. V., Crisp, A. H., & Gower, S. G. (1989). Anorexia nervosa and marriage. *International Journal of Eating Disorders, 8,* 275–284.

Hesselbrock, V. M., Hesselbrock, M. W., & Stabenau, J. R. (1985). Alcoholism in men patients subtyped by family history and antisocial personality. *Journal of Studies on Alcohol, 36,* 59–64.

Hoehn-Saric, R., Hazlett, R. L., & McLeod, D. R. (1993). Generalized anxiety disorder with early and late onset of anxiety symptoms. *Comprehensive Psychiatry, 34,* 291–298.

Hooley, J. M., & Hoffman, P. D. (1996). *Expressed emotion and borderline personality disorder.* Paper presented at the annual meeting of the Association for Advancement of Behavior Therapy, New York.

Hooley, J. M., Richters, J. E., Weintraub, S., & Neale, J. M. (1987). Psychopathology and marital distress: The positive side of positive symptoms. *Journal of Abnormal Psychology, 96,* 27–33.

Hooley, J. M., & Teasdale, J. D. (1989). Predictors of relapse in unipolar depressives: Expressed emotions, marital distress, and perceived criticism. *Journal of Abnormal Psychology, 98,* 229–237.

Horneffer, K. J., & Fincham, F. D. (1996). Attributional models of depression and marital distress. *Personality and Social Psychology Bulletin, 22,* 678–689.

Huen, R., & Maier, W. (1993). Morbid risks for major disorders and frequencies of personality disorders among spouses of psychiatric inpatients and controls. *Comprehensive Psychiatry, 34,* 137–143.

Huon, G. F. (1985). Bulimia: Therapy at a distance. In S. W. Touyz & P. J. Beumont (Eds.), *Eating disorders: Prevalence and treatment* (pp. 62–73). Baltimore: Williams & Wilkins.

Jacob, T., & Bremer, D. A. (1986). Assortative mating among men and women alcoholics. *Journal of Studies on Alcohol, 47,* 219–222.

Jacob, T., Dunn, N., & Leonard, K. E. (1983). Patterns of alcohol abuse and family stability. *Alcoholism: Clinical and Experimental Research, 7,* 382–385.

Jacob, T., & Leonard, K. E. (1988). Alcoholic-spouse interaction as a function of alcoholism subtype and alcohol consumption interaction. *Journal of Abnormal Psychology, 97,* 232–237.

Jacob, T., & Leonard, K. E. (1992). Sequential analysis of marital interaction involving alcoholic, depressed, and nondistressed men. *Journal of Abnormal Psychology, 101,* 647–656.

Jacob, T., Ritchey, D., Cvitkovic, J. F., & Blane, H. T. (1981). Communication styles of alcoholic and nonalcoholic families when drinking and not drinking. *Journal of Studies on Alcohol, 42,* 466–482.

Jacobson, N. S. (1989). The maintenance of treatment gains following social learning-based marital therapy. *Behavior Therapy, 20,* 325–336.

Jacobson, N. S., Fruzzetti, A. E., Dobson, K., Whisman, M., & Hops, H. (1993). Couple therapy as a treatment for depression: II. The effects of relationship quality and therapy on depressive relapse. *Journal of Consulting and Clinical Psychology, 61,* 516–519.

Jacobson, N. S., & Gurman, A. S. (Eds.). (1995). *Clinical handbook of couple therapy.* New York: Guilford Press.

Jacobson, N. S., Schmaling, K. B., & Holtzworth-Munroe, A. (1987). Component analysis of behavioral marital therapy: 2-year follow-up and prediction of relapse. *Journal of Marital and Family Therapy, 13,* 187–195.

Johnson, L., & Berndt, D. J. (1983). Preliminary investigation of bulimia and life adjustment. *American Journal of Psychiatry, 140,* 774–777.

Kantor, G. K., & Straus, M. A. (1987). The "drunken bum" theory of wife beating. *Social Problems, 34,* 213–230.

Karney, B. R., & Bradbury, T. N. (1995). The longitudinal course of marital quality and stability: A review of theory, method, and research. *Psychological Bulletin, 118,* 3–34.

Kelly, E. L., & Conley, J. J. (1987). Personality and compatibility: A prospective analysis of marital stability and marital satisfaction. *Journal of Personality and Social Psychology, 52,* 27–40.

Kenardy, J., Oei, T. P., & Evans, L. (1990). Neuroticism and age of onset for agoraphobia with panic attacks. *Journal of Behavior Therapy and Experimental Psychiatry, 21,* 193–197.

Kendler, K. S., Kessler, R. C., Walters, E. E., MacLean, C., Neale, M. C., Heath, A. C., & Eaves, L. J. (1995). Stressful life events, genetic liability, and onset of episode of major depression in women. *American Journal of Psychiatry, 152,* 833–842.

Kernberg, O. F. (1975). *Borderline conditions and pathological narcissism.* New York: Jason Aronson.

Kobak, R. R., & Hazan, C. (1991). Attachment in marriage: Effects of security and accuracy of working models. *Journal of Personality and Social Psychology, 60,* 861–869.

Kohut, H. S. (1977). *The restoration of the self.* New York: International Universities Press.

Lacey, J. H., Coker, S., & Birtchnell, S. A. (1986). Bulimia: Factors associated with its etiology and maintenance. *International Journal of Eating Disorders, 5,* 475–487.

Lavik, N. J. (1982). Marital status in psychiatric patients. *Acta Psychiatrica Scandinavica, 65,* 15–28.

Leonard, K. E. (1990). Marital functioning among episodic and steady alcoholics. In R. L. Collins, K. E. Leonard, & J. S. Searles (Eds.), *Alcohol and the family: Research and clinical perspectives* (pp. 220–243). New York: Guilford Press.

Leonard, K. E. (1993). Drinking patterns and intoxication in marital violence: Review, critique, and future directions for research. In S. E. Martin (Ed.), *Alcohol and interpersonal violence: Fostering multidisciplinary perspectives* (pp. 253–280). Rockville, MD: U.S. Department of Health and Human Services.

Leonard, K. E., & Blane, H. T. (1992). Alcohol and marital aggression in a national sample of young men. *Journal of Interpersonal Violence, 7,* 19–30.

Leonard, K. E., & Jacob, T. (1988). Alcohol, alcoholism, and family violence. In V. B. Van Hasselt, R. L. Morrison, A. S. Bellack, & M. Hersen (Eds.), *Handbook of family violence* (pp. 383–406). New York: Plenum Press.

Leonard, K. E., & Roberts, L. (1998). Marital aggression, quality, and stability in the first year of marriage: Findings from the Buffalo newlywed study. In T. N. Bradbury (Ed.), *The developmental course of marital dysfunction.* New York: Cambridge University Press.

Lewis, M. L. (1937). Alcoholism and family casework. *Social Casework, 35,* 8–14.

Maisto, S. A., O'Farrell, T. J., Connors, G. J., McKay, J. R., & Pelcovits, M. (1988). Alcoholics' attributions of factors affecting their relapse to drinking and reasons for terminating relapse episodes. *Addictive Behaviors, 13,* 79–82.

Manz, R., Deter, H.-C., & Herzog, W. (1992). Social support and long-term course of anorexia nervosa. In W. Herzog, H.-C. Deter, & W. Vandereycken (Eds.), *The course of eating disorders: Long-term follow-up studies of anorexia and bulimia nervosa* (pp. 323–336). Berlin: Springer-Verlag.

Merikangas, K. R. (1984). Divorce and assortative mating among depressed patients. *American Journal of Psychiatry, 141,* 74–76.

Merikangas, K. R., & Spiker, D. G. (1982). Assortative mating among in-patients with primary affective disorder. *Psychological Medicine, 12,* 753–764.

Minuchin, S., Rosman, B. L., & Baker, L. (1978). *Psychosomatic families: Anorexia nervosa in context.* Cambridge, MA: Harvard University Press.

Monteiro, W., Marks, I. M., & Ramm, E. (1985). Marital adjustment and treatment outcome in agoraphobia. *British Journal of Psychiatry, 146,* 383–390.

Moos, R. H., Finney, J. W., & Gamble, W. (1982). The process of recovery from alcoholism: II. Comparing spouses of alcoholic patients and matched community controls. *Journal of Studies on Alcohol, 43,* 888–909.

Moos, R. H., & Moos, B. S. (1984). The process of recovery from alcoholism: III. Comparing functioning of families of alcoholics and matched control families. *Journal of Studies on Alcohol, 45,* 111–118.

Murphy, C. M., & O'Farrell, T. J. (1994). Factors associated with marital aggression in male alcoholics. *Journal of Family Psychology, 8,* 321–335.

Norman, D. K., & Herzog, D. B. (1984). Persistent social maladjustment in bulimia: A one-year follow-up. *American Journal of Psychiatry, 141,* 444–446.

Noyes, R., Clancy, J., Woodman, C., Holt, C. S., Suelzer, M., Christiansen, J., & Anderson, D. J. (1993). Environmental factors related to the outcome of panic disorder: A seven-year follow-up study. *Journal of Nervous and Mental Disease, 181,* 529–538.

O'Farrell, T. J. (1990). Sexual functioning of male alcoholics. In R. L. Collins, K.

E. Leonard, & J. S. Searles (Eds.), *Alcohol and the family: Research and clinical perspectives* (pp. 244–271). New York: Guilford Press.

O'Farrell, T. J., & Birchler, G. R. (1987). Marital relationships of alcoholic, conflicted, and nonconflicted couples. *Journal of Marital and Family Therapy, 13,* 259–274.

O'Farrell, T. J., Choquette, K. A., & Birchler, G. R. (1991). Sexual satisfaction and dissatisfaction in the marital relationships of male alcoholics seeking marital therapy. *Journal of Studies on Alcohol, 52,* 441–447.

O'Farrell, T. J., Cutter, H. S. G., Hooley, J., & Fals-Stewart, W. (1996). *Expressed emotion and relapse in alcoholic patients.* Paper presented at the annual meeting of the Association for Advancement of Behavior Therapy, New York.

O'Kearney, R. (1996). Attachment disruption in anorexia nervosa and bulimia nervosa: A review of theory and empirical research. *International Journal of Eating Disorders, 20,* 115–127.

Oldham, J. M., Skodol, A. E., Kellman, H. D., Hyler, S. E., Doidge, N., Rosnick, L., & Gallaher, P. E. (1995). Comorbidity of Axis I and Axis II disorders. *American Journal of Psychiatry, 152,* 571–578.

Pan, H. S., Neidig, P. H., & O'Leary, K. D. (1994). Predicting mild and severe husband-to-wife physical aggression. *Journal of Consulting and Clinical Psychology, 62,* 975–981.

Pasch, L. A., & Bradbury, T. N. (1998). Social support, conflict, and the development of marital dysfunction. *Journal of Consulting and Clinical Psychology, 66,* 219–230.

Penn, D. L., & Mueser, K. T. (1996). Research update on the psychosocial treatment of schizophrenia. *American Journal of Psychiatry, 153,* 607–617.

Peter, H., & Hand, I. (1988). Patterns of patient–spouse interaction in agoraphobics: Assessment by Camberwell Family Interview (CFI) and impact on outcome of self-exposure treatment. In I. Hand & H. Wittchen (Eds.), *Panic and phobias: Vol. 2. Treatment and variables affecting course and outcome* (pp. 240–251). Berlin: Springer-Verlag.

Pollard, H., Pollard, H., & Corn, K. (1990). Panic onset and major events in lives of agoraphobics: A test of contiguity. *Journal of Abnormal Psychology, 98,* 318–321.

Pyle, R. L., Mitchell, J. E., & Eckert, E. D. (1981). Bulimia: A report of 34 cases. *Journal of Clinical Psychiatry, 42,* 60–64.

Regier, D. A., Farmer, M. E., Rae, D. S., Myers, J. K., Kramer, M., Robins, L. N., George, L. K., Karno, M., & Locke, B. Z. (1993). One-month prevalence of mental disorders in the United States and sociodemographic characteristics: The Epidemiologic Catchment Area study. *Acta Psychiatrica Scandinavica, 88,* 35–47.

Reich, J. H., Yates, W., & Nduaguda, M. (1989). Prevalence of DSM-III personality disorders in the community. *Social Psychiatry and Psychiatric Epidemiology, 24,* 12–16.

Repetti, R. L. (1989). Effects of daily workload on subsequent behavior during marital interaction: The roles of social withdrawal and spouse support. *Journal of Personality and Social Psychology, 57,* 651–659.

Riggs, D. A., Hiss, H., & Foa, E. B. (1992). Marital distress and the treatment of obsessive compulsive disorder. *Behavior Therapy, 23,* 585–597.

Roberts, J., Kassell, J., & Gotlib, I. H. (1995). Level and stability of self-esteem as predictors of depressive symptoms. *Personality and Individual Differences, 19,* 217–224.

Root, M. P. P. (1995). Conceptualization and treatment of eating disorders in couples. In N. S. Jacobson & A. S. Gurman (Eds.), *Clinical handbook of couple therapy* (pp. 437–457). New York: Guilford Press.

Root, M. P. P., Fallon, P., & Friedrich, W. N. (1986). *Bulimia: A systems approach to treatment.* New York: Norton.

Russell, G. F. M. (1979). Bulimia nervosa—An ominous variant of anorexia nervosa. *Psychological Medicine, 5,* 355–371.

Saklofske, D. F., Kelly, I. W., & Janzen, B. L. (1995). Neuroticism, depression, and depression proneness. *Personality and Individual Differences, 18,* 27–31.

Sanderson, W. C., Beck, A. T., & Beck, J. (1995). Syndrome comorbidity in patients with major depression or dysthymia: Prevalence of temporal relationships. *American Journal of Psychiatry, 147,* 1025–1028.

Saugstad, L. F. (1989). Social class, marriage, and fertility in schizophrenia. *Schizophrenia Bulletin, 15,* 9–43.

Schneier, F. R., Heckelman, L. R., Garfinkel, R., Campeas, R., Fallon, B. A., Gitow, A., Street, L., Del Bene, D., & Liebowitz, M. R. (1994). Functional impairment in social phobia. *Journal of Clinical Psychiatry, 55,* 322–329.

Schuckit, M. A., Tipp, J. E., & Kelner, E. (1994). Are daughters of alcoholics more likely to marry alcoholics? *American Journal of Drug and Alcohol Abuse, 20,* 237–245.

Scott, J., Williams, J. M. G., Brittleband, A., & Ferrier, I. N. (1995). The relationship between premorbid neuroticism, cognitive dysfunction, and persistence of depression: A 1-year follow-up. *Journal of Affective Disorders, 133,* 167–172.

Senchak, M., & Leonard, K. E. (1992). Attachment styles and marital adjustment among newlywed couples. *Journal of Social and Personal Relationships, 9,* 51–64.

Shea, M. T., Glass, D., Pilkonis, P., Watkins, J., & Docherty, J. (1987). Frequency and implications of personality disorders in a sample of depression outpatients. *Journal of Personality Disorders, 1,* 27–42.

Silberstein, L. R., Striegel-Moore, R. H., & Rodin, J. (1987). Feeling fat: A woman's shame. In H. B. Lewis (Ed.), *The role of shame in symptom formation* (pp. 89–108). Hillsdale, NJ: Erlbaum.

Slipp, S. (1995). Object relations marital therapy of personality disorders. In N. S. Jacobson & A. S. Gurman (Eds.), *Clinical handbook of couple therapy* (pp. 458–470). New York: Guilford Press.

Smith, A. L., & Weissman, M. M. (1992). Epidemiology. In E. S. Paykel (Ed.), *Handbook of affective disorders* (pp. 111–130). New York: Guilford Press.

Steinglass, P., Bennett, L. A., Wolin, S. J., & Reiss, D. (1987). *The alcoholic family.* New York: Basic Books.

Steinhausen, H.-C., & Seidel, R. (1992). A prospective follow-up study in early-onset eating disorders. In W. Herzog, H.-C. Deter, & W. Vandereycken (Eds.), *The course of eating disorders: Long-term follow-up studies of anorexia and bulimia nervosa* (pp. 108–117). Berlin: Springer-Verlag.

Steketee, G. (1988). Intra- and interpersonal characteristics predictive of long-term outcome following behavioral treatment of obsessive–compulsive disorders. In

I. Hand & H. Wittchen (Eds.). *Panic and phobias: Vol. 2. Treatment and variables affecting course and outcome* (pp. 221–232). Berlin: Springer-Verlag.

Steketee, G. (1993). Social support and treatment outcome of obsessive compulsive disorder at 9-month follow-up. *Behavioural Psychotherapy, 21,* 81–95.

Steketee, G., & Shapiro, L. J. (1995). Predicting behavioral treatment outcome for agoraphobia and obsessive compulsive disorder. *Clinical Psychology Review, 15,* 317–346.

Straus, M. A., & Gelles, R. J. (1990). *Physical violence in American families: Risk factors and adaptation to violence in 8,145 families.* New Brunswick, NJ: Transaction.

Striegel-Moore, R. H., Silberstein, L. R., Frensch, P., & Rodin, J. (1989). A prospective study of disordered eating among college students. *International Journal of Eating Disorders, 8,* 499–509.

Strober, M. (1984). Stressful life events associated with bulimia in anorexia nervosa: Empirical findings and theoretical speculations. *International Journal of Eating Disorders, 3,* 3–16.

Swift, W. J., & Wonderlich, S. A. (1988). Personality factors and diagnosis in eating disorders: Traits, disorders, and structures. In D. M. Garner & P. E. Garfinkel (Eds.), *Diagnostic issues in anorexia nervosa and bulimia nervosa* (pp. 112–165). New York: Brunner/Mazel.

Sykes, D. K., Leuser, B., Melia, M., & Gross, M. (1988). A demographic analysis of 252 patients with anorexia nervosa and bulimia. *International Journal of Psychosomatics, 35,* 5–9.

Van Buren, D. J., & Williamson, D. A. (1988). Marital relationships and conflict resolution skills of bulimics. *International Journal of Eating Disorders, 7,* 735–741.

Van den Broucke, S., & Vandereycken, W. (1989a). The marital relationships of patients with an eating disorder: A questionnaire study. *International Journal of Eating Disorders, 8,* 541–556.

Van den Broucke, S., & Vandereycken, W. (1989b). Eating disorders in married patients: Theory and therapy. In W. Vandereycken, E. Kog, & J. Vanderlinden (Eds.), *The family approach to eating disorders: Assessment and treatment of anorexia nervosa and bulimia* (pp. 333–346). New York: PMA.

Vandereycken, W. (1995). The families of patients with an eating disorder. In K. D. Brownell & C. G. Fairburn (Eds.), *Eating disorders and obesity: A comprehensive handbook* (pp. 219–223). New York: Guilford Press.

van Furth, E. F., van Strein, D. C., Maritna, L. M. L., van Son, M. J. M, Hendrickx, J. J. P., & van Engeland, H. (1996). EE and the prediction of outcome in adolescent eating disorders. *International Journal of Eating Disorders, 20,* 19–31.

Vaughn, C., & Leff, J. P. (1976). The measurement of expressed emotion in the families of psychiatric patients. *British Journal of Clinical and Social Psychology, 15,* 157–165.

Vitousek, K., & Manke, F. (1994). Personality variables and disorders in anorexia nervosa and bulimia nervosa. *Journal of Abnormal Psychology, 103,* 137–147.

Vose, R. H. (1981). *Agoraphobia.* London: Faber & Faber.

Waters, B. G., Marchenko, I., Abrams, N., Smiley, D., & Kalin, D. (1983). Assortative mating for major depressive disorder. *Journal of Affective Disorders, 5,* 9–17.

Weiss, R. L., & Heyman, R. E. (1990). Observation of marital interaction. In F. D. Fincham & T. N. Bradbury (Eds.), *The psychology of marriage* (pp. 87–119). New York: Guilford Press.

Wonderlich, S. A. (1995). Personality and eating disorders. In K. D. Brownell & C. G. Fairburn (Eds.), *Eating disorders and obesity: A comprehensive handbook* (pp. 171–176). New York: Guilford Press.

CHAPTER 7

———◆———

Parenting Styles and Psychopathology

MARIO CUSINATO

The influence of parents on their children is certainly enormous: They nourish and protect them; teach them to walk and talk; instill habits, aversions, and values; and provide some of the earliest models for social interaction and emotional regulation. Nothing could be more reasonable than to assume that parents form the personality of their children, in both a positive and a negative sense.

Laypeople and clinical professionals alike believe that a strong link exists between parents' rearing styles and children's development, personality, and pathology. References are copious on this subject, but studies often provide inconsistent results, discrepant conclusions, and anecdotal evidence. Some authors (McCrae & Costa, 1994) even use the expression "paradox of parental influence." In fact, studies attempting to provide better scientific bases show that parental influence has relatively little long-term effect on personality (Harrington, 1993; McClelland & Pilon, 1983; Reiss, Howe, Simmens, & Bussell, 1996). McCrae and Costa (1994) think that this paradox may be resolved on the basis of empirical generalization: "Child-rearing practices have little effect on basic tendencies in personality, but are a major influence on the individual's characteristic adaptations" (p. 120).

It is difficult to verify this assumption empirically because of theoretical and methodological problems. Most of the assumptions advanced in the literature make a strong appeal to common-sense beliefs, but they are oversimplified generalizations (McCrae & Costa, 1994, p. 6). The interactive influence of different rearing variables may be much more important for a child's psychological development than the effect of any single variable.

158

In this chapter, I first describe the key factors in parenting styles, and then consider various efforts to connect these styles in a linear fashion to negative child outcomes. I then discuss more complex theoretical models for interpreting links between parenting styles and child psychopathology. Finally, I consider strategies for investigating these links.

THREE KEY FACTORS IN PARENTING STYLE

Parental influence does not operate only through verbal communication or specific behaviors. Relationship channels are complex. For example, echoing and paralleling other authors (Broun, 1988; Higgins, 1990), L'Abate & Baggett (1997) suggest an "ERAAwC" model, which includes emotionality, rationality, activity, awareness, and context. In the continuity of everyday life, the actions of parental rearing take on a specific appearance and become an individual manner of being and acting; they turn to style. Many authors have created different models and assessment techniques to define parental styles. Besides specific peculiarities of such styles, we can identify three basic elements that we can label "factors," as they emerge chiefly from empirical inquiry.

The Warmth Factor

Of all the different aspects of parental behavior that have been found to influence the way children grow up, emotional warmth is consistently found to be the most important. Rollins and Thomas (1979) suggest that the degree of warmth in a parent–child relationship is best conceptualized and operationalized as the balance of supportive versus nonsupportive behaviors toward the child. Supportive behaviors include "praising, approving, encouraging, helping, cooperating, expressing terms of endearment, and physical affection" (p. 320). Nonsupportive behaviors include blaming, criticizing, punishing, threatening, ignoring the child, and expressing anger and negative evaluations of him or her. The variable emerges as a crucial factor no matter how it is measured, and it is directly connected with child self-esteem (Paulson, Hill, & Holmbeck, 1991; Roberts & Bengston, 1996; Fowler & Bulik, 1997; Kendler, Sham, & MacLean, 1997).

The Control Factor and Its Variables

Another universally acknowledged factor concerns control (Garber, Robinson, & Valentiner, 1997) even if it appears more complex than support; for this reason, researchers consider more control-related variables. Rollins and Thomas (1979) differentiate the *frequency* of control attempts from the *style* of control. Parents high on control frequency have rearing practices with many rules and a narrow calibration; they constantly find occasions to intervene in their children's ongoing activities with control attempts. On the other hand, parents with a low score on this variable turn out as being permissive and, to the extreme, negligent. The style of control attempts, however, is a variable that is logically independent of frequency; it concerns the type of intervention attempted, and ranges from coercion (the unilateral imposition of the parental will) to induction (the most egalitarian, reason-based attempt to induce voluntary compliance). The style dimension is not at all logically independent of the support dimension of warmth, so much so that Fowler and Bulik (1997) use the words "affectionless control," and makes the picture much more complex: "In fact, the indicators of nonsupport have a great deal in common with the indicators of coercion, and the descriptors of supportive parenting overlap considerably with the descriptors of the inductive style of parenting" (p. 216). However, when the overlapping content is removed, the style variable exhibits a continuum along which we can find at one pole the right to evaluate and direct the child, and at the other the right of the child to answer back to his or her parent; in the middle of the continuum, reciprocal respect can be placed.

The Consistency Factor

The degree of coherence and consistency in the various components of the messages exchanged between family members has been recognized as an important factor (Anderson & Fleming, 1986). Particularly in the child deviance literature, consistency of discipline and parental consensus on family values and expectations are viewed as key explanatory variables (Bahr, 1979). This factor is labeled and measured differently by various scholars; however, the root concept holds that the degree of internal consistency in the parental demands and evaluations of the child is an important issue in the child's performance (Broderick, 1993).

These three factors, variously considered and labeled, have been combined in family studies in order to specify different types of parental/family styles. For example, Olson (1989) has developed a "circumplex model" based on support and control concepts. Reiss (1989) has studied the impact of connection and disconnection patterns and applied them to families with adolescents recovering from serious psychiatric disorders (Reiss, Costell, Jones, & Berkman, 1980) or chronic somatic illness (Reiss, Gonzales, & Kramer, 1986). Steinglass, Bennett, Wolin, and Reiss (1987) have considered patterns of involvement and disengagement in alcoholic families, while Beavers has defined the patterns of closeness and tie preservation (Beavers & Voeller, 1983; Lewis, Beavers, Gossett, & Phillips, 1976). Recently L'Abate and Baggett (1997) have compared the parenting styles of Baumrind (1991)—authoritarian, permissive, authoritative, and refusing/unengaged—to the four selfhood positions derived from self–other relationship.

THE CONNECTION BETWEEN PARENTAL
REARING AND PSYCHOPATHOLOGY:
ATTEMPTS AT LINEAR EXPLANATIONS

The connection between parental rearing and child psychopathology has its roots in the universal experience that dysfunctional parental attitudes influence the development of psychopathology in the child's later life, and psychological research has highlighted this connection from the beginning. We can recall Freud (1905/1953), who believed that an excess of maternal affection spoils a child by making him or her "incapable in later life of temporarily doing without love or of being content with smaller amount of it" (p. 223). In accordance with the entire psychoanalytic tradition, exaggerated spoiling and extreme deprivation of affection may be the antecedents of the same maladaptive behavior (Adler, 1935/1956; Fenichel, 1945; Freud, 1926/1959). Explaining the basis of his attachment theory, Bowlby (1982) proposed a rather different opinion, even if he admitted that an overdependent, anxious attachment can also result from an excessively protective parental attitude and may discourage the child from learning to do things for himself or herself. However, overdependence usually develops as a result of the experience of the main attachment figure's unreliability, and ultimately of this figure's rejection. Starting from this model, further developments within attachment theory have linked the experiences of parental rearing with psychopathology. Thus Guidano (1987) has given a detailed account of various types of dysfunctional attachment and their implication for the occurrence of overt psychopathology. More recent contributions (Main, 1996; Waters, Posada, Crowell, & Lay, 1993) attempt to weigh the pros and cons of the relation between attachment theory and our understanding of disruptive behavior problems. Although the relevance of attachment to the understanding of the mechanisms of influence is emphasized, it is not accurate to interpret "every disruptive behavior as attachment-related or every attachment-related disruption as serving the same function" (Waters et al., 1993, p. 215). Specific theories have also been proposed for particular dysfunctions, such as antisocial behavior (Shaw & Bell, 1993).

At this point, we can take a cultural-level perspective and consider overprotection or "momism." This term originated in the sociological literature (Sebald, 1976), but has permeated the psychiatric literature as well. It refers to a mother's tendency to cushion and protect her child against any difficulty in his or her development to maturity; used and abused, the term ended up covering all kinds of dysfunctional maternal rearing practices, and was thus criticized for offering too simple an explanation of psychological problems (Erikson, 1963). In this respect, it is similar to the term "schizophrenogenic mother" (Fromm-Reichmann, 1949), another attempt at characterizing numerous dysfunctional aspects of maternal style. It combines overprotection, low nurture, and high control, to an extent that reveals many contradictions (Heilbrun, 1973; Parker, 1994). Paternal influence has also been examined, albeit to a lesser extent (Phares, 1992; Carratelli, Maggiulli, Ricceri, & Ruvutuso, 1993; Phares & Campes, 1993). A less close father–child relationship seems to predict later problem behavior, as specific inquiries have shown (Rothbaum, Schneider, Pott, & Beatty, 1995). On the whole, results of parental style studies (Alnaes & Torgersen, 1990; Borduin & Henggeler, 1987; Parker, 1983) have been modest and mostly nonsignificant as concerns paternal versus maternal rearing behavior in a variety of psychiatric and psychosomatic conditions. Nevertheless, when the father's and mother's negative or abusive behaviors add up, the connection to dysfunctional outcomes in offspring becomes stronger and often crucial (Norden, Klein, Donaldson, Pepper, & Klein, 1995); children perceiving their parents as manifesting symptoms have more behavior problems (Scherer, Mellow, Buych, & Anderson, 1996).

Punitiveness, lack of emotional warmth, and rejection may also be important background factors in the development of severe psychopathology, even in the absence of overprotection. For the most severe level, Miller (1990), drawing on Rutschky's (1977) work, uses the concept of "black pedagogy"—a pattern in which the child is defenseless and the parent can do what he or she desires, without fear of retaliation or revenge (Ceccarelli & Montesi, 1996).

MORE COMPLEX THEORETICAL MODELS CONNECTING PARENTAL STYLE AND PSYCHOPATHOLOGY

Accepting the axiom that individual behavior, personality, and pathology are products and reflections of family processes, researchers and scholars have strongly emphasized that the explanations are not as linear as some positions might allow us to suppose:

> By insisting adamantly that children's behaviors, personalities, and pathologies are the product of the styles of interaction in their families (and may trace their origins back for several generations, according to many of the theory's founders, such as Murray Bowen [1978] and Ivan Boszormenyi-Nagy and Gerardine Sparks [1973]), they fall into the trap of the linear explanation that systemic perspective was invented to avoid. (Broderick, 1993, p. 213)

The shift toward a more interactive, nonlinear modeling of the socialization process involves some problems that are not readily solved, and it is useful to go into more details. According to a linear connection, the influence of parenting styles on child development follows an environmental model of discontinuity, in which every developmental phase is produced by current context. An alternative position is that of considering child development as the disclosure of intrinsic characteristics, either preformed traits or epigenetically interactive qualities (Sameroff, 1983). Whereas the latter position is rather crude, an entirely environmental model runs the risk of stigmatizing parents and of nourishing their guilt, as studies on expressed emotion have done (Doane & Diamond, 1994). In such models, parental behavior appears to be the direct cause of child behavioral symptoms.

A first helpful step is offered by an interactionistic position, which combines the continuity given by the child with the possible discontinuity of experience. Anastasi (1958) is believed to be the author who introduced the meaningful shift toward an interactionistic conception when she pointed out that development may not continue outside its context. There is no logical reason to consider the development of an individual as independent of the environment. In fact, continuity cannot really be considered an attribute of the child, because every new achievement is a mixture of the child's intrinsic characteristics and of his or her experience. In this model, the concept of "risk" is more useful than that of "symptom" in order to interpret the connection between parenting styles and child development outcomes, as I will later consider in greater depth (Chase-Landsdale, Wakschlag, & Brooks-Gunn, 1993).

A more advanced formulation is offered by a transactional model (Sameroff & Chandler, 1975), which joins the respective contributions of child and environment with the context characteristics allowed by the child's nature. Different qualities and behaviors of the child trigger different responses from the environment. In this way, child development may be considered as a result of a dynamic interaction between the child and his or her experiences as supplied by the family and the social context. The innovation lies in the emphasis attributed by the child to the context, so that the experiences offered by the latter are not unrelated to the child. Negative transactions may be started by an atypical behavior of the child that a parent does not understand, or by a typical behavior of the child that the parent explains from a twisted perspective. This rationale may account for the process that leads to the development of particular parenting styles in which the child himself or herself plays an active and important role (Ge, Conger, Lorenz, Shanahan, & Elder, 1995). Of course, causal chains are always complex, so that in every inquiry a multidimensional model of the parent's and child's behavior seems more suitable. According to the steps of the development cycle and the level at which these are examined, different connections may be found, some of which will appear transactional and others will not. In some cases parents respond with love and affection to the child's every action, and in other cases they respond with anger and ill treatment to every behavior of the child. These responses are not examples of transaction, because the parent's prevailing interactive style is not modified by the child's behavior. In any case, we may expect that transactional processes characterize parent–child relationships.

The integration of many factors ruling development is bound by interactions with the regulatory systems that work at different levels of organization. The two most important of these systems are those that regulate the biological and social development. From conception to birth, the interactions with the biological system are prevalent; the period from birth to adulthood is characterized by the prevalence of the social system. Child development starts with biological regulation processes, but the controllers are in the social environment. These controllers modify the child's experience according to the changes resulting from his or her physical and behavioral development, and the result of these exchanges is an increase in the child's ability to regulate his or her biological and social behavior.

The transactional study of development shows the reciprocal role of the child's biological and social abilities. Nevertheless, it is useful to underline that the organization of experience, particularly if implicit, takes place according to models of family and cultural socialization that establish an "ecotype" similar to the biological "genotype" (Sameroff & Fiese, 1990). The ecotype is made up of subsystems interacting not only with the child but also among themselves. Even if the ecotype may be conceptualized at any time as separate from the child, changes in the abilities of the developing child become important events generating regulatory changes that probably represent important inputs to the growth of a development plan as the sequence of its basic steps. Recent genetic evidence suggests that the most important environmental influences on both normal and pathological development are those that are not shared by siblings in the same family (Reiss et al., 1995). In this way, a reciprocal interconnection may be identified among three regulatory systems: the genotype, ecotype, and phenotype (Sameroff, 1993).

Let us consider the ecotype system in connection with the phenotype. The experience of the developing child is made up in part of the beliefs, values, and personality of his or her parents; in part of the interaction models and transgenerational history of the family; and in part of socialization convictions and cultural regulations and support. At every level, development control is realized within the codes driving cognitive and socioemotional development. The family represents a large proportion of these social controllers (L'Abate, 1994a). In fact, it regulates the child's development in many ways, varying the level of explicit representation (Broderick, 1993). When individuals act as a part of the family, their behavior changes, although they are hardly ever conscious of it. Nevertheless, every individual makes his or her contribution to family interaction, so that the individualized interpretations given to codes by each parent are worth attention. These interpretations are largely conditioned by the coded interactions of the family, but each member idiographically appropriates them. These individual appropriations further condition the responses of each parent and of each child. Parenting style emerges from this multifactorial complexity as a concrete synthesis of many regulatory systems. The connection of parenting style with the outcomes of the offspring is likewise multifactorial, according to the principles of equifinality and equipotentiality (L'Abate, 1994a).

In this complex framework, the perspective offered by the concepts "at-risk child" and "resiliency" may be more useful than that of "psychopathology." The concept of "at-risk child" (Garmezy, 1993) or "individual vulnerability" (Perris, 1994) emphasizes the importance of psychosocial factors, besides those of a biological nature, as determinants. These terms define a status marked by a heightened likelihood for disorder at some time in the life span as a consequence of risk factors that may originate in genetic predisposition, dispositional personality attributes, harsh family circumstances, and/or negative environmental conditions. Negative parental styles may be considered as a principal element of risk; even if they are formed and reinforced within a vulnerability context for both offspring and parents, parenting styles seem independent of family structure (McFarlane, Bellissimo, & Norman, 1995).

A further aspect in the link between parental style and child psychopathology is the phenomenon of "resiliency," which has recently received increased attention (e.g., Magnusson & Casaer, 1993; Cicchetti & Cohen, 1995; Cowen et al., 1997). Although risk factors and disordered behavior deserve priority, it is obvious that normative development must be the baseline against which to evaluate deviations from that standard. Such a view helps to moderate premature interpretations of deviance. Thus, though life stressors are often evident in the lives of the mentally disordered, similar or identical events frequently occur in the lives of many adaptable people as well. Variations in responsiveness to stressful events have been a reason for initiating studies of protective factors that may serve to temper the effects of risk factors. The concept of "resiliency" or "stress resistance" was introduced to describe the maintenance of adequate behavior in the presence of major stressful life events. From the early case descriptions of resilient persons (Goertzel & Goerztel, 1962), efforts have been made to study the characteristics and background of accomplished persons who have been exposed to a variety of markedly stressful experiences, such as profound poverty in childhood, racial and ethnic prejudice, affect deprivation, physical and sexual abuse, a background of family mental disorder, physical and mental disability, and even family backgrounds and neighborhood settings that encourage delinquency and crime. Under all these constraining circumstances, some people have nevertheless overcome adversity and demonstrated functional competence over their life span. Although these outcomes reflect the reality of the phenomenon of resiliency, they can also serve as a basis for the systematic study of a specific trauma shared by groups of individuals and the varied outcomes that follow. The goal is the search for the attributes and underlying processes that are involved in the successful adaptation to disadvantaged and threatening circumstances (Masten, Best, & Garmezy, 1990).

Inputs to this new orientation have been multiple studies on children at risk for mental disorders because of possible family genetic status (Watt, Anthony, Wynne, & Rolf, 1984). The finding of a range of adaptability in these presumably at-risk offspring has increased the interest in resiliency research. The meaning of "resiliency" points to the tendency to rebound or recover and to similar concepts, but nothing suggests a context of "invulnerability" to stress; the term portrays an underlying process that allows an individual to return to a prior level of performance following a stressful imposition. Returning to that prior level is assumed to reflect a higher degree of competence or function—and it is this construct of enhanced competence, rather than the more popularized one of coping, that is the central element of research into the nature of resiliency (Garmezy & Masten, 1991). The low correlation rates between parental rearing styles and psychosocial adjustment or psychopathology in numerous empirical studies can find a useful explanation in the latest interesting orientations (Rosenstein & Horowitz, 1996; Cicchetti & Rogosch, 1997).

INVESTIGATION STRATEGIES

The theoretical concepts and models I have focused on above have become frames of reference in empirical investigations into the complex connection between parenting styles and children's negative or positive outcomes.

Garmezy (1993) notes that events with unremitting consequences over time may occur at various points of the life cycle; therefore, we can suitably use the concept of life span developmental psychopathology. To study the range of the temporal antecedents potentially implicated in psychopathology—in the present case, parental rearing styles—four research methods have been found useful: (1) case studies, (2) follow-back studies, (3) follow-up studies, and (4) follow-through research.

The case study method is a method of clinical retrospective inquiry in which single case studies serve as a basis for evaluating risk status and outcome. The use of this method has highlighted that explanations are based not only on genetic factors, but also on psychological responses to stress and on sociocultural elements that can influence mental disorder; the first such element is parental rearing style. Concrete proposals for using this method have already been defined and offered (L'Abate, 1994b; Miller & Crabtree, 1994). A series of case studies at the Yale Psychiatric Institute exemplifies the change processes in families of patients in a therapeutic setting with serious psychiatric disorders (Doane & Diamond, 1994). This research work has led to the identification of three family types—"high-intensity," "low-intensity," and "disconnected" families—and to the conclusion that attachment and warmth represent the basic relational variables between parents and children.

Follow-back studies are often retrospective reports based on societal records. Such studies are typically initiated when children's or adolescents' disordered behaviors warrant a search for records of their previous history (e.g., school records, court assessments, teacher judgments, peer relations data, and significant family data), which are examined for early signs of disorder.

Follow-up studies have a lengthy history. They typically involve evaluations of subjects' behavior and status at two time points: at an earlier age (usually childhood or adolescence) and, later, in adulthood. The method is not without research design problems. The selection of the at-risk group may predispose subjects in that group to negative outcomes. Often, also, follow-up research does not include adequate and comparable control cases matched with the subjects on all important attributes, and the selection of both subjects and controls may not actually be related to the explicitly specified selection criteria. In addition, the method does not allow a detailed accounting of the interim events and of the varying patterns of development and change occurring between selection and follow-up. Finally, if selection is based on early symptomatology, the processes that might account for the early onset of maladaptive behavior can no longer be examined with reliability in follow-up research. Although the method can provide data on outcomes of at-risk children, it cannot do so about the temporal developmental processes implied in good and poor outcomes.

In follow-through or longitudinal research, the researchers seek out a cohort of young individuals with a presumed risk status (often because of genetic or environmental factors in their life history) that may reflect a heightened probability of a negative outcome in adulthood. This method is a variant of the follow-up strategy, but an important difference is that it typically involves multiple evaluations of the cohort members as they reach various ages. The longitudinal study best delineates the phenomena of growth, the role of antecedent and concurrent significant experiences (both stressful and normative), and the impact of such experiences on the adaptational efforts of the cohort members. Such research may become even more powerful if data are gathered not only from this cohort of children but also from their parents and/or siblings, focusing on their relationships. It is the most powerful method of idiographic inquiry, in which various age/stage characteristics of children or adolescents moving toward adulthood can be investigated, with special attention given to developmental transitions and transformations, continuities and discontinuities in behavior, and shifts in status and adaptation over time.

Review studies (Burbach & Borduin, 1986; Brewin, Andrews, & Gotlib, 1993; Gerlsma, Emmelkamp, & Arrindell, 1990; Perris, 1994) have ascertained that research on early adverse family experiences and psychopathology has primarily utilized the follow-up method. Such adverse experiences have been implicated in the etiology of anxiety, depression, multiple personality disorder, schizophrenia, alcoholism, and eating disorders (Andrews, Brown, & Creasey, 1990; Gerslma et al., 1990; Goldstein, 1985; Holmes & Robins, 1988; Marton & Maharaj, 1994; Wilbur, 1984).

Within the range of psychiatric disturbances, those investigated most often have been depression and anxiety disorders. Patients with anxiety disorders are found to perceive their parents as less caring, more rejecting, and/or more overprotective than matched nonpsychiatric controls are found to do (Arrindell, Emmelkamp, Brilman, & Monsma, 1983; Ehiobuche, 1988; Gerslma et al., 1990). Furthermore, the fact that some specific links have been reported between particular subtypes of anxiety disorders and particular types of early experiences in these studies renders less tenable the hypothesis that reports of negative early experience are simply a function of a global negative response style. In studies with depressed patients, these clinical subjects have been compared with nonpsychiatric controls, and the former have reliably reported less adequate parenting (Crook, Raskin, & Eliot, 1981; Jacobson, Fasman, & DiMaschio, 1975; Parker, 1983; Kaslow, Deering, & Racusin, 1994). Inquiries with nonclinical subjects show that individuals who have experienced parental discord, little parental care and warmth, and hostile and abusive behaviors during childhood are at a greater risk of becoming depressed than are those who have not experienced such negative relationships.

Claims concerning the general unreliability of retrospective reports have been reviewed by Brewin et al. (1993) and Gerlsma (1994); recently, Schneewind and Ruppert (1998) have found the same weak reliability. Such claims concern the low reliability and validity of autobiographical memory in general, the presence of a general memory impairment associated with psychopathology, and the presence of specific mood-congruent memory biases associated with specific types of psychopathology.

The reviews of the available data on the accuracy of memory for early experiences do not support a reconstructive position (in which memory changes over time) as compared to a copy theory (in which the thoroughness of memory persists even after many years), because accuracy depends to a large extent on the characteristics of the events to be recalled. There is little evidence of a general deficit in memory associated with anxiety or depression; the data on personal memories that are available from naturalistic studies suggest that psychiatric patients' recall is as reliable as that of nonpatients. The studies offer little support for the claim that recall of childhood experiences is distorted by a depressed mood: "There is no evidence of a global response style ("blaming", "idealization") affecting the appraisal of all interpersonal relationships. Neither does social desirability in the classical sense affect questionnaire scores of parental behavior" (Brewin et al., 1993, p. 94). Both experimental and naturalistic studies reveal high stability in recall, even with changes in mood or clinical status. The test–retest reliability of accounts of early separations is similarly unrelated to the presence of psychiatric disorder (Finlay-Jones, Scott, Duncan-Jones, Byrne, & Henderson, 1981). Furthermore, patients' memories are in as much agreement with external criteria as are controls', whether the criteria be siblings' memories (Robins et al., 1985) or independent records, even if parents describe their own behavior in more positive terms than their offspring do (probably in order to shield their own role).

Therefore, claims that retrospective reports in general and those of psychiatric patients in particular are inherently unreliable are exaggerated. Nevertheless, it is clear that retrospective reports are subject to various limitations. The report process may be flawed by both internal and external factors. Social influences, childhood amnesia, and the simple fallibility of memory impose limitations on the accuracy of recall, and fear of the consequences of disclosure may create further disadvantages. However, provided that individuals are questioned about the occurrence of specific events or facts that they were old enough and sufficiently well placed to know about, the central features of their accounts are likely to be reasonably accurate. Because the influences on memory serve mainly to inhibit recall or disclosure, it is possible to conclude that reports confirming events should be given *more* weight than negative reports.

Researchers and clinicians agree that it is possible to enhance the recall of past experiences with more structured methods. Both laboratory and field studies of autobiographical memory (Bjork, 1989; Linton, 1986) suggest that assessments of past experience would be more reliable if they included inquiries about the occurrence of a range of specific events, rather than having subjects make global estimates of parental attitudes. Some authors (Brown & Rutter, 1966; Cannell & Kahn, 1968; Wolkind & Coleman, 1983) suggest that problems with retrospective recall, such as denial, forgetting, and bias, can be reduced with the use of specific interview techniques and an investigator-based approach to rating. Semistructured interview methods make it possible to elicit personal memories in response to general or specific recognition cues. Encouragement to report events in detail is also likely to help subjects to distinguish between memories of real and imagined experiences.

Self-report questionnaires that require respondents to make global judgments about the degree of rejection or overprotection they experienced appear useful to verify parental styles, as long as such measures are standardized and possess adequate psychometric properties (Gerlsma, 1994). In fact, the research field has benefited greatly from the development of several questionnaires for measuring offspring's perceptions in a standardized and reliable way. These include the Children's Reports of Parental Behavior Inventory, developed by Schaefer (1965) in the United States; the Parental Bonding Instrument, developed by Parker, Tupling, and Brown (1979) in Australia; and the EMBU (Swedish acronym for "My Memories of Upbringing") developed by Perris, Jacobsson, Linström, von Knorring, and Perris (1980) in Europe. These three questionnaires seem to be the most widely used and psychometrically best evaluated instruments (Gerlsma, 1994). For example, Gerlsma and Emmelkamp (1994) have conducted a meta-analysis on data from 39 studies, 17 of which had focused on child dysfunctions or difficulties (e.g., phobias, attempted suicide, depression, anxiety, drug addiction, and affective symptoms). In particular, the EMBU was recently used for a transcultural study in which data were obtained in 14 nations (Arrindell et al., 1994; van de Vijver & Poortinga, 1993). All these instruments have subscales measuring the key dimensions of parental rearing behavior, affection, and control. The combination of lack of affection and an excess of control is generally considered to be a vulnerability factor in the etiology of various psychological disorders (Parker, 1988; Bowlby, 1988; Perris, 1988).

Clinical interviewing affords many more opportunities for inquiring about past experience, because it allows investigators to elicit specific personal memories. Retrieving specific memories, as well as providing evidence for the validity (or invalidity) of global evaluations, is likely to generate contextual details that can in turn function as recognition cues for accessing additional memories. Interviewing in a clinical context may also allow more opportunities for subjects to overcome feelings of guilt and shame, and to report deeply distressing experiences such as assault and abuse. Nevertheless, clinical assessments could equally benefit from a structured interview with an emphasis on the retrieval of specific memories using predefined guidelines. Factual accounts that meet these criteria are likely to help place emotional reactions, both past and present, in their appropriate context; to contribute to the therapeutic store of "self-knowledge" (Liotti, 1988); and to give patients the opportunity to reconstruct deeply wounding and humiliating experiences for which they may continue to feel in some way responsible.

Longitudinal research is the most suitable way of studying the connections between parental styles and psychopathology. Nevertheless, reviewers (Brewin et al., 1993; Emmelkamp & Gerlsma, 1994; Magnusson & Casaer, 1993; Graves, Openshaw, Ascione, & Ericksen, 1997) regret the paucity of studies in which both children and their parents were assessed and the children were then followed into adulthood to identify early predictors of psychopathology. On the other hand, such studies are very complex, time-consuming, and energy-wasting, and also have to deal with the problem of sample attrition. Therefore, it is useful to pay attention to the planned longitudinal projects that have actually been carried out.

The *Inventory of Longitudinal Studies in the Social Sciences* (Young, Savola, & Phelps, 1991) reports 542 studies, 35 of which have focused specifically (although not exclusively) on the influence of child-rearing practices on offspring's development and adult outcomes. I have taken these 35 studies and catalogued them by project title, research leaders, time interval covered, type of subjects, number of subjects and attrition, and specific topics covered (see the Appendix to this chapter). These studies are interesting for many reasons, and they deserve closer consideration here.

Some of these inquiries were begun many years ago; for example, the Guidance Study by Huffine, Honzik, and Macfarlane (see Eichorn, Clausen, Haan, Honzik, & Mussen, 1981) was begun in 1928 and followed three-generation families over a period of 54 years. Some projects are still in progress, and new data are being gathered with the commitment of additional cohorts of researchers; this extension implies that interest in and support for longitudinal studies come not only from individuals, but also from scientific institutions. Some inquiries were planned to follow a large number of subjects. For example, Langner's Family Research Project started with 2,034 subjects; the Woodlawn Mental Health Longitudinal Community Epidemiological Project began with 1,770; the Adolescent Health Care Evaluation Study by Earls, Robins, and Stiffman started with 2,788. Furstenberg and Brooks-Gunn's Baltimore Study investigated four successive cohorts, covering over the various generations 1,328 subjects, although the core sample was eventually 1,034. Twelve of the 35 studies included both experimental and control groups. The interval between the gathering of the initial and the final data varied widely, with the shortest being 5 years (Adolescent Health Care Evaluation by Earls, Robins, & Stiffman and Understanding and Prediction of Delinquent Child Behavior by Patterson, Reid, & Dishion) and the longest being 54 years (the Guidance Study). The time interval for 15 studies was 15 years or more. Several of the inquiries included more than one cohort and thus obviously obtained more data. Eleven studies followed families and obtained data from parents and children; the other 24 studies followed the development of a family member with individual data. All the covered and tested topics are relevant to the influence of parental styles on offspring's development; some directly concern dysfunctional outcomes, but they are all meaningful as efforts to define the intergenerational dynamics of socialization.

By way of an example, let us consider a study begun by Sears in 1951 (Sears, Maccoby, & Levin, 1957) as a cross-sectional design, when 379 mothers were interviewed about their own and their spouses' parenting practices with their 5-year-old children. The subsample of offspring studied at age 41 was composed of 89 subjects; checks on the sampling indicated that the sample was representative of the original one. When the children were 5 years old, parenting measures concerned fathers' and mothers' warmth; mothers' strictness; punitiveness, and self-esteem; and children's sociability. Other measures, coded by two graduate students, concerned the families' social class and the difficulty of children's experience. About every 6 years, data waves were completed. When the children were 41 years old, the outcome measures were conventional social accomplishment, explanatory style, personality characteristics, adjustment, coping styles, and life satisfaction.

Some researchers who participated in the project (Franz, McClelland,

Weinberger, & Peterson, 1994) have elaborated specifically on the initial and the final data. Mothers' and fathers' initial views showed some overlap of parenting practices, with few differences. Correlations of the childhood and midlife data suggested that parenting was more influential than children's sociability in determining ability in close relationships at midlife: A warm father in childhood was associated with better social accomplishment in midlife, which in turn was correlated with several indicators of personal and interpersonal welfare. On the other side, maternal hostility, low maternal self-esteem, and difficult childhood experience appeared to be associated with an adult pessimistic explanatory style among men but not among women. Particularly for the men, we can speculate that these children acquired a pessimistic way of explaining events when they experienced traumas during childhood and their rearing was harsh and inconsistent. The differences found between men and women may have resulted from boys' and girls' different ways of acquiring explanatory styles.

> Whatever the dynamic, parenting made an important long-term difference in the lives of the adults in this sample. Over a period of 36 years, the children of warm, affectionate fathers, and boys with warm mothers and less stressful childhood years were more likely to be well adjusted adults who, at age 41, were mentally healthy, coping adequately, and psychosocially mature. (Franz et al., 1994, p. 141)

Over and over again, reviewers emphasize that research efforts and results in this area are only at a preliminary stage (Brewin et al., 1993; Dornbusch, Ritter, Leiderman, Roberts, & Fraleigh, 1987; Garmezy, 1993). They seem chiefly to be considering data collection. Probably this is correct, if we take into account that parental styles are evolving remarkably in accordance with major sociocultural changes (Scabini, 1995; Schneewind & Ruppert, 1998). But it is also timely to work at the meta-analytic level, in order not to waste a tremendous harvest of information (Gerlsma & Emmelkamp, 1994). Some reliable landmarks are just around the corner, and they will be a great help in organizing more prompt interventions, in addition to increasing our knowledge (van IJzendoorn, Juffer, & Duyvesteyn, 1995; Joiner & Wagner, 1996; van IJzendoorn & Bakermans-Kranenburg, 1996).

REFERENCES

Adler, A. (1956). *The individual psychology of Alfred Adler* (H. L. Ansbacher & R. R. Ansbacher, Eds. and Trans.). New York: Harper & Row. (Original work published 1935)

Alnaes, R., & Torgersen, S. (1990). Parental representation in patients with major depression, anxiety disorder, and mixed conditions. *Acta Psychiatrica Scandinavica, 81,* 518–522.

Anastasi, A. (1958). Heredity, environment, and the question "How?" *Psychological Review, 75,* 81–95.

Anderson, S. A., & Fleming, W. A. (1986). Late adolescents' identity formation: Individuation from the family of origin. *Adolescence, 21,* 785–796.

Andrews, B., Brown, G. W., & Creasey, L. (1990). Intergenerational links between psychiatric disorder in mothers and daughters: The role of parenting experiences. *Journal of Child Psychology and Psychiatry, 31,* 1115–1129.

Arrindell, W. A., Emmelkamp, P. M. G., Brilman, E., & Monsma, A. (1983). Psychometric evaluation of an inventory for assessment of parental rearing practices: A Dutch form of the EMBU. *Acta Psychiatrica Scandinavica, 67,* 163–177.

Arrindell, W. A., Perris, C., Eisemann, M., van der Ende, J., Gaszner, P., Iwawaki, S., Maj, M., & Zhang, J. (1994). Parental rearing behavior from a cross-cultural perspective: A summary of data obtained in 14 nations. In C. Perris, W. A. Arrindell, & M. Eisemann (Eds.), *Parenting and psychopathology* (pp. 145–172). New York: Wiley.

Bahr, S. J. (1979). Family determinants and effects of deviance. In W. R. Burr, R. Hill, F. I. Ney, & I. L. Reiss (Eds.), *Contemporary theories about the family* (Vol. 1, pp. 615–644). New York: Free Press.

Baumrind, D. (1991). The influence of parenting style on adolescent competence and substance use. *Journal of Early Adolescence, 11,* 56–95.

Beavers, W. R., & Voeller, M. N. (1983). Family models: Comparing and contrasting the Olson circumplex model with the Beavers system model. *Family Process, 22,* 85–97.

Bjork, R. A. (1989). Retrieval inhibition as an adaptive mechanism in human memory. In H. L. Roediger & F. I. M. Craik (Eds.), *Varieties of memory and consciousness* (pp. 309–330). Hillsdale, NJ: Erlbaum.

Borduin, C. M., & Henggeler, S. W. (1987). Post-divorce mother–son relations of delinquent and well-adjusted adolescents. *Journal of Applied Developmental Psychology, 8,* 273–288.

Boszormenyi-Nagy, I., & Sparks, G. (1973). *Invisible loyalties: Reciprocity in intergenerational family therapy.* New York: Harper & Row.

Bowen, M. (1978). *Family therapy in clinical practice.* New York: Jason Aronson.

Bowlby, J. (1982). *Attachment and loss: Vol. 1. Attachment.* New York: Basic Books.

Brewin, C. R., Andrews, B., & Gotlib, I. H. (1993). Psychopathology and early experience: A reappraisal of retrospective reports. *Psychological Bulletin, 113,* 82–98.

Broderick, C. B. (1993). *Understanding family process.* Newbury Park, CA: Sage.

Broun, B. G. (1988). The BASK model of dissociation: Part I. *Dissociation, 1,* 4–23.

Brown, G. W., & Rutter, M. (1966). The measurement of family activities and relationships: A methodological study. *Human Relations, 19,* 241–263.

Burbach, D. J., & Borduin, C. M. (1986). Parent–child relations and the etiology of depression: A review of methods and findings. *Clinical Psychology Review, 6,* 133–153.

Cannell, C. F., & Kahn, R. O. (1968). Interviewing. In O. Lindzey & E. Aronson (Eds.), *Handbook of social psychology* (Vol. 2, pp. 526–595). Reading, MA: Addison-Wesley.

Carratelli, T. J., Maggiulli, O., Ricceri, F., & Ruvutuso, A. (1993). Ruolo e funzioni del padre nelle relazioni del bambino autistico con il suo ambiente primario: Riflessioni da un setting osservativo diagnostico [Role and function of fathers in the child's relation to his or her primary environment: Reflections from a diagnostic observation setting]. *Psichiatria dell'Infanzia e dell'Adolescenza, 60,* 241–249.

Ceccarelli, G., & Montesi, M. (1996). A study on black pedagogy. In M. Cusinato (Ed.), *Research on family resources and needs across the world* (pp. 321–340). Milan: LED.

Chase-Landsdale, P. L., Wakschlag, L. S., & Brooks-Gunn, J. (1993). A psychological perspective on the development of caring in children and youth: The role of the family. *Journal of Adolescence, 18,* 515–556.

Cicchetti, D., & Cohen, D. J. (Eds.). (1995). *Developmental psychopathology: Vol. 1. Theory and methods.* New York: Wiley-Interscience.

Cicchetti, D., & Rogosch, F. A. (1997). The role of self-organization in the promotion of resilience in maltreated children. *Development and Psychopathology, 9,* 797–815.

Cowen, E. L., Wyman, P. A., Work, W. C., Kim, J. Y., Fagen, D. B., & Magnus, K. B. (1997). Follow-up study of young stress-affected and stress-resilient urban children. *Development and Psychopathology, 9,* 565–577.

Crook, T., Raskin, A., & Eliot, J. (1981). Parent–child relationships and adult depression. *Child Development, 52,* 950–957.

Doane, J. A., & Diamond, D. (1994). *Affect and attachment in the family.* New York: Basic Books.

Dornbusch, S. M., Ritter, P. L., Leiderman, H., Roberts, D. F., & Fraleigh, M. J. (1987). The relation of parenting style to adolescent school performance. *Child Development, 58,* 1244–1257.

Ehiobuche, I. (1988). Obsessive–compulsive neurosis in relation to parental child-rearing patterns amongst Greek, Italian, and Anglo-Australian subjects. *Acta Psychiatrica Scandinavica, 78,* 115–120.

Eichorn, D. H., Clausen, J. A., Haan, N., Honzik, M., & Mussen, P. H. (Eds.). (1981). *Present and past in middle life.* New York: Academic Press.

Erikson, E. H. (1963). *Childhood and society* (2nd ed.). New York: Norton.

Fenichel, O. (1945). *The psychoanalytic theory of neurosis.* New York: Norton.

Finlay-Jones, R., Scott, R., Duncan-Jones, P., Byrne, D., & Henderson, S. (1981). The reliability of reports of early separations. *Australian and New Zealand Journal of Psychiatry, 15,* 27–31.

Fowler, S. J., & Bulik, C. M. (1997). Family environment and psychiatric history in women with binge-eating disorder and obese control. *Behaviour Change, 14,* 106.

Franz, C. E., McClelland, D. C., Weinberger, J., & Peterson, C. (1994). Parenting antecedents of adult adjustment: A longitudinal study. In C. Perris, W. A. Arrindell, & M. Eisemann (Eds.), *Parenting and psychopathology* (pp. 127–144). New York: Wiley.

Freud, S. (1953). Three essays on the theory of sexuality. In J. Strachey (Ed. and Trans.), *The standard edition of the complete psychological works of Sigmund Freud* (Vol. 7, pp. 125–243). London: Hogarth Press. (Original work published 1905)

Freud, S. (1959). Inhibitions, symptoms, and anxiety. In J. Strachey (Ed. and Trans.), *The standard edition of the complete psychological works of*

Sigmund Freud (Vol. 20, pp. 75–175). London: Hogarth Press. (Original work published 1926)

Fromm-Reichmann, F. (1949). Notes on the development of treatment of schizophrenics by psychoanalytic psychotherapy. *Psychiatry, 11,* 263–273.

Garber, J., Robinson, N. S., & Valentiner, D. (1997). The relation between parenting and adolescent depression: Self-worth as a mediator. *Journal of Adolescent Research, 12,* 12–33.

Garmezy, N. (1993). Developmental psychopathology: Some historical and current perspectives. In D. Magnusson & P. Casaer (Eds.), *Longitudinal research on individual development: Present status and future perspectives* (pp. 95–126). New York: Cambridge University Press.

Garmezy, N., & Masten, A. S. (1991). The protective role of competence indicators in children at risk: The research for antecedents of schizophrenia. Part I: Conceptual models and research methods. In E. M. Cummings, A. L. Greene, & K. H. Karraker (Eds.), *Life-span developmental psychology: Perspectives on stress and coping* (pp. 151–174). Hillsdale, NJ: Erlbaum.

Ge, X., Conger, R. D., Lorenz, F. O., Shanahan, M., & Elder, G. H. (1995). Mutual influences in parent and adolescent psychological distress. *Developmental Psychology, 31,* 406–419.

Gerlsma, C. (1994). Parental rearing styles and psychopathology: Notes on the validity of questionnaires for recalled parental behavior. In C. Perris, W. A. Arrindell, & M. Eisemann (Eds.), *Parenting and psychopathology* (pp. 75–105). New York: Wiley.

Gerlsma, C., & Emmelkamp, P. M. G. (1994). How large are gender differences in perceived parental rearing styles?: A meta-analytic review. In C. Perris, W. A. Arrindell, & M. Eisemann (Eds.), *Parenting and psychopathology* (pp. 55–74). New York: Wiley.

Gerlsma, C., Emmelkamp, P. M. G., & Arrindell, W. A. (1990). Anxiety, depression, and perception of early parenting: Connotation of two parental rearing style questionnaires. *Personality and Individual Differences, 12,* 551–555.

Goertzel, V., & Goerztel, M. G. (1962). *Cradles of eminence.* Boston: Little, Brown.

Goldstein, M. J. (1985). Family factors that antedate the onset of schizophrenia and related disorders: The results of a fifteen-year prospective longitudinal study. *Acta Psychiatrica Scandinavica, 71,* 7–18.

Graves, R. B., Openshaw, D. K., Ascione, F. R., & Ericksen, S. L (1997). Demographic and parental characteristics of youthful sexual offenders. *International Journal of Offender Therapy and Comparative Criminology, 40,* 300–317.

Guidano, V. F. (1987). *Complexity of the self.* New York: Guilford Press.

Harrington, D. M. (1993). Child-rearing antecedents of suboptimal personality: Exploring aspects of Alice Miller's concept of poisonous pedagogy. In D. C. Funder, R. D. Parke, C. Tomlinson-Keasey, & K. Widaman (Eds.), *Studying lives through time: Personality and development* (pp. 289–313). Washington, DC: American Psychological Association.

Heilbrun, A. B. (1973). *Aversive maternal control: A theory of schizophrenic development.* New York: Wiley.

Higgins, E. T. (1990). Personality, social psychology, and person–situation relations: Standards and knowledge activation as a common language. In L. A. Pervin

(Ed.), *Handbook of personality: Theory and research* (pp. 301–338). New York: Guilford Press.

Holmes, S. J., & Robins, L. N. (1988). The role of parental disciplinary practices in the development of depression and alcoholism. *Psychiatry, 51,* 24–35.

Jacobson, S., Fasman, J., & DiMaschio, A. (1975). Deprivation in the childhood of depressed women. *Journal of Nervous and Mental Disease, 160,* 5–14.

Joiner, T. E., & Wagner, K. D. (1996). Parental, child-centered attribution and outcome: A meta-analytic review with conceptual and methodological implications. *Journal of Abnormal Child Psychology, 24,* 37–52.

Kaslow, N. J., Deering, C. G., & Racusin, G. R. (1994). Depressed children and their families. *Clinical Psychology Review, 14,* 39–59.

Kendler, K. S., Sham, P. C., & MacLean, C. J. (1997). The determinants of parenting: An epidemiological, multi-informant, retrospective study. *Psychological Medicine, 27,* 549–563.

L'Abate, L. (1994a). *A theory of personality development.* New York: Wiley.

L'Abate, L. (1994b). *Family evaluation: A psychological approach.* Thousand Oaks, CA: Sage.

L'Abate, L., & Baggett, M. S. (1997). *The self in the family.* New York: Wiley.

Lewis, J. M., Beavers, W. R., Gossett, J. T., & Phillips, V. A. (1976). *No single thread: Psychological health in family systems.* New York: Brunner/Mazel.

Linton, M. (1986). Ways of searching and the contents of memory. In D. C. Rubin (Ed.), *Autobiographical memory* (pp. 50–67). Cambridge, England: Cambridge University Press.

Liotti, G. (1988). Attachment and cognition: A guideline for the reconstruction of early pathogenic experiences in cognitive psychotherapy. In C. Perris, I. M. Blackburn, & H. H. Perris (Eds.), *Cognitive psychotherapy: Theory and practice* (pp. 62–79). Berlin: Springer-Verlag.

Magnusson, D., & Casaer, P. (Eds.). (1993). *Longitudinal research on individual development: Present status and future perspectives.* New York: Cambridge University Press.

Main, M. (1996). Introduction to the special section on attachment and psychopathology: 2. Overview of the field of attachment. *Journal of Consulting and Clinical Psychology, 64,* 237–243.

Marton, P., & Maharaj, S. (1994). Family factors in adolescent unipolar depression. *Canadian Journal of Psychiatry, 38,* 373–382.

Masten, A. S., Best, K. M., & Garmezy, N. (1990). Resilience and development: Contribution from the study of children who overcome adversity. *Development and Psychopathology, 2,* 425–444.

McClelland, D. C., & Pilon, D. A. (1983). Sources of adult motives in patterns of parent behavior in early childhood. *Journal of Personality and Social Psychology, 62,* 480–488.

McCrae, R. R., & Costa, P. T. (1994). The paradox of parental influence: Understanding retrospective studies of parent–child relations and adult personality. In C. Perris, W. A. Arrindell, & M. Eisemann (Eds.), *Parenting and psychopathology* (pp. 107–125). New York: Wiley.

McFarlane, A. H., Bellissimo, A., & Norman, G. R. (1995). Family structure, family functioning, and adolescent well-being: The transcendent influence of parental style. *Journal of Child Psychology and Psychiatry, 36,* 847–864.

Miller, A. (1990). *L'infanzia rimossa [Childhood removed].* Milan: Garzanti.

Miller, W. L., & Crabtree, B. F. (1994). Clinical research. In N. K. Denzin & Y. S. Lincoln (Eds.), *Handbook of qualitative research* (pp. 340–352). Thousand Oaks, CA: Sage.

Norden, K. A., Klein, D. N., Donaldson, S. K., Pepper, C. M., & Klein, L. M. (1995). Reports of the early home environment in DSM-III-R personality disorders. *Journal of Personality Disorders, 9,* 213–223.

Olson, D. H. (1989). *The circumplex model: Systematic assessment and treatment of families.* New York: Hawthorn Press.

Parker, G. (1983). *Parental overprotection: A risk factor in psychological development.* New York: Grune & Stratton.

Parker, G. (1988). Parental style and parental loss. In A. S. Henderson & G. D. Burrows (Eds.), *Handbook of social psychiatry* (pp. 15–25). Amsterdam: Elsevier.

Parker, G. (1994). Parental bonding and depressive disorders. In M. C. Sperling & W. H. Berman (Eds.), *Attachment in adults: Clinical and developmental perspectives* (pp. 299–312). New York: Guilford Press.

Parker, G., Tupling, H., & Brown, L. B. (1979). A Parental Bonding Instrument. *British Journal of Medical Psychology, 52,* 1–10.

Paulson, S. F., Hill, J. P., & Holmbeck, G. N. (1991). Distinguishing between closeness and parental warmth in family with seventh-grade boys and girls. *Journal of Early Adolescence, 11,* 276–293.

Perris, C. (1988). A theoretical framework for linking the experience of dysfunctional parental rearing attitudes with manifest psychopathology. *Acta Psychiatrica Scandinavica, 78,* 93–110.

Perris, C. (1994). Linking the experience of dysfunctional parental rearing with manifest psychopathology: A theoretical framework. In C. Perris, W. A. Arrindell, & M. Eisemann (Eds.), *Parenting and psychopathology* (pp. 3–34). New York: Wiley.

Perris, C., Jacobsson, L., Linström, H., von Knorring, L., & Perris, H. (1980). Development of a new inventory for assessing memories of parental rearing behaviour. *Acta Psychiatrica Scandinavica, 61,* 265–274.

Phares, V. (1992). Where's Poppa?: The relative lack of attention to the role of fathers in child and adolescent psychopathology. *American Psychologist, 47,* 656–664.

Phares, V., & Campes, B. E. (1993). Fathers and developmental psychopathology. *Current Directions in Psychological Sciences, 2,* 162–165.

Reiss, D. (1989). The represented and practicing family: Contrasting visions of family continuity. In A. Sameroff & R. Emde (Eds.), *Relationship disturbances in early childhood: A developmental approach* (pp. 191–220). New York: Basic Books.

Reiss, D., Costell, R., Jones, C., & Berkman, H. (1980). The family meets the hospital: A laboratory forecast of the encounter. *Archives of General Psychiatry, 34,* 141–154.

Reiss, D., Gonzales, S., & Kramer, N. (1986). Family process, chronic illness, and death: On the weakness of strong bonds. *Archives of General Psychiatry, 43,* 795–804.

Reiss, D., Hetherington, E. M., Plomin, R., Howe, G. W., Simmens, S. J., Henderson, S. H., O'Connor, T. J., Bussell, D. A., Anderson, E. R., & Law, T. (1995). Genetic questions for environmental studies: Differential parenting and psychopathology in adolescence. *Archives of General Psychiatry, 52,* 925–936.

Reiss, D., Howe, G. W., Simmens, S. J., & Bussell, D. A. (1996). Genetic questions for environmental studies: Differential parenting and psychopathology in adolescence. *Annual Progress in Child Psychiatry and Child Development, 29,* 206–235.

Roberts, R. E. L., & Bengston, V. L. (1996). Affective ties to parents in early adulthood and self-esteem across 20 years. *Social Psychology Quarterly, 59,* 96–106.

Robins, L., Schoenberg, S. P., Holmes, S. J., Ratcliff, K. S., Benham, A., & Works, J. (1985). Early home environment and retrospective recall. *American Journal of Orthopsychiatry, 55,* 27–41.

Rollins, B. C., & Thomas, D. L. (1979). Parental support, power, and control techniques in the socialization of children. In W. R. Burr, R. Hill, F. I. Ney, & I. L. Reiss (Eds.), *Contemporary theories about the family* (Vol. 1, pp. 317–364). New York: Free Press.

Rosenstein, D. S., & Horowitz, H. A. (1996). Adolescent attachment and psychopathology. *Journal of Consulting and Clinical Psychology, 64,* 244–253.

Rothbaum, F., Schneider, R. K., Pott, M., & Beatty, M. (1995). Early parent–child relationships and later problem behavior: A longitudinal study. *Merrill–Palmer Quarterly, 41,* 133–151.

Rutschky, K. (Ed.). (1977). *Schwarze Pädagogik [Black pedagogy].* Berlin: Ullstein.

Sameroff, A. J. (1983). Developmental systems: Contexts and evolution. In P. H. Mussen (Series Ed.) & W. Kessen (Vol. Ed.), *Handbook of child psychology: Vol. 1. History, theory, and methods* (4th ed., pp. 237–294). New York: Wiley.

Sameroff, A. J. (1993). Development models and risks. In C. H. Zeanah (Ed.), *Handbook of infant mental health* (pp. 3–12). New York: Guilford Press.

Sameroff, A. J., & Chandler, M. J. (1975). Reproductive risk and the continuum of caretaking casualty. In F. D. Horowitz, E. M. Hetherington, S. Scarr-Salapatek, & G. Siegel (Eds.), *Review of child development research* (Vol. 4, pp. 187–244). New York: Cambridge University Press.

Sameroff, A. J., & Fiese, B. H. (1990). Transactional regulation and early intervention. In S. J. Meisels & J. P. Shonkoff (Eds.), *Handbook of early childhood intervention* (pp. 199–191). New York: Cambridge University Press.

Scabini, E. (1995). *Psicologia sociale della famiglia [Social psychosociology of the family].* Turin: Bollati Boringhieri.

Schaefer, E. S. (1965). A configurational analysis of children's reports of parent behavior. *Journal of Consulting Psychology, 29,* 552–557.

Scherer, D. G., Mellow, T., Buych, D., & Anderson, C. (1996). Relation between children's perceptions of maternal mental illness and children's psychological adjustment. *Journal of Clinical Child Psychology, 25,* 156–169.

Schneewind, K. A., & Ruppert, S. (1998). *Personality and family development. An intergenerational longitudinal comparison.* Mahwah, NJ: LEA.

Sears, R. R., Maccoby, E. E., & Levin, H. (1957). *Patterns of child-rearing.* Evanston, IL: Row, Peterson.

Sebald, H. (1976). *Momism: The silent disease of America.* Chicago: Nelson Hall.

Shaw, D. S., & Bell, R. Q. (1993). Developmental theories of parental contributors to antisocial behavior, *Journal of Abnormal Child Psychology, 21,* 493–518.

Steinglass, P., Bennett, L. A., Wolin, S. J., & Reiss, D. (1987). *The alcoholic family.* New York: Basic Books.

van de Vijver, F. J. R., & Poortinga, Y. H. (1993). Cross-cultural generalization and universality. *Journal of Cross-Cultural Psychology, 13,* 387–408.

van-IJzendoorn, M. H., & Bakermans-Kranenburg, M. J. (1996). Attachment representations in mothers, fathers, adolescents, and clinical groups: A meta-analytic search for normative data. *Journal of Abnormal Child Psychology, 24,* 37–52.

van IJzendoorn, M. H., Juffer, F., & Duyvesteyn, M. G. C. (1995). Breaking the intergenerational cycle of insecure attachment: A review of the effects of attachment-based interventions on maternal sensitivity and infant security. *Journal of Child Psychology and Psychiatry, 36,* 225–248.

Waters, E., Posada, G., Crowell, J., & Lay, K. (1993). Is attachment theory ready to contribute to our understanding of disruptive behavior problems? *Development and Psychopathology, 5,* 215–224.

Watt, N. F., Anthony, E. J., Wynne, L. C., & Rolf, J. E. (Eds.). (1984). *Children at risk for schizophrenia: A longitudinal perspective.* Cambridge, England: Cambridge University Press.

Wilbur, C. B. (1984). Multiple personality and child abuse: An overview. *Psychiatric Clinics of North America, 7,* 3–7.

Wolkind, S., & Coleman, E. (1983). Adult psychiatric disorder and childhood experiences: The validity of retrospective data. *British Journal of Psychiatry, 142,* 188–191.

Young, C. H., Savola, K. L., & Phelps, E. (1991). *Inventory of longitudinal studies in the social sciences.* Newbury Park, CA: Sage.

APPENDIX. Summary of Longitudinal Studies on Parenting Styles and Child Development Outcomes

Study	Research leaders	Years covered	Subjects	n (and attrition)	Topics covered and tested
St. Louis Risk Research Project	Anthony, E., & Worland, J.	1967–1982	Schizophrenic families Manic families Physically ill families Normal control families	100→62 60→35 78→47 130→80	Extent to which children from families with a psychotic parent developed clearly defined psychopathology
Family Socialization and Developmental Competence Project	Baumrind, D.	1968–1980	Nonclinic families	134→89	Influence of contrasting patterns of parental authority on the development of instrumental competence and dysfunction throughout childhood and adolescence
Bethesda Longitudinal Study of Early Child and Family Development	Bell, R. Q., Ryder, R. G., & Halverson, C. F.	1964–1973	Nonclinic spouses	875→132	Sequence of events from early marriage by which social, emotional, and cognitive behaviors develop in the young child
Longitudinal Study of Three-Generation Families	Bengtson, V. L., & Gatz, M.	1971–1989	Three- and four-generation families; children followed over a period of 18 years	827→741	Changes and continuity in family relationships and their consequences for individual mental illness
Harvard Child Maltreatment Project	Cicchetti, D., & Ross, G.	1980–1985	Maltreating families	200→150	Etiology, intergenerational transmission, and developmental sequelae of child maltreatment
Longitudinal Study of Adaptation to Remarriage in Stepfamilies	Hetherington, E. M., & Clingempeel G.	1981–1988	Stepfamilies Nondivorced nuclear control group	210→180	Remarriage and the dynamic process of family reorganization over the 6-year period following remarriage, as well as children's development

Study	Authors	Years	Sample	N	Focus
A Longitudinal Study of Ego and Cognitive Development	Block, J., & Block, J. H.	1969–1990	Two cohorts of children	128→102	Parental child-rearing attitudes and values; child socioemotional development
The Harlem Longitudinal Study of Black Youth	Brunswick, A. F.	1968–1990	African American youth (12–18 years old)	668→200	Peer and parent influences, self-esteem, personality characteristics
Colorado Adoption Project	DeFries, J. C., Plomin, R., & Fulkes, D. W.	1977–1988	245 adoptive families 245 control families	490→459	Genetic and environmental influences on behavioral development
Virginia Longitudinal Study of Divorce	Hetherington, E. M., Cox, M., & Cox, R.	1971–1980	Divorced families Nondivorced families	72→42 72→59	Responses to the family crisis of divorce and their effects on child outcome
Understanding and Prediction of Delinquent Child Behavior	Patterson, G. R., Reid, J. B., & Dishion, T. J.	1984–1989	Males from selected high-risk fourth-grade classrooms	206→203	Influence of family structure and relations on children's antisocial behavior, substance use, and depression
Rochester Longitudinal Study	Sameroff, A. J., Seifer, R., Zax, M., & Barocas, R.	1970–1988	Women with a history of mental illness Women with no history of mental illness	337→180	Women's birth experiences and cognitive, psychomotor, emotional, and social functioning of their offspring
Epidemiologic Study of Behavior Problems in Children	Earls, F., & Garrison, W.	1974–1983	Children (1–3 years old; four cohorts)	523→134	Acute and chronic stress in families; developmental progress and problems
Adolescent Health Care Evaluation Study	Earls, F., Robins, L., & Stiffman, A.	1984–1989	Adolescents (13–18 years old; two cohorts)	2,788→650	Home environment and family history; physical/mental health and substance abuse
Mother–Child Research Project	Egeland, B., & Sroufe, A.	1975–1989	Primiparous women	267→190	Child maltreatment and developmental psychopathology

(continued)

APPENDIX (*continued*)

Project	Authors	Years	Sample	N	Focus
The New York High-Risk Project	Erlenmeyer-Kimling, L.	1971–1987	Children of schizophrenic and depressed parents Children of normal parents	206→191	Genetic factors in biobehavioral, psychosocial, and clinical deviance; environmental aspects of resiliency
The Baltimore Study: Adolescent Parenthood and Transmission of Social Disadvantage	Furstenberg, F. F., & Brooks-Gunn, J.	1966–1986	Three-generation families followed over a period of 20 years	1,328→1,034	Pregnant teenagers' attitudes about their children and their family relationships
The UCLA High-Risk Project	Goldstein, M. J.	1964–1979	Disturbed adolescents followed over a period of 15 years	64→51	Parental communication deviance, family role structure, and thought disorders
The Early Training Project	Gray, S., & Klaus, R.	1962–1976	Children with educational disadvantages (four cohorts)	90→86	Parental attitudes; child social disorders and resiliency
Adolescence and Family Development Project	Hauser, S. T., Power, S., Jacobson, A., & Noam, G. G.	1978–1991	Adolescents (14–16 years old) Psychiatric hospitalized adolescents (14–16 years old) Diabetic adolescents (14–16 years old)	76→17 70→15 55→42	Family interaction, parental rearing, and adolescent psychosocial development
A Longitudinal Study of the Consequences of Child Abuse	Herrenkohl, R. C., & Herrenkohl, E. C.	1975–1982	Maltreated children (1 to 6 years old) Control children (1 to 6 years old)	439→152 250→201	Maltreatment of children, influence of welfare agencies, and child development
Development of Aggressive Behavior	Huesmann, C. T., & Eron, L. D.	1960–1981	Children (8 years old) followed over a period of 21 years	875→632	Child aggression, peer relations, and child-rearing factors
Guidance Study	Huffine, C., Honzik, M., & Macfarlane, J. W.	1928–1982	Three-generation families followed over a period of 54 years	248→157	Parental counseling and preschool children's problems

Study	Investigator	Years	Sample	N	Focus
Houston Parent–Child Development Center Project	Johnson, D. L.	1971–1989	Mexican American Families with a 1-year-old child (eight cohorts)	390→127	Mothers' child-rearing, social support, and behavioral problems
Intergenerational Transmission of Deviance	Kandel, D.	1971–1990	Adolescents (14–17 years old) followed over a period of 19 years	1,661→1,160	Marital and parental histories, parent–child interactions, and problem behaviors and delinquency
The Woodlawn Mental Health Longitudinal Community Epidemiological Project	Kellam, S., Ensminger, M., & Branch, J.	1964–1975	Children (6 years old) followed over a period of 11 years (three cohorts)	1,770→939	Developing family structure and relationships; child psychological well-being
The Family Research Project	Langner, T. S.	1966–1972	Children (6–18 years old) followed over a period of 16 years (two cohorts)	2,034→1,393	Child-rearing practices and development of child psychological disorders
The Iowa HABIT Project	Loney, J., Paternite, C. E., & Langhorne, J. E.	1967–1989	Outpatients of psychiatrical clinics (6–12 years old) followed over a period of 22 years	135→77	Parental child-rearing styles and development of child behavior problems
Cambridge–Somerville Youth Study	McCord, J.	1936–1976	High-risk children (4–11 years old) / Low-risk children (4–11 years old)	253→235 / 253→235	Parental antisocial characteristics; child social behaviors and resiliency
Trajectories of Health and Illness: A Longitudinal Follow-Up Study of Child Psychiatric Patients	Noam, G. G.	1984–1990	Adolescents with psychiatric illness followed over a period of 6 years (two cohorts)	229→94	Family functioning and stress; child social adjustment level
A Study of Child Rearing and Child Development in Normal Families and Families with Affective Disorders	Radke-Yarrow, M.	1980–1991	Families with affective disorders / Normal families	80→60 / 50→30	Child-rearing practices and child development

(continued)

APPENDIX (*continued*)

Patterns of Child Rearing	Sears, R., Maccoby, E., & Levin, H.	1951–1989	Children (5 years old) followed over a period of 26 years	379→89	Child-rearing practices and child development and problems
New York Longitudinal Study	Thomas, A., Chess, S., Lerner, J., & Lerner, R.	1956–1988	White European American children (1–6 years old) from 84 families; White European American mentally retarded children (5–11 years old); Puerto Rican children (1–7 years old)	133→131 52→52 97→97	Family structure and parent–child relationships; development of clinical symptomatology and social problems
The Stony Brook High-Risk Project	Weintraub, S.	1971–1982	Children of schizophrenic parents; Children of depressed parents; Children of bipolar parents; Children of normal parents	80→44 54→48 134→54 136→65	Parental psychological adjustment and psychopathology; child psychological problems
University of Rochester Child and Family Study	Wynne, L., & Cole, R.	1972–1980	Children (4–10 years old) and their parents (six cohorts)	278→216	Parental mental disorders and child functioning level

CHAPTER 8

⟹·◇·⟸

Intergenerational Relationships in Modern Families

VICTOR G. CICIRELLI

In past years, a standard definition of "family" was accepted by society as a whole. The U.S. Bureau of the Census (1991) has defined a family as two or more persons residing together and related by birth, marriage, or adoption. A family so defined is granted certain legal privileges by society, and it also assumes certain obligations important to its functioning as a social unit. In the United States, the privileges include such things as tax breaks for children, family medical insurance, Social Security benefits, rights of inheritance, right to consent to medical treatment for family members, and so on. The obligations include such things as maintaining a household, dividing household tasks, supporting and protecting children, providing a legacy for the family, and the like.

A standard definition of family sets a boundary, making it clear which individuals are included or excluded as family members, and thus identifying the family unit. Until recently, the family as defined above has been represented by the traditional two-generation or nuclear family, where family members live together in the same household performing the necessary functions to survive as a unit, with the father as sole breadwinner while the mother stays home and rears the children. Current conceptions of the traditional family include modified parental roles with careers for both father and mother. Complementary to the nuclear family are the connections to other close family members in direct lineage (known as the "modified extended family," including children, grandchildren, and the father's and mother's families of origin) and to more remote relatives (known as the "kin network"). These wider conceptions of family include "collateral kin" (family members of the same generation), as well as "ascending kin" and "descending kin" (family members of different generations). In earlier decades, whether members of the extended family and kin network lived close by in different households or at a distance because of migration, their lifestyles were still relatively similar because a relatively homogeneous Western culture existed, with similar norms and values for everyone.

However, in the 1990s it has become impossible to provide a standard definition of the family. Rapid advances in science and technology, economic and industrial changes, and social and cultural changes have produced a fragmented and heterogeneous society with multiple and conflicting values and norms. In the multicultural society now existing, the phrase "a typical family" is an oxymoron (Peterson, 1996).

Individuals in modern society have developed new groupings to satisfy emerging needs and desires (Marciano & Sussman, 1992). These have led to new household and living arrangements along with alternative lifestyles. However, such groups no longer fit the older definition of a family. At the present time, there is confusion as to whether these groups can be considered families. For one thing, their legal privileges and societal obligations are not determined, nor is it clear who is consistently included or excluded as a family member. For example, many individuals no longer spend most of their lives in one type of grouping: They may marry, divorce, remain single for a while, become part of a cohabiting couple, then remarry, and so on.

Perhaps such situations would be only a minor problem if the traditional family type represented most members of society; however, the traditional family has shrunk from its formerly dominant position in society until it is now a minority type itself. More important, these newer groups are becoming the dominant forms of social units. Such confusion points to the necessity of revising or expanding the definition of family to fit present-day realities.

A MODERN DEFINITION OF "FAMILY"

It would seem that a more modern definition would regard the family as a disjunctive concept, defined in terms of different and multiple criteria. A given family type would not have to embody all the criteria, but might fit some of the criteria and not others.

As a first step, "family" may be defined as a household of related or unrelated individuals (or a combination of both) who have an exclusive relationship with each other of long duration, and who have a commitment to provide love, care, and nurturance to each other. Such a definition goes beyond the present legal criteria, and places importance on psychosocial or cultural criteria.

One might even go beyond this to state that a family consists of two or more individuals who have a commitment to nurture and protect each other in an exclusive and durable relationship. This eliminates the restriction that a family necessarily lives in the same household. With modern rapid transportation and communications, there can be frequent communication between family members and participation in each other's lives without having to reside in the same physical space, such as a household.

In short, the criteria for defining a family should be broadened or extended to include social and cultural criteria. This would recognize the sense in which many groupings of people with differing values and norms consider themselves families in a multicultural society, regardless of whether marriage is involved. Such factors as a common household, living arrangements, and alternative lifestyles could be included among the attributes used to define a family.

Within this framework, we can define "family" as a group of individuals existing (1) when two individuals are legally married; *or* (2) when two or more individuals are genetically connected; *or* (3) when one or more individuals are legally adopted by an adult; *or* (4) when unmarried and unrelated individuals share a household and living arrangements of long duration and exclusivity, with a relationship characterized by love and commitment; *or* (5) when unmarried and unrelated individuals share a relationship with love and commitment, but do not share the same household; *or* (6) an individual lives alone but interacts, participates, and communicates in a committed relationship with one or more individuals with genetic commonality.

Such a broad definition allows us to regard various groupings of individuals as specific (albeit diverse) family types, and provides a common ground for dealing with them. It eliminates the necessity of talking about household and living arrangements and alternative lifestyles as separate from families. Instead, we can utilize the latter to help define specific types of families, such as the multigenerational family, the single-parent family, the heterosexual cohabitant family, the reconstituted or blended family, the childless family, the singlehood "family," the homosexual cohabitant family, and the communal family.

GENERATIONAL STRUCTURE OF THE FAMILY

Before proceeding further, we must take into consideration another factor in relation to the family—that is, its generational structure. The notion of "generational structure" involves the use of genetic criteria in defining a family, but in a somewhat larger and more elaborate context.

Individuals may be related by blood or adoption to others in the same generation (collateral kin, such as siblings and cousins); they may also be related to others in different generations (ascending and descending kin, such as parents and children). Whereas intragenerational relationships exist within a single generation, intergenerational relationships can extend over two or more generations to include multigenerational relationships (as found in three-, four-, and even five-generation families with grandparents and grandchildren, great-grandparents and great-grandchildren, and even great-great-grandparents and great-great-grandchildren). Extending the genetic criteria to intergenerational relationships in a defining a family involves a merging of the concepts of "family," "extended family," and "kin network." Obviously, on the interpersonal level, some relationships between individuals in this enlarged conception of family will be remote and rather meaningless, but a pool of family members exists from which certain individuals are selected for closer relationships. This notion of "family" bears some resemblance to Antonucci and Akiyama's (1994) concept of "convoy"—the network of individuals who are close and important to a person over time, providing supportive relationships.

It is assumed that in any family, some generational structure or organization exists; this allows us to extend the concept of family even to singlehood, paradoxical as that may seem. A person living alone but in close communication with a sibling, a mother, and so on has a family (by genetic definition) that influences his or her life through the quality of interpersonal relationships. It is also assumed that different types of generational organizations or structures can exist, and that they are related to the quality of the interaction and interpersonal relationships between family members. For example, if an individual has connections to a sibling, a grandparent, and an uncle, there will be a different quality of interaction and interpersonal relationship in each case. In this view of the family, we are concerned with the different generational structures that link various family members and that are related to differences in the quality of interpersonal relationships.

In the remainder of this chapter, my objectives are (1) to identify and describe various existing family types according to this broad definition of "family," noting any differences in the generational structure of various family types; (2) to determine any differences in the quality of interpersonal relationships that empirical studies may suggest; and (3) to bring out possible implications of the family types for the mental health of family members.

MODERN FAMILY TYPES

Before each family type is discussed in turn, the reader is reminded that no one type of family constitutes a majority of the population. Also, an individual's membership in a given type of family may change over time as relationships change. Marriage, divorce, widowhood, separation, birth or death of children, cohabitation, "coming out" as a homosexual, and the like can all signal transition into a different family type.

Multigenerational Family

The multigenerational family is an emerging family type that has received much publicity in recent years, because the increasing life span of older people allows for an increase in the number of generations within a family. The two-generation family is the nuclear type. The three-generation family involves both intra- and intergenerational structure, and is reasonably common. What are now emerging from individuals' greater life expectancies are four- and five-generation families. This increase in the number of generations also increases the complexity of the intergenerational connections within a family. As noted above, we can think in terms of grandparents, great-grandparents, and great-great-grandparents, and of grandchildren, great-grandchildren, and great-great-grandchildren.

As such, the multigenerational family represents the prototype of an aging family with unique characteristics. It consists of many individuals with a long relationship history with one another; individuals in the same role for extended periods of time (e.g., a woman may occupy the role of mother for 70 years or more); individuals added to the family through births and marriages; older individuals facing unique developmental tasks, such as retirement, widowhood, and chronic illness; and individuals dealing with new and complex family relationships as the family continues to evolve over long time periods. From the viewpoint of the great- or great-great-grandparents themselves, there seem to be certain benefits: Multigenerational relationships can give them a sense of greater longevity and perhaps a feeling of symbolic immortality as their lineage continues to expand, and their newer descendants can sometimes stimulate their lives with new activities, although there may be too great a distance between them in age or geography for the latter to happen (Doka & Mertz, 1988). Also, multigenerational families may have benefits for the family as a whole, because additional generations are available to care for grandchildren and to provide more stability and wisdom to the family. On the other hand, the greater longevity associated with multigenerational families also increases the burden of providing care for so many older generations in their declining years. A further problem is associated with a trend toward fewer children in each generation as a consequence of decreased fertility, resulting in a verticalization of family structure (the "beanpole" family), with more generations but fewer people in a generation (Bengtson, Rosenthal, & Burton, 1990).

However, there is evidence to indicate that the beanpole multigenerational family may not be the rapidly growing family type that Bengtson et al. (1990) originally suggested. On the contrary, recent evidence seems to indicate that although three-generation families are common, the frequency of four- and five-generation families is low and is increasing very little. Only for individuals in their 90s is there a slight increase in multigenerational families at the present time, with fewer than half reporting four or more generations (Farkas & Hogan, 1995; Johnson & Troll, 1996). Whether this is to be a predominant family type of the future is still uncertain; however, Uhlenberg (1995) pointed out that the drop in fertility in the United States after 1965 will not have a major impact on the families of the elderly for several more decades.

Single-Parent Family

The single-parent family can consist of either a father and child or a mother and child (although the mother–child family is far more common). As a result of the high divorce rate and the increase in unwed mothers, this is one of the fastest-growing family types. It is estimated that half of young children in the United States in the 1990s will spend some time in a one-parent family before reaching the age of 18, because of divorced or unwed parents (Bumpass, 1990).

In a single-mother family, both mother and children tend to suffer for lack of income, and may have to depend on other relatives for help. This may lead to intragenerational structures involving the mother's siblings and cousins, as well as intergenerational structures involving the children's grandparents (and perhaps also great-aunts and great-uncles), who are likely to have more financial resources than the single mother. Depending on whether contact with the child's father and the father's family of origin is maintained, the structure of the single-mother family may be rather complex. As the family ages, additional generations of the family may also be present.

A variant of the single-parent family is the grandparent–grandchild family. As of the 1990 census (Atchley, 1994), some 5% of U.S. children lived with grandparents (without parents in the household) in situations where the parents were deceased or were incapacitated by severe problems. Grandparents serving as surrogate parents were found more frequently among ethnic minorities.

Reconstituted or Blended Family

"Reconstituted" or "blended" families are formed when two previously divorced or widowed individuals marry, with one or both having children from a prior liaison. According to Glick (1989), more than two-thirds of divorced men and women eventually remarry, thus forming blended families. The blended family is a stepfamily with varying numbers of steprelatives; it can be exceedingly complex, particularly when blended families have been formed in more than one generation or when a number of previous marriages are involved. Similarly, the variety of generational structures possible in this family type can be very large, involving intragenerational stepsiblings and other stepkin, as well as a variety of intergenerational blood relatives and steprelatives: parents, grandparents, children, and so on.

Heterosexual Cohabitant Family

Basically, "cohabitation" is voluntary choice by two individuals to live together. They may be sexually active or celibate, in a temporary or permanent relationship, and with or without children. The cohabiting partners may have no desire to become married, or they may perceive the cohabitation as a steppingstone to a common-law or otherwise legal marriage.

For young people, cohabitation is often called "trial marriage," "shacking up," "living together," "concubinage," and so on (Buunk & van Driel, 1989). Heterosexual cohabitation occurs with high frequency among young adults, especially among the less educated; in a recent national survey of sexual practices, some 90% of women in the 20-to-29 age group were in some kind of partnership, whereas only half were married (Laumann, Gagnon, Michael, & Michaels, 1994).

For the elderly, cohabitation may occur for financial reasons (e.g., they may lose Social Security or other pension income if they remarry) or the resistance of the partners' families to the marriage (e.g., adult children may dislike a proposed new spouse or may fear the loss of their inheritance).

For younger cohabitants, the intragenerational structure may involve relationships with each partner's siblings and other collateral kin. The intergenerational structure may involve connections with each partner's parents, grandparents, and children (if they exist). Among older cohabitants, the intergenerational structure may involve connections with each partner's children and grandchildren. (If cohabitation follows previous marriages and blended families, obviously generational structures will be very complex, as each partner brings complex family structures to the cohabitation.)

Homosexual Cohabitant Family (Gays and Lesbians)

In addition to many younger individuals who have openly declared their homosexuality, there are many older individuals who have "come out of the closet," perhaps leaving their traditional families behind in order to express their homosexuality. Obviously, not all homosexuals are involved in steady relationships; many live as singles, changing partners as expedient or desired. However, a number of homosexuals form rather stable couples, and the partners live for long periods committed to each other; these homosexual couples can be regarded as a type of family. One can consider such homosexual cohabitation as a family if the partners have a serious commitment to each other, regardless of the existence of legal sanction. One or both partners may have children or grandchildren, either from previous marriages or by adoption.

Openly homosexual adults make up only a small portion of the U.S. population—2.8% for gays and 1.4% for lesbians (Laumann et al., 1994). However, from 40% to 60% of gay men and from 45% to 80% of lesbian women are involved in close, steady relationships with a single partner (Peplau & Cochran, 1990). About half of the gay couples and three-fourths of the lesbian couples live together and may be said to constitute families. Many of these unions are of more than 10 years' duration, with stability as great as that of heterosexual couples (Blumstein & Schwartz, 1983).

The potential intragenerational structure of the family involves the siblings and collateral kin of each partner, while the potential intergenerational structure includes parents, grandparents, and possibly children and grandchildren. However, the extent to which the potential generational structures become shared, real family relationships depends on the degree to which each homosexual partner is accepted by his or her own and the other's family members.

Singlehood "Family"

Most adults spend some portion of their lives as single individuals without a spouse (or a cohabiting partner) and without children, as a result of personal choice, career demands, lack of opportunity, divorce, or widowhood (Macklin, 1987). This is a small group of people; approximately 10% of older people have never married (Huyck, 1994). To view singlehood as a "family" may seem puzzling. But, given our previous criteria, singles living alone can still be regarded as a family because most have some blood relationships (intragenerational ties with siblings or cousins and/or intergenerational ties with parents, grandparents, aunts, uncles, nieces, and nephews). In this sense, other relatives serve as substitutes for some of the roles typically filled by a spouse, children, or deceased parents. Single individuals still have a position within a family; it may differ from the traditional nuclear family unit, but family roles still exist.

Childless Family

The childless family consists of a couple without children. Among young couples, possibilities for children may still exist, but for older couples childlessness is a permanent state. According to Johnson and Troll (1996), about one-third of elders over age 70 are childless, but these authors did not distinguish between those who were married and those who were widowed or divorced.

The intragenerational structure of the childless family may include the siblings and cousins of each spouse. The intergenerational structure may include each spouse's parents and grandparents, as well as possibly nieces and nephews.

Communal Family

A "communal" family consists of a group of individuals who voluntarily share a household and the tasks involved, and have a commitment to help and protect each other. Among the elderly, communal families can be very important to help them avoid nursing homes or other institutions, and they may maintain close relationships with each other. Each person in a communal family may have both intragenerational and intergenerational kin; for the most part, such relationships are not shared with others in the communal family.

INTERGENERATIONAL RELATIONSHIPS IN VARIOUS FAMILY TYPES

In this portion of the chapter, the nature of intergenerational relationships within the family is examined for each of the various family types previously discussed. As an extension of the genetic criteria for determining the definition of "family," it provides a basis for considering diverse groups as specific family types. However, and more important, my hypothesis is that the quality of interpersonal relationships among family types is greatly influenced by generational structure as manifested by intragenerational and intergenerational relationships. In other words, both the number and kind of family relationships within the generational structure are associated with the quality of interpersonal relationships, which in turn influences the mental health of family members. In short, the present model is as follows: Generational structure (number and kinds of existing relatives genetically connected to family members) influences the quality of the family members' interpersonal relationships, which in turn influences mental health. (Obviously there will be a reciprocal relationship.) Unfortunately, the studies and data available to document this model are extremely limited.

Multigenerational Family

The generational structure in a multigenerational family can be quite complex, and, obviously, the quality of interpersonal relationships will vary with particular family members. However, the generational structure itself should lead to certain expectations between generations that will influence the quality of interpersonal relationships.

As pointed out earlier, families of more than three generations are relatively uncommon. In terms of family relationships, the greatest amounts of contact and exchange of assistance occur between adjacent generations (parents and children), falling off rapidly as the intergenerational distance increases (Mangen, Bengtson, & Landry, 1988; Uhlenberg, 1995). Nevertheless, some degree of relationship between family members separated by two or more generations exists, especially between grandparents and grandchildren. There is a large literature on grandparental relationships—too large to summarize here (see Cherlin & Furstenberg, 1986; Kornhaber, 1996).

Because grandparents' relationships with grandchildren vary widely, there have been attempts to classify grandparents according to grandparenting style (e.g., Neugarten & Weinstein, 1964; Robertson, 1977; Kivnick, 1982). One important dimension that emerges in all the typologies is the degree to which grandparents desire to be, or are, involved with their grandchildren.

Relationships with grandparents can continue well into the grandchildren's adulthood, until the grandparents' death. According to Roberto and Stroes (1995), some 89% of their college student sample had at least one living grandparent. The students' contact with their grandmother was monthly or less, but they did visit, seek advice, help with chores, and in general enjoyed the relationship. Relationships with grandmothers were rated as stronger than those with grandfathers. Using a somewhat older sample (ranging in age from 18 to 51), Hodgson (1995) found that most respondents maintained relationships and felt quite close to at least one grandparent, with proximity and closeness of feeling the main reasons for contact. In general, relationships with grandmothers were seen as closer than those with grandfathers, and were particularly close if a grandparent had acted as a surrogate parent at some point earlier in life.

In general, relationships between young grandchildren and grandparents are mediated by the children's parents (King & Elder, 1995; Kornhaber, 1996; Mangen et al., 1988; Robertson, 1977). The quality of the grandchild–grandparent relationship in general depends on the quality of the parent–grandparent relationship and the grandparent's perceived supportiveness toward the parent, as well as on the quality of the parent's relationship with the child. Positive mediating relationships with the parent are more important for the child's relationships with paternal grandparents than for those with maternal grandparents.

Similarly, a child's parents (or grandparents) may foster relationships between the child and a great-grandparent (Doka & Mertz, 1988; Wentowski, 1985). Although the frequency of contact with great-grandparents reported in these studies depended on the distance involved, the elders' health, and the closeness of the relationships with the middle two generations, most great-grandmothers viewed the relationship very positively, seeing it as symbolic of family success and vitality. They saw great-grandparenthood as similar to being a grandparent, except that contact and the kinds of activities they could undertake with their great-grandchildren were limited by their declining physical strength. As with grandparenthood, great-grandparental relationships varied from close to remote.

Blended or Reconstituted Family

In general, family relationships are more difficult in the blended family. Family relationships become more voluntary as the size and complexity of the generational structure increases, and tend to be weakened overall (Cooney, 1994). Compared to members of intact families, stepfamily members have less contact, poorer relationship quality, and less family support over the long term; this effect is greater for father–stepmother remarriages than for mother–stepfather remarriages (White, 1994).

Relationships with grandparents in a blended family depend to a great extent on whether a grandparent's adult child is a grandchild's custodial parent. If the grandparent disapproves of the custodial adult child's divorce, the relationship with the grandchild may be weakened. If the adult child is not the custodial parent, then the child's relationship with the grandparent depends on the extent of visitation granted by the custodial parent; some grandparents have taken legal action to seek visitation rights (Kornhaber, 1996).

A child in a blended family may have as many four grandparents and four stepgrandparents. Depending on the age of the child when the remarriage took place and whether the child resides with a particular stepgrandparent's adult child, the child's relationship as a young adult with that stepgrandparent may be stronger or weaker (Trygstad & Sanders, 1995). If a stepgrandparent has not accepted the divorce or the new marriage, this will have negative effects on the relationship with the stepgrandchild. In general, the relationship is pleasant but neutral, with little exchange of support. Stepgrandparent relationships are better when the adult child's remarriage has occurred after widowhood than after divorce.

Single-Parent Family

As noted above, single parenthood can result from out-of-wedlock births, as well as from divorce and widowhood; in general, it is more common among low-income families (particularly African Americans). Although a sizable proportion of divorcees remarry, singlehood remains a permanent status for those who do not. Overall, children who grew up in a family with a single divorced parent had weaker relationships in all aspects of family solidarity in adulthood (White, 1994); this effect was stronger for the noncustodial parent.

Many grandparents are concerned about losing contact with grandchildren after parents divorce; this is especially true for paternal grandparents after a son has divorced. Because custody of children typically goes to the mother, the relationship with the mother and maternal grandparents continues, but up to a third of children of divorce have little or no contact with fathers or paternal grandparents (Booth & Amato, 1994; Cooney, 1994). When parental divorce occurs in midlife, custody is not an issue, but children's relationships with fathers diminish while their relationships with mothers continue relatively unchanged (Cooney, 1994).

In a large number of cases where their adult child becomes a single parent, grandparents provide considerable assistance to their child and become quite involved in the care of grandchildren (Bengtson et al., 1990), either within a three-generation household or from a distance. In one study, maintaining communication and good family relationships with both the younger and older generation were important factors in subjects' functioning successfully as single parents (Olson & Haynes, 1993).

Increasingly, grandparents are taking over a new and important role— that is, helping to raise grandchildren when parents are unable or unwilling to do so (Giarrusso, Silverstein, & Bengtson, 1996; Jendrek, 1994; Minkler & Roe, 1996). This may be a satisfying role for those grandparents who want to be more actively involved with their grandchildren, but it is often a great burden for those grandparents who have limited resources or poor health. They may want to maintain more of a distance from grandchildren, but feel a sense of obligation to provide care when their own children have failed in their parental duties. Although stressed by their responsibilities, the grandparents serving as surrogate parents in the absence of parents also find positive qualities in their relation with their grandchildren; they love the grandchildren and feel very attached to them.

Heterosexual Cohabitant Family

Most heterosexual cohabitations are relatively short-lived, leading either to breakups or to marriage. Long-term cohabitations (i.e., ones lasting more than 10 years) are relatively infrequent (Blumstein & Schwartz, 1983). Because there is relatively less social stigma attached to heterosexual cohabitation today than in earlier times (Ganong, Coleman, & Maples, 1990), relationships with parents and other family members are likely to be maintained, but may be strained by these relatives' reservations about the cohabitation arrangement (Buunk & van Driel, 1989). Buunk and van Driel found that cohabiting women indicated strained relationships with parents more than did men; in some cases there was severe family conflict. However, cohabitation appeared to be both more stable and more acceptable if the partners were older and if they had been previously married.

Homosexual Cohabitant Family

Perhaps more than in any other type of family, intergenerational relationships may be absent or strained in gay or lesbian families (Fullmer, 1995).

Although both partners may have living parents and grandparents from their families of origin, and some may have children and grandchildren (from previous heterosexual unions or through adoption), the homosexual cohabitants may be rejected by members of the extended family. This is particularly the case for older homosexuals, of whom from 14% to 59% (as reported in previous literature) have children (Quam & Whitford, 1992); a major concern for them is fear of rejection by children and grandchildren. For most, relationships with children and grandchildren are not close, but they are somewhat better for lesbians than for gay men. A further concern for gay or lesbian parents is how to inform children of their sexual orientation, particularly when such parents have custody of the children (Allen & Demo, 1995; Fullmer, 1995).

Whether or not homosexuals can expect care from family members should they need it is another question, although many aging gays and lesbians depend on families for support. Lesbians face potential family conflicts in middle age, at a time when daughters are normally expected to provide care to elderly parents (Warshow, 1991). A parent who does not accept a lesbian daughter's lifestyle and partner may also be unwilling to accept needed help.

Singlehood "Family"

For some people, singlehood is a state of long duration, often lasting for the individuals' entire adult lives. However, many singles have lived with family members (parents, siblings, etc.) all their adult lives and have close family relationships (Rubinstein, 1987; Rubinstein, Alexander, Goodman, & Luborsky, 1991). Despite being childless, older singles have indirect descending kin; almost 60% of Rubinstein et al.'s (1991) sample had key relationships with nieces and nephews.

Childless Family

Childless couples who have living parents or grandparents tend to have relationships with them similar to those in traditional families. However, with no direct descendants, childless couples tend to form special relationships with certain nieces and nephews.

Communal Family

Little is known about the intergenerational relationships of adults living in communal families with their biological families. If they have living family members, their relationships with them may be expected to be less close than those of other family types.

IMPLICATIONS OF INTERGENERATIONAL
RELATIONSHIPS FOR MENTAL HEALTH

That earlier generations of the family affect the mental health of later generations is well known, given the hereditary patterns of a number of mental and physical diseases (e.g., bipolar disorders); psychosocial transmission of certain behavior patterns in intergenerational relationships can occur as well (Kornhaber, 1996). Narcissistic, distant, abusive, and insensitive grandparents produce dysfunctional family relationships. By the same token, good intergenerational relationships can promote good mental health.

Various family types may be related to differences in the quality of relationships between family members. For example, relationships within traditional multigenerational families are likely to be closer than the intergenerational relationships of cohabiting homosexual families, in view of frequent family rejection of the homosexual lifestyle. However, regardless of the type of family, existing research makes clear that maintaining close intergenerational relationships within the family contributes to better mental health (Antonucci & Akiyama, 1994). Some family types may promote mental health more than others, depending upon various aspects of the relationships. In some family types, the degree of attachment may be greater and relationships may be closer or warmer, in comparison to other family types characterized by more distant and uncaring relationships. One factor may be negative cultural stereotypes associated with less traditional family types: Married adults and children whose parents are married are viewed more favorably than those who are divorced, unmarried, cohabiting, and so on (Ganong et al., 1990). Such stereotypes influence how individuals of different family types view themselves, resulting in lower self-esteem, depression, and so on. In addition, individuals of different family types may encounter social problems related to their family status, such as rejection of cohabiting families by others. Also, certain family types (e.g., single-parent families) are likely to have diminished economic resources, with indirect effects on the physical and psychological well-being of family members. In one study, single mothers who lived with or near their extended families were less likely to be depressed and upset than were those who lived at a distance (Wagner, 1993). Gay and lesbian couples may experience reduction of stress and better psychological well-being if they disclose their homosexuality to their kin, but they risk other threats to well-being (e.g., reduced self-esteem) if disclosure leads to rejection and alienation (Fullmer, 1995).

Problems experienced by a member of one generation can negatively affect members of another generation. A recent study by Pillemer and Suitor (1991) showed that when an adult child had emotional problems, health problems, or substance use problems, or was under serious stress, elderly parents reported more depression symptomatology. Similarly, later-life divorce or widowhood of elderly parents can negatively affect the relationship with adult children (particularly for elderly fathers), leading to reduced well-being (Aquilino, 1994).

Are Less Traditional Family Types Harmful to Mental Health?

Despite some evidence showing increased incidence of poor mental health among certain family types, a good deal of controversy still exists as to whether the traditional family type is the norm and other family types (e.g., the single-parent family and the blended family) are deviations that have led to negative mental health consequences for family members. Popenoe (1992) sees the traditional family has having been weakened over recent decades, becoming smaller and less stable. Whereas marriages that endure provide emotionally rewarding relationships for family members, broken marriages may lead to a poorer quality of life for both children and adults. Others (Cohler & Altergott, 1994; Fassel, 1992b; Orthner, 1992) see the traditional family type as outmoded and very much in transition today, with norms and values that no longer apply.

We might ask whether the traditional nuclear family was ever predominant, or whether it should have ever been used as a standard to judge an effectively functioning family group. In earlier decades of the 20th century, in many families there were extramarital affairs, extreme father domination, incest, child abuse, neglect, alcoholism, delinquency, divorce, and so on; there was often little love or nurturing of the children. In short, having two parents, with the mother in the home as a full-time parent for the children, was not in itself a guarantee of a functional family. Indeed, the fact that large numbers of present-day adult children who grew up in traditional families have not emulated them (witness the increase in other family types) may indicate that the traditional family is fundamentally flawed as a norm for today's social realities (Popenoe, 1992).

Whether other family types are necessarily associated with dysfunctional outcomes is also open to question. For example, increased poverty has been associated with the single-parent family, which in turn has had a negative effect on children, leading to subsequent societal problems (Elshtain, 1997). Other studies have shown harm to children in divorced single-parent families or adjustment problems in newly reconstituted families (e.g., Wallerstein & Blakeslee, 1992). However, Skolnick and Rosencranz (1997) assert that much research in this area has methodological limitations (lack of adequate control groups, correlational rather than causal designs, etc.), and that it paints a darker picture of the single-parent family than the results actually justify. Single-parent families may not be the cause of children's problems, but both may be caused by underlying social conditions. Other scholars in the area view divorce (and subsequent single-parent or reconstituted families) not as deviant, but as necessary and positive reactions to family situations that were no longer viable because of changing conditions (Ahrons & Rodgers, 1992;

Fassel, 1992a). Passel views divorce as a stimulus for positive growth of children in many families; it often leads to increased independence and resilience, access to a wide range of feelings, and the ability to walk away from unhealthy relationships and accept change. With regard to blended or reconstituted families, which are often seen as a source of problems, there may indeed be difficult adjustments when children and adults from two previously broken families come together to form a new family in a single household. However, adjustments are made within a few years, and most family members achieve a satisfactory lifestyle.

In studies of the effects of various family types on the family members, the effects of the generational structure of the family have not been made clear. In the single-parent family, the generational structure may include grandparents and members of the ex-spouse's family who are available to provide help. Indeed, the role of grandparents is often increased in such families, in comparison to the traditional family (Robertson, 1994). In the blended family, the generational structure may include an enlarged and positive support system. Cohabitation and singlehood as family types may be quite functional on their own; however, their generational structures may reinforce healthy functioning. Similarly, gay, lesbian, and communal family types may receive support from their generational structures. Certainly we should not conclude that these family types represent a failure of family life, with deleterious effects on family members, without consideration of how the generational structure influences family functioning. The point is that these alternative family types may deviate from the norm of the traditional family type, but they are not necessarily destroying their members and society.

The concept of the true multigenerational family is still emerging, and whether it proves to be functional or dysfunctional depends on the number of members of additional generations in such a family, as well as their competence level and resources. With regard to alternative family types, these family forms have been emerging for a long time and will continue to do so. Increasing acceptance will lead to greater use of generational connections and more functional families. From an evolutionary viewpoint, it may be that new family types represent attempts to adjust to changing circumstances. Changes are taking place in society, industry, global economies, religion, government, and the culture, making adaptive changes in the family necessary. Some family subtypes may prove highly functional and others dysfunctional in particular settings. What is needed is research to identify the factors that lead to successful functioning of members in the various family types in particular circumstances, as well as the factors associated with dysfunctional outcomes.

Clinical Interventions

Mental health problems arise among individuals representing all family types; given present evidence, it is not clear that particular family types are intrinsically dysfunctional for family members, whereas other family types promote better mental health. According to Skolnick and Rosencranz (1997), children from a conflict-filled traditional family can have worse problems than children of divorced parents. It is recognized, however, that individuals in certain family types may be subject to various stressors to a greater degree than those in other family types. For example, an unwed single mother may face social stigma and lack of social support, as well as economic problems. A gay or lesbian may also experience social stigma and rejection by family members and the wider society. A child in a blended family may experience the stress of adjusting to a new stepparent and stepsiblings, in addition to trying to maintain a relationship with the noncustodial parent. However, stress does not in itself imply poor mental health. According to Antonucci and Akiyama (1994), social support from family members helps to buffer the individual against stress and to promote psychological well-being. On the other hand, the quality of social relationships with family members, rather than the structural characteristics of the family, is the essential factor in well-being. Having family members who get on an individual's nerves can lead to depression or other mental health problems, just as having family members who are verbally or physically abusive can do so.

When an individual is viewed as having sufficiently troublesome symptomatology to warrant clinical intervention, the therapist needs first to look at the developmental stage of the target individual, and then to examine the generational structure of the family. In addition to the type of family and the particular generational structure, whether the target individual is a child, an adolescent, a young adult, a middle-aged adult, or an elderly person is important if the therapist is to anticipate the future developmental needs and the developmental trajectory of the individual and the family as a whole (Jameson & Alexander, 1994).

Dealing with the individual within the family implies some kind of family systems model for therapy (Jameson & Alexander, 1994; Qualls, 1994). The therapist needs to identify the basic themes of the family, and the functions and behavior patterns of each member as these are exhibited in interactions between family members. Within this framework, various therapeutic techniques can be applied; the therapist can work with key family members to help the individual within the family.

Different approaches may need to be considered when any mental health intervention is planned, depending on the type of family involved. Whatever intervention is planned, key family members from the generational structure (such as grandparents) should be included in family therapy. Furthermore, any application of family therapy should take place within the socioeconomic/cultural context within which the family is embedded. The task is to find ways to maximize the individual's psychological well-being and to develop more meaningful relationships with family members within the constraints of the family's particular context. Improvement of mental health through family intervention should first consider what approaches might be most effective with different family structures and family members, relative to their degree of adaptation to their changing environment.

CONCLUSIONS

At the present time, there is no standard definition of "family"; a multicultural society has led to various housing and living arrangements and alternative lifestyles for groups of individuals that no longer fit the traditional definition of the term. This creates confusion, because the privileges and obligations of the traditional family are not applied to these newer groups. In this chapter, a general concept of "family" that includes the new groups as specific types of families has been advanced. A coherent scheme also makes it possible to study and understand these types of families from similar psychological principles, and to develop or use appropriate mental intervention strategies to help them when needed. From this perspective, various family types can be viewed as representing different contexts or settings for individuals in relationships. It is the present concept of family relationships that provides the common link. Furthermore, this more general conception of the family reduces the distinction among "family," "extended family," and "kin network"; they are all regarded as aspects of perceived relationships between family members. These relationships should always be considered in studying different family types.

Finally, both intragenerational and intergenerational (including multigenerational) structures must be considered relative to each family type— that is, the number and kinds of family members involved, especially those family members defined in terms of genetic criteria. It is assumed that the generational structures themselves are important factors—not only in helping to define types of families, but also in influencing the quality of interpersonal relationships. For example, multigenerational families may have difficulty in maintaining a satisfactory quality of relationships between various generations, because of the large cohort differences; reconstituted families may have a great dissipation of the quality of relationships, because of the existence of many additional family members with reduced commitment to each other; homosexual cohabitant families may have weak intergenerational attachments, as a result of rejection by kin and a poor quality of relationships in a vertical family structure; and so on. Communal families may build close relationships between core family members as a substitute for relationships with blood family members; cohabitant heterosexual families may have more temporary generational structures in relation to their shared families, as the cohabitant relationship itself may be more temporary; singlehood "families" may be alone in their living arrangements but may enjoy close intragenerational and intergenerational relationships.

Overall, relationships are closer between individuals in the same or adjacent generations, but become weaker as the number of steps between generations increases. Typically, relationships with parents are closer than those with grandparents; relationships with great-grandparents, although they may be valued, are not as close as those with grandparents.

The type of family may be partially defined and/or related to a particular generational structure, which in turn is related to the quality of interpersonal relationships among family members. Mental health and illness may vary with the particular family type. The therapist should be aware of the kinds of relationships implied by a client's family type; in particular, he or she should consider the kinds of generational structures involved, and try to discern how they may be influencing the quality of the client's interpersonal relationships.

Much research is needed regarding such issues—for example, which family members are most willing to commit themselves to help, and can provide guidance and mentoring beyond financial help. Clearly, much further research is needed in these areas to determine which generational structures best buffer family members against mental dysfunction.

REFERENCES

Ahrons, C. R., & Rodgers, R. H. (1992). Divorce is normal. In V. Wagner (Ed.), *Family in America: Opposing viewpoints* (pp. 92–99). San Diego, CA: Greenhaven Press.

Allen, K. R., & Demo, D. H. (1995). The families of lesbians and gay men: A new frontier in family research. *Journal of Marriage and the Family, 57,* 111–127.

Antonucci, T. C., & Akiyama, H. (1994). Convoys of social relations: Family and friendships within a life span context. In R. Blieszner & V. H. Bedford (Eds.), *Aging and the family: Theory and research* (pp. 355–371). Westport, CT: Praeger.

Aquilino, W. S. (1994). Later life divorce and widowhood: Impact on young adults' assessment of parent–child relations. *Journal of Marriage and the Family, 56,* 908–922.

Atchley, R. C. (1994). *Social forces and aging* (7th ed.). Belmont, CA: Wadsworth.

Bengtson, V. L., Rosenthal, C., & Burton, L. (1990). Families and aging: Diversity and heterogeneity. In R. H. Binstock & L. K. George (Eds.), *Handbook of aging and the social sciences* (3rd ed., pp. 263–287). San Diego, CA: Academic Press.

Blumstein, P., & Schwartz, P. (1983). *American couples: Money, work, sex.* New York: Morrow.

Booth, A., & Amato, P. R. (1994). Parental marital quality, parental divorce, and relations with parents. *Journal of Marriage and the Family, 56,* 21–34.

Bumpass, L. L. (1990). What's happening to the family?: Interactions between demographic and institutional change. *Demography, 26,* 279–286.

Buunk, B. P., & van Driel, B. (1989). *Variant lifestyles and relationships.* Newbury Park, CA: Sage.

Cherlin, A., & Furstenberg, F. (1986). *The new American grandparent: A place in the family.* New York: Basic Books.

Cohler, B. J., & Altergott, K. (1994). The family of the second half of life: Connecting theories and findings. In R. Blieszner & V. H. Bedford (Eds.), *Aging and the family: Theory and research* (pp. 59–94). Westport, CT: Praeger.

Cooney, T. M. (1994). Young adults' relations with parents: The influence of parental divorce. *Journal of Marriage and the Family, 56,* 45–56.

Doka, K. J., & Mertz, M. E. (1988). The meaning and significance of great-grand-parenthood. *The Gerontologist, 28, 192–197.*

Elshtain, J. B. (1997). Single-parent families contribute to the breakdown of society. In. K. L. Swisher (Ed.), *Single-parent families* (pp. 53–59). San Diego, CA: Greenhaven Press.

Farkas, J. I., & Hogan, D. P. (1995). The demography of changing intergenerational relationships. In V. L. Bengtson, K. W. Schaie, & L. M. Burton (Eds.), *Adult intergenerational relations: Effects of social change* (pp. 1–18). New York: Springer.

Fassel, D. (1992a). Divorce may not harm children. In V. Wagner (Ed.), *Family in America: Opposing viewpoints* (pp. 115–119). San Diego, CA: Greenhaven Press.

Fassel, D. (1992b). The traditional family is obsolete. In V. Wagner (Ed.), *Family in America: Opposing viewpoints* (pp. 33–39). San Diego, CA: Greenhaven Press.

Fullmer, E. M. (1995). Challenging biases against families of older gays and lesbians. In G. C. Smith, S. S. Tobin, E. A. Robertson-Tchabo, & P. W. Power (Eds.), *Strengthening aging families: Diversity in practice and policy* (pp. 90–119). Thousand Oaks, CA: Sage.

Ganong, L. H., Coleman, M., & Maples, D. (1990). A meta-analytic review of family structure stereotypes. *Journal of Marriage and the Family, 52,* 287–297.

Giarrusso, R., Silverstein, M., & Bengtson, V. L. (1996). Family complexity and the grandparent role. *Generations, 20*(1), 17–23.

Glick, P. C. (1989). The family life cycle and social change. *Family Relations, 38,* 123–129.

Hodgson, L. G. (1995). Adult grandchildren and their grandparents: The enduring bond. In J. Hendricks (Ed.), *The ties of later life* (pp. 155–170). Amityville, NY: Baywood.

Huyck, M. H. (1994). Marriage and close relationships of the marital kind. In R. Blieszner & V. H. Bedford (Eds.), *Aging and the family: Theory and research* (pp. 181–200). Westport, CT: Praeger.

Jameson, P. B., & Alexander, J. F. (1994). Implications of a developmental family systems model for clinical practice. In L. L'Abate (Ed.), *Handbook of developmental family psychology and psychopathology* (pp. 392–411). New York: Wiley.

Jendrek, M. P. (1994). Grandparents who parent their grandchildren: Circumstances and decisions. *The Gerontologist, 34,* 206–216.

Johnson, C. L., & Troll, L. (1996). Family structure and the timing of transitions from 70 to 103 years of age. *Journal of Marriage and the Family, 58,* 178–187.

King, V., & Elder, G. H., Jr. (1995). American children view their grandparents: Linked lives across three rural generations. *Journal of Marriage and the Family, 57,* 165–178.

Kivnick, H. Q. (1982). *The meaning of grandparenthood.* Ann Arbor, MI: UNI Research.

Kornhaber, A. (1996). *Contemporary grandparenting.* Thousand Oaks, CA: Sage.

Laumann, E. O., Gagnon, J. H., Michael, R. T., & Michaels, S. (1994). *The social organization of sexuality: Sexual practices in the United States.* Chicago: University of Chicago Press.

Macklin, E. D. (1987). Nontraditional family forms. In M. B. Sussman & S. K. Steinmetz (Eds.), *Handbook of marriage and the family* (pp. 371–397). New York: Plenum Press.

Mangen, D. J., Bengtson, V. L., & Landry, P. H., Jr. (Eds.). (1988). *Measurement of intergenerational relations.* Newbury Park, CA: Sage.

Marciano, T., & Sussman, M. B. (1992). The definition of family is expanding. In V. Wagner (Ed.), *Family in America: Opposing viewpoints* (pp. 40–46). San Diego, CA: Greenhaven Press.

Minkler, M., & Roe, K. M. (1996). Grandparents as surrogate parents. *Generations, 20*(1), 34–38.

Neugarten, B. L., & Weinstein, K. K. (1964). The changing American grandparent. *Journal of Marriage and the Family, 26,* 299–304.

Olson, M. R., & Haynes, J. A. (1993). Successful single parents. *Families in Society: The Journal of Contemporary Human Services, 74,* 259–267.

Orthner, D. K. (1992). The family is in transition. In V. Wagner (Ed.), *Family in America: Opposing viewpoints* (pp. 25–32). San Diego, CA: Greenhaven Press.

Peplau, L. A., & Cochran, S. D. (1990). A relationship perspective on homosexuality. In D. P. McWhirter, S. A. Sanders, & J. M. Reinisch (Eds.), *Homosexuality, heterosexuality: Concepts of sexual orientation* (pp. 321–349). New York: Oxford University Press.

Peterson, K. S. (1996, November 27). "Typical" family is a modern-day oxymoron. *USA Today,* p. 4D.

Pillemer, K., & Suitor, J. J. (1991). "Will I ever escape my child's problems?": Effects of adult children's problems on elderly parents. *Journal of Marriage and the Family, 53,* 585–594.

Popenoe, D. (1992). The family is in decline. In V. Wagner (Ed.), *Family in America: Opposing viewpoints* (pp. 17–24). San Diego, CA: Greenhaven Press.

Qualls, S. H. (1994). Clinical interventions with later-life families. In R. Blieszner & V. H. Bedford (Eds.), *Aging and the family: Theory and research* (pp. 474–487). Westport, CT: Praeger.

Quam, J. K., & Whitford, G. S. (1992). Adaptation and age-related expectations of older gay and lesbian adults. *The Gerontologist, 32,* 367–374.

Roberto, K. A., & Stroes, J. (1995). Grandchildren and grandparents: Roles, influences, and relationships. In J. Hendricks (Ed.), *The ties of later life* (pp. 142–153). Amityville, NY: Baywood.

Robertson, J. F. (1977). Grandmotherhood: A study of role concepts. *Journal of Marriage and the Family, 39,* 165–174.

Robertson, J. F. (1994). Grandparenting in an era of rapid change. In R. Blieszner & V. H. Bedford (Eds.), *Aging and the family: Theory and research* (pp. 243–260). Westport, CT: Praeger.

Rubinstein, R. L. (1987). Never married elderly as a social type: Re-evaluating some images. *The Gerontologist, 27,* 108–114.

Rubinstein, R. L., Alexander, B. B., Goodman, M., & Luborsky, M. (1991). Key relationships of never married, childless older women: A cultural analysis. *Journal of Gerontology, 46,* S270–S277.

Skolnick, A., & Rosencranz, S. (1997). The harmful effects of single-parent families are exaggerated. In K. L. Swisher (Ed.), *Single-parent families* (pp. 62–70). San Diego, CA: Greenhaven Press.

Trygstad, D. W., & Sanders, G. F. (1995). The significance of stepgrandparents. In J. Hendricks (Ed.), *The ties of later life* (pp. 209–223). Amityville, NY: Baywood.

Uhlenberg, P. (1995). Commentary: Demographic influences on intergenerational relations. In V. L. Bengtson, K. W. Schaie, & L. M. Burton (Eds.), *Adult intergenerational relations: Effects of social change* (pp. 19–25). New York: Springer.

U.S. Bureau of the Census. (1991). *Household and family characteristics, March 1991* (Publication No. AP-20-458). Washington, DC: U.S. Government Printing Office.

Wagner, R. M. (1993). Psychosocial adjustments during the first year of single parenthood: A comparison of Mexican-American and Anglo women. *Journal of Divorce and Remarriage, 19*(1–2), 12–33.

Wallerstein, J. S., & Blakeslee, S. (1992). Divorce harms children. In V. Wagner (Ed.), *Family in America: Opposing viewpoints* (pp. 108–114). San Diego, CA: Greenhaven Press.

Warshow, J. (1991). Eldercare as a feminist issue. In B. Sang, J. Warshow, & A. J. Smith (Eds.), *Lesbians of midlife: A creative transition* (pp. 65–72). San Francisco: Spinsters.

Wentowski, G. (1985). Older women's perceptions of great-grandparenthood: A research note. *The Gerontologist, 25,* 593–596.

White, L. (1994). Growing up with single parents and stepparents: Long-term effects on family solidarity. *Journal of Marriage and the Family, 56,* 935–948.

CHAPTER 9

⸺⬦⸺

Comprehensive Assessment of Family Functioning

ROBERT W. HEFFER
DOUGLAS K. SNYDER

Family psychologists are obliged to render assessment, evaluation, and diagnosis in a competent and ethical manner (American Psychological Association, 1985, 1992). As a profession, psychology expends great effort toward delineating standards for the development and application of tests and methods used to quantify human beliefs and experiences (American Educational Research Association, American Psychological Association, & National Council on Measurement in Education, 1987; Board of Professional Affairs, 1987).

Although controversy persists regarding the relative benefits of an individual-focused, diagnostic approach versus a system-focused, process-oriented approach to family assessment (Carlson, Hinkle, & Sperry, 1993; Sporakowski, 1995; Strong, 1993), most authors acknowledge the importance of thorough training of family therapists in assessment and diagnosis (Benson, Long, & Sporakowski, 1992; Hohenshil, 1993; Waldo, Brotherton, & Horswill, 1993). However, Boughner, Hayes, Bubenzer, and West (1994) reported that a mere 39% of the marital and family therapists they surveyed used any standardized instruments regularly. Moreover, despite the proliferation of measures of marital and family functioning, most suffer from inadequate attention to psychometric features, and few are in widespread use (Schumm, 1990).

In its broadest context, "assessment" implies a systematic information-gathering process (L'Abate, 1994; Witt, Elliott, Gresham, & Kramer, 1988). Given this definition, even family therapists who eschew standardized measurement techniques assess families regularly. Family therapists consistently gather information by way of clinical interviews; observe clients' behavior; and obtain self-report information regarding clients' beliefs, affect, perceptions, and relationships (Kaslow & Celano, 1995). In evaluating family functioning, all family therapists adopt implicit or explicit models of assessment. What are these models? Do models stemming from different theoretical orientations have comparable merit in the assessment of families? How aware of their assessment models are family therapists? Do such models need to be explicit?

In addressing these issues, we advocate a comprehensive approach to assessing family functioning that has utility for practitioners and researchers alike. First, we discuss issues that are fundamental to evaluating families. Next, we examine a comprehensive assessment model that we and our colleagues have proposed elsewhere (Snyder, Cavell, Heffer, & Mangrum, 1995). Finally, we provide a case example integrating the principles and procedures articulated in this chapter.

FOUNDATIONS OF FAMILY ASSESSMENT

The Personal Model of the Family Therapist

The context of the therapist–client relationship must be considered in the assessment of families. Clients' expectations and beliefs regarding the assessment and therapeutic process, previous experiences involving a confidante or authority figure, and current level of distress coalesce with a therapist's life history, professional development, and personal model of assessment and intervention to shape the nature and course of the client–therapist relationship. Because the therapist is the presumed "expert" in the relationship, his or her personal model will significantly affect the process and expected outcomes of assessment and intervention with families; therefore, this model should be made explicit.

As described by Barnett and Zucker (1990), a therapist's personal model refers to "the various assumptions, whether deliberate, informal, or intuitive, that guide professional behaviors" (p. 102). Furthermore, therapists "are guided by personal theories regarding their own behavior and the behavior of clients" (p. 128). We contend that every professional has a theoretical perspective, whether or not it is well articulated or acknowledged. Specific clinical judgments, decisions, and actions emerge from broad conceptual perspectives mediated by one's personal application of a theoretical orientation or integration of multiple orientations. Explicit recognition of one's personal model allows potential sources of error in assessment and treatment decisions to be addressed more readily. In addition, an effective conceptual model requires sufficient flexibility to adapt to the unique situations presented by families, but the theoretical framework must not be so diffuse that the assessment process lacks structure.

We believe that a psychologist's personal model influences alternative conceptualizations of family functioning and the specific steps taken in the assessment–intervention process. Therefore, we articulate here the assumptions and principles that guide our evaluations of families.

Assessment Is a Continual Hypothesis-Testing Process

Predicated on our personal commitment to an integrated scientist/practitioner model of practice, we recommend a hypothesis-testing approach to assessing families. Specifically, the first task in assessing families is to pose questions or hypotheses regarding family functioning. In a fashion similar to conducting a research study, plans are developed to systematically gather information that will answer the assessment questions with as much clarity and certainty as possible. Once the assessment information is obtained and scrutinized, the assessor actively formulates how family transactions proceed within a socioecological context and conform with theoretical conceptualizations (Bronfenbrenner, 1986; Fiese & Sameroff, 1992). During this phase in the assessment process, the assessor should be particularly attentive to a general tendency to notice information that confirms currently held hypotheses, and to ignore evidence that disconfirms hypotheses. Arkes (1981) has argued that the clinical decision process is enhanced when alternative hypotheses are considered tenable for as long as possible. The next phase is to explore the assessment findings with the family, emphasizing the implications for treatment planning (Baucom & Epstein, 1990). When therapy emerges explicitly from assessment information, the developing and monitoring of measurable treatment goals are facilitated.

Family Assessment Is Unique

Family assessment is distinct from assessments that are individual-focused. For example, most adults in individual therapy are self-referred and acknowledge, at some level, personal responsibility for disclosing information and bringing about change. In contrast, participants in family assessment often initially accentuate a need for change in *other* family members. Because of the number of information sources in family assessment, different family members' expectancies regarding the pace and complexity of the assessment process need to be calibrated. A benefit of family assessment is the opportunity to observe the interpersonal exchanges of family members directly, and to contrast family members' subjective appraisals of the referral problem.

We promote a family-focused assessment process. Common characteristics across and within families should not diminish a therapist's appreciation for the unique constellation of a given family or for the distinct influence of a given member on family functioning. Consideration of the therapist's own influence on the family, and sensitivity to how his or her own expectations and values affect the assessment process, are paramount. Family case formulations are generated in a socioecological context. Moreover, rather than highlighting only deficits to be ameliorated, assessment needs to emphasize family strengths as vehicles for change in therapy. Finally, we note that family assessors must frequently advocate for families that need auxiliary services resulting from disabilities or financial hardship (Sachs, 1994; Turnbill & Turnbill, 1994).

Assessment Is Driven by Theory

Theoretical conceptualizations underlying the assessment process substantially affect decisions concerning what to assess and how to translate findings into recommendations for intervention (Jacob & Tennenbaum, 1988). Filsinger (1983) noted that "most assessment techniques are ... linked, to some degree, to specific theoretical orientations and may do a better job of measuring some concepts than others" (p. 19). It is incumbent on the family assessor to remain alert to his or her personal and theoretical approach to families and its ramifications for assessment and therapy processes. Independent of one's own personal model, the family assessor must take care to select instruments that have sound psychometric properties and clinical utility (Snyder & Rice, 1996).

Assessment Is Driven by Empiricism

Steeped in a scientist-practitioner tradition, we look to empiricism to direct and inform our clinical practice. A family assessor can understand families in an objective manner (Cavell & Snyder, 1991), while acknowledging that his or her interpretations are influenced by both personal and theoretical perspectives. Alternative models of assessment have been articulated in both the clinical and the research literature. For example, family narratives can be evaluated via conversation analysis, although this method is more labor-intensive than those typically employed (Gale, 1996). In addition, family assessment can be bolstered by the application of single-case design methodology to monitor therapy progress and to define therapy outcomes (Dickey, 1996). Continual development of evaluation skills is a goal of a competent and ethical family assessor. Admittedly, a commitment to empirically based assessment is not for the timid; ongoing retooling of assessment skills is an endeavor that requires tenacity.

Assessment Considers Socioecological and Developmental Contexts

Throughout the family assessment process, the assessor must attend to the socioecological context of the referral question and the reciprocal influences inherent in the client–therapist relationship (Ross, 1977). In addition, an accurate case formulation includes an appreciation for the developmental context of individuals within the dyad or family *and* of the dyad or family system itself as a unique entity. For example, referral issues involving frequent child oppositional behavior, nocturnal enuresis, and aggression toward peers will certainly be interpreted differently if the "problem child" is 3 years old versus 15 years old. "Without [a developmental] context, ideally derived from both theory and normative data, it is extremely difficult to anticipate whether the behavior is likely to change, over what period of time, to what degree, and in what direction" (Jacob & Tennenbaum, 1988, p. 7).

Likewise, the family unit itself may be conceptualized as progressing along a developmental continuum. For example, according to Hill and Mattessich (1979), families share enough commonality that their development across the life span can be charted in predictable stages. Changes in family development are marked by the emergence and alteration over time of norms, roles, and other family characteristics necessary for the persistence of the family as a social system. The interrelatedness of individuals within a family necessitates that changes in role behaviors for one member result in changes for other family members as well. New stages in family development accompany significant alterations in the positions and role behaviors of individual members. For example, additional family positions are generated by the birth or adoption of a member, whereas loss of positions is experienced when a member dies, loses a job, or leaves the marriage.

Assessment Includes Multiple Levels and Multiple Perspectives

Multilevel, multiperspective assessment has been encouraged throughout the family assessment literature (Cromwell & Peterson, 1981; Kaslow & Celano, 1995; L'Abate, 1994). As we have described elsewhere (Snyder et al., (1995), several levels of assessment may be delineated: (1) individuals, (2) dyads, (3) nuclear families, (4) extended family systems and related systems interfacing with the immediate family, and (5) community and cultural systems. We typically begin assessment at an intermediate level of analysis (i.e., the dyad or family level) and then proceed concomitantly toward the individual level and broader systemic levels. For example, the impact on the family of parents' working outside the home (Shellenberger & Hoffman, 1995) and the extent to which a school system interacts with a family system (Fine, 1995) are grist for the family assessment mill. At each level of assessment, gleaning perspectives from interview or other self-report measures is paramount. Within families, reports from all members must be assimilated. Reports from significant others outside the family (e.g., teachers, extended family members, medical care personnel) should be pursued when relevant, and integrated as well.

Specific Steps in the Family Assessment Process

Assessment and intervention processes are an iterative, recursive blend of evaluation, hypothesis formulation, intervention, observation of effects, and intervention adjustments. In fact, some (Selvini Palazzoli, Boscolo, Cecchin, & Prata, 1980; Tomm, 1988) have framed the assessment process itself as a therapeutic intervention, because it involves collaboration, interpretation, and corrective feedback among therapist and family members. Furthermore, assessment is integral to appropriate interventions; without adequate assessment, even structured therapeutic approaches can be misapplied. First, a clear understanding of family needs is developed through assessment. Only then should specific interventions be recommended or applied.

Table 9.1 outlines specific steps in the family assessment process. These steps require varying amounts of resource allocation, depending on the nature of the referral question and the unique features of the client family. Each step is accompanied by the iterative hypothesis-testing approach described previously. In addition, the socioecological and developmental contexts of the referral questions are considered concurrently at each step of the assessment process.

A COMPREHENSIVE FAMILY ASSESSMENT MODEL

The intricacies of family assessment compel the assessor to adopt a comprehensive conceptual model, in which multiple assessment techniques are employed to garner information from multiple system levels and informants across conceptually distinct but overlapping domains. Drawing from Grotevant and Carlson (1989) and Jacob and Tennenbaum (1988), we (Snyder et al., 1995) have proposed a comprehensive model for assessing families in which assessment constructs are organized into five domains: (1) cognitive; (2) affective; (3) communication and interpersonal; (4) structural and developmental; and (5) control, sanctions, and related behaviors. Assessment data across domains are gathered via multiple assessment strategies, primarily self-report and observational techniques; these strategies include both formal (i.e., more structured and psychometrically focused) and informal (i.e., less structured and more clinically focused) procedures. The assessment techniques across domains are used to evaluate each of five system levels: (1) individuals, (2) dyads, (3) the nuclear family, (4) the extended family system, and (5) community and cultural systems.

As depicted in Figure 9.1, the nuclear family system is defined as two or more individuals involved in one or more dyadic relationships. Each dyad is interrelated and instrumental to other dyadic relationships. The extended family system—including parents' respective families of origin, as well as close relationships with others from work, school, or the neighbor-

TABLE 9.1. Steps in the Family Assessment Process

Throughout: Continually form and test hypotheses.

 1. Review referral information.
 2. Interview the family.
 3. Observe family behavior.
 4. Conduct standardized assessments.
 5. Gather information from outside the family, when relevant.
 6. Organize and review all data.
 7. Integrate data from a theoretical perspective.
 8. Develop recommendations.
 9. Write an integrated report.
10. Meet with the family:
    a. Discuss formulation of family strengths and difficulties.
    b. Establish intervention goals.
    c. Recommend specific interventions.
11. Implement recommendations.
12. Engage in continual reassessment and reformulation throughout treatment.

hood—is the immediate socioecological context for the nuclear family. Similarly, a more extensive community or cultural system constitutes a more distal but still influential socioecological context for both the nuclear and extended family systems. Roles across system levels vary (e.g., parents of the nuclear family serve as children in their families of origin), based on the developmental context of individual family members (Erikson, 1968), the family itself (Gerson, 1995), and the specific culture in which the family is embedded (Slonim, 1991). In our model, culture is defined as the "set of attitudes, values, beliefs, and behaviors shared by a group of people, communicated from one generation to the next via language or some other means of communication" (Matsumoto, 1997, pp. 4–5). For example, in this model an individual family member's cognitions (i.e., intelligence, aptitude, capacity for self-reflection, insight, and self-view) are intertwined with assumptions, standards, expectancies, and attributions regarding relationships (Baucom, Epstein, Sayers, & Sher, 1989) espoused by the nuclear and extended family, as well as with the values and norms promulgated by the culture and community systems.

Implementing such a comprehensive family assessment model can be a daunting challenge. How are decisions made about where to start, where to proceed, when to probe, and when to remain nondirective? The fact that a family being assessed often resembles a spinning top only serves to complicate the assessment endeavor further. One strategy we have found appealing is to think of this assessment model as a Windows®-style computer software management system, the assessment levels and domains as interfacing programs, and the assessment techniques as the mouse. Of course, the "spinning" family is the 3.5-inch diskette on which the assessor is currently working!

Our own family assessment experiences are akin to having all the interfacing programs running concurrently, but using the Windows® fea-

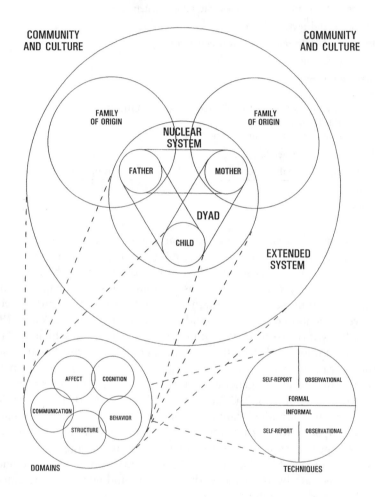

FIGURE 9.1. Comprehensive model for assessing family functioning. The five levels in the model are (1) individuals, (2) dyads, (3) nuclear family, (4) extended family, and (5) community and cultural systems. Each level may be assessed via multiple techniques (i.e., formal and informal self-report and observational techniques) across five overlapping domains. The domains include (1) cognitive; (2) affective; (3) communication and interpersonal; (4) structural and developmental; and (5) control, sanctions, and related behaviors. From Snyder, Cavell, Heffer, and Mangrum (1995). Copyright 1995 by the American Psychological Association. Reprinted by permission.

ture to call to the foreground specific levels and domains at a given phase of the assessment. Multiple hypotheses are generated and entertained as some specific windows are kept running in the background, while details of other, currently opened windows are examined. Determining how to proceed is based partly on the referral issues and partly on the assessor's personal model of assessment and training. For example, one of us initially approaches families from a couple perspective, whereas the other first formulates family cases from a view of parent–child relationships. In either approach the same levels and domains are typically assessed, but the sequence of windows' opening and closing varies.

Although intended to offer a comprehensive method for assessing family functioning, this model does not aim to be prescriptive or rigid. The program is designed to supply ample random-access memory, to offer flexibility in data processing, and to be user-friendly! Similarly, this chapter does not provide an exhaustive list of specific procedures to evaluate individuals, families, or systems. Other recent sources are available to readers seeking more extensive descriptions of individual and family assessment procedures (Butcher, 1997; Fredman & Sherman, 1987; Grotevant & Carlson, 1989; L'Abate, 1994; L'Abate & Bagarozzi, 1993; Robinson, Shaver, & Wrightman, 1991; Touliatos, Perlmutter, & Straus, 1990). Additional resources are recommended for readers who may be relatively less attuned to child-focused family assessment (Hughes & Baker, 1990; Kamphaus & Frick, 1996; La Greca, 1990; Witt, Cavell, Heffer, Carey, & Martens, 1988; Witt, Heffer, & Pfeiffer, 1990).

We have selected several assessment techniques for each of the system levels in our comprehensive model (see Table 9.2). Selections have been based on the popularity of a given procedure, its psychometric underpinnings (Snyder & Rice, 1996), and its treatment evaluation utility (Hayes, Nelson, & Jarrett, 1987). As shown in Table 9.2, the degree to which these procedures evaluate specific domains of functioning varies across system levels. Moreover, although some instruments are placed within a given system level, information pertaining to other levels may be supplied as well. For example, the Child Behavioral Checklist (CBCL; Achenbach, 1991) and the Behavior Assessment System for Children (BASC; Reynolds & Kamphaus, 1992) both provide parent, child, and teacher reports of child behavior and adjustment at home and at school. In general, assessment procedures that tap more global functioning of individuals or families have been chosen over measures restricted to narrower aspects of functioning (e.g., depression, anxiety).

Assessing Individual Family Members

Individual family members' ability to understand psychological or behavioral concepts, capacity for self-reflection and insight, cognitive style and attitudes, and educational or occupational skills capture the attention of

TABLE 9.2. Selected Techniques Applied to the Comprehensive Model for Assessing Family Functioning

Level and domain assessment questions	Selected assessment techniques
Individuals	
How may cognitive style or abilities influence family members' responses to therapy or each other?	Wechsler scales (Sattler, 1992)
	Attributional Style Questionnaire (Peterson & Villanova, 1988)
	Children's Attributional Style Questionnaire (Fielstein et al., 1985)
What dimensions of adult individual emotional or behavioral functioning influence family functioning? Which, if any, warrant separate treatment? Which reflect strengths?	Minnesota Multiphasic Personality Inventory—2 (Butcher et al., 1989; Butcher & Williams, 1992)
	Millon Clinical Multiaxial Inventory—III (Millon et al., 1994)
	NEO Personality Inventory—Revised (Costa & McCrae, 1992)
	Symptom Checklist 90—Revised (Derogatis, 1994)
	California Personality Inventory (Gough, 1996; McAllister, 1996)
	Schedule for Affective Disorders and Schizophrenia (Endicott & Spitzer, 1978)
	Diagnostic Interview Schedule (Robins et al., 1981)
What dimensions of child/adolescent individual emotional or functioning influence family functioning? Which, if any, warrant separate treatment? Which reflect strengths?	CBCL (Achenbach, 1991, 1992)
	BASC (Reynolds & Kamphaus, 1992)
	Minnesota Multiphasic Personality Inventory—Adolescent (Archer, 1992; Butcher et al., 1992)
	Millon Adolescent Clinical Inventory (Millon et al., 1993)
	Personality Inventory for Children (Lachar, 1990)
	Personality Inventory for Youth (Lachar & Gruber, 1995a, 1995b)
	Schedule for Affective Disorders and Schizophrenia for School-Age Children (Ambrosini et al., 1989; Chambers et al., 1985)
	Diagnostic Interview Schedule for Children—Revised (Shaffer et al., 1993; Frick et al.,1994)
Dyads	
What are the sources and levels of distress or satisfaction and communication patterns in the marriage or the parent–child relationship(s)?	Marital Satisfaction Inventory—Revised (Snyder, 1997; Snyder & Costin, 1994)
	Sexual Functioning Inventory (Derogatis & Melisaratos, 1979)
	Marital Interaction Coding System—Global (Weiss & Tolman, 1990)
	Rapid Couples Interaction Coding System (Krokoff et al., 1989)
	Parent–Adolescent Interaction Coding System (Robin & Weiss, 1980)
	Dyadic Parent–Child Interaction Coding System (Eisenstadt et al., 1993; Eyberg & Robinson, 1983)
	Family Interaction Coding System (Patterson, 1982)
What relationship expectations and attributions exist among family members?	Relationship Attribution Measure (Fincham & Bradbury, 1992)
	Relationship Belief Inventory (Eidelson & Epstein, 1982)
	Child Report of Parental Behavior Inventory (Schludermann & Schludermann, 1983)

(continued)

Level and domain assessment questions	Selected assessment techniques
Nuclear family system	
How do family members perceive the quality of family relationships? How effectively does the family respond to daily challenges and crises?	Family Environment Scale (Moos & Moos, 1994) Children's Version: Family Environment Scale (Pino et al., 1984) Family Adaptation and Cohesion Evaluation Scales III (Olson et al., 1985; Olson, 1986) Family Assessment Measure (Skinner et al., 1984) Parenting Stress Index, third edition (Abidin, 1990)
How is the family organized along dimensions of affect, authority, and control? How do family members influence each other?	Family Behavior Interview (Robin & Foster, 1989) Genogram (McGoldrick & Gerson, 1985) Family Hierarchy Test (Madanes et al., 1980) Hutchins Behavior Inventory (Hutchins, 1992) Child Rearing Practices Report (Roberts et al., 1984; Kochanska et al., 1989) O'Leary–Porter Scale (Porter & O'Leary, 1980) Alabama Parenting Questionnaire (Frick, 1990; Shelton, Frick, & Wooton, 1996) Home Observation for Measurement of the Environment (Caldwell & Bradley, 1994)
Extended family system	
How do family members function in work or school settings?	Devereux Scales of Mental Disorders (Naglieri et al., 1994) Devereux Behavior Rating Scale—School Form (Naglieri et al., 1993) Comprehensive Behavior Rating Scale for Children (Neeper et al., 1990) Peer nominations and ratings (Gresham & Little, 1993) BASC Student Observation System (Reynolds & Kamphaus, 1992) CBCL Direct Observation Form (Achenbach, 1995) Observations of peer interactions (Dodge, 1983)
To what extent do relationships with extended family members serve as sources of support or stress? How are sources of support or stress shared among family members?	Ways of Coping Questionnaire (Folkman & Lazarus, 1988; Lazarus & Folkman, 1984) Interpersonal Support Evaluation List (Cohen et al., 1985) Social Networks Interview (Garbarino & Sherman, 1980) Social Networks of Youth (Garbarino & Kapadia, 1986) Survey of Children's Social Support (Dubow & Ullman, 1989) Dialogues About Families (Reid & Ramey, 1992)
Community and culture system	
To what extent do family members access community resources? How are community resources perceived by family members?	Neighborhood and Community Assessment (Garbarino & Sherman, 1980) Eco-map (Hartman, 1979, 1995) Systematic Ecological Problem Solving (Cantrell & Cantrell, 1980, 1985) Mothers' Activity Checklist (Kelley & Carper, 1988) Community Interaction Checklist (Wahler, 1980)
To what extent to family members identify with a particular ethnic heritage?	Behavioral Acculturation Scale (Szapocznik et al., 1980) Cultural Assessment of Emotions (Castillo, 1997) Cultural Assessment for DSM-IV (Kleinman, 1992)

the thorough family assessor. School-related difficulties for children or adolescents often warrant assessment of basic intellectual ability and academic achievement via classroom observations or standardized measures of individual cognitive abilities. Furthermore, the content, intensity, and mutability of each family member's emotional functioning affect that person's responsiveness to other family members and to the therapist as well. The capacities to relate warmly to others and to engage in goal-directed negotiation are critical elements of a family member's interpersonal style (Beavers, Hampson, & Hulgus, 1985), as is the capacity for behavioral self-control (i.e., deferring immediate impulses toward self-gratification, either for other persons' benefit or for preferred delayed rewards for oneself).

Although the issue is somewhat controversial in family therapy circles (Benson et al., 1992), comprehensive family assessment may warrant a *Diagnostic and Statistical Manual of Mental Disorders,* fourth edition (DSM-IV) diagnosis (American Psychiatric Association, 1994) reflecting individual psychopathology, maladjustment, and degree of stress. However, with the recent inclusion of the Global Assessment of Relationship Functioning Scale in the DSM-IV appendices, family assessors can supplement the diagnosis of family members with ratings of problem solving, organization, and emotional climate of the family (American Psychiatric Association, 1994; Denton, 1993).

Assessing Dyads

Inconsistencies in cognitive and affective functioning between the members of a dyad are particularly relevant to family assessment (Snyder, Lachar, Freiman, & Hoover, 1991). For example, relationship distress frequently derives from differences in expectations between husband and wife, or between parent and teenage son or daughter. Furthermore, a spouse's depressive symptoms consistently predict poorer response to marital therapy, perhaps because the depressed partner's low energy level and hopelessness impede efforts toward relationship change (Snyder, Mangrum, & Wills, 1993). Inconsistencies at broader system levels may assume prominence in a family where members at one generational level strive to blend in with peers adopting a predominant or mainstream culture, while members of an older generation in the same home labor to preserve the distinguishing customs reflecting their ethnic heritage.

The role of communication patterns in family functioning is well established (Jacobson, 1992; O'Leary, 1987; Reid, 1978). When communication is coercive (Patterson, 1982) or characterized by a differential distribution of power (Huston, 1983), dyadic interactions become particularly conflictual (Margolin, Michelli, & Jacobson, 1988). In fact, nonverbal expression of negative affect between members of a couple is a robust predictor of relationship dissatisfaction (Gottman, 1979). In contrast, nondistressed couples tend to accentuate positive aspects of the relationship and tolerate differences in assumptions and expectations (Baucom et al., 1989). The association of relationship satisfaction and acceptance or capacity to forgive among dyads in families is gaining increased attention in the clinical and research literatures (Smedes, 1984; Sofield, Juliano, & Hammett, 1990).

Assessing Nuclear Families

The nuclear family is more than a conglomeration of dyadic relationships; it has a unique structure and hierarchy. For example, Fiese and Sameroff (1992) describe the concept of "family code," which dictates the expected behavior of family members in a variety of settings. A family code incorporates the family's belief system, defines the family as distinct from other families, and structures or organizes family daily routines. The family code may be considered a system of family definitions that serve as guidelines for a family's behavior, much as society regulates its citizens' behavior through various levels of normative consensus in a cultural code. Components of a family code are (1) "family paradigms" (i.e., global belief systems defining the family's social world); (2) "family stories" (i.e., narratives and interpretations that transmit values that distinguish a given family); and (3) "family rituals" (i.e., customs organizing the family's daily routines). The distinctive quality of each family underscores the value of using observations of family interactions to establish an understanding of family functioning.

As noted earlier, the family should be viewed as a dynamic entity from a life-span developmental conceptualization. Gerson (1995) has explicitly extended this family developmental approach by proposing three family life phases, each divided into two stages. During the "coupling" phase, individuals typically proceed from the unattached young adult stage to the family formation stage. A subsequent "expansion" phase includes stages defined by families with young children and families with adolescents. Finally, tasks of launching children and moving on in later life encompass the "contraction" phase. Crises in family life occur when a family struggles with a particular life stage or when progression to the next stage is overly challenging. Dissatisfaction, conflict, and negativity may result when family members contend with each other during crises; when members collaborate, families typically experience satisfaction, efficacy, and encouraging interactions in response to crises.

Assessing Extended Family Systems

Significant persons in a family's extended system can either enhance or detract from family functioning. For example, when social supports are absent or are perceived as intrusive (Wahler, 1980), the coping of individual family members and the nuclear family itself are negatively affected. Figley (1989) has described how extended systems function as family stressors when conflicts erupt over expectations of the parents' families of origin regarding parenting practices. Furthermore, successes or failures in school or work settings can set the tone for family interactions at home (Fine, 1995; Shellenberger & Hoffman, 1995).

When perceived as satisfactory and desired, social support from persons in a family's extended system greatly facilitates family coping and adaptation, particularly during crises (Quittner, 1992). Such support has the potential to fortify nuclear family relationships in day-to-day functioning as well. The kind of regular support that typifies a therapist's interactions with families qualifies the therapist as part of the family's extended system. Because a family assessor becomes part of the family network, the assessor must be vigilant regarding his or her influence on alterations in family functioning and the assessment process itself (Ross, 1977).

Assessing Community and Culture Systems

Family assessors have long called for consideration of ethnic and cultural heritage when therapists are evaluating, conceptualizing, and intervening with families from diverse backgrounds (Hansen & Falicov, 1983; McGoldrick, Giordano & Pearce, 1996). Recommendations have been made regarding the meaning of psychological and interpersonal phenomena across world cultures (Castillo, 1997; Matsumoto, 1997), as well as relevant considerations for psychological assessment of racial and ethnic minorities in the United States (Boyd-Franklin, 1989; Gray-Little, 1997; Okazaki & Sue, 1997; Velásquez, 1997). Concentrated effort has been exerted within the assessment literature to promote methods for incorporating the unique experiences and perspectives of persons of varying cultural experiences into psychological evaluations (Slonim, 1991; Vargas & Willis, 1994). However, substantial work remains to be done in this area (Dana, 1994). Of the multiple systems proposed in our comprehensive family assessment model, the community and cultural system has the fewest formal assessment options for the family assessor.

CASE EXAMPLE

As we have noted, all psychological assessment occurs within a context. The individual, couple, or family seeking services from a psychologist exists in a social context that is relationship-based. Examples of interpersonal relationships include a family member's relationship to a family of origin, a partner, biological children or stepchildren, siblings, extended family members, peers, and authority figures at work. In addition, consideration of relationships among referral issues and such socioecological variables as the demands and values of the community in which a family lives, the ethnic culture of origin, and the dominant culture is integral to successful family assessment and intervention.

An example of how interpersonal and socioecological variables intertwine may be demonstrated by the case of a 26-year-old Hispanic woman, Rosa, who was self-referred for insomnia. During the initial interview, Rosa reported significant marital conflict. She and her husband, Gustavo (age 32), both subsequently agreed to participate in a more comprehensive family assessment. Family members in the home included Gustavo, Rosa, her 8-year-old son from a previous marriage (Carlos), a 4-year-old daughter (Anna), and a 6-month-old daughter (Maria). Rosa's first husband had died unexpectedly of a heart attack when Carlos was 1 year old. She met and married Gustavo (his only marriage) when Carlos was 3 years old. Specific problem areas for the couple included lack of trust and effective communication, frequent verbal conflict, and substantial differences regarding the parenting of the children, particularly Carlos. In addition, the baby, Maria, was born with an immunological disorder that rendered her extremely susceptible to infections. The pediatrician recommended that Maria be kept indoors and away from nonfamily members as much as possible for the first year of life. Maria's health problems resulted in growth deficiencies, for which she received an additional diagnosis of "failure to thrive."

Dysfunctional interpersonal relationships were described by the couple in both their marital and their parental roles. Interactions among the children and adults in the home were adversely affected by parental disagreements. Moreover, issues surrounding Rosa's unemployment since Maria's birth (she had previously worked as a bank clerk) and her role as Maria's primary caregiver were prominent sources of disharmony. The salient socioecological variables in this case included educational, religious, and ethnic differences between husband and wife. Although both were Hispanic and bilingual (with Spanish as their primary language), Rosa had been raised in the southwestern United States, whereas Gustavo had been raised in Mexico until age 14, when his family immigrated to the United States. In addition, Rosa had completed a 2-year vocational/technological degree and aligned herself with an evangelical Protestant church, whereas Gustavo had graduated from high school and espoused traditional Roman Catholic beliefs. The couple's values, attitudes, and expectations regarding marriage, parenting, and employment were colored by their respective cultures of origin and life experiences. Other challenges for this couple included issues of cultural identification and assimilation into the dominant culture of their community. Although both acknowledged that family discord had existed for several years, Rosa and Gustavo asserted that problems in the family had been tolerable until the birth and subsequent health problems of Maria 6 months earlier.

Initially, the family assessment consisted only of clinical interviews (Karpel, 1994). Because Rosa and Gustavo did not appear to require extensive personality evaluation, they both completed the Symptom Check-list 90—Revised (SCL-90-R; Derogatis, 1994) to screen for psychopathology. Rosa's SCL-90-R profile indicated symptoms of mild depression and somatization; Gustavo's profile suggested problems associated with anxiety and anger management. The couple also completed the Marital Satisfaction Inventory—Revised (MSI-R; Snyder, 1997) to assess key features of the marital relationship. The MSI-R profile confirmed moderate levels of relationship distress for both partners, with particular discontent regarding problem solving and leisure time together, as well as conflict over child rearing issues.

To assess the individual functioning of 8-year-old Carlos, Rosa and Gustavo independently completed the CBCL (Achenbach, 1991), and his third-grade teacher completed the Teacher Report Form. The teacher reported problems primarily in the areas of attention, concentration, and social withdrawal. She also noted that Carlos's grades had been dropping consistently since the previous school year. A subsequent school observation and teacher consultation resulted in school-based assessment and interventions to ameliorate a mild reading disability.

Rosa's CBCL report for Carlos suggested only mild internalizing problems at home. In contrast, Gustavo's CBCL report indicated his perception that Carlos was exhibiting significant externalizing problems. An interview with Carlos confirmed that he was dissatisfied with his school performance and was eager to get the assistance he needed to read more effectively. He also reported that he wanted to get along better with his stepfather and was uncertain why they argued so much. An interview with Anna disclosed that she was very happy to have a baby sister, but was sad that the baby was sick. Anna reported that she wanted her family to stop fighting and to "have fun again." She was pleased to be able to stay home with her mother and Maria while Carlos was at school and her father worked as a produce manager in a grocery store.

In-session observations of parent–child interactions (Eyberg & Robinson, 1983) indicated that both parents were nurturant toward Anna and responded firmly and calmly to her few instances of misbehavior. In contrast, Gustavo struggled to relate positively with Carlos, and he seemed annoyed and critical when his stepson did not comply with instructions immediately. Carlos's behavior during the observation (and his usual behavior at home, as determined via careful probes during clinical interviews)was typically not excessively oppositional or defiant with Gustavo. When a genogram (McGoldrick & Gerson, 1985) and eco-map diagrams (Hartman, 1995) were used with the family, a picture emerged of a somewhat socially isolated family in which neither Gustavo nor Carlos felt affectively connected with each other, and Rosa felt alone and responsible for the family's well-being. A follow-up with social networks interviews (Garbarino & Kapadia, 1986; Garbarino & Sherman, 1980) revealed that even prior to Maria's birth, the family had had few social supports. The families of origin for Rosa and Gustavo both lived over 700 miles away, and the family had not developed strong ties in the community because, the spouses said, they each attended different churches. Given the unique stress of caring for a chronically ill infant, Gustavo and Rosa also completed the Questionnaire on Resources and Stress (QRS; Holroyd, 1987), which measures the impact of an ill or disabled member on the family. Gustavo and Rosa expressed significant stress associated with excessive time demands, lack of social support, apprehension about Maria's poor health, and limited social activities.

The assessor incorporated the assessment data into a theoretical context by referring to the literature on pediatric chronic illness (Kazak, Segal-Andrews, & Johnson, 1995; Wallander & Thompson, 1995; Wood, 1995). Such literature indicates that family functioning is altered substantially when an ill or disabled child is added to the nuclear family system, especially when the illness is life-threatening or seriously affects the child's growth and development (Heffer & Kelley, 1994). Additional readings on the influence of a Hispanic heritage on psychological and family functioning bolstered the assessment of cultural factors contributing to the case formulation (Castillo, 1997; Szapocznik, Kurtines, & Fernandez, 1980).

The family assessment findings were discussed with Gustavo and Rosa, and a treatment plan was proposed. Family strengths were emphasized as a foundation for potential improvement in family functioning. For example, Gustavo was supported for his willingness to discuss his concerns with the assessor and to follow up with treatment recommendations, which ran counter to the gender role stereotypes of many Hispanic men. Similarly, Rosa was encouraged for her stamina under tremendous personal and family pressures. Carlos's eagerness to perform well in school and Anna's gentle spirit were noted as well. Furthermore, care was taken to describe the tragedy of Maria's illness as an opportunity for the family to learn how to work together to overcome extremely difficult circumstances.

Couple therapy (Baucom & Epstein, 1990) was recommended for Rosa and Gustavo to enhance the quality of their marital relationship and communication patterns. Sessions were also planned for the family in which improving satisfaction with parent–child interactions would be the objective (Webster-Stratton, 1994). Although Maria was already being served by an early intervention program in the community, Rosa and Gustavo had not taken full advantage of the respite care and auxiliary support services offered there. Through consultation with the program staff, the family began receiving respite care for Maria both during their weekly therapy appointments and for 1 day per week, which allowed Rosa time to complete necessary errands and to spend some time alone with Anna. Child care was also provided during the monthly parent support group that Rosa and Gustavo began attending at the program center.

Consultation with Maria's pediatrician clarified for the parents some questions they had about her prognosis and the limitations on contact with nonfamily members. Consultation with Maria's nurse practitioner also identified steps Rosa and Gustavo could take to improve the child's physical growth. Along the lines suggested Eisenstadt, Eyberg, McNeil, Newcomb, and Funderbunk (1993), Rosa and Gustavo also agreed to spend several hours each week engaging in mutually pleasant activities with Carlos. Finally, the parents were assisted in collaborating more effectively with school personnel and obtaining appropriate educational services for Carlos.

At regular intervals throughout the family intervention, less formal assessment techniques (e.g., interviews, family observations, consultation with medical and school personnel) were used to monitor therapy progress. Near the final therapy session, more formal assessment techniques (e.g., the SCL-90-R, MSI-R, CBCL, and QRS, as well as structured observations of parent–child interactions) were readministered to document positive treatment outcomes.

CONCLUSION

Comprehensive assessment of families across multiple levels and domains is critical to effective intervention. We advocate an evaluation strategy that targets a range of functioning from the individual to the broader cultural level, and that uses both formal and informal assessment techniques. Important sources of data include subjective phenomenology as well as objective behavioral indicators. Both assessment and intervention are facilitated by explicit theoretical approaches that incorporate a socioecological perspective. Equally important is the personal model of the assessor, which guides the evaluation process and shapes clinical judgments. Assessment of family functioning is a continual hypothesis-testing process interwoven with clinical interventions to monitor progress toward therapeutic goals and reformulate treatment strategies.

REFERENCES

Abidin, R. (1990). *Parenting Stress Index manual* (3rd ed.). Charlottesville, VA: Pediatric Psychology Press.

Achenbach, T. M. (1995). *Child Behavior Checklist Direct Observation Form and 5–18 Profile*. Burlington: University of Vermont, Department of Psychiatry.

Achenbach, T. M. (1991). *Integrative guide for the 1991 CBCL/4–18, YSR, and TRF Profiles*. Burlington: University of Vermont, Department of Psychiatry.

Achenbach, T. M. (1992). *Manual for the Child Behavior Checklist/2–3 and 1992 Profile*. Burlington: University of Vermont, Department of Psychiatry.

Ambrosini, P. J., Metz, C., Prabucki, K., & Lee, J. (1989). Videotape reliability of the third revised edition of the K-SADS. *Journal of the American Academy of Child and Adolescent Psychiatry, 28,* 723-728.

American Educational Research Association, American Psychological Association,

& National Council on Measurement in Education. (1987). *Standards for educational and psychological testing.* Washington, DC: American Psychological Association.

American Psychiatric Association. (1994). *Diagnostic and statistical manual of mental disorders* (4th ed.). Washington, DC: Author.

American Psychological Association. (1985). *Standards for educational and psychological tests.* Washington, DC: Author.

American Psychological Association. (1992). *Ethical principles of psychologists and code of conduct.* Washington, DC: Author.

Archer, R. P. (1992). *MMPI-A: Assessing adolescent psychopathology.* Hillsdale, NJ: Erlbaum.

Arkes, H. R. (1981). Impediments to accurate clinical judgment and possible ways to minimize their impact. *Journal of Consulting and Clinical Psychology, 49,* 323–330.

Barnett, D. W., & Zucker, K. B. (1990). *The personal and social assessment of children.* Boston: Allyn & Bacon.

Baucom, D. H., & Epstein, N. (1990). *Cognitive-behavioral marital therapy.* New York: Brunner/Mazel.

Baucom, D. H., Epstein, N., Sayers, S., & Sher, T. G. (1989). The role of cognitions in marital relationships: Definitional, methodological, and conceptual issues. *Journal of Consulting and Clinical Psychology, 57,* 31–38.

Beavers, W. R., Hampson, R. D., & Hulgus, Y. F. (1985). The Beavers systems approach to family assessment. *Family Process, 24,* 398–405.

Benson, M. J., Long, J. K., & Sporakowski, M. J. (1992). Teaching psychopathology and the DSM-III-R from a family systems perspective. *Family Relations, 41,* 135–140.

Board of Professional Affairs, Committee on Professional Standards, American Psychological Association. (1987). General guidelines for providers of services. *American Psychologist, 42,* 1–12.

Boughner, S. R., Hayes, S. F., Bubenzer, D. L., & West, J. D. (1994). Use of standardized assessment instruments by marital and family therapists: A survey. *Journal of Marital and Family Therapy, 20,* 69–75.

Boyd-Franklin, N. (1989). *Black families in therapy: A multisystems approach.* New York: Guilford Press.

Bronfenbrenner, U. (1986). Ecology of the family as a context for human development: Research perspectives. *Developmental Psychology, 22,* 723–742.

Butcher, J. N. (Ed.). (1997). *Clinical personality assessment: Practical approaches.* New York: Oxford University Press.

Butcher, J. N., Dahlstrom, W. G., Graham, J. R., Tellegen, A., & Kaemmer, B. (1989). *MMPI-2: Manual for administration and scoring.* Minneapolis: University of Minnesota Press.

Butcher, J. N., & Williams, C. (1992). *Essentials of MMPI-2 and MMPI-A interpretation.* Minneapolis: University of Minnesota Press.

Butcher, J. N., Williams, C., Graham, J. R., Archer, R., Tellegan, A. M., Ben-Porath, Y. S., & Kaemmer, B. (1992). *MMPI-A: Manual for administration, scoring, and interpretation.* Minneapolis: University of Minnesota Press.

Caldwell, B. M., & Bradley, R. H. (1994). Environmental issues in developmental follow-up research. In S. L. Friedman & H. C. Haywood (Eds.), *Developmen-*

tal follow-up: Concepts, domains, and methods (pp. 235–256). New York: Academic Press.

Cantrell, M. L., & Cantrell, R. P. (1985). Assessment of the natural environment. *Education and Treatment of Children, 8,* 275–295.

Cantrell, R. P., & Cantrell, M. L. (1980). Ecological problem solving: A decision making heuristic for prevention–intervention education strategies. In J. Hogg & P. Mittler (Eds.), *Advances in mental handicap research* (Vol. 1, pp. 267–301). New York: Wiley.

Carlson, J., Hinkle, J. S., & Sperry, L. (1993). Using diagnosis and DSM-III-R and IV in marriage and family counseling and therapy: Increasing treatment outcomes without losing heart and soul. *The Family Journal, 1,* 308–312.

Castillo, R. J. (1997). *Culture and mental illness: A client-centered approach.* Pacific Grove, CA: Brooks/Cole.

Cavell, T. A., & Snyder, D. K. (1991). Iconoclasm versus innovation: Building a science of family therapy—Comment on Moon, Dillon, and Sprenkle. *Journal of Marital and Family Therapy, 17,* 167–171.

Chambers, W. J., Puig-Antich, J., Hirsch, M., Paez, P., Ambrosini, P., Tabrizi, M. A., & Davies, M. (1985). Test–retest reliability of the Schedule for Affective Disorders and Schizophrenia for School-Age Children, Present Episode. *Archives of General Psychiatry, 42,* 696–702.

Cohen, S., Mermelstein, R., Kamarck, R., & Hoberman, H. M. (1985). Measuring the functional components of social support. In I. G. Sarason & B. R. Sarason (Eds.), *Social support: Theory, research, and applications* (pp. 73–94). Dordrecht, The Netherlands: Nijhoff.

Costa, P. T., & McCrae, R. R. (1992). *Revised NEO Personality Inventory (NEO-PI-R) and NEO Five Factor Inventory (NEO-FFI) professional manual.* Odessa, FL: Psychological Assessment Resources.

Cromwell, R. E., & Peterson, G. W. (1981). Multisystem–multimethod assessment: A framework. In E. E. Filsinger & R. A. Lewis (Eds.), *Assessing marriage: New behavioral approaches* (pp. 38–54). Beverly Hills, CA: Sage.

Dana, R. H. (1994). Testing and assessment ethics for all persons: Beginning and agenda. *Professional Psychology: Research and Practice, 4,* 349–354.

Denton, W. H. (1993, December). Assessment of relational functioning to be optional in the DSM-IV. *Family Therapy News,* p. 28.

Derogatis, L. R. (1994). *Symptom Checklist 90—Revised (SCL-90-R): Administration, scoring, and procedures manual* (3rd ed.). Minneapolis: National Computer Systems.

Derogatis, L. R., & Melisaratos, N. (1979). The DSFI: A multidimensional measure of sexual functioning. *Journal of Sex and Marital Therapy, 5,* 244–281.

Dickey, M. H. (1996). Methods for single-case experiments in family therapy. In D. H. Sprenkle & S. M. Moon (Eds.), *Research methods in family therapy* (pp. 264–285). New York: Guilford Press.

Dodge, K. A. (1983). Behavioral antecedents of peer social status. *Child Development, 54,* 1386–1399.

Dubow, E. F., & Ullman, D. G. (1989). Assessing social support in elementary school children: The Survey of Children's Social Support. *Journal of Clinical Child Psychology, 18,* 52–64.

Eidelson, R. J., & Epstein, N. (1982). Cognition and relationship maladjustment:

Development of a measure of dysfunctional relationship beliefs. *Journal of Consulting and Clinical Psychology, 50,* 715–720.

Eisenstadt, T. H., Eyberg, S. M., McNeil, C. B., Newcomb, K., & Funderbunk, B. (1993). Parent–child interaction therapy with behavior problem children: Relative effectiveness of two stages and overall treatment outcome. *Journal of Clinical Child Psychology, 22,* 42–51.

Endicott, J., & Spitzer, R. L. (1978). A diagnostic interview: The Schedule for Affective Disorders and Schizophrenia. *Archives of General Psychiatry, 35,* 837–844.

Erikson, E. H. (1968). *Identity, youth, and crisis.* New York: Norton.

Eyberg, S. M., & Robinson, E. A. (1983). Dyadic Parent–Child Interaction Coding System: A manual. *Psychological Documents, 13, ? ,* (Ms. No. 2582).

Fielstein, E., Klein, M. S., Fischer, M., Hanon, C., Kchuger, P., Schneider, M. J., & Leitenberg, H. (1985). Self-esteem and causal attributions for success and failure in children. *Cognitive Therapy and Research, 9,* 381–398.

Fiese, B. H., & Sameroff, A. J. (1992). Family context in pediatric psychology: A transactional perspective. In M. C. Roberts & J. L. Wallander (Eds.), *Family issues in pediatric psychology* (pp. 239–260). Hillsdale, NJ: Erlbaum.

Figley, C. R. (1989). *Treating stress in families.* New York: Brunner/Mazel.

Filsinger, E. E. (1983). Assessment: What it is and why it is important. In E. E. Filsinger (Ed.), *Marriage and family assessment: A sourcebook for family therapy* (pp. 11–22). Beverly Hills, CA: Sage.

Fincham, F. D., & Bradbury, T. N. (1992). Assessing attributions in marriage: The Relationship Attribution Measure. *Journal of Personality and Social Psychology, 62,* 457–468.

Fine, M. J. (1995). Family–school intervention. In R. H. Mikesell, D. D. Lusterman, & S. H. McDaniel (Eds.), *Integrating family therapy: Handbook of family psychology and systems theory* (pp. 481–495). Washington, DC: American Psychological Association.

Folkman, S., & Lazarus, R. S. (1988). *Manual for the Ways of Coping Questionnaire.* Palo Alto, CA: Consulting Psychologists Press.

Fredman, N., & Sherman, R. (1987). *Handbook of measurements for marriage and family therapy.* New York: Brunner/Mazel.

Frick, P. J. (1990). *The Alabama Parenting Questionnaire.* Tuscaloosa: University of Alabama.

Frick, P. J., Lahey, B. B., Christ, M. G., Applegate, B., Kerdyck, L., Ollendick, T., Hynd, G. W., Garfinkle, B., Greenhill, L., Biedernman, J., Barkley, R. A., McBurnett, K., Newcorn, J., & Waldman, I. (1994). DSM-IV field trials for the disruptive behavior disorders. *Journal of the American Academy of Child and Adolescent Psychiatry, 33,* 529–539.

Gale, J. (1996). Conversation analysis: Studying the construction of therapeutic realities. In D. H. Sprenkle & S. M. Moon (Eds.), *Research methods in family therapy* (pp. 107–124). New York: Guilford Press.

Garbarino, J., & Kapadia, S. (1986). Ecological assessment procedures. In H. M. Knoff (Ed.), *The assessment of child and adolescent personality* (pp. 451–486). New York: Guilford Press.

Garbarino, J., & Sherman, D. (1980). High-risk neighborhoods and high-risk families: The human ecology of child maltreatment. *Child Development, 51,* 188–198.

228   DIMENSIONS OF FAMILY STRUCTURE

Gerson, R. (1995). The family life cycle: Phases, stages and crises. In R. H. Mikesell, D. D. Lusterman, & S. H. McDaniel (Eds.), *Integrating family therapy: Handbook of family psychology and systems theory* (pp. 91–111). Washington, DC: American Psychological Association.

Gottman, J. M. (1979). *Marital interactions: Experimental investigations.* New York: Academic Press.

Gough, H. G. (1996). *Revised California Personality Inventory (CPI) manual* (3rd ed.). Palo Alto, CA: Consulting Psychologists Press.

Gray-Little, B. (1997). The assessment of psychopathology in racial and ethnic minorities. In J. N. Butcher (Ed.), *Clinical personality assessment: Practical approaches* (pp. 140–157). New York: Oxford University Press.

Gresham, F. M., & Little, S. G. (1993). Peer-referenced assessment strategies. In T. H. Ollendick & M. Hersen (Eds.), *Handbook of child and adolescent assessment* (pp. 165–179). Needham Heights, MA: Allyn & Bacon.

Grotevant, H. D., & Carlson, C. I. (1989). *Family assessment: A guide to methods and measures.* New York: Guilford Press.

Hansen, J. C., & Falicov, C. J. (1983). *Cultural perspectives in family therapy.* Rockville, MD: Aspen.

Hartman, A. (1979). *Finding families: An ecological approach to family assessment in adoption.* Beverly Hills, CA: Sage.

Hartman, A. (1995). Diagrammatic assessment in family relationships. *Families in Society, 76,* 111–112.

Hayes, S. C., Nelson, R. O., & Jarrett, R. B. (1987). The treatment utility of assessment: A functional approach to evaluating assessment quality. *American Psychologist, 42,* 963–974.

Heffer, R. W., & Kelley, M. L. (1994). Nonorganic failure to thrive: Developmental outcomes and psychosocial assessment and intervention issues. *Research in Developmental Disabilities, 15,* 247–268.

Hill, R., & Mattessich, P. (1979). Family development theory and life-span development. In P. B. Baltes & O. G. Brim (Eds.), *Life-span development and behavior* (Vol. 2, pp. 161–204). New York: Plenum Press.

Hohenshil, T. H. (1993). Teaching the DSM-III-R in counselor education. *Counselor Education and Supervision, 32,* 267–275.

Holroyd, J. (1987). *Questionnaire on Resources and Stress—for families with chronically ill or handicapped members.* Austin, TX: Pro-Ed.

Hughes, J. N., & Baker, D. B. (1990). *The clinical child interview.* New York: Guilford Press.

Huston, T. L. (1983). Power. In H. H. Kelley, E. Berscheid, A. Christensen, J. H. Harvey, T. L. Huston, G. Levinger, E. McClintock, L. A. Peplau, & D. R. Peterson (Eds.), *Close relationships* (pp. 169–219). New York: Freeman.

Hutchins, D. E. (1992). *Hutchins Behavior Inventory.* Palo Alto, CA: Consulting Psychologists Press.

Jacob, T., & Tennenbaum, D. L. (1988). *Family assessment: Rationale, methods, and future directions.* New York: Plenum Press.

Jacobson, N. S. (1992). Behavioral couple therapy: A new beginning. *Behavior Therapy, 23,* 493–506.

Kamphaus, R. W., & Frick, P. J. (1996). *Clinical assessment of child and adolescent personality and behavior.* Needham Heights, MA: Allyn & Bacon.

Karpel, M. A. (1994). *Evaluating couples: A handbook for practitioners.* New York: Norton.

Kaslow, N. J., & Celano, M. P. (1995). The family therapies. In A. S. Gurman & S. B. Messer (Eds.), *Essential psychotherapies: Theory and practice* (pp. 343–402). New York: Guilford Press.

Kazak, A. E., Segal-Andrews, A. M., & Johnson, K. (1995). Pediatric psychology research and practice: A family/systems approach. In M. C. Roberts (Ed.), *Handbook of pediatric psychology* (2nd ed., pp. 84–104). New York: Guilford Press.

Kelley, M. L., & Carper, L. B. (1988). The Mothers' Activity Checklist: An instrument for assessing pleasant and unpleasant events. *Behavioral Assessment, 10,* 331–341.

Kleinman, A. (1992). How important is culture for DSM-IV? In J. E. Mezzich, A. Kleinmen, H. Fabrega, B. Good, G. Johnson-Powell, K. M. Lin, S. Manson, & D. Parron (Eds.), *Cultural proposals for DSM-IV: Submitted to the DSM-IV Task Force by the Steering Committee, NIMH Group on Culture and Diagnosis* (pp. 7–28). Pittsburgh: University of Pittsburgh.

Kochanska, G., Kuczynski, L., & Radke-Yarrow, M. (1989). Correspondence between mothers' self-reported and observed child rearing practices. *Child Development, 60,* 56–63.

Krokoff, L. J., Gottman, J. M., & Hass, S. D. (1989). Validation of a global Rapid Couples Interaction Scoring System. *Behavioral Assessment, 11,* 65–79.

L'Abate, L. (1994). *Family evaluation: A psychological approach.* Thousand Oaks, CA: Sage.

L'Abate, L., & Bagarozzi, D. (1993). *Sourcebook of marriage and family evaluation.* New York: Brunner/Mazel.

La Greca, A. M. (1990). *Through the eyes of the child.* Needham Heights, MA: Allyn & Bacon.

Lachar, D. (1990). *Multidimensional description of child personality: A manual for the Personality Inventory for Children.* Los Angeles: Western Psychological Services.

Lachar, D., & Gruber, C. P. (1995a). *Personality Inventory for Youth (PIY) manual: Administration and interpretation technical guide.* Los Angeles: Western Psychological Services.

Lachar, D., & Gruber, C. P. (1995b). *Personality Inventory for Youth (PIY) manual: Technical guide.* Los Angeles: Western Psychological Services.

Lazarus, R. S., & Folkman, S. (1984). *Stress, appraisals, and coping.* New York: Springer.

Madanes, C., Dukes, J., & Harben, H. T. (1980). Family ties of heroin addicts. *Archives of General Psychiatry, 43,* 889–894.

Margolin, G., Michelli, J., & Jacobson, N. S. (1988). Assessment of marital dysfunction. In A. S. Bellack & M. Hersen (Eds.), *Behavioral assessment* (pp. 441–489). New York: Pergamon Press.

Matsumoto, D. (1997). *Culture and modern life.* Pacific Grove, CA: Brooks/Cole.

McAllister, L. (1996). *A practical guide to CPI interpretation* (3rd ed.). Palo Alto, CA: Consulting Psychologists Press.

McGoldrick, M., & Gerson, R. (1985). *Genograms in family assessment.* New York: Norton.

McGoldrick, M., Giordano, J., & Pearce, J. K. (Eds.). (1996). *Ethnicity and family therapy* (2nd ed.). New York: Guilford Press.

Millon, T., Millon, C., & Davis, R. (1993). *Manual for the Millon Adolescent Clinical Inventory.* Minneapolis: National Computer Systems.

Millon, T., Millon, C., & Davis, R. (1994). *Manual for the Millon Clinical Multiaxial Inventory—III.* Minneapolis: National Computer Systems.

Moos, R. H., & Moos, B. S. (1994). *Family Environment Scale manual: Development, application, and research.* Palo Alto, CA: Consulting Psychologists Press.

Naglieri, J. A., LeBuffe, P. A., & Pfieffer, S. I. (1993). *Devereux Behavior Rating Scales-School Form.* San Antonio, TX: Psychological Corporation.

Naglieri, J. A., LeBuffe, P. A., & Pfieffer, S. I. (1994). *Devereux Scales of Mental Disorders.* San Antonio, TX: Psychological Corporation.

Neeper, R., Lahey, B. B., & Frick, P. J. (1990). *Comprehensive Behavior Rating Scale for Children.* San Antonio, TX: Psychological Corporation.

Okazaki, S., & Sue, S. (1997). Cultural considerations in psychological assessment of Asian-Americans. In J. N. Butcher (Ed.), *Clinical personality assessment: Practical approaches* (pp. 107–119). New York: Oxford University Press.

O'Leary, K. D. (1987). *Assessment of marital discord: An integration for research and clinical practice.* Hillsdale, NJ: Erlbaum.

Olson, D. H. (1986). Circumplex model VII: Validation studies and FACES III. *Family Process, 25,* 337–351.

Olson, D. H., Portner, J., & Lavee, Y. (1985). *FACES III.* (Available from Family Social Science, University of Minnesota, St. Paul, MN 55108)

Patterson, G. R. (1982). *Coercive family process.* Eugene, OR: Castalia.

Peterson, C., & Villanova, P. (1988). An expanded Attributional Style Questionnaire. *Journal of Abnormal Psychology, 97,* 87–89.

Pino, C. J., Simons, N., & Slawinowski, M. J. (1984). *Children's Version: Family Environment Scale.* Palo Alto, CA: Consulting Psychologists Press.

Porter, B., & O'Leary, K. D. (1980). Marital discord and childhood behavior problems. *Journal of Abnormal Child Psychology, 8,* 287–295.

Quittner, A. L. (1992). Re-examining research on stress and social support: The importance of contextual factors. In A. M. La Greca, L. J. Siegel, J. L. Wallander, & C. E. Walker (Eds.), *Stress and coping in child health* (pp. 85–118). New York: Guilford Press.

Reid, J. B. (Ed.). (1978). *A social learning approach to family intervention: Vol. 2. Observation in home settings.* Eugene, OR: Castalia.

Reid, M., & Ramey, S. L. (1992). *Dialogues About Families administration manual: Interviews with children and parents about themselves, their families, goals and values, and social networks.* Seattle: Child Development and Mental Retardation Center, University of Washington.

Reynolds, C. R., & Kamphaus, R. W. (1992). *BASC: Behavioral Assessment System for Children manual.* Circle Pines, MN: American Guidance Service.

Roberts, G. C., Block, J. H., & Block, J. (1984). Continuity and change in parents' childrearing practices. *Child Development, 55,* 586–597.

Robin, A. L., & Foster, S. L. (1989). *Negotiating parent–adolescent conflict.* New York: Guilford Press.

Robin, A. L., & Weiss, J. G. (1980). Criterion-related validity of behavioral and self-report measures of problem-solving communication skills in distressed and nondistressed parent–adolescent dyads. *Behavioral Assessment, 2,* 339–352.

Robins, L. N., Helzer, J. E., Croughan, J., & Ratcliff, K. S. (1981). The National Institute of Mental Health Diagnostic Interview Schedule: Its history, characteristics, and validity. *Archives of General Psychiatry, 38,* 381–389.

Robinson, J. P., Shaver, P. R., & Wrightman, L. S. (1991). *Measures of personality and social psychological attitudes.* San Diego, CA: Academic Press.

Ross, L. (1977). The intuitive psychologist and his shortcomings: Distortions in the attribution process. In L. Berkowitz (Ed.), *Advances in experimental social psychology* (Vol. 10, pp. 54–73). New York: Academic Press.

Sachs, P. R. (1994). Working with individuals with disabilities: What the family therapist needs to know. *The Family Psychologist, 10,* 19–22.

Sattler, J. M. (1992). *Assessment of children* (3rd ed., rev.). San Diego, CA: Jerome M. Sattler, Publisher.

Schumm, W. R. (1990). Evolution of the family field: Measurement principles and techniques. In J. Touliatos, B. F. Perlmutter, & M. A. Straus (Eds.), *Handbook of family measurement techniques* (pp. 23–36). Newbury Park, CA: Sage.

Selvini Palazzoli, M., Boscolo, L., Cecchin, G., & Prata, G. (1980). Hypothesizing—circularity—neutrality: Three guidelines for the conductor of the session. *Family Process, 19,* 3–12.

Schludermann, S., & Schludermann, E. (1983). Sociocultural change and adolescents' perceptions of parental behaviors. *Developmental Psychology, 19,* 674–685.

Shaffer, D., Schwab-Stone, M., Fisher, P., Cohen, P., Piacentini, J., Davies, M., Conners, C. K., & Regier, D. (1993). The Diagnostic Interview Schedule for Children—Revised Version (DISC-R): Preparation, field testing, interrater reliability, and acceptability. *Journal of the American Academy of Child and Adolescent Psychiatry, 32,* 643–650.

Shellenberger, S., & Hoffman, S. S. (1995). The changing family–work system. In R. H. Mikesell, D. D. Lusterman, & S. H. McDaniel (Eds.), *Integrating family therapy: Handbook of family psychology and systems theory* (pp. 461–479). Washington, DC: American Psychological Association.

Shelton, K. K., Frick, P. J., & Wooton, J. (1996). Assessment of parenting practices in families of elementary school-age children. *Journal of Clinical Child Psychology, 25,* 317–329.

Skinner, H. A., Steinhauer, P. D., & Santa-Barbara, J. (1984). *The Family Assessment Measure: Administration and interpretation guide.* Toronto: Addiction Research Foundation.

Slonim, M. (1991). *Children, culture, and ethnicity: Evaluating and understanding the impact.* New York: Garland Press.

Smedes, L. B. (1984). *Forgive and forget: Healing the hurts we don't deserve.* San Francisco: Harper & Row.

Snyder, D. K. (1997). *Manual for the Marital Satisfaction Inventory—Revised.* Los Angeles: Western Psychological Services.

Snyder, D. K., Cavell, T. A., Heffer, R. W., & Mangrum, L. F. (1995). Marital and family assessment: A multifaceted, multilevel approach. In R. H. Mikesell, D. D. Lusterman, & S. H. McDaniel (Eds.), *Integrating family therapy: Handbook of family psychology and systems theory* (pp. 163–182). Washington, DC: American Psychological Association.

Snyder, D. K., & Costin, S. (1994). The Marital Satisfaction Inventory. In M. E. Maruish (Ed.), *Use of psychological testing for treatment planning and outcome assessment* (pp. 322–351). Hillsdale, NJ: Erlbaum.

Snyder, D. K., Lachar, D., Freiman, K. E., & Hoover, D. W. (1991). Toward the actuarial assessment of couples' relationships. In J. P. Vincent (Ed.), *Advances in family intervention, assessment, and theory* (Vol. 5, pp. 89–122). London: Jessica Kingsley.

Snyder, D. K., Mangrum, L. F., & Wills, R. M. (1993). Predicting couples' response to marital therapy: A comparison of short- and long-term predictors. *Journal of Consulting and Clinical Psychology, 61,* 61–69.

Snyder, D. K., & Rice, J. L. (1996). Methodological issues and strategies in scale development. In D. H. Sprenkle & S. M. Moon (Eds.), *Research methods in family therapy* (pp. 216–237). New York: Guilford Press.

Sofield, L., Juliano, C., & Hammett, R. (1990). *Design for wholeness: Dealing with anger, learning to forgive, building self-esteem.* Notre Dame, IN: Ave Maria Press.

Sporakowski, M. J. (1995). Assessment and diagnosis in marriage and family counseling. *Journal of Counseling and Development, 74,* 60–74.

Strong, T. (1993). DSM-IV and describing problems in family therapy. *Family Process, 32,* 249–253.

Szapocznik, J., Kurtines, W. M., & Fernandez, T. (1980). Bicultural involvement in Hispanic American youths. *International Journal of Intercultural Relations, 4,* 353–365.

Tomm, K. (1988). Interventive interviewing: Part III. Intending to ask lineal, circular, strategic, or reflexive questions? *Family Process, 27,* 1–15.

Touliatos, J., Perlmutter, B. F., & Straus, M. A. (Eds.). (1990). *Handbook of family measurement techniques.* Newbury Park, CA: Sage.

Turnbill, H. R., & Turnbill, A. P. (1994). How changing norms and forms affect family therapists' legal obligations. *The Family Psychologist, 10,* 19–22.

Vargas, L. A., & Willis, D. J. (1994). Introduction to the special section: New directions in the treatment and assessment of ethnic minority children and adolescents. *Journal of Clinical Child Psychology, 23,* 2–4.

Velásquez, R. J. (1997). The assessment of Hispanic clients. In J. N. Butcher (Ed.), *Clinical personality assessment: Practical approaches* (pp. 120–139). New York: Oxford University Press.

Wahler, R. G. (1980). The insular mother: Her problems in parent–child treatment. *Journal of Applied Behavior Analysis, 13,* 273–294.

Waldo, M., Brotherton, W. D., & Horswill, R. (1993). Integrating DSM-III-R training into school, marriage and family, and mental health counselor preparation. *Counselor Education and Supervision, 32,* 332–342.

Wallander, J. L., & Thompson, R. J. (1995). Psychosocial adjustment of children with chronic physical conditions. In M. C. Roberts (Ed.), *Handbook of pediatric psychology* (2nd ed., pp. 124–141). New York: Guilford Press.

Webster-Stratton, C. (1994). Advancing videotape parent training: A comparison study. *Journal of Consulting and Clinical Psychology, 62,* 583–593.

Weiss, R. L., & Tolman, A. O. (1990). The Marital Interaction Coding System— Global (MICS-G): A global companion to the MICS. *Behavioral Assessment, 12,* 271–294.

Witt, J. C., Cavell, T. A., Heffer, R. W., Carey, M. P., & Martens, B. K. (1988). Child self-report: Interviewing techniques and rating scales. In E. S. Shapiro & T. R. Kratochwill (Eds.), *Behavioral assessment in schools: Approaches to classification and intervention* (pp. 384–454). New York: Guilford Press.

Witt, J. C., Elliott, S. N., Gresham, F. M., & Kramer, J. J. (1988). *Assessment of special children: Tests and the problem-solving process*. Glenview, IL: Scott, Foresman.

Witt, J. C., Heffer, R. W., & Pfeiffer, J. (1990). Structured rating scales: A review of self-report and informant rating processes, procedures, and issues. In C. R. Reynolds & R. W. Kamphaus (Eds.), *Handbook of psychological and educational assessment in children: Vol. 2. Personality, behavior, and context* (pp. 364–394). New York: Guilford Press.

Wood, B. L. (1995). A developmental biopsychosocial approach to the treatment of chronic illness in children and adolescents. In R. H. Mikesell, D. D. Lusterman, & S. H. McDaniel (Eds.), *Integrating family therapy: Handbook of family psychology and systems theory* (pp. 437-455). Washington, DC: American Psychological Association.

VARIETIES OF INDIVIDUAL AND FAMILY PSYCHOPATHOLOGY

CHAPTER 10

⬥

Destructive Parentification in Families: Causes and Consequences

GREGORY J. JURKOVIC

Family members are emotionally bonded by their mutual concern, loyalty, and trust. When these bonds are exploited or breached, various relational problems and disorders—traditionally ascribed to individuals—are the result. One of the most common, albeit often hidden, imbalances in the exchange of caring in families involves a process referred to in the literature as "destructive parentification" (Boszormenyi-Nagy, 1987; Boszormenyi-Nagy & Krasner, 1986; Boszormenyi-Nagy & Spark, 1973). Destructively parentified children assume excessive responsibility for other family members and often for the family as a whole. Their caretaking efforts are neither acknowledged nor supported. Similar dynamics characterize couple relationships in which one or both partners induce the other to enact a parentified role.

Changes in the postmodern American family have heightened children's risk for destructive parentification. For example, the rates of cohabitation, divorce, single parenting, out-of-wedlock births, and homeless families have risen significantly. Moreover, the traditional two-parent family, which once was the norm, is overtaxed emotionally and economically and is struggling to survive, frequently without the benefit of extended family ties. Deteriorating neighborhoods, joblessness, inadequate social services, and insufficient resources for diverse family forms are further stranding parents and couples in U.S. society. As a result, children are increasingly being called upon to serve as a primary support system for their parents, siblings, and families. Although this is often adaptive for the

237

family, the parentification process, particularly in its most destructive form, may significantly disrupt children's development and functioning (Jurkovic, 1997).

The dynamics associated with parentification have been the focus of a theoretically diverse group of investigators over the years. As early as 1948, Schmideberg observed that emotionally deprived parents may unconsciously regard their children as parental figures. Other individual- and family-oriented psychodynamic writers, as well as researchers guided by family systems theory, role theory, models of codependency, anthropology, developmental psychology, and attachment theory, have referred to kindred processes. Such constructs as "role reversal" (Morris & Gould, 1963), "parental child" (Minuchin, Montalvo, Guerney, Rosman, & Schumer, 1967; Minuchin, 1974), "spousification" (Sroufe & Ward, 1980), and "compulsive caregiving" (Bowlby, 1979) all relate to parentification. (See Jurkovic, 1997, for further discussion of these and associated constructs.)

The early work of Boszormenyi-Nagy, Minuchin, Bowlby, and others has drawn increasing scholarly attention to the plight of parentified individuals and their families. Although most of the literature in this area consists of clinical descriptions and theoretical formulations, a growing data base exists that is enriching our understanding of destructively parentifying relational processes. After briefly considering definitional problems, this chapter draws from the empirical work conducted to date to highlight causes and consequences of parentification.

DEFINING "PARENTIFICATION"

"By definition," according to Boszormenyi-Nagy and Spark (1973), "parentification implies the subjective distortion of a relationship as if one's partner or even children were his [or her] parent" (p. 151). Whether such distortions are destructive, however, is dependent on their relational consequences and ethical significance within the balance of give and take in the family.

Within Boszormenyi-Nagy's framework, the parentified family member's role is not limited to overt caretaking, as it is in Minuchin's (1974) description; rather, it may include various role activities and processes that appear to protect or satisfy the object needs of the parentifier. For example, immature or irresponsible behavior by a child that distracts a parent from his or her depression can be seen as a form of caretaking. The implication is that any unfair relational dynamic, regardless of the overt behaviors involved, potentially signifies a destructive parentification process. "Ironically," according to Karpel (1976), "the concept of parentification has . . . been as over-burdened as the child it often describes" (p. 166).

Clearly, the conceptual boundaries of Boszormenyi-Nagy's definition of parentification must be more carefully drawn if the construct is to have specific referents and to be investigated empirically. Toward this end, Karpel (1976) distinguished "functional" and "ethical" levels of the parentification process. The former involves overt caretaking behaviors that do not require a high degree of clinical inference to discern. Individuals who are committed to and concerned about their partners or parents, but are not overfunctioning in an overtly protective, caretaking, or responsible fashion, are referred to by Karpel as "loyal objects." The children mentioned earlier who seem to be engaging in distracting misbehavior to help a depressed parent fall into the class of loyal objects. Whereas all parentified individuals are loyal objects, not all loyal objects are parentified.

The ethical level of parentification refers to the balance of fairness in the family. The destructiveness of the parentification process turns in Boszormenyi-Nagy's theory on the degree to which the parentified individual's actions are appropriately acknowledged, supported, and reciprocated. Because of the inherent asymmetry of the parent–child relationship, it is assumed from an ethical perspective that children's contributions to the family should not exceed their developmental capacity or equal those of the parents.

Although Karpel has helped to delimit the parentification construct, he has not captured all of its multivalent features. In an effort to define parentification more comprehensively, while at the same time increasing its specificity and operationalizability, I have recently proposed an elaboration of the properties of the parentified family member's role (degree of overtness, type of role assignments, extent of responsibility, object of concern, laterality of caretaking) and the context within which this role is embedded (developmental stage, internalization, boundaries, social legitimacy, ethicality). Ongoing attempts to operationalize parentification through various self-report, projective, interview, and observational methods are increasingly incorporating these properties (see Jurkovic, 1997).

CAUSES

Investigators in the area of parentification have explored causal agents that span multiple levels of analysis, ranging from variables at an ontogenetic level to macrosystemic influences.

Parental Background

Ontogenetically, it can be adduced that the quality of the parent–child relationship is grounded in the parent's experiences of being parented as a child. Suggestive evidence for this linkage has emerged in studies of abused and neglected children, many of whom possess parentified attributes. Retrospective empirical investigations of the parents of these children have revealed a history of various abuses and privations in their own families of origin. The data from prospective studies, however, are less clear (see Rutter, 1989).

Investigators have begun to evaluate intergenerational continuities in parenting problems for youngsters whose maltreatment is restricted primarily to a destructive form of parentification. Sroufe and Ward (1980), for example, serendipitously discovered a phenomenon, which they termed "spousification," in the course of investigating the disciplinary actions of mothers of young children. They observed that when some of the mothers needed attention, support, or reassurance, they turned to their children, whom they physically overstimulated. Follow-up investigation revealed signs of sexual misuse and deprivation in the backgrounds of these mothers. (See also Sroufe, Jacobvitz, Mangelsdorf, DeAngelo, & Ward, 1985.)

Relatedly, Burkett (1991) observed family interactions and found that mothers with a history of sexual abuse were more self-focused than were nonabused women. The children of the abused mothers were also more parent-focused than the control children. Further reflecting a reversal of parent–child roles, striking differences emerged between the two groups of mothers in a semistructured parenting interview. The mothers who had been maltreated reported using their children as primary companions and emotional caretakers to a much greater extent than did the comparison women. For example, one of the maltreated mothers described her relationship with her 9-year-old daughter as follows (quoted in Burkett, 1991, p. 429):

> It's her and I, and sometimes I get support from her, and I'm not sure if she's old enough to give it. I forget that she's a child, especially when I'm confiding in her, I'm talking to her at an adult level, and I forget that she's not an adult. I've decided I can't confide in her like she's another adult because she just can't keep it to herself.

On the basis of observational and questionnaire data, Jacobvitz, Morgan, Kretchmar, and Morgan (1991) discovered that grandmothers' memories of overprotection in their families of origin were related to a pattern of role reversal and intrusiveness with their adult daughters. Similarly, the daughters' memories of overprotection during childhood, or their current unaffectionate and enmeshed relationships with their mothers (including parentification), predicted their intrusive care of their own infants. Moreover, their reports of overprotection were related to a generalized distrust of others, which in turn forecast their own parental intrusiveness when their infants were 9 months old. This study provides some of the best empirical evidence to date for intergenerational continuity of boundary disturbances, although it appears that these disturbances may assume different forms: overprotection, role reversal (or parentification), and intrusiveness.

Attachment

The family histories of many parents who were parentified or who parentify their own children intimate disruptions in their attachment to primary caretakers. Just as sexual abuse can be seen as the intergenerational transmission of an insecure attachment (Alexander, 1992), so can destructive forms of parentification. Parents with unmet attachment needs often look to their children to gratify these needs, particularly if their partners have failed them in this regard. The children may accommodate their parents to maintain affectional ties that otherwise would not be available to them. Paradoxically, by serving as attachment figures for their parents, they satisfy their own needs for proximity and connection—however insecurely (Bowlby, 1980).

Main and Cassidy (1988) found that infants who appeared disorganized and disoriented with their caregivers (evidence of an attachment disturbance) exhibited signs of parentification later in their development. Older children in families may also become caregivers and even supplemental attachment figures for their younger siblings, in the event of separation from parental figures or loss of a family member (Ainsworth, 1989). Evidence of such potentially adaptive kinship bonds also exists in the absence of trauma (Stewart, 1983; Stewart & Marvin, 1984).

Parental Cognitions and Attitudes

The transgenerational transmission of destructive parentification and related parent–child dysfunction may also be mediated by cognitive processes (see, e.g., Bowlby, 1979; Newberger & White, 1989). A number of studies of populations at risk for parentifying children provide indirect evidence for this hypothesis. Newberger (1977) found that in comparison to a matched group of nonabusive parents, parents with a recent history of having abused their children scored significantly lower on her semistructured interview measure of Parental Awareness. The responses of the abusive group revealed tendencies to view children as projections of their own experiences and to infuse their conceptions of the parental role with their own personal wishes and needs. Characteristic of the "egoistic" stage in Newberger's coding scheme, this orientation has also been observed by others interested in parentification (e.g., Karpel, 1976; Minuchin et al., 1967). Newberger also reported, however, that half of the abusive parents reasoned as high as the comparison group at some point in the interview, suggesting that they had the capacity to conceive of the parenting process in mature ways. Further exploration led Newberger to hypothesize that severe stress and problems of survival compromised the reasoning abilities of these parents.

From a developmental perspective, it is plausible that the reasoning of young parents, especially teenagers with children, would also reveal considerable egoistic thinking about family roles and processes. Such thinking is consistent with the expressed parentifying wishes of many unwed teenage mothers to give birth to children who will love and nurture them. The stress and social constriction resulting from having children while negotiating adolescence also probably retard teenagers' sociocognitive development. Some support for this hypothesis can be found in a study conducted by Jelley (1980). In comparison to a matched group of low-income African American adolescents without children, those with children reasoned at an egoistic level on Newberger's measure to a significantly greater degree.

Other investigators (Fox, Baisch, Goldberg, & Hochmuth, 1987; Hanson, 1990) also discovered that in comparison to adult normative data, pregnant adolescents scored in the less mature range on all four scales (Corporal Punishment, Developmental Expectations, Empathy, Role Reversal) of Bavolek's (1984) Adult–Adolescent Parenting Inventory (AAPI). In Hanson's sample, composed mostly of European American adolescents, 29% of the scores on the AAPI Role Reversal scale were exceptionally low, placing them at high risk of parentifying their children. Although only 5% of the African American adolescents scored as low in Fox et al.'s study, the number (23%) of European American adolescents with low Role Reversal scores in their sample approached that in Hanson's group. Thus, it appears that parenting attitudes about parentification differ as a function of ethnic/racial background—an observation that is discussed further later in this section.

Inspection of Bavolek's normative data on the AAPI for different groups reveals that abused adolescents obtained less mature scores on the Role Reversal scale than either the adults or the nonabused adolescents. This finding also points to the putative role of parenting attitudes as a mediating variable in the relation of parental deprivation and abuse to the parentification of children.

Developmental Capacity to Care

Another ubiquitous ontogenetic process that figures importantly in the parentification process is children's developing ability to take care of family members—an ability that destructively parentifying parents exploit. Drawing from the developmental theorizing and studies of Stern (1985) and others (see, e.g., Zahn-Waxler & Robinson, 1995), I have speculated that by the end of the first year of life children are attuned to their parents' feelings and intentions, and increasingly sacrifice aspects of their development to meet the parentifying demands of family members (Jurkovic, 1997).

Bridgeman (1983) has empirically documented the performance of helping and nurturing actions by children as young as 18 months during play with their parents. In addition, Rheingold (1982) found a high incidence of unsolicited helping behavior on the part of the youngest children in her sample (aged 18–30 months) (see also Rheingold, Hay, & West, 1976). Of note is that these data were collected in a laboratory environment. Naturalistic observations in children's homes have revealed beneficent behavior in even younger children, particularly in reaction to parents' emotional needs (e.g., Zahn-Waxler & Kochanska, 1988; Zahn-Waxler & Robinson, 1995).

Stressors

Serious and prolonged stress in the family often leads to the parentification of one or more of its members. Researchers have examined this phenomenon across a variety of stressors. For example, over four decades ago Bossard and Boll (1956) found that oldest children, particularly girls, in large families tended to assume significant responsibilities in the home.

Dawson (1980) discovered that children of single parents were assigned more household management tasks than their counterparts in two-parent families were. Indeed, based on his large-scale study in this area, Weiss (1979) had earlier reported that children in single-parent families were often defined as "junior partners." Fry and Trifiletti's (1983) factor analysis of interview data from 150 adolescents in single-parent families revealed four stress-causing dimensions: role reversal, family conflict and distress, parents' affective states, and adolescent disharmony.

Marital stress is another probable determinant of parentification in children. Longitudinal data collected by Cummings, Zahn-Waxler, and Radke-Yarrow (1981, 1984) indicated that even 2-year-olds actively attempted to stop or mediate parental conflict and to console the emotionally injured party. Two years later these same youngsters were observed to be practicing similar intervention strategies, although more efficaciously. Perhaps related to the adaptiveness of their mediating role, they also appeared less distressed.

Children whose parents suffer from various forms of psychopathology are also often conscripted into a parentified role. For example, we, along with others, have discovered more evidence of childhood parentification in college students with alcoholic parents than in students from nonalcoholic families (Chase, Deming, & Wells, 1998; Goglia, Jurkovic, Burt, & Burge-Callaway, 1992).

Zahn-Waxler and her colleagues (see Zahn-Waxler & Kochanska, 1988; Zahn-Waxler & Robinson, 1995) have found that children become overinvolved in the problems of parents with major depression and bipolar disorders. In one study, depressed and well mothers were prompted to simulate sadness and concern in the presence of their 2- and 3-year-olds. Toddlers exhibited significantly more frequent comforting responses, and significantly more types of such responses, toward depressed than toward nondepressed mothers. There are suggestions, however, that many children who become overinvolved at an early age in the emotional problems of their parents engage in more avoidant and distancing behaviors later in childhood (Zahn-Waxler, Kochanska, Krupnick, & McKnew, 1990).

Sociocultural Factors

In evaluating the significance of the different determinants discussed thus far, it is important to consider the moderating effect of the sociocultural context of children's parentified activities. For example, cross-cultural research has revealed that sibling caretaking is common and is appropriately defined and supervised in many societies (see Super & Harkness, 1981, 1982; Weisner & Gallimore, 1977). One investigative team (Harrison, Wilson, Pine, Chan, & Buriel, 1990) found that older siblings in African American, Asian Pacific American, Native American, and Hispanic families are routinely assigned child care responsibilities in the home. Although this practice is partly an adaptation of ethnic minority families to their stressful situation within larger society, it also derives from a long-standing intergenerational world view that values loyalty, cooperation, and kinship ties. It also reflects the fact that some cultures and subcultures regard children as responsible beings very early in their lives (Rehberg & Richman, 1989).

Gender is another potentially important moderating variable in this area. Related to gender role socialization patterns, girls in the United States and other countries around the world are typically overrepresented in an overt caretaking capacity in their families (see Goglia et al., 1992; Weisner & Gallimore, 1977; Whiting & Edwards, 1973; Wolkin, 1984). Although female college students scored higher than their male cohorts on a self-report measure of parentification in our study (Goglia et al., 1992), the two groups did not differ on Walsh's (1979) projective measure of child-as-mate and child-as-parent boundary distortions. We speculated, in part, that although males are as involved and concerned about family members as females, they may express their concern differently—for example, as loyal objects.

CONSEQUENCES

As with research in the area of causation, empirical exploration of the multilateral effects of parentification has been limited. Nonetheless, the data base in this area has illuminated both positive and negative outcomes for the parentified child, as well as for other members of his or her family.

Parentified Children

Personality Functioning

The relation of parentification to various personality dimensions and traits has been the focus of a number of studies. For example, as part of his study of Kenyan families, Ember (1973) found that boys whose work included tasks (e.g., child care) usually assigned to girls exhibited more traditionally feminine social behaviors than boys who were not given such tasks. It is possible that parentification, particularly if it involves child care and expressive responsibilities, encourages an androgynous gender role orientation in boys, while fostering a more extreme, traditionally feminine one in girls. Further testing of this hypothesis is needed.

Other researchers have found that children's involvement in household work does not appear to covary with teacher ratings of responsibility and dependability at school (Elder, 1974; Harris, Clark, Rose, & Valasek, 1963). However, cross-cultural studies of prosocial behavior have provided evidence of beneficial effects. Whiting and Whiting (1975), for example, found that the most altruistic children in their samples included those whose work was extensive and directly benefited the family (e.g., collecting firewood, cooking, babysitting). Caring for babies was significantly related to nurturance toward peers in Ember's (1973) research of Kenyan children. Weiss's (1979) research on single-parent households in the United States also suggests that because of their vital contribution to familial functioning, children in these families are more responsible, independent, and attuned to adult values and worries than their cohorts in two-parent families are.

The single parents and adolescents interviewed by Weiss (1979), however, also reported a number of concerns. Parents' regrets that their youngsters' childhood and teenage years had not been less stressful were echoed by the adolescent respondents. Having learned to share their parents' problems and uncertainties, the latter experienced less security. One of the adolescent girls in this sample said, "You don't have, not necessarily the childhood, but you don't have the freedom of not worrying about things, about money" (quoted in Weiss, 1979, p. 106). Weiss's findings also indicate that an adolescent's development is less likely to be compromised by living in a single-parent household if (1) the adolescent's earlier needs for nurturance have been met, and (2) parental support and investment continue to be provided. Younger children in these families, however, are in danger of being destructively parentified because of developmental limitations in their ability to cope with a junior partner role. Goodnow (1988) similarly concluded that children feel less exploited if they perceive that their work assignments—however demanding—are necessary, are shared with their parents, and can be completed autonomously.

Investigating 1,208 adolescents in the Boston area, Gore, Aseltine, and Colten (1993) discovered that in families experiencing significant stress, girls who were very involved in their mothers' problems and who scored high on an interpersonal involvement scale reported more symptoms of depression than did boys with the same profile. According to the researchers, because of the greater emphasis on relationships in the socialization of girls than in that of boys, the latter's involvement in their mothers' difficulties may not have been as emotionally upsetting. The stability of these gender differences will be addressed by Gore and his colleagues in planned follow-up interviews of the participants until their young adult years.

Cross-sectional data collected by Wolkin (1984) indicate that the long-term effects of excessive parentification may be similar for males and females. Self-report parentification scores in a sample of college undergraduates correlated positively with indices of depression and dependency on the Minnesota Multiphasic Personality Inventory. One gender difference did emerge, however: Scores on the Self-Acceptance scale of the California Psychological Inventory and on the parentification instrument were positively related for females but not for males. Perhaps the congruence of the females' responsibilities as a child with gender role expectations provided them with some measure of self-esteem in the face of the negative emotional effects of destructive parentification.

Johnston, Gonzalez, and Campbell (1987) collected data indicating that the gender of the parent with whom the child reverses roles is a factor in this area as well. In an effort to predict the effects of entrenched postdivorce custody disputes on an ethnically diverse group of children (aged 4–11 years), they examined a number of independent variables, including the degree of role reversal. Interestingly, the results demonstrated that role reversal with fathers was directly related to withdrawn, uncommunicative behavior at baseline, whereas role reversal with mothers was inversely correlated with such behavior; however, the latter finding attained statistical significance only at the 2-year follow-up. Unfortunately, Johnston et al. did not evaluate the moderating roles of gender and age of the child.

Also interested in cross-gender boundary problems, including parent–child overinvolvement and role reversal, Fullinwider-Bush and Jacobvitz (1993) found in a collegiate sample that women reporting such problems in their paternal relationships showed little interest on a measure of personal identity in even establishing an identity. Weak mother–daughter boundaries, on the other hand, were related to a premature commitment to family values and beliefs—an externally based identity orientation. In general, it appears that growing up in a household marked by poor parent–child boundaries undermines womens' ability to explore self-definitional issues that lead to the development of an autonomous ego identity. Whether the same is true for males warrants investigating as well.

In a more recent study with college women, Jacobvitz and Bush (1996) discovered two family patterns of past and current boundary dissolution: (1) fathers with emotionally distant marriages who seek intimacy with their daughters (father–daughter alliance), and (2) mothers who triangulate their daughters into their conflicted marriages (mother–daughter triangulation). Regression analyses revealed that childhood father–daughter alliance contributes to depression, anxiety, and low self-esteem, whereas current mother–daughter triangulation contributes to anxiety.

Jones and Wells (1996) tested the hypothesis that childhood parentification underlies the development of self-defeating, narcissistic, and compulsive personality characteristics. They assumed that a child is induced to assume a parentified role by suppressing autonomous strivings either to take care of the parent's physical or emotional needs (masochistic or self-defeating parentification) or to become the parent's idealized self-projection (narcissistic parentification). The parentified individual's perfectionism and ritualized need for control through caretaking activities were viewed as evidence of compulsivity. For both the male and female college students in their sample, Jones and Wells's expectations were confirmed, except for the hypothesized relation between parentification and compulsive tendencies.

Finally, in a study that Godsall, Emshoff, Jurkovic, Anderson, and Stanwick (in press) conducted recently with adolescents of substance abusing and non-substance-abusing parents, parentification proved to be a more powerful predictor of self-esteem than the other variables studied, including the family's substance abuse status. The degree of destructive parentification was inversely related to positive self-regard.

Peer Relations

Some of the adolescents in Weiss's (1979) study described themselves as "loners." Although they were not isolated, their involvement in the peer culture appeared limited. Dawson (1980) also found that the increased responsibility of children in single-parent families was associated with less sociability. Other adolescents interviewed in Weiss's (1979) study reported that their peers viewed them as unusually serious and mature. One girl reported that she functioned in the role of "Dear Abby" for her friends. The nature of these adolescents' peer relationships, however, did not appear to hurt their self-esteem. Rather, aware that they were more responsible than their peers from two-parent households, they described themselves as highly competent. Yet Weiss noted that their responses also reflected envy of youngsters with fewer responsibilities.

A strikingly different picture, however, emerged for children in Weiss's sample who at a young age assumed considerable responsibility at home, served as support figures for overwhelmed and sometimes depressed parents, and cared for themselves throughout much of the day. Socially isolated and lacking in spontaneity and playfulness with age-mates, they were viewed by Weiss as being "precocious and oddly self-reliant."

Developmental precursors to the social behaviors observed by Weiss are suggested in an interesting data set collected by Zahn-Waxler and her colleagues (Cummings, Iannotti, & Zahn-Waxler, 1985; Zahn-Waxler, Cummings, Iannotti, & Radke-Yarrow, 1984). Two-year-olds of mothers with major depression became more anxious and preoccupied when confronted with distress in others, including peers, than toddlers of well mothers did. They also exhibited a heightened level of sensitivity and an overcontrolled, precociously polite manner of interacting with playmates.

In another longitudinal study of 5- and 6-year-old boys, who lived in high-conflict homes with one parent having a history of bipolar disorder and the other a history of major depression, Zahn-Waxler, McKnew, Cummings, Davenport, and Radke-Yarrow (1984) found evidence at follow-up of continuing problems in emotional regulation. However, in comparison to control children, the target children were more sensitive to interpersonal discord and better able to generate solutions, including peacemaking strategies, in conflict situations.

Consistent with the findings of Zahn-Waxler and her colleagues, Valleau, Bergner, and Horton (1995) more recently found that college students with a history of parentification reported a pattern of interpersonal relating that involved excessive caretaking. In contrast to nonparentified students, those scoring high in parentification endorsed such items on a caretaker survey as "I tend to place the needs of others before my own needs in relationships," and "It is very hard for me to 'let go' in situations where I see others in difficulty, especially if I believe they are not handling things well."

Sociocognitive Development

In addition to the socioemotional effects of parentification, Goodnow (1988) speculates that children's household responsibilities affect their cognitive development and orientation toward learning. For example, a friend may be defined by a parentified child not only as a playmate, but also as a potential work partner who can share in the discharge of chores (Super & Harkness, 1986). The friendship conceptions of many parentified youngsters whose responsibilities preempt peer involvement may also be immature. Although this hypothesis has not been directly tested, Dean, Malik, Richards, and Stringer (1986) have studied the interpersonal conceptions of abused and neglected children. They assumed that the demands in the families of these children for caretaking and for curtailment of social contacts interfere with basic conditions for parent–child complementarity and reciprocity between peers. As expected, they found that in comparison to nonmaltreated controls, young maltreated children (6–8 years of age) construed peer relationships in less reciprocal terms.

Dean et al. (1986) also discovered that in relation to parental figures, the maltreated youngsters were more likely to portray children as being kind and helpful. However, they were less likely than those in the nonmaltreated group to represent parents as reciprocating the kindness of children. They conceptualized parental unresponsiveness as being their fault. Such an overgeneralized sense of responsibility, which may contribute to a pathogenic form of guilt, has also been observed by Zahn-Waxler and her colleagues in even younger children (see Zahn-Waxler & Robinson, 1995). Dean et al. concluded that from the perspective of attachment theory (Bowlby, 1980), such a conception is part of a representational view serving to maintain their physical and emotional closeness to parental figures.

The way children are assigned tasks by their parents may also affect their learning style (Goodnow, 1988). It is plausible that if children are given support and reasonable autonomy, then they can learn to work independently while remaining open to help, not only at home but in other contexts (such as school). On the other hand, as Goodnow points out, parents whose socialization patterns in general are status-oriented and nonreciprocal are likely to require their children to discharge their duties servilely. They learn that "all learning and all interactions follow a strictly hierarchical, order-and-obey pattern" (Goodnow, 1988, p. 17).

Because the demands of their work load at home may conflict with academic tasks, it is probable that parentified children also often experience role strain and perform poorly in school. Suggestive evidence for this observation was found in a recent study by Chase et al. (1998). Compared to a group of students regularly admitted to college, students admitted on a provisional basis, because of marginal high school grades and Scholastic Aptitude Test scores, reported more signs of destructive parentification. This effect was even more pronounced for students whose parents were problem drinkers.

On the other hand, in his studies of achievement motivation in children, McClelland (1961) discovered that many of the boys subjected to early expectations for caretaking developed a "conscientiousness syndrome." McClelland's findings suggested a type of achievement-oriented boy "who may indeed form the backbone of the civil service, but . . . is not likely to be found in the front line of entrepreneurs in the country" (p. 348). Weiss (1979) speculates that young parentified children of single parents, rather than becoming rule-bound employees, may as adults work more independently and creatively than individuals who did not have as much early responsibility. Yet they may be at risk for experiencing increasing job dissatisfaction, as they discover that their work, however rewarding, cannot fulfill unmet dependency needs.

We have pointed to the same risk for helping professionals, many of whom have functioned in a parentified capacity in their families of origin (Jurkovic, 1997; Jurkovic, Jessee, & Goglia, 1991). It appears that the occupational choice of these individuals is often coextensive with their childhood role, serving as a central feature in their self-definition and relationships with others. Interested in this dynamic, Sessions (1986) asked groups of clinical psychology graduate students and advanced undergraduates in engineering to report their degree of parentification while growing up. As expected, the psychology students were significantly more parentified than the engineering majors.

Other Family Members

What are the effects of parentification processes on other members of the parentified child's family? A number of studies, many of which were conducted several decades ago, are relevant to this question. For example,

Essman and Deutsch (1979) collected data suggesting that older siblings in the role of parent surrogate are insensitive to their younger siblings' feelings. Students in 10th through 12th grades were presented with hypothetical situations involving a younger sibling and were asked to respond to various queries about the situation from the perspective of an older sibling. Ninety-two percent of the responses of these adolescents were coded as "ineffective" (i.e., not communicating their own or their sibling's feelings).

It is likely, therefore, that the sibling relationships and the socioemotional and cognitive development of younger charges of parentified children are negatively affected. Indeed, ethnographic accounts indicate that siblings under the care of slightly older siblings lacking well-defined personalities are impeded in their ability to self-differentiate. This outcome may be less problematic, however, in societies that do not emphasize personal achievement and autonomy (Mead, 1928/1961; Weisner & Gallimore, 1977). If parents, extended family, and other adults in the community are available to structure and to supervise the caretaking activities of the older siblings, then fewer deleterious effects would also be expected.

Cross-cultural investigations further suggest that children who are significantly parented by older siblings experience less separation anxiety and more motivation to affiliate with others (Weisner & Gallimore, 1977). The peers with whom they have the opportunity to affiliate, however, are likely to be limited largely to those of their older sibling caretakers (Mead, 1928/1961). They may also have less access to potentially positive interactions with parental figures. Yet, because they are not the primary target of their parents' parentifying and often stultifying demands, another potential benefit for the younger siblings is that they are freer to develop normally (Miller, 1979/1981). This observation has not been evaluated empirically, however. Clearly, more questions are being raised about the sibling subsystem of parentified children than we have data to address at this point.

Even fewer data are available to enable us to evaluate the impact of the parentification process on the parents and the family as a whole. Some investigators have concluded that parentification decreases parental role strain and stress (Weisner & Gallimore, 1977; Weiss, 1979). On the other hand, Minuchin et al. (1967) have observed that parents are likely to experience increasing competition for control and leadership in the family from their parentified offspring.

CONCLUSIONS

What was an empirical *terra incognita* for many years is slowly being charted by investigators from various disciplines. The data have confirmed a number of clinically based observations and suppositions about the parentification process, while at the same time extending our knowledge base in this area. It is becoming increasingly apparent that destructive parentification underlies many different forms of family and individual dysfunction.

Empirical investigation of the determinants of parentification has established a number of promising leads. Understandably, researchers are still largely attempting to account for variance—that is, to identify variables that are related to and predictive of parentification. Further work along these lines would benefit from consideration of issues discussed in the clinical literature on parentification (see Jurkovic, 1997). For example, the collusive role of the nonparentifying parent has not been examined empirically. Nor has parentification in couples. For example, continuous with their role as children, parentified individuals often form codependent relationships with addicted, narcissistic, or otherwise needy partners. Their codependency appears driven, in part, by the hope that they can change their partners' behavior.

Although the data do not support the construction of elaborate causal models at this point, they suggest various primary, moderating, and mediating variables that may help explain the transgenerational transmission of destructive parentification. For example, it is plausible that some type of deprivation, abuse, or serious boundary violation in the parent's background (primary determinant) leads to parentifying attitudes and cognitions (mediators), which in turn result in the destructive parentification of one of the children. Social legitimacy, the availability of a nurturing adult partner, and the age and sex of the child all probably play a moderating role in this putative pathway.

The parentification process appears to have multiple effects of a negative as well as a positive nature on parentified children and other family members. It is important, however, not to assume simple cause–effect connections in this area. An unhealthy outcome observed at one time point may remit later in the child's development, in the event of significant changes in the family or in the child's extrafamilial relationships. Transactions between various predictor and outcome variables can also adversely affect one another over time. For example, marital stress that conduces to the parentification of one of the children may further intensify problems in the parents' relationship, which places greater demands on the child, who perhaps becomes even more socially isolated. Alternatively, as discussed earlier, parentified children's marital interventions may be stress-reducing for both them and their parents.

To evaluate the complexity of the etiological relationships considered in this chapter will require more causal modeling and prospective studies. Such studies, particularly if they incorporate various moderating and mediating variables at multiple levels of analysis, promise to shed light on (1) the conditions under which the parentification process is adaptive or maladaptive for different family members and subsystems, including the next generation; and (2) the mechanisms responsible for these outcomes.

252   INDIVIDUAL AND FAMILY PSYCHOPATHOLOGY

REFERENCES

Ainsworth, M. D. S. (1989). Attachments beyond infancy. *American Psychologist, 44,* 709–716.

Alexander, P. C. (1992). Application of attachment theory to the study of sexual abuse. *Journal of Consulting and Clinical Psychology, 60,* 185–195.

Bavolek, S. J. (1984). *Handbook for the Adult–Adolescent Parenting Inventory (AAPI).* Schaumburg, IL: Family Development Associates.

Bossard, J. H. S., & Boll, E. S. (1956). *The large family system.* Philadelphia: University of Pennsylvania Press.

Boszormenyi-Nagy, I. (1987). *Foundations of contextual therapy.* New York: Brunner/Mazel.

Boszormenyi-Nagy, I., & Krasner, B. R. (1986). *Between give and take: A clinical guide to contextual therapy.* New York: Brunner/Mazel.

Boszormenyi-Nagy, I., & Spark, G. M. (1973). *Invisible loyalties: Reciprocity in intergenerational family therapy.* New York: Harper & Row.

Bowlby, J. (1979). *The making and breaking of affectional bonds.* London: Tavistock.

Bowlby, J. (1980). *Attachment and loss: Vol. 3. Loss, sadness, and depression.* New York: Basic Books.

Bridgeman, D. L. (1983). Benevolent babies: Emergence of the social self. In D. L. Bridgeman (Ed.), *The nature of prosocial development: Interdisciplinary theories and strategies* (pp. 95–112). New York: Academic Press.

Burkett, L. P. (1991). Parenting behaviors of women who were sexually abused as children in their families of origin. *Family Process, 30,* 421–434.

Chase, N. D., Deming, M. P., & Wells, M. (1998). Parentification, parental alcoholism, and academic status among young adults. *American Journal of Family Therapy, 26,* 105–114.

Cummings, E. M., Iannotti, R. J., & Zahn-Waxler, C. (1985). Influence of conflict between adults on the emotions and aggression of young children. *Developmental Psychology, 21,* 495–507.

Cummings, E. M., Zahn-Waxler, C., & Radke-Yarrow, M. (1981). Young children's responses to expressions of anger and affection by others in the family. *Child Development, 52,* 1274–1282.

Cummings, E. M., Zahn-Waxler, C., & Radke-Yarrow, M. (1984). Developmental changes in children's reactions to anger in the same family. *Developmental Psychology, 21,* 747–760.

Dawson, F. (1980). *The parental child in single and dual parent families.* Unpublished master's thesis, Georgia State University.

Dean, A. L., Malik, M. M., Richards, W., & Stringer, S. A. (1986). Effects of parental maltreatment on children's conceptions of interpersonal relationships. *Developmental Psychology, 22,* 617–626.

Elder, G. (1974). *Children of the Great Depression.* Chicago: University of Chicago Press.

Ember, C. (1973). Female task assignment and the social behavior of boys. *Ethos, 1,* 424–439.

Essman, C. S., & Deutsch, F. (1979). Siblings as babysitters: Responses of adolescents to younger siblings in problem situations. *Adolescence, 14,* 411–420.

Fox, R. A., Baisch, M. J., Goldberg, B. D., & Hochmuth, M. C. (1987). Parenting attitudes of pregnant adolescents. *Psychological Reports, 61,* 403–406.

Fry, P. S., & Trifiletti, R. J. (1983). An exploration of the adolescent's perspective: Perceptions of major stress dimensions in the single-parent family. *Journal of Psychiatric Treatment and Evaluation, 5,* 101–111.

Fullinwider-Bush, N., & Jacobvitz, D. B. (1993). The transition to young adulthood: Generation boundary dissolution and female identity development. *Family Process, 32,* 87–103.

Godsall, R., Emshoff, J., Jurkovic, G., Anderson, L., & Stanwick, T. (in press). Why some kids do well in bad situations: The effects of parentification. *International Journal of the Addictions.*

Goglia, L. R., Jurkovic, G. J., Burt, A. M., & Burge-Callaway, K. G. (1992). Generational boundary distortions by adult children of alcoholics: Child-as-parent and child-as-mate. *American Journal of Family Therapy, 20,* 291–299.

Goodnow, J. J. (1988). Children's household work: Its nature and function. *Psychological Bulletin, 103,* 5–26.

Gore, S., Aseltine, R. H., & Colten, M. E. (1993). Gender, social-relational involvement, and depression. *Journal of Research on Adolescence, 3,* 101–125.

Hanson, R. A. (1990). Initial parenting attitudes of pregnant adolescents and a comparison with the decision about adoption. *Adolescence, 25,* 629–643.

Harris, D. E., Clark, K. E., Rose, A. M., & Valasek, F. (1963). The relationship of children's home duties to an attitude of responsibility. *Child Development, 25,* 29–33.

Harrison, A. O., Wilson, M. N., Pine, C. J., Chan, S. Q., & Buriel, R. (1990). Family ecologies of ethnic minority children. *Child Development, 61,* 347–362.

Jacobvitz, D. B., & Bush, N. F. (1996). Reconstructions of family relationships: Parent–child alliances, personal distress, and self-esteem. *Developmental Psychology, 32,* 732–743.

Jacobvitz, D. B., Morgan, E., Kretchmar, M. D., & Morgan, Y. (1991). The transmission of mother–child boundary disturbances across three generations. *Development and Psychopathology, 3,* 513–527.

Jelley, G. (1980). *Parental awareness in black teenage mothers: A cognitive-developmental study.* Unpublished master's thesis, Georgia State University.

Johnston, J. R., Gonzalez, R., & Campbell, L. E. G. (1987). Ongoing postdivorce conflict and child disturbance. *Journal of Abnormal Child Psychology, 15,* 493–509.

Jones, R. A., & Wells, M. (1996). An empirical study of parentification and personality. *American Journal of Family Therapy, 24,* 145–152.

Jurkovic, G. J. (1997). *Lost childhoods: The plight of the parentified child.* New York: Brunner/Mazel.

Jurkovic, G. J., Jessee, E. H., & Goglia, L. R. (1991). Treatment of parental children and their families: Conceptual and technical issues. *American Journal of Family Therapy, 19,* 302–314.

Karpel, M. A. (1976). Intrapsychic and interpersonal processes in the parentification of children. *Dissertation Abstracts International, 38,* 365. (University Microfilms No. 77-15090)

Main, M., & Cassidy, J. (1988). Categories of response to reunion with the parent at age 6: Predictable from infant attachment classifications and stable over a 1-month period. *Developmental Psychology, 24,* 415–426.

McClelland, D. C. (1961). *The achieving society.* Princeton, NJ: Van Nostrand.

Mead, M. (1961). *Coming of age in Samoa: A psychological study of primitive youth for Western civilization.* New York: Morrow. (Original work published 1928)

Miller, A. (1981). *The drama of the gifted child* (R. Ward, Trans.). New York: Basic Books. (Original work published 1979)

Minuchin, S. (1974). *Families and family therapy.* Cambridge, MA: Harvard University Press.

Minuchin, S., Montalvo, B., Guerney, B. G., Rosman, B., & Schumer, F. (1967). *Families of the slums.* New York: Basic Books.

Morris, M. G., & Gould, R. W. (1963). Role reversal: A necessary concept in dealing with the "battered child syndrome." *American Journal of Orthopsychiatry, 33,* 298–299.

Newberger, C. M. (1977). Parental conceptions of children and child-rearing: A structural–developmental analysis. *Dissertation Abstracts International, 38,* 6123. (University Microfilms No. 78-08622)

Newberger, C. M., & White, K. M. (1989). Cognitive foundations for parental care. In D. Cicchetti & V. Carlson (Eds.), *Child maltreatment: Theory and research on the causes and consequences of child abuse and neglect* (pp. 302–316). New York: Cambridge University Press.

Rehberg, H. R., & Richman, C. L. (1989). Prosocial behavior in preschool children: A look at the interaction of race, gender, and family composition. *International Journal of Behavioral Development, 12,* 385–401.

Rheingold, H. L. (1982). Little children's participation in the work of adults: A nascent prosocial behavior. *Child Development, 53,* 114–125.

Rheingold, H. L., Hay, D. F., & West, M. J. (1976). Sharing in the second year of life. *Child Development, 47,* 1148–1158.

Rutter, M. (1989). Intergenerational continuities and discontinuities in serious parenting difficulties. In D. Cicchetti & V. Carlson (Eds.), *Child maltreatment: Theory and research on the causes and consequences of child abuse and neglect* (pp. 317–348). New York: Cambridge University Press.

Schmideberg, M. (1948). Parents as children. *Psychiatric Quarterly, 22*(Suppl.), 207–218.

Sessions, M. (1986). Influence of parentification on professional role choice and interpersonal style. *Dissertation Abstracts International, 47,* 5066. (University Microfilms No. 87-06815)

Sroufe, L. A., Jacobvitz, D., Mangelsdorf, S., DeAngelo, E., & Ward, M. J. (1985). Generational boundary dissolution between mothers and their preschool children: A relationship systems approach. *Child Development, 56,* 317–332.

Sroufe, L. A., & Ward, J. J. (1980). Seductive behavior of mothers of toddlers: Occurrence, correlates, and family origins. *Child Development, 51,* 1222–1229.

Stern, D. (1985). *The interpersonal world of the infant.* New York: Basic Books.

Stewart, R. B. (1983). Sibling attachment relationship: Child–infant interactions in the strange situation. *Developmental Psychology, 19,* 192–199.

Stewart, R. B., & Marvin, R. S. (1984). Sibling relations: The role of conceptual perspective-taking in the ontogeny of sibling caregiving. *Child Development, 55,* 1322–1332.

Super, C. M., & Harkness, S. (1981). Figure, ground, and gestalt: The cultural context of the active individual. In R. M. Lerner & N. A. Busch-Rossnagel (Eds.), *Individuals as producers of their development: A life-span perspective* (pp. 69–86). New York: Academic Press.

Super, C. M., & Harkness, S. (1982). The infant's niche in rural Kenya and metropolitan America. In L. L. Adler (Ed.), *Cross-cultural research at issue* (pp. 47–55). New York: Academic Press.

Super, C. M., & Harkness, S. (1986). The developmental niche: A conceptualization of the interface of child and culture. *International Journal of Behavioral Development, 9,* 545–569.

Valleau, M. P., Bergner, R. M., & Horton, C. B. (1995). Parentification and caretaker syndrome: An empirical investigation. *Family Therapy, 22,* 157–164.

Walsh, F. W. (1979). Breaching of family generation boundaries by schizophrenics, disturbed, and normals. *International Journal of Family Therapy, 1,* 254–275.

Weisner, T. S., & Gallimore, R. (1977). My brother's keeper: Child and sibling caretaking. *Current Anthropology, 18,* 169–190.

Weiss, R. S. (1979). Growing up a little faster: The experience of growing up in a single parent household. *Journal of Social Issues, 35,* 97–111.

Whiting, B., & Edwards, C. P. (1973). A cross-cultural analysis of sex differences in the behavior of children aged three through eleven. *Journal of Social Psychology, 91,* 171–188.

Whiting, B., & Whiting, J. W. (1975). *Children of six cultures.* Cambridge, MA: Harvard University Press.

Wolkin, J. R. (1984). Childhood parentification: An exploration of long-term effects. *Dissertation Abstracts International, 45,* 2707. (University Microfilms No. 84-24601)

Zahn-Waxler, C., Cummings, E. M., Iannotti, R. M., & Radke-Yarrow, M. (1984). Young offspring of depressed parents: A population at risk for affective problems. In D. Cicchetti & K. Schneider-Rosen (Eds.), *New directions for child development: No. 26. Childhood depression* (pp. 81–105). San Francisco: Jossey-Bass.

Zahn-Waxler, C., & Kochanska, G. (1988). The origins of guilt. In R. Dienstbier & A. Thompson (Eds.), *Nebraska Symposium on Motivation: Vol. 36. Socioemotional development* (pp. 222–258). Lincoln: University of Nebraska Press.

Zahn-Waxler, C., Kochanska, G., Krupnick, J., & McKnew, D. (1990). Patterns of guilt in children of depressed and well mothers. *Developmental Psychology, 26,* 51–59.

Zahn-Waxler, C., McKnew, D., Cummings, E., Davenport, Y., & Radke-Yarrow, M. (1984). Problem behaviors and peer interactions of young children with a manic–depressive parent. *American Journal of Psychiatry, 141,* 236–240.

Zahn-Waxler, C., & Robinson, J. (1995). Empathy and guilt: Early origins of feelings of responsibility. In J. P. Tangney & K. W. Fischer (Eds.), *Self-conscious emotions: The psychology of shame, guilt, embarrassment, and pride* (pp. 143–173). New York: Guilford Press.

CHAPTER 11

═══◆═══

Marital Processes
and Depression

STEVEN R. H. BEACH
FRANK D. FINCHAM

In the past decade, marital and family therapists have shown considerable interest in co-occurring marital discord and depression. Clinically, the typical presentation is that of spouses who want marital therapy because they have a variety of problems and difficulties, including communication, bickering, lack of sex, difficulties with their children, and concern that their marriage is falling apart. Rather quickly, however, the clinician may notice that one of the spouses—usually the wife—is also depressed. In many cases, it is likely that she has been experiencing depressed mood for several months or more; that she no longer finds pleasure in the things she used to enjoy; that she is not sleeping well and feels tired all the time; and that she alternates among feeling worthless, being harshly self-critical, and wishing she were dead. The importance of understanding the relationship between marital problems on the one hand and the psychopathology of depression on the other is highlighted by such cases.

Because the situation described above is familiar to most therapists who work with couples, empirically informed guidelines for working with such couples are needed. This chapter therefore examines research on the etiology and treatment of depression in the context of marriage. The chapter is organized into three sections. The first identifies targets for intervention that might both enhance marital satisfaction and alleviate depression, by examining how relationship processes can initiate and maintain depression. In the second section, we turn from the possible treatment implications of etiology and maintenance to examine directly the

256

efficacy of marital interventions for working with depressed spouses. The final section summarizes the implications of our analysis.

RELATIONSHIP PROCESSES IN THE INITIATION AND MAINTENANCE OF DEPRESSIVE SYMPTOMS

The processes that may initiate and maintain depression in marriage are complex. In this section, we illustrate how relationship processes can be used to identify targets for intervention.

Marital Satisfaction as a Target for Intervention When One Spouse Is Depressed

One way to intervene for a couple presenting with marital discord and depression may be to enhance the marital satisfaction of both partners. Increasing marital satisfaction may influence level of depression if marital satisfaction and depression are strongly related, if marital dissatisfaction precedes depressive episodes, and if marital satisfaction plays a causal role in the chain of events leading to depression. We examine each of these assumptions in turn.

Are Marital Satisfaction and Depression Strongly Related?

A large body of empirical evidence encompassing a wide array of research designs and assessment strategies shows a robust association between depressive symptomatology and marital distress (for a review, see Beach, Smith, & Fincham, 1994). Representative of the epidemiological portion of this literature is a finding from the Epidemiologic Catchment Area research data (representing over 3,000 interviews; Regier et al., 1984) that there was a 25-fold increase in the relative risk of major depression for people reporting themselves to be in unhappy marriages (Weissman, 1987). Representative of those studies using standard self-report questionnaires, O'Leary, Christian, and Mendell (1993) found a 10-fold increase in risk for depression among discordant relative to nondiscordant spouses in a sample of 328 newly married couples. Furthermore, these authors found that the association between depressive symptomatology and marital discord remained significant even after the partners' levels of both depressive symptomatology and marital discord were controlled for. A representative study from the literature on married persons presenting for therapy for their depression (Roy, 1987) showed that 66.3% of women and 71.4% of males indicated that they had marital problems which preceded the onset of their depression. Finally, in a study of couples presenting for marital therapy (Beach, Jouriles, & O'Leary, 1985) about half had at least one spouse reporting elevated levels of depressive symptoms (Beck Depression Inventory scores > 14).

As suggested by these four examples, the concurrent relationship between marital discord and depression is robust across samples, stages of family development, and definitions of the two constructs. In addition, recent research has continued to replicate this relationship across measures and samples (e.g., Assh & Byers, 1996; Demo & Acock, 1996; Johnson & Jacobs, 1997; Thompson, Whiffin, & Blain, 1995; Vega et al., 1996; Vinokur, Price, & Caplan, 1996; Zelkowitz & Milet, 1996).

Does Marital Discord Precede Depression?

It is important to remember that no matter how robust the correlation between marital discord and depression, it does not speak to the issue of their temporal relation. Does marital discord precede depression or vice versa?

A number of authors have examined the longitudinal association between marital relationship variables and depression. Some authors conceptualize marital events as stressors and examine their relation to later depression. For example, Christian-Herman, O'Leary, and Avery-Leaf (1997) recruited 50 women who had recently experienced a significant negative marital event, such as physical abuse or discovery of a trust violation. Women were excluded from the sample if they had ever had a major depressive episode, because these researchers were interested in whether negative marital events would create an increased risk for a major depressive episode. Thirty-six percent of the women experiencing recent negative marital events were clinically depressed, as assessed by the Structured Clinical Interview for DSM-III-R. This level of depression far exceeds the point prevalence rate of depression for women generally (7–8%; American Psychiatric Association, 1987). Similarly, in a clinical sample presenting with both marital discord and depression, 70% of depressed and maritally discordant women believed that their marital discord preceded their depression; 60% of these women believed that their marital discord was the primary cause of their depression (O'Leary, Risso, & Beach, 1990). Thus, marital variables appear important in understanding the onset of major depression.

In some studies, marital variables have been examined as moderators of the stress–depression relationship. In their longitudinal work, Brown and Harris (1978, 1986) have examined the effect of marital conflict on depression. They found that negative marital interactions (e.g., arguing, strain, violence, and coldness) at the time of the initial interview predicted much greater vulnerability to depression. Indeed, women confronted with a severe difficulty or negative life event were more than three times as likely to become depressed if their marriage had been characterized by negative marital interaction. This provided rather striking evidence of the marital context's exerting an influence on the stress–depression relationship.

Data showing that marital discord precedes depression (see also Beach

& O'Leary, 1993a) do not, of course, preclude instances of depression leading to marital discord or instances in which they are unrelated. For example, a recent longitudinal study of newlyweds implicates premarital dysphoria in husbands as a precursor of later spousal marital discord for both spouses (Beach & O'Leary, 1993b). Similarly, recent data presented by Gotlib, Lewinsohn, and Seeley (1996) suggest that experiencing an episode of depression during adolescence is associated both with earlier age at marriage and with decreased satisfaction with subsequent marriage. Likewise, recent work on stress-generation (e.g., Davila, Bradbury, Cohan, & Tochluk, 1997) and reassurance seeking (e.g., Joiner & Metalsky, 1995) highlight possible mechanisms linking depression to later marital problems. At the same time, there is recent work to indicate that marital quality may be unrelated to recurrences of severe depression (Paykel, Cooper, Ramana, & Hayhurst, 1996). As such results make clear, there is evidence showing that marital discord precedes depression, evidence to show that depression precedes marital discord, and evidence that in extreme cases the two may be unrelated.

Does Level of Marital Satisfaction Cause Changes in Depressive Symptomatology?

The evidence on concurrent and longitudinal associations is consistent with either an effect of marital discord on depression, the reverse, or a bidirectional pattern of causation. To tease apart these possibilities, we and our colleagues have investigated a range of causal models (Beach et al., 1995; Fincham, Beach, Harold, & Osborne, 1997) .

In a longitudinal study using a national random probability sample of women working full-time ($n = 577$), Beach et al. (1995) found a significant effect of marital satisfaction on depressive symptomatology 1 year later. Women who endorsed low levels of marital satisfaction showed greater depressive symptoms, even after the relationship between marital satisfaction and depression at the initial assessment was controlled for. Accordingly, there is evidence that the prospective effect of marital satisfaction on depression for women may be generalizable to a broad cross-section of working women.

We (Fincham et al., 1997) used a series of complementary causal models to probe the relationship of marital satisfaction and depression in a sample of 150 newlywed couples assessed at two points separated by an 18-month interval. Couples were recruited from marriage license records to increase generalizability of the results. Estimating causal parameters in a series of models made it possible to examine possible causal effects over time, to investigate possible mediation of longitudinal effects through concurrent effects, and to examine possible bidirectional effects.

Replicating earlier work, we found that both marital satisfaction and depressive symptomatology were relatively stable in early marriage and were clearly related to each other both cross-sectionally and longitudinally. When initial levels of each variable were controlled for (via a cross-lagged stability model), there were significant cross-lagged effects for husbands from earlier marital satisfaction to later depressive symptomatology and from earlier depressive symptomatology to later marital satisfaction. The only effects for wives were from earlier marital satisfaction to later depressive symptomatology. These gender differences emerged more strongly when causal relationships were modeled that controlled for mediation of longitudinal effects through stability and concurrent effects. In particular, for wives there was a significant prospective effect of marital satisfaction on later depressive symptomatology, whereas for husbands there was a significant effect of depressive symptomatology on later marital satisfaction. Finally, when possible concurrent, reciprocal effects between marital satisfaction and depressive symptomatology were examined (via nonrecursive models), an effect of depressive symptomatology on marital satisfaction emerged for men, but an effect of marital satisfaction on depressive symptomatology emerged for women.

These results (Fincham et al., 1997) are clinically important for several reasons. They confirm long-held suspicions that the marital discord model of depression may be more relevant to a relationship in which it is the wife who is depressed. Because women are often perceived as being more relationship-oriented than men, and may often feel greater responsibility for resolution of relationship difficulties, they may experience greater vulnerability to marital stressors than do men. Conversely, because men may more commonly respond to dysphoric feelings by denigrating relationships or by withdrawing, depressive symptoms may more commonly influence later marital satisfaction among men. This is clinically important, because it means that interventions designed to increase marital satisfaction may prove relatively more effective in decreasing depressive symptomatology among women than among men. Careful review of the pattern of results across different causal models for women also provides interesting clues regarding the likely time frame of effects of marital satisfaction on depressive symptomatology. In particular, contrasting the magnitude of effect estimates for the cross-lagged versus the nonrecursive models suggests that the effect of marital satisfaction on depressive symptoms for women may occur over a relatively shorter time frame than the 18-month lag used in this investigation. This is supportive of marital intervention for depression, as it suggests that marital interventions may have the potential to produce effects on depression in the time frame customary for marital therapy.

Taken together, the results reviewed here suggest that for women marital satisfaction often plays an etiological role in the development of depressive symptoms, and that interventions designed to increase marital satisfaction may play a useful role in alleviating their depressive symptomatology. However, increasing felt marital satisfaction is not the only target for intervention suggested by research on relationship processes and depression.

Avoidance of Conflict and Constructive Engagement as Targets for Intervention

A common clinical observation is that depressed individuals show problematic patterns of problem solving. Often, in work with a married couple in which one partner is depressed, it becomes apparent that the spouses avoid "real" issues and spend their time focusing on minor details or vague general complaints. Also, the depressed spouse often may not express needs clearly or may fail to make requests for the partner to change. Alternatively, the depressed spouse may ask primarily for reductions in negative partner behavior instead of asking for increases in desired behavior, or may make vague global requests that would seem overwhelming to almost any partner. To the extent that there are observable problems in communication and not just perceived problems, that difficulty in dealing with conflict is related to increased depressive behavior, and that depressed persons have an identifiable aversion to direct engagement in areas of disagreement, a strong case may be made for use of problem-solving communication training as a component of marital therapy for depression. We therefore examine data on problem solving and its relationship to depression and depressive symptomatology.

Are Difficulties in Marital Problem Solving Associated with Depression?

Hinchliffe, Hooper, and Roberts (1978) found that couples with a depressed spouse showed greater conflict, tension, and negative expressiveness in their interactions than did nondepressed control couples. Interestingly, the depressed patients in this study were more verbally productive and laughed more often with a stranger than they did with their spouses; these findings highlight the importance of the marital system in understanding depression. Consistent with these results, Hautzinger, Linden, and Hoffman (1982) showed that communication patterns in couples with a depressed spouse were more disturbed than in couples without a depressed partner. Spouses of depressed partners seldom agreed with their partners, often offered help in an ambivalent manner, and often evaluated their depressed partners negatively.

In a similar vein, Arkowitz, Holliday, and Hutter (1982) found that following interactions with their wives, husbands of depressed women reported feeling more hostile than did husbands of psychiatric and nonpsychiatric control subjects. Comparable findings were reported by Kahn, Coyne, and Margolin (1985), who found that couples with a depressed spouse were more sad and angry following marital interactions, and experienced each other as more negative, hostile, mistrusting, and detached than did nondepressed couples. Kowalik and Gotlib (1987) had depressed and nondepressed psychiatric outpatients and nondepressed nonpsychiatric controls participate in an interactional task with their spouses while simultaneously coding both the intended impact of their own behavior and their perception of their spouses' behavior. The communications of the depressed patients were more intentionally negative and less intentionally positive than the communications of nondepressed controls.

Ruscher and Gotlib (1988) examined the marital interactions of mildly depressed persons from the community, and found that couples in which one partner was depressed emitted a greater proportion of negative verbal and nonverbal behaviors than did nondepressed control couples. Gotlib and Whiffen (1989) reported that the interactions of depressed male and female psychiatric inpatients and their spouses were characterized by negative affect and hostility. Finally, McCabe and Gotlib (1993) examined perceptions and actual problem-solving behaviors of couples in which the wife was either clinically depressed (depressed couples) or nondepressed (nondepressed couples). Depressed couples, and particularly depressed wives, perceived their family lives to be more negative than did nondepressed couples; the depressed couples also perceived their interactions to be more hostile, less friendly, and more dominated by their partners than did nondepressed couples. Moreover, depressed wives became increasingly negative in their verbal behavior over the course of the interaction.

Clearly, there is evidence that couples in which one partner is depressed have difficulties with marital communication, and that these difficulties are manifested in problem-solving discussions. We consider next the possibility that potential conflict and partner aggression elicit a constellation of "depressive" behaviors (including self-derogation, physical and psychological complaints, and displays of depressed affect), and that these behaviors are higher among depressed persons than among their nondepressed partners or community controls (Biglan et al., 1985; Nelson & Beach, 1990; Schmaling & Jacobson, 1990). Importantly, these are behaviors that make depressed persons look more depressed to others, and may result in their viewing themselves as more depressed.

What Is the Relationship between Depressive Behavior and Partner Verbal Aggression?

In their pioneering study, Biglan et al. (1985) found that in couples in which the wives were both depressed and maritally discordant, depressive behavior had the effect of suppressing subsequent aggressive responses from the husbands. In a subsequent study, Schmaling and Jacobson (1990) compared four groups of couples: nondepressed/nondiscordant, nondepressed/discordant, depressed/nondiscordant, and depressed/discordant. They found that spouses responded differently to depressive than to aggressive behavior. Discordant spouses tended to reciprocate aggressive behavior, whereas depressive behavior did not increase aggressive behavior on the part of spouses. In a third study, Nelson and Beach (1990) compared the marital interactions of three groups of couples: nondepressed/nondiscordant, nondepressed/discordant, and depressed/discordant. Again, depressed and aggressive behavior were found to be functionally distinct. In this study, depressive behavior was found to suppress aggressive responding by spouses and to do so most strongly in the nondepressed/discordant group. Taken together, the results of these three studies suggest that depressive behavior is functionally distinct from aggressive behavior.

Although this line of research is clear in highlighting the potential functional significance of "depressive" behavior (i.e., that it does not elicit partner verbal aggression), it does not explain the reason for higher levels of depressive behavior in the depressed group. This explanation requires some understanding of the different motivations that may inform the behavior of depressed and nondepressed partners.

An initial finding by Schmaling and Jacobson (1990) provides some clues regarding motivational differences. They note that depressive behavior, as defined by the Oregon research group, was elevated for depressed wives during a problem-focused discussion, but not during a discussion of "how their day had gone." This suggests that depressive behavior is elicited by a conflictual task, but not by a neutral task involving interaction with the spouse. This finding underscores the linkage of marital conflict and displays of depressive symptomatology among the depressed.

In a follow-up to the Schmaling and Jacobson (1990) study, Schmaling, Whisman, Fruzzetti, and Truax (1991) examined the behavior of 100 couples as they attempted to decide which problem areas to discuss during an upcoming videotaped problem-solving discussion. Schmaling et al. found that husbands' attempts to involve the interviewer and wives' active summarizing of proposed topics for discussion predicted wives' level of depression. In both cases, more active behavior was associated with less depression in the wives. This result fits well with findings by Christian, O'Leary, and Vivian (1994) indicating that among discordant couples, depression was associated with poorer self-reported problem-solving skills in both husbands and wives.

These studies suggest that something in the relational behavior of couples with a depressed spouse elicits and maintains prototypically "depressive" behavior. Interestingly, this behavior is most strongly elicited in the context of tasks with the potential to generate "conflict." In these situations, couples with a depressed member appear least able to solve problems effectively. Also, it appears that "depressive" responses are functionally distinct from "aggressive" responses, in that they do not elicit partner retaliation. Although these studies indicate that problem solving is compromised in depression and that a focus on problem-solving training seems warranted, they do little to identify the obstacles to good joint problem solving in couples with a depressed partner. One possibility that has been explored in a preliminary manner is that depressed spouses are more averse to partner hostility or anger, and that this leads them to avoid situations (such as problem solving) that provide a context in which partner anger and verbal aggression are more likely.

Is Depressive Symptomatology Associated with Aversion to Partner Aggression?

Jones and Katz (1998) carried out a preliminary attempt to examine this possibility. In their study, 285 women in dating relationships were asked to imagine a series of scenarios in which they had a disagreement with their partners. They were asked what their goal vis-à-vis partner anger would be, whether they would engage in various behaviors (assertive vs. depressive responses), and whether engaging in "depressed" behavior would be effective in either suppressing partner anger or resolving the problem. Respondents reported a greater probability of engaging in depressive behavior if a partner remained angry during the discussion for a long time than if the conflict was brief. In addition, women with higher levels of depressive symptoms were more likely than other women to report that they would engage in depressive behavior during conflict situations. Further, women reported an expectation that depressive behavior would suppress partner anger, but those with greater depressive symptoms also reported expecting depressive behavior to resolve dating conflict. Finally those who expected depressive behavior to both suppress and resolve dating conflict were the most likely to report engaging in depressive behavior during prolonged conflict situations. Accordingly, it appears that depressive behavior during conflict may be related to expectations regarding its impact on the partner.

Do Partner Criticism and Arguments with the Partner Influence Onset or Relapse of Depression?

If partner criticism and the potential for conflict with the partner are pivotal contexts in eliciting depressive behavior, one might expect such contexts to elicit depressive episodes. Alternatively, it might be that such contexts are consequential only for increasing level of distress, but not for pushing partners over the threshold of diagnosable depression. In an early examination of these issues, Vaughn and Leff (1976) found that depressives were particularly vulnerable to family tension and to hostile statements made by family members, and Schless, Schwartz, Goetz, and Mendels (1974) demonstrated that this vulnerability to marriage- and family-related stresses persisted after depressed patients recovered. Likewise, Hooley, Orley, and Teasdale (1986) found that levels of "expressed emotion," an index in which implied criticism of the partner figures prominently, predicted relapse of depression. Hooley (1986; Hooley & Teasdale, 1989) also found a high rate of negative comments in the spouses of depressed patients, and demonstrated that this high rate of criticism predicted relapse in the patients.

In a more recent investigation, Mundt, Fiedler, Ernst, and Backenstrab (1996) found that although elevated levels of "covert criticism" predicted relapse only for a subgroup of their patients with endogenous depression, relapsing couples showed a greater overall propensity to have long chains of negative marital interaction. Accordingly, it appears that the marital criticism and the potential negativity of conflict with the partner may be related to onset of depressive episodes, not just to increased level of distress (see also Marks, Wieck, Checkley, & Kumar, 1996).

It has also been found that negative marital events often precede the onset of depressive symptoms (Paykel & Cooper, 1992). Paykel et al. (1969) and Paykel and Tanner (1976), for example, used semistructured interviews of hospitalized patients to examine event occurrence and timing. In both cases, marital arguments and other stressors preceded depression, and they were especially prominent during the month preceding depression onset.

Taken together, the data on depressed versus nondepressed differences in problem-solving ability, the ability of conflict contexts to elicit depressive behavior, differences in goals and perceived consequences of depressive behavior among the more dysphoric, and the ability of conflict to precipitate depressive episodes are clear: They appear to establish a potentially important role for avoidance of conflict in the production and maintenance of depression. Depressed partners display characteristic patterns of dysfunctional problem-solving communication. However, these are most clearly manifested when conflict is present or may be present. Under these circumstances, depressed partners may be more likely to want to avoid conflict and may see depressive behavior as more effective in resolving conflict. Indeed, increases in arguments and partner criticism may play a role in precipitating a depressive episode. To the extent that couples can be given an alternative to nonproductive bickering and fighting—that is, problem-solving communication—this pattern of depressive behavior to avoid conflict should be undercut substantially. Accordingly, it appears reasonable to hypothesize that successful problem-solving communication training should reduce the frequency of depressive behavior.

Positive Spouse Behavior as a Potential Target of Intervention

So far, we have focused on negatively valenced behavior as a target for intervention. This is in keeping with the marital discord model (Beach, Sandeen, & O'Leary, 1990), which identifies a lack of positive (supportive) behavior and an excess of negative (stressful) behavior in the marriage as influencing level of depression, with much or all of the effect being mediated by level of marital dissatisfaction. Recently, however, alternative pathways from marriage to depressive symptomatology have been proposed. In particular, self-verification theory has been identified as a source of hypotheses about processes that may increase depressive symptoms even in the context of "good" relationships. Because such processes should be independent of those identified in the marital discord model, they may suggest new or additional points of clinical intervention with depressed/discordant spouses. Accordingly, we examine partner verification of negative self-beliefs and the potential role of nonjudgmental, supportive listening in alleviating depressive symptoms.

Partner Verification of Negative Self-Beliefs as a Potential Target

Self-verification theory (Swann, 1983) suggests that people may often seek and show a preference for partner feedback that confirms their self-view. This has the effect of directing those with low self-esteem to seek out and prefer negative feedback about the self. On the one hand, as with other forms of self-verification, the recipient should feel more positive about the source. On the other, negative self-verification may also increase subjective certainty regarding one's negative attributes (e.g., Pelham & Swann, 1994), and thereby render one's negative self-view more stable (e.g., Swann & Predmore, 1985). Accordingly, negative self-verification should intensify the depressogenic effects of negative self-views, providing an insidious avenue of negative marital influence on depressive symptoms. For example, without conflict, the nondepressed partner may agree with and underscore the depressed partner's perception of the self as dependent or lacking, thus helping to maintain that partner's depressive symptomatology.

The relationship of partner verification processes to depressive symptoms was investigated by Katz and Beach (1997). They examined both direct and indirect effects of self-verification on depressive symptoms. As in prior research, self-verification had a positive effect on relationship satisfaction. Because marital satisfaction was inversely related to depressive symptoms, this resulted in an overall inverse relationship between self-verification and depression. However, as predicted, the effect of negative self-views was intensified when these were verified by the partner. Interestingly, the effect applied to both dating and married samples. Accordingly, as hypothesized by Katz and Beach (1997), there were effects of marriage on depressive symptoms that were not mediated by marital dissatisfaction.

How might this "insidious" partner effect on depression be countered? To better understand how "positive" partner behavior might be rendered more constructive, we briefly examine recent work on the facilitation of intimacy.

Increasing Intimacy and Facilitative Self-Disclosure

In her book on the psychology of intimacy, Prager (1995) highlights a number of interaction patterns that contribute to felt intimacy and closeness to a partner. Facing the other person, leaning toward the other, smiling and/or nodding as the other talks, making eye contact, and maintaining an "open," relaxed posture all convey involvement and intensify feelings of intimate connection between partners. Accordingly, wherever such nonverbal factors are subculturally appropriate, it may be useful to attend to them in working with depressed persons and their spouses.

Verbal self-disclosure has long been viewed as a hallmark of intimacy (Derlega & Chaikin, 1975). And as relationship satisfaction increases, self-disclosure may increase as well. Of course, self-disclosure may carry both benefits and potential risks. In particular, self-disclosure of a negative view of the partner could be one source of negative verification. Although such revelations may further increase the felt closeness of the relationship, they may nonetheless undermine efforts to resolve a depressive episode. Accordingly, it may be important to foster self-disclosure that verifies positive aspects of the partner, or that at least implicitly verifies the partner's worth without verifying his or her negative self-beliefs.

Likewise, self-disclosures that include both facts and one's own feelings about a situation are likely to be viewed as more intimate (Howell & Conway, 1990). For a discordant couple with a depressed partner, however, affectively laden self-disclosures are likely to be predominantly "angry." Because "angry" self-disclosures powerfully elicit anger from the partner, such an approach carries the strong risk of escalating negative interaction. It may be useful, therefore, in working with a depressed couple to encourage sharing of the spouses' reactions to events and exploring of emotional reactions that go beyond "anger." In particular, if the nondepressed spouse can be led to express feelings of loss, loneliness, or hurt that may have led to earlier expressions of anger, this may help both spouses feel closer to each other (cf. Greenberg & Johnson, 1988; Jacobson & Christiansen, 1996). In this way, they may be led to explore in an intimate way even events or issues that have been problematic for them. At the same time, such intimate disclosures may be more likely to verify partner strengths, and less likely to verify partner weaknesses, than are "angry" disclosures aimed at punishing the partner.

It appears, then, that negative self-disclosure may be particularly problematic in a couple with a depressed partner, and that increasing nonjudgmental listening may be a first step to counteracting this area of difficulty. Thus, another approach to treatment is to increase positive spouse behavior, particularly the nondepressed partner's listening and intimate self-disclosure, while encouraging the same in the depressed partner.

Of course, etiology does not necessarily predict treatment. At present, there are no tests of the efficacy of such highly tailored approaches to marital intervention with depression. However, there is outcome research that has examined the efficacy of marital therapy in the treatment of depression. Although the outcome research does not address all the issue raised by our review of the basic literature, it does provide a window on whether marital interventions should be considered promising approaches in working with depressed persons.

DO EFFICACIOUS MARITAL TREATMENTS INFLUENCE DEPRESSION?

Treatment Outcome Research

A number of case studies and group comparisons have examined spousal involvement in therapy and its potential utility in alleviating depressive symptomatology (e.g., Friedman, 1975; Hafner, Badenoch, Fisher, & Swift, 1983; Lewinsohn & Shaw, 1969; Lewinsohn & Shaffer, 1971; McLean, Ogston, & Grauer, 1973). More recently, four outcome studies have examined reasonably well-specified marital therapies for depression and compared their effectiveness to that of widely used individual therapies. These studies support the hypothesis that conjoint marital therapy can be as effective in the treatment of depression as alternative individual approaches when it is applied to couples that are maritally discordant and contain a depressed member. Each is reviewed in turn.

In the first of these studies, Beach and O'Leary (1992; O'Leary & Beach, 1990) randomly assigned 45 couples to either individual cognitive therapy (CT), conjoint behavioral marital therapy (BMT), or a 15-week waiting-list condition. To be included in the study, both partners had to score in the discordant range on the Dyadic Adjustment Scale (DAS) and to present themselves as being discordant.

The primary finding was that CT and BMT were equally effective in reducing depression symptoms, and that both were clearly superior to the waiting-list control group. However, only BMT improved the marital relationship, and there were large differences among the three conditions in marital outcome. At the termination of therapy, BMT produced a statistically significant (20-point) increase in DAS scores over the pre-therapy scores. However, wives in the CT and waiting-list groups showed little change (-2 and 1 scale points, respectively).

In the second study, Jacobson, Dobson, Fruzzetti, Schmaling, and Salusky (1991) randomly assigned 60 married women who had been diagnosed as depressed to either individual CT, BMT, or a treatment combining BMT and CT. Couples were not selected for the presence of marital discord. Accordingly, it was possible to examine directly whether BMT would be helpful for depressed/maritally nondiscordant people. Jacobson et al. (1991) found that the marital intervention was not helpful for alleviating depression in the absence of marital discord (i.e., among people with DAS scores greater than 97). However, in the half of the sample that reported some marital discord, the results were consistent with O'Leary and Beach's (1990; Beach & O'Leary, 1992) findings: BMT was as effective as CT in reducing depression. Furthermore, only BMT resulted in significant improvement in marital adjustment among depressed/discordant couples. Finally, CT was also effective in reducing depressive symptomatology among the depressed/discordant. Thus, the Jacobson et al. (1991) study also suggests the possibility that BMT, applied to an appropriate population, may be as effective as individual approaches in relieving the episode of depression, as well as more effective in enhancing marital functioning.

In the third study (Foley, Rounsaville, Weissman, Sholomaskas, & Chevron, 1989), 18 depressed outpatients were randomly assigned to either individual interpersonal psychotherapy (IPT; Klerman, Weissman, Rounsaville, & Chevron, 1984) or a newly developed couple format version of IPT. Individual IPT is designed to handle marital disputes, so the use of a conjoint format required relatively minor changes. Nevertheless, the intervention was structured to include a focus on conjoint communication training, making it similar to BMT. This study differed from the two studies already reviewed by including husbands ($n = 5$) in addition to wives ($n = 13$), rather than a sample composed entirely of wives.

Foley et al. (1989) found that participants in both treatments exhibited a significant reduction in symptoms of depression, but they found no differential improvement on measures of depressive symptomatology between the two groups. The interventions also produced equal enhancement of general social functioning. On the other hand, at session 16, participants receiving couple IPT reported marginally higher marital satisfaction scores (Short Marital Adjustment Test; Locke & Wallace, 1959) and scored significantly higher on one subscale of the DAS.

In the fourth study, Emanuels-Zuurveen and Emmelkamp (1996) randomly assigned 27 depressed outpatients to either individual cognitive-behavioral therapy or communication-focused marital therapy. As in Foley et al. (1989), the sample for this study included both depressed husbands ($n = 13$) as well as depressed wives ($n = 14$). Participants in both treatments exhibited a significant reduction in depressive symptom, and there was no differential improvement between the two groups. In contrast, there was a significant, differential effect of treatment on marital outcomes, with the marital therapy condition producing substantially greater gains in marital satisfaction. In addition, there was a significant reduction in the depressed patient's criticism of the nondepressed partner only among those receiving marital therapy. Thus, this investigation replicated the pattern obtained in each of the three earlier studies: equivalent outcome for when the focus is depressive symptoms, better outcome in marital therapy when the focus is marital functioning.

In sum, studies designed to test the efficacy of established marital therapy approaches in relieving depressive symptomatology have produced results that are quite encouraging. Although the interventions used did not target every potential point of marital intervention, and so may underestimate the maximum effect that could be obtained using marital approaches, they produced sufficiently strong results to encourage additional work with marital interventions.

Is It Possible to Predict Who Will Do Better
in Marital Therapy for Depression?

Another important clinical issue that may influence treatment decisions is that of differential response to treatment and the potential to identify in advance clients who will do better or worse in a given type of treatment. Several attempts have been made to examine these issues. A first attempt was made by Beach and O'Leary (1992), using factors that represented pretherapy cognitive dysfunction and pretherapy marital dysfunction. Wives receiving CT showed a very strong predictive relationship between the marital factor and outcome in the predicted direction: A better pretreatment marital environment predicted better outcome in CT. Conversely, more dysfunctional thinking also predicted better outcome in CT, albeit not as robustly as pretreatment marital environment did. Thus, within a population of persons interested in maintaining their marriages but having problems with both marital discord and depression, having a more negative view of the partner and the relationship, along with less evidence of a depressogenic thinking style, was predictive of residual depressive symptomatology for wives receiving CT.

O'Leary et al. (1990) addressed the question using a clinically immediate and intuitively appealing predictor of outcome—namely, depressed patients' accounts of the temporal order of, and causal relationship between, their marital problems and their depression. Women entering the treatment protocol were asked which problem came first, marital discord or depression. The correlation between temporal order ratings and residualized gains in marital satisfaction were high in the CT condition ($r = -.65$, $p < .001$). However, for BMT subjects the correlations were nonsignificant. Depressed patients who reported that their marital problems came before their depression had poor marital outcomes if they were assigned to CT, but positive marital outcomes if they were assigned to BMT. Conversely, those patients reporting that depression preceded their marital discord did about equally well in either condition. The ratings were not significantly related to change in depressive symptomatology.

In brief, then, it does appear possible to say something about couples who will do better and benefit uniquely from being involved in marital therapy. There seems to be good reason for preceding with marital therapy for cases in which (1) the depressed partner is relatively more concerned about marital problems than about the depression, or (2) the marital problems are viewed as having preceded and perhaps caused the depressive symptoms, or (3) the cognitive and other "individual" symptoms seem less salient than do the marital problems. In these cases, clients may benefit as much from marital therapy as from individual approaches for their depression, and may benefit considerably more in terms of their marital relationships. Alternatively stated, persons with discordant relationships who receive marital therapy may often experience improvement in depression, regardless of whether their depression came before or after the start of their marital problems; however, persons with more long-standing marital problems who receive individual therapy may find their marital problems worsening even as their depression improves.

Marital Processes and Depression: What about Depressed Men?

There are considerably more data about the effect of marital therapy on the depressive symptoms of women than about its efficacy as an approach with men. This reflects the facts that women are more frequently depressed, and that men may be less likely to request marital therapy in response to their own depressive symptomatology. Lower frequency of requesting marital therapy may, of course, be a reflection of gender role constraints for men. However, the longitudinal data suggest that for men marital satisfaction may be better conceptualized as a likely casualty of depression than as a cause of depression. What are the salient issues when the depressed spouse is a man? Is there a role for marital therapy in such cases?

Gender roles give rise to clear differences in expectations regarding behavior among men and women. Men are more likely to use direct influence strategies to "make" others change (e.g., reward, coercion, appeal to expertise; Howard, Blumstein, & Schwartz, 1986). In addition, men are also expected to show more calmness in a crisis and to be able to "stand up to others." The internalization of these expectations may lead men to view interpersonal conflict in terms of competition and "winning," or may lead them to withdraw (or attempt to do so) when conflict might cause them to "lose their cool" (Gottman, 1994). Such tendencies should make men less likely to take responsibility for marital discord and more likely to minimize the seriousness of partner concerns. Finally, men may also be more likely to engage in distracting behaviors when they notice dysphoric feelings, to avoid personal blame for any deterioration in their own satisfaction, and to leave noxious interpersonal situations in order to repair their mood (Nolen-Hoeksema, 1987). Thus, men may be relatively less likely to become dysphoric in response to marital problems, and more prone to withdraw from and denigrate close relationships when they are dysphoric.

If so, a marital therapist may find it difficult to work with a couple in which the husband is depressed, and may find it useful to suggest individually oriented interventions to help the husband work on individual issues before beginning to focus on changing marital behavior. In particular, it may be relatively more important for the depressed man to focus on reducing the felt need to blame the partner for his dysphoria, and to find ways to better care for himself. Work with the wife during this time might focus on finding ways to reduce her involvement in verifying his feelings of low self-worth. Once some progress has been made in dealing with the depression, marital work might be expected to proceed more rapidly.

Summary

So, when the therapist is confronted with a couple asking for marital therapy in which one or both spouses are depressed, what is the most useful approach to working with this constellation of problems? We hope that we are now in a better position to answer this pivotal clinical question.

When should a therapist proceed to do marital therapy? It appears that for clients in which the marital problems came first, or seem more compelling and important to the couple, marital therapy may provide a relatively better constellation of outcomes than individual approaches. When should a therapist refer for individual treatment? If the depressed spouse is male, or if the dysfunctional beliefs and individual concerns seem more pronounced than do the marital concerns, the results of individual therapy may be as good as marital therapy; thus, it may be reasonable to start with individual treatment approaches first. Indeed, it may make marital work easier, should such work still be necessary later in the treatment process.

CONCLUSION

In concluding this chapter, we address two treatment issues that have not yet been discussed in our analysis. The first concerns medication, and the second relates to subclinical depression; each is discussed in turn.

What about Medication?

The possible additive effects produced by combining marital therapy with medication for depression need to be investigated. Friedman's (1975) study hinted at the possibility of additive benefits, and the literature on IPT indicates strong potential additive effects of an interpersonally focused intervention in combination with antidepressant medication (Klerman, DiMascio, Weissman, Prusoff, & Paykel, 1974; Rounsaville, Klerman, & Weissman, 1981; Weissman, Klerman, Prusoff, Sholomskas, & Padian, 1981). Within a maritally discordant population, the combination of marital therapy and antidepressant medication may prove particularly powerful and synergistic. It is particularly important to determine the parameters governing better and worse responses to combinations of antidepressant medication and marital therapy. For example, it would be of interest to know whether marital therapy for depression works better when it starts before or after the depressed spouse begins a course of antidepressant treatment. Likewise, we might wonder whether the timing of the two components of treatment has any effect on maintenance of gains. Currently, there is little to guide us on these matters. At most, we can say that combination treatments seem likely to work well and are not contra-indicated by any existing studies.

What about Subclinical Depression?

Although much of the attention among marital therapy researchers has been directed toward understanding the role of marital therapy in the treatment of the clinical syndrome of depression, there has been increasing recognition that subclinical levels of depression pose a significant and costly health problem in their own right (Wells et al., 1989). Persons with significant but nonclinical levels of depressive symptomatology showed substantially poorer performance at work and at home, compared to persons with a variety of chronic ailments (Wells et al., 1989) and to less depressed persons (Beach, Martin, Blum, & Roman, 1993). Given the high rate of episodes of heightened depressive symptomatology (Weissman, Bruce, Leaf, Florio, & Holzer, 1991), the cost of subclinical levels of depressive symptoms may surpass that of diagnosable episodes of depression. Elevated symptoms of depression also constitute a significant risk factor for the development of a first episode of major depression (Horwath, Johnson, Klerman, & Weissman, 1992), and may lead both to heightened reactivity to stressors in general (Hammen, Mayol, deMayo, & Marks, 1986) and to heightened reactivity to marital discord in particular (Beach & O'Leary, 1993b). Accordingly, reducing subclinical levels of depressive symptomatology may prove helpful in reducing the risk of future episodes. Together, these considerations suggest that it may prove cost-effective to identify, and provide marital therapy for, persons who are maritally discordant and experiencing subclinical levels of depression. Because higher levels of depressive symptomatology are associated with greater gains in marital therapy (Jacobson, Follette, & Pagel, 1986), this may be a population that would be particularly responsive to marital therapy.

Final Comments

Marital therapy has demonstrated efficacy as a treatment or a component of treatment for depression. As currently constituted, marital therapy seems most appropriate for couples in which marital problems are relatively pronounced, the wife is the depressed partner, marital problems are seen as having preceded the onset of the depression, and dysfunctional beliefs related to depression seem less pronounced. Accordingly, there may be little reason for marital therapists to refer such cases routinely for individual treatment. When marital therapy is selected as a treatment, it may be useful to use as a guide a manual associated with successful prior outcome research (e.g., Beach et al., 1990). However, therapists should not be afraid to address additional issues and further tailor the approach to fit particular clients. In this chapter, we have highlighted a number of key issues that may be pivotal in fully addressing marital processes that can contribute to the maintenance or exacerbation of depression. These issues may provide the key to further enhancing marital interventions for depression and creating a new generation of interventions for co-occurring marital discord and depression.

ACKNOWLEDGMENTS

Support for this chapter was provided by Grant No. SBR-9511385 from the National Science Foundation to Steven R. H. Beach and by grants from the Nuffield Foundation, the National Health Service, and the Economic and Social Research Council of Great Britain to Frank D. Fincham. These grants are gratefully acknowledged.

REFERENCES

American Psychiatric Association. (1987). *Diagnostic and statistical manual of mental disorders* (3rd ed., rev.). Washington, DC: Author.

Arkowitz, H., Holliday, S., & Hutter, M. (1982, November). *Depressed women and their husbands: A study of marital interaction and adjustment.* Paper presented at the 16th Annual Convention of the Association for Advancement of Behavior Therapy, Los Angeles.

Assh, S. D., & Byers, E. S. (1996). Understanding the co-occurence of marital distress and depression in women. *Journal of Social and Personal Relationships, 13,* 537–552.

Beach, S. R. H., Harwood, E. M., Horan, P. M., Katz, J., Blum, T. C., Martin, J. K., & Roman, P. M. (1995, November). *Marital effects on depression: Measuring the longitudinal relationship.* Paper presented at the 29th Annual Convention of the Association for Advancement of Behavior Therapy, Washington, DC.

Beach, S. R. H., Jouriles, E. N., & O'Leary, K. D. (1985). Extramarital sex: Impact on depression and commitment in couples seeking marital therapy. *Journal of Sex and Marital Therapy, 11,* 99–108.

Beach, S. R. H., Martin, J. D., Blum, T. C., & Roman, P. M. (1993). Subclinical depression and role fulfillment in domestic settings: Spurious relationships, imagined problems, or real effects? *Journal of Psychopathology and Behavioral Assessment, 15,* 113–128.

Beach, S. R. H., & O'Leary, K. D. (1992). Treating depression in the context of marital discord: Outcome and predictors of response for marital therapy vs. cognitive therapy. *Behavior Therapy, 23,* 507–528.

Beach, S. R. H., & O'Leary, K. D. (1993a). Marital discord and dysphoria: For whom does the marital relationship predict depressive symptoms? *Journal of Social and Personal Relationships, 10,* 405–420.

Beach, S. R. H., & O'Leary, K. D. (1993b). Dysphoria and marital discord: Are dysphoric individuals at risk for marital maladjustment? *Journal of Marital and Family Therapy, 19,* 355–368.

Beach, S. R. H., Sandeen, E. E., & O'Leary, K. D. (1990). *Depression in marriage: A model for etiology and treatment.* New York: Guilford Press.

Beach, S. R. H., Smith, D. A., & Fincham, F. D. (1994). Marital interventions for depression: Empirical foundation and future prospects. *Applied and Preventive Psychology, 3,* 233–250.

Biglan, A., Hops, H., Sherman, L., Friedman, L. S., Arthur, J., & Osteen, V. (1985). Problem solving interactions of depressed women and their spouses. *Behavior Therapy, 16,* 431–451.

Brown, G. W., & Harris, T. (1978). *Social origins of depression: A study of psychiatric disorders in women.* New York: Free Press.

Brown, G. W., & Harris, T. (1986). Establishing causal links: The Bedford College studies of depression. In H. Katschnig (Ed.), *Life events and psychiatric disorders: Controversial issues* (pp. 107–187). Cambridge, England: Cambridge University Press.

Christian, J. L., O'Leary, K. D., & Vivian, D. (1994). Depressive symptomatology in maritally discordant women and men: The role of individual and relationship variables. *Journal of Family Psychology, 8,* 32–42.

Christian-Herman, J., O'Leary, K.D., & Avery-Leaf, S. (1997). *The impact of severe negative life events in marriage on depression.* Manuscript submitted for publication.

Davila, J., Bradbury, T. N., Cohan, C. L., Tochluk, S. (1997). Marital functioning and depressive symptoms: Evidence for a stress generation model. *Journal of Personality and Social Psychology, 73,* 849–861.

Demo, D. H., & Acock, A. C. (1996). Singlehood, marriage, and remarriage: The effects of family structure and family relationships on mothers' well-being. *Journal of Family Issues, 17,* 388–407.

Derlega, V. J., & Chaikin, A. L. (1975). *Sharing intimacy.* Englewood Cliffs, NJ: Prentice-Hall.

Emanuels-Zuurveen, L., & Emmelkamp, P. M. G. (1996). Individual behavioral-cognitive therapy v. marital therapy for depression in maritally distressed couples. *British Journal of Psychiatry, 169,* 181–188.

Fincham, F. D., Beach, S. R. H., Harold, G., T., & Osborne, L. N. (1997). Marital satisfaction and depression: Different causal relationships for men and women? *Psychological Science, 8,* 351–357.

Foley, S. H., Rounsaville, B. J., Weissman, M. M., Sholomaskas, D., & Chevron, E. (1989). Individual versus conjoint interpersonal therapy for depressed patients with marital disputes. *International Journal of Family Psychiatry, 10,* 29–42.

Friedman, A. (1975). Interaction of drug therapy with marital therapy in depressive patients. *Archives of General Psychiatry, 32,* 619–637.

Gotlib, I. H., Lewinsohn, P. M., & Seeley, J. R. (1996, November). *Consequences of depression during adolescence: Marital status and marital functioning in early adulthood.* Paper presented at the 30th Annual Convention of the Association for Advancement of Behavior Therapy, New York.

Gotlib, I. H., & Whiffen, V. E. (1989). Depression and marital functioning: An examination of specificity and gender differences. *Journal of Abnormal Psychology, 98,* 23–30.

Gottman, J. M. (1994). *What predicts divorce?* Hillsdale, NJ: Erlbaum.

Greenberg, L. S., & Johnson, S. M. (1988). *Emotionally focused therapy for couples.* New York: Guilford Press.

Hafner, R. J., Badenoch, A., Fisher, J., & Swift, H. (1983). Spouse-aided versus individual therapy in persisting psychiatric disorders: A systematic comparison. *Family Process, 22,* 385–399.

Hammen, C., Mayol, A., deMayo, R., & Marks, T. (1986). Initial symptom levels and the life-event–depression relationship. *Journal of Abnormal Psychology, 95,* 114–122.

Hautzinger, M., Linden, M., & Hoffman, N. (1982). Distressed couples with and without a depressed partner: An analysis of their verbal interaction. *Journal of Behavior Therapy and Experimental Psychology, 13,* 307–314.

Hinchliffe, M., Hooper, D., & Roberts, F. J. (1978). *The melancholy marriage.* New York: Wiley.

Horwath, E., Johnson, J., Klerman, G. L., & Weissman, M. M. (1992). Depressive symptoms as relative and attributable risk factors for first-onset major depression. *Archives of General Psychiatry, 49,* 817–823.

Hooley, J. M. (1986). Expressed emotion and depression: Interactions between patients and high- versus low-expressed emotion spouses. *Journal of Abnormal Psychology, 95,* 237–246.

Hooley, J. M., Orley, J., & Teasdale, J. D. (1986). Levels of expressed emotion and relapse in depressed patients. *British Journal of Psychiatry, 148,* 642–647.

Hooley, J. M., & Teasdale, J. D. (1989). Predictors of relapse in unipolar depressives: Expressed emotion, marital distress, and perceived criticism. *Journal of Abnormal Psychology, 98,* 229–237.

Howard, J. A., Blumstein, P., & Schwartz, P. (1986). Sex, power, and influence tactics in intimate relationships. *Journal of Personality and Social Psychology, 51,* 102–109.

Howell, A., & Conway, M. (1990). Perceived intimacy of expressed emotion. *Journal of Social Psychology, 130,* 467–476.

Jacobson, N. S., & Christiansen, A. (1996). *Couple therapy: An integrative approach.* New York: Norton.

Jacobson, N. S., Dobson, K., Fruzzetti, A. E., Schmaling, D. B., & Salusky, S. (1991). Marital therapy as a treatment for depression. *Journal of Consulting and Clinical Psychology, 59,* 547–557.

Jacobson, N. S., & Follette, W. C., & Pagel, M. (1986). *Predicting who will benefit from behavioral marital therapy. Journal of Consulting and Clinical Psychology, 54,* 518–522.

Johnson, S. L., & Jacob, T. (1997). Marital interactions of depressed men and women. *Journal of Consulting and Clinical Psychology, 65,* 15–23.

Joiner, T. E., Jr., & Metalsky, G. I. (1995). A prospective test of an integrative interpersonal theory of depression: A naturalistic study of college roommates. *Journal of Personality and Social Psychology, 69,* 778–788.

Jones, D., & Katz, J. (1998). *Accounting for the use of distressed behavior during dating conflict: Effects of depressed mood, dating quality, and expected consequences of distressed behavior.* Manuscript submitted for publication.

Kahn, J., Coyne, J. C., & Margolin, G. (1985). Depression and marital disagreement: The social construction of despair. *Journal of Social and Personal Relationships, 2,* 447–461.

Katz, J., & Beach, S. R. H. (1997). Self-verification and depression in romantic relationships. *Journal of Marriage and the Family, 59,* 903–914.

Klerman, G. L., DiMascio, A., Weissman, M. M., Prusoff, B. A., & Paykel, E. S. (1974). Treatment of depression by drugs and psychotherapy. *American Journal of Psychiatry, 131,* 186–191.

Klerman, G. L., Weissman, M. M., Rounsaville, B. J., & Chevron, E. S. (1984). *Interpersonal psychotherapy of depression.* New York: Basic Books.

Kowalik, D. L., & Gotlib, I. H. (1987). Depression and marital interaction: Concordance between intent and perception of communication. *Journal of Abnormal Psychology, 96,* 127–134.

Lewinsohn, P. M., & Shaffer, M. (1971). Use of home observations as an integral part of the treatment of depression: Preliminary report and case studies. *Journal of Consulting and Clinical Psychology, 37,* 87–94.

Lewinsohn, P. M., & Shaw, D. A. (1969). Feedback about interpersonal behavior as an agent of behavior change: A case study in the treatment of depression. *Psychotherapy and Psychosomatics, 17,* 82–88.

Locke, H. J., & Wallace, K. M. (1959). Short marital adjustment and prediction tests: Their reliability and validity. *Marriage and Family Living, 21,* 231–235.

Marks, M., Wieck, A., Checkley, S., & Kumar, C. (1996). How does marriage protect women with histories of affective disorder from post-partum relapse? *British Journal of Medical Psychology, 69,* 778–788.

McCabe, S. B., & Gotlib, I. H. (1993). Interactions of couples with and without a depressed spouse: Self-report and observations of problem-solving situations. *Journal of Social and Personal Relationships, 10,* 589–599.

McLean, P. D., Ogston, K., & Grauer, L. (1973). A behavioral approach to the treatment of depression. *Journal of Behavior Therapy and Experimental Psychiatry, 4,* 323–330.

Mundt, C., Fiedler, P., Ernst, S., & Backenstrab, M. (1996). Expressed emotion and marital interaction in endogenous depressives. In C. Mundt, M. J. Goldstein, K. Hahlweg, & P. Fiedler (Eds.), *Interpersonal factors in the origin and course of affective disorders* (pp. 240–256). London: Gaskell.

Nelson, G. M., & Beach, S. R. H. (1990). Sequential interaction in depression: Effects of depressive behavior on spousal aggression. *Behavior Therapy, 12,* 167–182.

Nolen-Hoeksema, S. (1987). Sex differences in unipolar depression: Evidence and theory. *Psychological Bulletin, 101,* 259–282.

O'Leary, K. D., & Beach, S. R. H. (1990). Marital therapy: A viable treatment for depression and marital discord. *American Journal of Psychiatry, 147,* 183–186.

O'Leary, K. D., Christian, J. L., & Mendell, N. R. (1994). A closer look at the link between marital discord and depressive symptomatology. *Journal of Social and Clinical Psychology, 14,* 1–9.

O'Leary, K. D., Christian, J. L., & Mendell, N. R. (1993). A closer look at the link between marital discord and depressive symptomatology. *Journal of Social and Clinical Psychology, 14,* 1–9.

O'Leary, K. D., Risso, L. P., & Beach, S. R. H. (1990). Attributions about the marital discord/depression link and therapy outcome. *Behavior Therapy, 21,* 413–422.

Paykel, E. S., & Cooper, Z. (1992). Life events and social stress. In E. S. Paykel (Ed.), *Handbook of affective disorders* (2nd ed., pp. 149–170). New York: Guilford Press.

Paykel, E. S., Cooper, Z., Ramana, R., & Hayhurst, H. (1996). Life events, social support, and marital relationships in the outcome of severe depression. *Psychological Medicine, 26,* 121–133.

Paykel, E. S., Myers, J. K., Dienelt, M. N., Klerman, G. L., Lindenthal, J. J., & Pepper, M. P. (1969). Life events and depression: A controlled study. *Archives of General Psychiatry, 21,* 753–760.

Paykel, E. S., & Tanner J. (1976). Life events, depressive relapse, and maintenance treatment. *Psychological Medicine, 6,* 481–485.

Pelham, B. W., & Swann, W. B. (1994). The juncture of intrapersonal and interpersonal knowledge: Self-certainty and interpersonal congruence. *Personality and Social Psychology Bulletin, 20,* 349–357.

Prager, K. J. (1995). *The psychology of intimacy.* New York: Guilford Press.

Regier, D. A., Myers, J. K., Kramer, M., Robins, L. N., Blazer, D. G., Hough, R. L., Eaton, W. W., & Locke, B. Z. (1984). The NIMH Epidemiologic Catchment Area program: Historical context, major objectives, and study population characteristics. *Archives of General Psychiatry, 41,* 934–941.

Rounsaville, B. J., Klerman, G. L., & Weissman, M. M. (1981). Do psychotherapy and pharmacotherapy of depression conflict?: Empirical evidence from a clinical trial. *Archives of General Psychiatry, 38,* 24–29.

Roy, A. (1987). Five risk factors for depression. *British Journal of Psychiatry, 150,* 536–541.

Ruscher, S. M., & Gotlib, I. H. (1988). Marital interaction patterns of couples with and without a depressed partner. *Behavior Therapy, 19,* 455–470.

Schless, A. P., Schwartz, L., Goetz, C., & Mendels, J. (1974). How depressives view the significance of life events. *British Journal of Psychiatry, 125,* 406–410.

Schmaling, K. B., & Jacobson, N. S. (1990). Marital interaction and depression. *Journal of Abnormal Psychology, 99,* 229–236.

Schmaling, K. B., Whisman, M. A., Fruzzetti, A. E., & Truax, P. (1991). Identifying areas of marital conflict: Interactional behaviors associated with depression. *Journal of Family Psychology, 5,* 145–157.

Swann, W. B. (1983). Self-verification: Bringing social reality into harmony with the self. In J. Suls & A. G. Greenwald (Eds.), *Social psychology perspectives* (Vol. 2, pp. 33–66). Hillsdale, NJ: Erlbaum.

Swann, W. B., & Predmore, S. C. (1985). Intimates as agents of social support: Sources of consolation or despair? *Journal of Personality and Social Psychology, 49,* 1609–1617.

Thompson, J. M., Whiffin, V. E., & Blain, M. D. (1995). Depressive symptoms, sex, and perceptions of intimate relationships. *Journal of Social and Personal Relationships, 12,* 49–66.

Vaughn, C. E., & Leff, J. P. (1976). The influence of family and social factors on the course of psychiatric illness: A comparison of schizophrenic and depressed neurotic patients. *British Journal of Psychiatry*, *129*, 125–137.

Vega, B. R., Canas, F., Banyon, C., Franco, B., Graell, M., Santodomingo, J. (1996). Interpersonal factors in female depression. *European Journal of Psychiatry*, *10*, 16–24.

Vinokur, A. D., Price, R. H., & Caplan, R. D. (1996). Hard times and hurtful partners: How financial strain affects depression and relationship satisfaction of unemployed persons and their spouses. *Journal of Personality and Social Psychology*, *71*, 166–179.

Wells, K. B., Stewart, A., Hays, R. D., Burnam, M. A., Rogers, W., Daniels, M., Berry, S., Greenfield, S., & Ware, J. (1989). The functioning and well being of depressed patients: Results from the Medical Outcomes Study. *Journal of the American Medical Association*, *262*, 914–919.

Weissman, M. M. (1987). Advances in psychiatric epidemiology: Rates and risks for major depression. *American Journal of Public Health*, *77*, 445–451.

Weissman, M. M., Bruce, M. L., Leaf, P. J., Florio, L. P., & Holzer, C. (1991). Affective disorders. In L. N. Robins & D. A. Regier (Eds.), *Psychiatric disorders in America: The Epidemiological Catchment Area study* (pp. 53–80). New York: Free Press.

Weissman, M. M., Klerman, G. L., Prusoff, B. A., Sholomskas, D., & Padian, N. (1981). Depressed outpatients one year after treatment with drugs and/or interpersonal psychotherapy (IPT). *Archives of General Psychiatry*, *38*, 51–55.

Zelkowitz, P. M., Millet, T. H. (1996). Post-partum psychiatric disorders: Their relationship to psychological adjustment and marital satisfaction in the spouses. *Journal of Abnormal Psychology*, *105*, 281–285.

CHAPTER 12

Schizophrenia
and the Family

IAN R. NICHOLSON

DEFINITION AND DIAGNOSIS

Schizophrenia has been known for thousands of years. As early as 1400 B.C., Sanskrit writings described people who would now be diagnosed with schizophrenia (Doran, Brier, & Roy, 1986). Some medical historians have reviewed the lives of such historical figures as Socrates or William Blake, attempting to find evidence for the presence of schizophrenia in earlier eras (e.g., Zilboorg, 1941). German and French psychiatric texts in the 19th century include several references to variants of schizophrenia (Wilkinson, 1987). Modern definitions began, however, near the beginning of the 20th century.

In 1898, Emil Kraepelin developed a diagnostic system that included the category of "dementia praecox." This new category grouped together three similar but previously separate forms of disorder: "catatonic," "hebephrenic," and "paranoid." Common to these forms were several symptoms, including progressive mental deterioration (i.e., dementia) and an onset during puberty or adolescence (i.e., praecox). These common symptoms allowed the forms to be organized under than one major category. Kraepelin revised his categories several times in the years that followed. In the last version, he described it as "a series of states, the common characteristic of which is a peculiar destruction of the internal connections of the psychic personality. The effects of this injury predominate in the emotional and volitional spheres of mental life" (1913/1919, p. 3).

While Kraepelin was revising his texts, Eugen Bleuler's (1911/1950) text on schizophrenia appeared. It made a major impact at its publication, for several reasons. First, Bleuler introduced the term "schizophrenia" to overcome the difficulties inherent in the term "dementia praecox." Employing this term allowed him to emphasize the disintegration of personality due to a loosening of associations, which he viewed as the most important characteristic of the disorder. In 1912, the term was first employed in an English-language medical journal, *The Lancet* (Simpson & Weiner, 1989); it has been used ever since. Second, Bleuler reinforced Kraepelin's categories and also added a fourth category, "simple schizophrenia." Third, he posited that the group of schizophrenias could be viewed as a single clinical entity, as all four categories shared four primary characteristics. These characteristics, which have since become known as "the four A's," were disorders of association, autism, ambivalence, and affect. There have been several diagnostic systems in the United States and across the world since the time of Kraepelin and Bleuler (Stengel, 1959). However, Bleuler's view dominated most theory and research on schizophrenia from the publication of the 1950 English translation of his text until the development of the third edition of the American Psychiatric Association's *Diagnostic and Statistical Manual of Mental Disorders* (DSM-III) in 1980 (Andreasen, 1989; Cromwell, 1975).

The current diagnostic system used in the United States is the fourth edition of this manual (DSM-IV; American Psychiatric Association, 1994). Similar to the DSM-III, it is based on the idea of defining multiple, separate disorders according to operational criteria based (for the most part) on descriptive psychopathology, rather than inferences or criteria from a disorder's presumed causation or etiology (Klerman, 1983). For the diagnosis of schizophrenia, there are two primary diagnostic criteria and four additional criteria that serve to separate it from other disorders. To meet the first criterion, a person must display, for most of a 1-month period, two or more symptoms from a list of five. These symptoms are (1) delusions; (2) hallucinations; (3) disorganized speech (e.g., incoherence or frequent loosening of associations); (4) extremely disorganized behavior or catatonia; and (5) negative symptoms (i.e., flattened affect, impoverished thinking, lack of goal-directed behavior).

There are two exceptions to this mandatory "two-symptom rule." The first is a case where a hallucination involves a voice that continually comments on the person's thoughts or behaviors, or where it involves two or more voices talking with each other. The second exception is a case where a delusion can be described as "bizarre." The difference between a bizarre and a nonbizarre delusion involves whether the delusion is physically possible (e.g., "My spouse is unfaithful to me," "I am being followed by organized crime") or physically impossible (e.g., "Aliens are controlling my brain by rays shot through all electric lights," "I am pregnant with the race horse Secretariat"). If either of these two exceptions is present, then only one symptom is required for a diagnosis.

The second criterion requires major dysfunction. For a meaningful portion of time since the onset of the disorder, at least one important area of functioning must be markedly below levels evident prior to the disorder. The definition of "functioning" is broad, including such areas as work, self-care, or relationships. The only exception to this criterion is for a childhood/adolescent onset. In these instances, there only needs to be evidence that the person has not reached expected levels of achievement at school, at work, or in relationships. When both diagnostic criteria are met, then a diagnosis of some disorder can be made.

However, to rule out other disorders, four other criteria must be met. First, there must be continuous signs of disorder for at least 6 months. If not, then a person is usually diagnosed as having a schizophreniform disorder (1–6 months) or a brief psychotic disorder (less than 1 month). Second, the person cannot have had a significant major mood episode (depressive, manic, or mixed) during the same period as the psychotic symptomatology. If such an episode has been present, then a diagnosis of a mood disorder with psychotic features or a schizoaffective disorder is often made. Third, the disturbance must not be due to the direct physiological effects of a substance (e.g., narcotics, medication side effect) or a medical condition (e.g., epilepsy, Cushing's syndrome). In these instances, a diagnosis of a substance-related or substance-induced disorder or a psychotic disorder due to a general medical condition may be made. Fourth, if the person has a preexisting pervasive developmental disorder (e.g., autistic disorder), then additional prominent delusions or hallucinations must also be present. If these criteria are met, then and only then can the diagnosis of schizophrenia be made.

Two additional aspects of schizophrenic symptomatology must also be outlined before one can begin to discuss the role of the family with the disorder. First, the DSM-IV describes four subtypes of the disorder, defined by the predominant symptomatology at the time of the diagnosis ("paranoid," "disorganized," "catatonic," and "undifferentiated"). Although many theorists recognize that these are not different disorders, they are identifiable typologies that can be used to describe many patients (Heinrichs, 1993; Nicholson & Neufeld, 1993). These differences, particularly the difference between paranoid and nonparanoid schizophrenias, have been very useful in research (McGlashan & Fenton, 1991). For example, paranoid schizophrenics have been found to have higher levels of social competence than nonparanoid schizophrenics (Dobson & Neufeld, 1987).

A second aspect of symptomatology is another popular method of subtyping the symptoms: "positive" and "negative" (Crow, 1980). Positive symptoms are those that are in excess of normal functioning (e.g., hallucinations, bizarre behavior), whereas negative symptoms are seen as a loss of functioning (e.g., emotional emptiness, lack of interest in self-care). This subdivision has also been very useful in many respects for both research and clinical work (Harvey & Walker, 1987). Although schizophrenia may be a single disorder, recognizing that there are many possible ways that the disorder can present itself will be useful in understanding the many ways it can affect patients and their families.

THE COSTS OF SCHIZOPHRENIA

Financial Costs

The lifetime prevalence for schizophrenia in the United States is usually estimated to be between 0.5% and 1.0% (American Psychiatric Association, 1994). That is, given a population estimate of 265 million, between 1,325,000 and 2,650,000 people in the United States will have had a diagnosis of schizophrenia, now or in the past. Many more males than females are diagnosed with the disorder, with a male–female ratio of between 1.5:1 and 2:1 (Goldstein, Santangelo, Simpson, & Tsuang, 1990). Schizophrenia also tends to be a chronic disorder; few people who develop it ever escape its diagnosis. As a result, the incidence rate is comparatively low, with only an estimated 1 in 10,000 people being newly diagnosed each year. That is, approximately 26,500 new cases will be diagnosed in the United States this year.

The economic costs of schizophrenia to society have been analyzed several times over the years (e.g., Fein, 1958; McGuire, 1991). In a recent analysis, Wyatt, Henter, Leary, and Taylor (1995) estimated the cost of schizophrenia in the United States at $65 billion per year. This included $18.6 billion in direct costs, such as inpatient hospital care, outpatient care, nursing home care, intermediate/domiciliary care, medication, concomitant drug/alcohol use treatment, supported living (e.g., halfway houses), shelters, crime-related facilities (including jails and prisons), suicide, research, and specialized training for professionals. There were also approximately $46.5 billion in indirect costs, including lost productivity from patients in institutions, lost productivity due to premature mortality from suicide, lost nonmonetary production (e.g., housework), lost productivity from unemployment or decreased work performance, and lost productivity from family caregivers.

The economic costs due to lost productivity by families were estimated by Wyatt et al. (1995) at $7 billion. The family caregivers of schizophrenics are usually parents who take care of their adult children. Wyatt et al. recognized that many of these parents would have gone back to school to upgrade their skills or returned to work when their children left the home. Even those caregivers who are employed are more likely to take time off work to look after actively symptomatic patients. Families also often have to bear many of the direct costs listed above, and their share of these has been estimated at more than $2 billion (Rupp & Keith, 1993).

Family Burden

There are noneconomic but equally important costs of schizophrenia for these families, and these are increasingly being acknowledged by mental health professionals (e.g., Bellack & Mueser, 1993; Vaccaro, Young, & Glynn, 1993). Deinstitutionalization in the United States has resulted in ever-increasing numbers of schizophrenics' needing family support and very often having to live with their parents (Backer & Richardson, 1989). It is estimated that more than 65% of the care given to mentally ill persons in the United States is provided by family members (Lamb, 1984). Often parents and other relatives are involved not out of love or kindness, but out of a sense of duty or responsibility (sometimes even legal responsibility). Many families resent "what appears to be a de facto decision by practitioners and policy makers that families should serve as the major caregiving institution" (Hatfield, Spanoil, & Zipple, 1987, p. 224). The severity and complexity of schizophrenia result in very stressful lives for the families involved (Noh & Turner, 1987). Things become even more difficult for many families as the schizophrenic patients and their caregivers age. A survey done by the California Alliance for the Mentally Ill in the early 1980s reported that the average age of a family caregiver was 59 years (William, Williams, Sommer, & Sommer, 1986).

For severe mental illness, Lefley (1989) has described the highly stressful family burdens as both "objective burdens" related to practical problems (e.g., medical bills) and "subjective burdens" relating to the psychological stress (e.g., reduction or elimination of leisure activities). Many of these are consistent with the chronic burdens experienced by the families of individuals with other chronic disabilities. These burdens include financial strain, disruptions in household activities, altered relationships with other family members and friends, and limited social activities. These stressors are the results of increased attention to a patient and decreased time available for other activities. However, there are many other strains that are specific to severe mental illness. These strains include cycles of symptom exacerbation and remission, failure of patients to develop age-appropriate functioning in many areas, and dealing with the ever-changing mental health care systems. Social barriers are built up against these families because of the stigma against mental patients. In crises, these caregivers may have to deal not only with mental health care providers, but also with emergency services and the police. Moreover, they may have to deal with patients' symptoms and may have to fear for their physical safety during these times. These negative broad stressors affect not only the caregivers but the entire family.

Lefley (1989) has also pointed out that behavioral management is an ongoing source of tension in the families of patients with major mental illness. Families often need to live with unpredictable, abusive, aggressive, or assaultive behaviors. The patients can often run into interpersonal problems with family friends and neighbors. As well, both the positive symptoms (such as paranoia and bizarre behaviors) and the negative symptoms (such as lack of emotional connectedness, poor self-care, and apathy) can be significant unpredictable stressors for a family to cope with on a continuing basis.[1]

THE FAMILY AND THE MENTAL
HEALTH CARE PROVIDERS

With these stressors, one might assume that mental health care providers are sources of relief for families. However, many studies have shown that such care providers constitute another source of stress for the families of schizophrenics (e.g., Holden & Levine, 1982). Kazarian and Vanderheyden (1992) reviewed the literature and developed a summary of the reasons cited for the negative attitudes of families toward mental health care providers. For example, families report that the providers focus on patients' pathology and deficits, and ignore the patients as whole persons. Families also experience a lack of empathy for what they are going through, and a lack of respect for the hard work and effort that they put forth on a daily basis. Moreover, families also believe that the providers are unwilling to educate them, do not give them adequate emotional support, fail to let them participate in treatment planning for the patients, and fail to give them assistance in dealing with the patients on a daily basis. As a result, the family members often feel isolated from both the treatment and the providers. According to Kazarian and Vanderheyden, a major underlying factor for these problems is the perceived tendency to blame the family for the onset and course of the disorder.

There is strong support for the validity of these concerns. Early psychodynamic theories often put the blame for the development of schizophrenia on a patient's mother. For example, Harry Stack Sullivan (1929) believed that an anxious mother passes her anxiety on to her son or daughter. This child then tries to deal with anxiety and develops a fragmented system of the self. Lustful thoughts that develop in teenage years cannot be dealt with in this disorganized system; panic develops, and the system begins to fall apart. Sullivan saw schizophrenia as the result of the system's reorganizing itself to establish meaning.

There have been several other psychoanalytic and psychodynamic

---

[1]The interested reader is referred to the "First Person Accounts" series in the National Institute of Mental Health's journal *Schizophrenia Bulletin*. This regular series is written by patients, ex-patients, and family members to describe for mental health professionals the issues and difficulties they confront. Contributions from the perspectives of several different types of relatives are available (e.g., a spouse in Anonymous, 1994; a sibling in Brown, 1996; a parent in Kagigebi, 1995).

models and studies from a variety of perspectives, and most attribute some factors in the etiology of schizophrenia to the family (Arieti, 1957; Hartmann, 1953; Klein, 1948; Lidz, Cornelison, Fleck, & Terry, 1957). One of the most famous theorists has been Frieda Fromm-Reichman (1948), who coined the phrase "schizophrenogenic mother." This term was used to describe the cause of schizophrenia as a mother whose interpersonal style is so bizarre and negative that the disorder develops as the only way the child can cope with his or her reality. Even while more modern theories of stress and vulnerability were being developed, the phrase continued to be used in them (e.g., Meehl, 1962). It has now often been replaced by the "schizophrenogenic family," which lays the blame on the entire family (Perris, 1989). Even though the view that schizophrenia is a neurological or neurochemical disorder is now widely accepted (Johnson, 1989), this has not eliminated the belief that the family is the cause of the disorder from the minds of many mental health professionals (Backer & Richardson, 1989).

EXPRESSED EMOTION

Development of the Concept

One of the few benefits of the emphasis once placed on the family's role in the development of schizophrenia was research on family interactions and their relation to exacerbations of the disorder. Concepts examined in this research have included "communication deviance," a multidimensional construct pertaining to the clarity of a relative's communications (Wynne & Singer, 1963), and "affective style," a measure of both a relative's verbal and emotional behaviors (Doane, Falloon, Goldstein, & Mintz, 1985). The construct that has engendered the most interest and research, however, has been "expressed emotion" (EE).

Brown, Birley, and Wing (1972) are credited with originating the concept of EE. These authors assessed 101 patients with schizophrenia from two hospitals in England between early 1966 and summer 1968. The assessment included eight types of interviews with patients and the family members with whom they lived (parents, spouses, or siblings). A family member's response was coded not only for what had happened in the home, but also for the relative's feelings about the event. Five areas of emotional response were rated: (1) number of critical comments about someone else in the home, (2) hostility, (3) dissatisfaction, (4) warmth, and (5) emotional overinvolvement (i.e., unusually marked concern about the patient). An overall classification of EE was developed, based on the number of critical comments, marked overinvolvement, and hostility; 45 of the 101 families were described as "high-EE" and the other 56 as "low-EE." The patients were followed up for 9 months to see who would have a significant exacerbation of their symptoms. The authors then compared the 35 relapsing patients with the 66 nonrelapsing patients to learn whether there were differences in the emotional levels of their families.

Brown et al. (1972) found that 58% of the high-EE patients relapsed, compared with a relapse rate of only 16% for the low-EE patients. There was also a significant positive relation between relapses and the number of critical comments, hostility, and parental overinvolvement. There was a curvilinear relation with warmth, in which those with a middle range were less likely to relapse; those who were high in warmth were also high in emotional overinvolvement, whereas those low in warmth were often highly critical. Dissatisfaction was related to relapse in the high-EE group but not in the low-EE group. The relation between EE and relapse was independent of other factors that also affected relapse, such as lack of regular medication or acceptance of admission. Brown et al. concluded that "a high degree of emotion expressed by relatives at the time of key admission was found to be strongly associated with symptomatic relapse during the nine months following discharge" (1972, p. 253).

This study was then replicated by Vaughn and Leff (1976a), but was extended in some important ways. Thirty-seven schizophrenic patients and their families were assessed and followed for 9 months. Vaughn and Leff found high hostility to be consistently present, with high numbers of critical remarks; as a result, ratings of high or low EE were based solely on number of critical comments and emotional overinvolvement. Nonetheless, high EE was related to relapse, and this relation was independent of other social and clinical factors.

A subsequent analysis of this data also led Vaughn and Leff (1981) to conclude that a high-EE relative differs from a low-EE relative in four general response patterns. First, they said, the high-EE relative shows an unwillingness to allow the schizophrenic patient autonomy, becoming highly intrusive into several parts of his or her life. Second, the high-EE relative is more likely to have strong emotional reactions (anger or acute distress) to the patient's behavior. Third, the high-EE relative often views the patient as fully responsible for his or her behavior, and doubts that the schizophrenic has a legitimate illness. Fourth, the high-EE relative has little tolerance for the symptomatic behavior of schizophrenia and expects the patient to behave in a "normal" manner. These conclusions led Vaughn and Leff to suggest that patients' families should be assessed, in order to allow mental health professionals to predict who is "at the greatest risk for relapse and most in need of protective medication and clinical support" (1981, p. 44).

Criticism of the Concept

The concept of EE has been assessed in many studies in the last 20 years. Several reviews of this research have all supported the basic idea that high EE is related to relapse in schizophrenia (Bebbington & Kuipers, 1994b; Lefley, 1992; Kavanagh, 1992; Miklowitz, 1994; Vaughn, 1989). Yet there are problems with the concept, and these have has led to opposition to it from some critics (e.g., Hatfield et al., 1987; Jenkins & Karno, 1992; Kanter, Lamb, & Loeper, 1987). Acknowledging that it has been highly criticized and has many problems, Bellack and Mueser (1993) nonetheless wrote that "rumors of its death are premature and the preponderance of data still supports the construct" (p. 325). It is still important, however, to note what these criticisms are and what has been done about some of them.

Some criticisms of EE are common to research into many other areas of psychopathology. For example, gender differences have been brought up as an area of concern by several authors (e.g., Hogarty, 1985). However, though there has been a preponderance of male schizophrenics with high-EE families, there are also higher numbers of male schizophrenics in many studies (Kavanagh, 1992). A recent reanalysis of data by Bebbington and Kuipers (1994b) from several studies found that although there was a higher relapse rate for male schizophrenics, "EE significantly predicts relapse both in males and females. Moreover, [the statistical analyses] suggest that the association is equally strong in the two sexes" (p. 712). Yet, a recent study by Davis, Goldstein, and Nuechterlein (1996) found that EE did not predict relapse in their sample of female schizophrenics. Davis et al. found that the males were more likely to be harshly criticized than the females, and they believed that this had significant influence on the EE in the family.

Another common criticism in psychopathology research is cultural bias, and this issue has been raised to question the validity and generalizability of EE (e.g., Jenkins & Karno, 1992). Whereas English and U.S. studies usually report high-EE rates between 40% and 60%, other studies from different countries report much lower rates (13% in Scotland, reported by McReadie & Robinson, 1987; 23% in India, reported by Leff et al., 1987). Bebbington and Kuipers (1994b), reviewing the results of several of these studies, agreed that there were differences in some studies in the ratios of high-EE and low-EE relatives. Nonetheless, the relation between EE and relapse was present, regardless of geographic location (Japan in Mino, Inove, Tanaka, & Tsuda, 1997). The few studies that failed to find a relapse were not restricted to any geographic regions. Bebbington and Kuipers concluded that although the expression of emotion may be different in different cultures, the evidence suggests that high EE in any culture is related to relapse in schizophrenia.

A criticism common in many areas of research, not just psychopathology, is the representativeness of the studies' samples. In Lefley's (1992) review of the EE research, she concluded that "throughout the literature there is also a strong suggestion of antecedent differences in patients, including but not limited to current medication status, that may be correlates of relatives' expressed emotion and also predisposing to relapse" (p. 593). Some studies have investigated such possible differences and found that EE continued to be a strong predictor of a relapse (Linszen et al.,

1997). Kavanagh's (1992) review acknowledged that there may be questions about the representativeness of the samples. Nonetheless, he did not believe that factors affecting the sample (e.g., refusal rates for refusal to participate, non-English-speaking patients) did not significantly affect the internal validity of the studies and their overall conclusions. Kavanagh also pointed out, however, that such factors did suggest that "the EE literature is based on a subset of the schizophrenia population" (p. 604).

On the other hand, the EE–relapse effect has been shown not to be unique to families and schizophrenia. A small group of studies has found that the EE level of staff members at a facility where a schizophrenic is living can predict the patient's response to treatment (Ball, Moore, & Kuipers, 1992; Higson & Kavanagh, 1988) and reflect his or her level of symptomatology (Snyder, Wallace, Moe, & Liberman, 1994). As well, most other studies have found that high-EE is related to the successful management of disorders as diverse as major depression (Hooley, Orley, & Teasdale, 1986), bipolar disorder (Priebe, Wildgrube, & Muller-Oerlinghausen, 1989), "mental handicap" (Greedharry, 1987), obesity (Flanagan & Wagner, 1991), and eating disorders (Szmukler, Eisler, Russell, & Dare, 1985). It has also been found to be more likely in families of children referred to a mental health clinic than on a nonclinical comparison group of families (Kershner, Cohen, & Coyne, 1996). Taken together, these studies support the notion that high family EE may not be related to schizophrenia onset or relapse specifically. Instead, it may be a common factor in all psychopathology and perhaps even physical illness (Kuipers, 1992).

One of the recognized specific problems found in EE research is the inherent instability of the EE typology (high vs. low). Although the view that EE type is a stable family characteristic is assumed by many mental health professionals, research has not supported this view (Falloon, 1988; Hatfield et al., 1987; Mintz, Liberman, Miklowitz, & Mintz, 1987). EE has been described, instead, as a "snapshot" of family functioning at the time of the assessment (Smith & Birchwood, 1990). There is also a common pattern to EE typology instability. For example, Goldstein et al. (1989), in a study of EE in 36 families, found that 9 out of 22 high-EE families (41%) became low-EE families at an 8-week follow-up reassessment. However, most of the low-EE families remained low-EE families (11 of 14, or 79%) at the time of the reassessment, and few became high-EE families (3 of 14, or 21%). This pattern of change is not thought to be due to a statistical regression of extreme scores toward the mean because of the inequality of the shifts (Kavanagh, 1992). Although there are several other possibilities, such as measurement error, a reversion of type, or a genuine fluidity in the construct, the exact reason for this pattern is not known (Smith & Birchwood, 1990). Kuipers and Bebbington (1988) have hypothesized three basic family EE patterns. The first pattern is that there are some very high-EE families that have difficulty with any stress, and this group remains high-EE at the reassessment. The second group of families consists of good copers who deal with all problems with little expression of negative emotions, and this group remains low-EE. The third group of families consists of those who are usually low-EE except at times of severe stress (e.g., when a schizophrenic family member is very symptomatic or is hospitalized) at which times they become high-EE families. While this model is likely, given the known relation between stress and schizophrenia, it has yet to be adequately investigated.

The artificial dichotomizing of EE into the high and low categories has also not been investigated to determine its appropriateness (Hatfield et al., 1987; King & Dixon, 1996). Nonetheless, it has been widely accepted as the standard in EE research. There are benefits to the use of categories in mental health work, even when an underlying dimension is recognized. For example, the use of categories increases convenience in the communication between professionals (Meehl & Golden, 1982) and is more consistent with the disease model of much of psychopathology (Klerman, 1989). Several clinicians see the addition of further dimensions in such areas as "unnecessary complexity" (Feighner & Herbstein, 1987). Nonetheless, dimensional models are becoming increasingly important in all areas of psychopathology (Barlow, 1991). For example, dimensions are superior in measuring change and are more efficient in the prediction of patient outcome (Lorr, 1986). They are also less likely to result in a "halo effect"; that is, the behaviors exhibited by a person being categorized are less likely to be seen as a predetermined stereotype (Frances, 1982). It has been argued that the argument between dimensions and categories is actually a political one between psychiatrists on the biological/categorical side and psychologists on the continuum/dimensional side (Blashfield & Livesley, 1991).

There are more than professional political issues at stake, however, in assigning families to either the high-EE or low-EE category. The categorizing (or "labeling") of families as one type or the other can have serious negative effects. Those categorized as high-EE are more likely to be seen as "problem families" or "bad families" by many mental health professionals working with them (Hatfield et al., 1987; Lefley, 1992). This leads to more blaming of such families by the professionals working with the patients. On the other side of the issue, being categorized as low-EE may result in less emphasis being placed on the needs of such families, compared with those of high-EE families (Kuipers & Bebbington, 1988; Smith & Birchwood, 1990). It has been suggested that some low-EE families tend to use distancing and disengagement as strategies to cope with a schizophrenic relative, and that this tends to support negative symptoms, such as social withdrawal and poor social adjustment (Birchwood & Smith, 1987). Such families may also be willing to accept more significant levels of psychopathology (which may need to be addressed by mental health professionals), may not express appropriate levels of anger or control, may not set appropriate limits on a patient's behavior, may experience more apathy toward a patient, and may feel more pressure to keep a patient out of the hospital (Hatfield et al., 1987). The factor causing a family to fall into one of these two categories may only be one comment said or unsaid during the assessment interview, which puts its score either above or below a cutoff level. The problems of families' being described as either high-EE or low-EE are too important to be left undiscussed because of political disagreements between professional groups.

The major problem with the EE research, however, has been the interpretation of the correlation between high EE and relapse. In their original EE research study, Brown et al. (1972) wrote that they "cannot specify the direction of cause and effect, but the fact that a decrease in expressed emotion at follow-up accompanies an improvement in the patients' behaviour strongly suggests that there is a two-way relationship" (p. 255). They also wrote that they were "unable to comment on claims that factors in the relatives' personality and handling of the patient as a child cause the first onset of the illness, except to say that the fact that expressed emotion acts as strongly in marital partners as in parents argues for a reactive rather than a causal model" (p. 255). Nonetheless, many mental health professionals have taken the existence of the relation between high EE and relapse as evidence supporting schizophrenia as the result of a negative upbringing or a hostile family environment. For example, in a discussion of the stress–schizophrenia relation for the *Annual Review of Psychology,* Fowles (1992) argues that EE research lends itself to the interpretation that an exacerbation of symptomatology for a schizophrenic is the result of a family's high EE and that the relation does not go in the other direction. Other authors, however, have argued that the relation between family EE and relapse is interactive (Greenley, 1986; Koenigsberg & Handley, 1986). Some have even gone to the extent of developing theoretical models with feedback loops for the relations between stress in the family environment and symptomatology in schizophrenia (e.g., Ciompi, 1989; Kavanagh, 1992).

Considerable research does support an interactive view of the relation between family EE and relapse. For example, most of the recent research on symptomatology levels and EE status has suggested interaction between the two (e.g., Glynn et al., 1990; Mavreas, Tomaras, Karydi, Economou, & Stefanis, 1992). As well, there is evidence suggesting that EE level is related to the level of burden on relatives resulting from the patients' disorder (Jackson, Smith, & McGorry, 1990; Scazufca & Kuipers, 1996). EE also has not been shown to predict relapse in patients at the time of their initial diagnosis, but only after they have had significant time to be with their families (Stirling et al., 1991). Likewise, a "poorer illness course" has been seen as possibly causing high EE (Parker, Johnston, & Hayward, 1988), as has a greater tendency toward odd and disruptive behavior by patients when recently discharged (Rosenfarb, Goldstein, Mintz, & Nuechterlein, 1995; Woo, Goldstein, & Nuechterlein, 1997). Taken together, these and similar studies have led most researchers and theorists to conclude that EE reflects the families' methods of coping with the stress caused by the patients' schizophrenia.

The Relation between EE and Stress

The relation between EE and stress is quite complex, as is the link between stress and schizophrenia. Although there is evidence that the stress caused by a patient's schizophrenia is reflected by increases in EE, it has been widely hypothesized that high EE is also a stressor for schizophrenics (e.g., Hans & Marcus, 1987; Nuechterlein, 1987). There are several models for the relation between stress and vulnerability to schizophrenia. The first major article on the topic, by Zubin and Spring (1977), attempted to synthesize a number of models from several different areas of research. Their eventual model "proposed that each of us is endowed with a degree of vulnerability that under suitable circumstances will express itself in an episode of schizophrenia" (p. 109). The vulnerability level results from a genetic endowment that is then influenced early in life by major life events and biological circumstances. The vulnerability level results in a "tolerance threshold" for each individual. If a person's stress is below the threshold, than the individual can absorb the stress. If it is above the threshold, however, than an episode of schizophrenia will develop. This model has had a major impact on research and theorizing since it was first developed.

Although the Zubin and Spring model has significant strengths, many questions and criticisms have been raised (Nicholson & Neufeld, 1989). For example, does symptomatology result in additional stress on the schizophrenic patient (either directly or indirectly)? Do the patient's coping mechanisms affect the stress and the vulnerability, and, if so, what is the mechanism? Because of these and other concerns, we (Nicholson & Neufeld, 1992) have developed the "dynamic vulnerability perspective" for understanding the relation between stress and schizophrenia (see Figure 12.1). This model emphasizes the dynamic and interactional perspective on the relations among stress, symptomatology, and vulnerability. A patient's abilities to appraise stressful situations accurately and to cope adequately with the stressors are also part of the dynamic vulnerability perspective; both affect and are affected by both the stressors and the symptoms. Also, this perspective proposes not only that the symptomatology can result in stress (e.g., the stress from a family's strong emotional reactions to a significant increase in a patient's bizarre behavior), but that a stressor can result in an increase in symptomatology. Formal quantitative models based on the dynamic vulnerability perspective have been developed to show the significant, repetitive mutual escalation of these interactive components (Neufeld & Nicholson, 1991). The dynamic vulnerability perspective has also been used to describe the effects of family interventions in schizophrenia as having their influence on both stressors and coping skills (Yank, Bentley, & Hargrove, 1993).

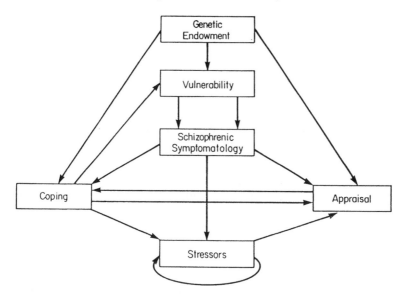

FIGURE 12.1. The dynamic vulnerability perspective of the relation between stress and schizophrenia. From Nicholson and Neufeld (1992). Copyright 1992 by American Orthopsychiatric Association. Reprinted by permission.

Some of the strongest evidence for a relation between high EE and stress in schizophrenics is the psychophysiological arousal research by Tarrier and colleagues. Tarrier, Vaughn, Lader, and Leff (1979) compared the nonspecific skin conductance responses (a measure of general psychophysiological arousal) of remitted schizophrenics who were living in the community in two conditions. First, each patient was measured while interacting with a neutral person (the experimenter) for 15 minutes. A second 15-minute measurement was then taken while the patient was interacting with a key relative. The responses suggested that arousal was higher during interaction with the family member than during interaction with the experimenter. The patients with high-EE families also had higher arousal levels than the patients with low-EE families. Sturgeon, Turpin, Kuipers, Berkowitz, and Leff (1984) used the same strategy to assess schizophrenics while hospitalized. They found that in these circumstances, the schizophrenics with high-EE families had consistently higher arousal levels, even when talking to the experimenter. Tarrier (1991a) assessed patients from families that changed from high-EE (while symptomatic) to low-EE when assessed at a 9-month follow-up. The results suggested that when this change occurred, there was a concomitant change in schizophrenics' arousal in the presence of a relative. Tarrier and Barrowclough (1989) found that those patients who relapsed had higher arousal in the presence of a relative than did those who failed to relapse in 9 months. Taken together, these and other similar studies have been interpreted as showing links among symptomatology levels, stress, arousal, and EE (Tarrier & Turpin, 1992).

FAMILY INTERVENTIONS

If there is one primary benefit to the EE research, it has been the increased emphasis on family interventions with schizophrenics. Dozens of studies have been conducted (with various levels of methodological rigor) in the last 20 years on the efficacy of different forms of family interventions and family psychoeducational programs, with effects on relapse lasting at least 8 years (Tarrier, Barrowclough, Porceddu, & Fitzpatrick, 1994). Several guides and handbooks for mental health professionals outline programs with documented efficacy (e.g., Anderson, Reiss, & Hogarty, 1986; Falloon, Boyd, & McGill, 1984). There have also been many reviews of the research, which have generally reached the same conclusion: "There is an impressive body of evidence suggesting that family interventions are efficacious at delaying if not preventing relapse for persons with schizophrenia who have significant family contact" (Dixon & Lehman, 1995, p. 641). These studies have also shown that the average per-patient treatment costs decrease significantly after the addition of these family interventions (e.g., Tarrier, Lownson, & Barrowclough, 1991). Yet, except for a lack of research support for the benefits of stand-alone family psychoeducation (Kazarian & Vanderheyden, 1992; Lam, 1991), there is no evidence for any differential benefits between forms of family intervention (Schooler, Keith, Severe, & Matthews, 1995).

Common Components of Interventions and Mechanisms of Effectiveness

Because of the repeatedly demonstrated efficacy of different forms of family interventions, several reviews have looked for the common components of these programs (Bellack & Muesser, 1993; Dixon & Lehman, 1995; Lam, 1991; Leff, 1994a; Mari & Streiner, 1994; Penn & Mueser, 1996; Schooler et al., 1995; Vaccaro et al., 1993). Although no two of these reviews have decided upon a consistent listing of the important components that are similar across studies, five elements have been mentioned in most if not all of the reviews:

1. *Family psychoeducation.* Though it is generally agreed that family psychoeducation programs are not sufficient for change, they are listed in several reviews as necessary for change to occur. Common to psychoeducation programs is information related to diagnosis, symptomatology, etiological theories, course, treatment, and management issues. Less common to these programs is information relating to premorbid functioning,

early signs of the disorder, epidemiology, community resources, and legal issues (Kazarian & Vanderheyden, 1992). One of the most important effects of this education is the lowering of family members' expectations of what they can expect from the patients to more realistic levels (Leff, 1994b).

2. *Family members as part of the treatment team.* Several authors have pointed out that when family members learn what can be expected of them and how they can help patients, they become an important part of treatment teams. According to some authors, giving families the sense that they are not alone in their struggle with their schizophrenic relatives, and giving them the sense that they are understood, may be the most important effects of these treatment strategies (Hatfield et al., 1987).

3. *Changes in family functioning.* Beyond the effects on families of these earlier elements, interventions aimed specifically at family functioning are usually incorporated into the programs. These interventions can include addressing within-family communication styles and changing patterns of household EE. In many interventions, the primary aim is the lowering of family EE.

4. *Cognitive-behavioral orientation.* Although the language and the focus of the interventions may differ between studies, the use of an orientation with an emphasis on behavioral and cognitive strategies is common. These interventions share such aims as focusing on the here and now, focusing on practical and behavioral goals, teaching problem-solving skills, providing social skills training, and employing both cognitive restructuring techniques and behavioral techniques.

5. *Medication compliance.* Improved medication compliance is sometimes a secondary product of the other elements, but it is often a focus of particular importance in family interventions, and special emphasis is placed on this issue throughout all aspects of the interventions. The evidence shows that medication compliance is the necessary foundation upon which all the rest of treatment appears to depend; without it, the remaining interventions are of little practical efficacy (Breslin, 1992; Falloon, 1992).

When these five components of psychosocial family interventions are embedded in a comprehensive psychiatric rehabilitation program, they have consistently been effective in reducing the relapse of schizophrenia (Vaccaro et al., 1993). Possible mechanisms by which the relapse reductions have been achieved in the family interventions have been proposed in several recent reviews (Bellack & Mueser, 1993; Dixon & Lehman, 1995; Liberman, 1994; Mari & Streiner, 1994). Four types of mechanisms have been described in these and other reviews:

1. *Decrease in family EE.* Since high EE has been the target of several studies, the reduction of the "emotional temperature" (Liberman, 1994) of a stressful family environment has often been taken as an indicator of a successful intervention (e.g., Leff et al., 1990).

2. *Increase in the families' quality of life.* Recent studies have suggested that relapse may be lessened because the families' quality of life has been enhanced. For example, Falloon and Pederson (1985) found that their family intervention resulted in reductions in family distress, less subjective burden in the families, fewer disruptions in activities, and possibly fewer physical and mental health problems.

3. *Increased medication compliance.* Another possible reason for decreased relapse is the enhanced compliance with medications found in some studies. For example, Hogarty et al. (1986) found that 77% of schizophrenics in family interventions were compliant with their medication, whereas only 43% of the control schizophrenics were compliant. Though their analysis showed that there were treatment effects beyond medication compliance, there was a significant effect of compliance.

4. *Increased attention from the treatment team.* Lam (1991) hypothesized that another mechanism having an effect on relapse was an increase in the amount or quality of treatment team contact. Some studies have indicated an increase in the number of sessions patients and families have with the team because of the family therapy. It is also possible that the increase in family–team alliance permits both to "intervene more promptly or frequently at an earlier stage before a full-blown relapse [has] set in" (Lam, 1991, p. 434). More recent studies may have attempted to keep contact between the treatment teams and the families similar for the treatment and control groups, but research has not addressed the quality of the relation. Since enhancing this relation has been a focus for many treatment programs, it is likely that some of the effect on reduced relapse is due to this factor. Although the differential impact of this and the other factors has not been assessed, it is likely that all four factors are involved to some degree in the decreased relapse rates.

It is important to point out the one form of family intervention that has *not* been successful in decreasing relapse in schizophrenia. Psychodynamic interventions have been described in two studies, and neither intervention was shown to be more effective than standard care (Köttgen, Sonnichsen, Mollenhauser, & Jurth, 1984; McFarlane, 1994). Although there continues to be theorizing on the psychoanalytic models for psychological interventions with the families of schizophrenics (Alanen, 1994), the available evidence supports the view that this is one form of treatment that does not have any additional benefit for patients and their families (Dixon & Lehman, 1995; Leff, 1994b).

Criticism of Family Interventions

Even with this consistent success, there are important criticisms about the reliability and validity of these research studies. The criticisms tend to fall into two general categories. First, there are concerns about the generalizability of the results. Several authors have pointed out that one criterion for acceptance of a family into many of these treatment groups has been that the family must be high-EE. As a result, it is questionable whether the results can be generalized to low-EE families (Kuipers & Bebbington, 1988; Lam, 1991). Some more recent studies have worked at including low-EE families and tend to report similar results as long as there are similar levels of contact between patients and their families (Dixon & Lehman, 1995). There is even some evidence that the addition of a family intervention to a low-EE family may actually increase relapse by increasing family stress (Linszen et al., 1996). It is still unsure, however, whether the best approaches for these two groups of families are the same or different (e.g., McFarlane et al., 1995). To avoid the problem of high-EE versus low-EE families, Leff (1994b) developed a set of four guidelines for identifying the families in greatest need of intervention: (1) There are frequent arguments in families that lead to some type of verbal or physical violence; (2) families often call the police; (3) patients are on maintenance dosages of medication but relapse at a frequency of more than once a year; and (4) families frequently contact the hospital staff for either reassurance or information. Leff has argued that when these guidelines are used, measuring EE is not necessary. Nonetheless, as highlighted by Breslin (1992), only compliant families are included in these studies, regardless of EE level. Moreover, many patients either do not live with their families or have little contact with them. Thus, these findings are encouraging, but their interpretation must be tempered by the possible lack of widespread generalizability.

Second, there are concerns about the lack across different studies of a clear, acceptable definition of "relapse" in schizophrenia (Mari & Streiner, 1994). Most definitions have included a recurrence of symptoms in patients who had previously become symptom-free, or a significant exacerbation of low-level initial symptomatology (e.g., both of these criteria were used in Hogarty et al., 1991). Different studies have used change in symptom level, but with one of several different possible time frames (e.g., 1 week in Falloon et al., 1982; 3 weeks in Hogarty et al., 1986). Relapse has also been defined as a change in how a patient is managed, such as rehospitalization or substantial medication changes (e.g., Goldstein, Rodnick, Evans, May, & Steinberg, 1978). Studies have often employed a variety of different criteria, and a schizophrenic patient has been defined as having relapsed if he or she has met any one of them. Furthermore, many investigators assess a number of other variables as well, but there is no consistency in what else is assessed (e.g., disruption in family activities in Falloon & Pederson, 1985; family cohesiveness in Mills & Hansen, 1991; level of EE in Leff et al., 1990). With no standard reference for outcome assessment, studies cannot often be compared with one another, and the extent to which specific results have been replicated is thus unclear.

AREAS FOR FUTURE RESEARCH

As the reviews of the EE research and the family intervention research have both suggested, some general findings are well replicated. However, other areas have been underinvestigated. First, there are questions about how to assess EE. The standard measure is the Camberwell Family Interview (CFI; Vaughn & Leff, 1976b). The CFI is a semistructured interview that is conducted with individual key relatives without the patient present. Each relative is asked by a neutral, nonjudgmental interviewer about the patient's history and symptoms, as well as his or her relationship with the patient. The interview is taped and later scored by a trained EE rater. Several studies have reported strong reliability for these ratings, along with good validity when all key relatives are assessed.

While accepting that the CFI has been supported in several studies, Kazarian (1992) has pointed out three problems with the measure. First, the use of nonvocal aspects of speech in the ratings has been criticized. Second, the CFI interviews are very time-consuming, with the interview for each family member lasting between 30 and 60 minutes and an even greater amount of time required for the rating of each separate interview. Third, the interviewers and raters require several months of training to achieve the necessary reliability and validity. In Kazarian's opinion, these administrative shortcomings of the CFI limit its widespread clinical application.

As a result of these problems, several alternative measures have been developed to assess EE (Kazarian, 1992). For example, the Five Minute Speech Sample (Magana et al., 1986) has been increasingly employed in recent years. In this measure, a key relative is instructed to speak about the patient for 5 minutes. The speech is then sampled and coded via a system similar to that of the CFI. There has been support for the use of this measure as a brief screening device (Malla, Kazarian, Barnes, & Cole, 1991). Another measure specific to EE has been the Level of Expressed Emotion Scale (Cole & Kazarian, 1988). This scale consists of 60 questions developed to assess the various important aspects of EE. It has also been shown to have good reliability and validity in schizophrenic samples (Cole & Kazarian, 1993; Kazarian, Malla, Cole, & Baker, 1990). Questionnaires aimed at a patient's views of family EE may become more important, as one study found that patients' *perceptions* of criticism were more predictive of their outcome at 1 year than relatives' EE as assessed through a speech sample (Tompson et al., 1995). It is for these reasons, among others, that the measurement of EE is seen as an important area for future research (Kavanagh, 1992).

Another important area for future research is determining the important aspects of therapy. Penn and Mueser (1996) have described the quest for these as the search "to establish criteria for the minimum amount of treatment" (p. 612) for which one can reasonably expect a treatment response. There have been some important findings in recent years. For example, many investigators now see 9 months of treatment to be all that is necessary for reducing the number of critical comments, whereas reducing overinvolvement may require 2 years of treatment (Leff et al., 1990). Recent research also suggests that multiple-family interventions may be more effective than single-family interventions, particularly for high-EE families (McFarlane et al., 1995). Moreover, better results may be obtained when the patients are involved in some portion of the family interventions (Vaughan et al., 1992). There is no evidence, however, about whether treatment is best delivered in the clinic or in the family home (Randolph et al., 1994). It has also been suggested that treatments are only effective because they give the family the message that *under no circumstances should the patient be hospitalized,* and this results in higher family burden but lower relapse (Hatfield et al., 1987). Despite these and other similar initial findings and questions, there needs to be much more research on what the most cost-efficient methods of delivering treatment are and how they have their effects.

Related to these research issues is the question of who are the best families to have in which therapy. For example, there is now some evidence that even low-EE families can benefit from some interventions (Randolph et al., 1994). However, psychoeducation has also found to be more necessary among high-EE families than among low-EE families, who are likely to have a greater knowledge of schizophrenia (Cozolino, Goldstein, Nuechterlein, West, & Snyder, 1988). Research also supports greater effects if patients are young and have a shorter treatment history (Lam, 1991). It has been pointed out that if a patient is experiencing an acute exacerbation of his or her symptoms, then the family will be more likely to become involved (Tarrier, 1991b). Solomon, Draine, Mannion, and Meisel (1996) found that families who have less exposure to and support from other families of patients with severe mental disorders are more likely to show an increase in their sense of self-efficacy after group psychoeducation than after an individualized consultation.

Symptomatic differences among patients may also have an impact on the best choice of family intervention. The problem of negative symptoms has usually been ignored in research on symptom relapse (Lefley, 1992). Since these symptoms are not as "psychotic"-like, family members may be likely to ascribe them to a patient's personal qualities rather than to the disorder (Harrison & Dadds, 1992). Although there is some limited evidence that changes in these symptoms are possible through psychoeducation (Goldman & Quinn, 1988), it is unclear whether family interventions can have any impact on future changes in these symptoms or the families' attributions toward them. Some research shows that the EE reactions of families differ according to the patients' symptoms. Ivanovic, Vuletic, and Bebbington (1994) reported that the families of paranoid schizophrenics were more likely to be critical toward the patients, whereas the families of disorganized schizophrenics were more likely to be overinvolved with the patients. As this brief overview indicates, there are several differences between families and among patients that can have an effect on the family–patient relationship. There is little research, however, on how these differences may relate to the question of which family interventions would be the most effective.

Several questions relating to low-EE families also remain to be answered. It is unclear by what mechanism low EE has its effect on patients' relapse rates. Does low EE have a protective effect on the patient (Mintz et al., 1987), or does it reflect high unexpressed emotions (Hatfield et al., 1987)? Should the high-EE response by families be considered the norm for this type of situation, as suggested by some reviewers? If this is the case, then have low-EE families developed a strategy of distancing themselves from the patients that serves to isolate the patients, reinforcing negative symptoms (Smith & Birchwood, 1990)? Or, as suggested by other reviewers, does a low-EE family response reflect strong coping, and should low-EE families be studied to determine why they have not developed into high-EE families (Kavanagh, 1992)? Does increasing patients' contact with low-EE families protect them against relapse (Bebbington & Kuipers, 1994a)? In any case, the low-EE family is not as well understood or investigated as the high-EE family, and this leaves some aspects of our understanding of high EE lacking.

Another possible area for future research is the effect of "family" interventions on "nonfamilies." As pointed out earlier, several studies have suggested that a schizophrenic who lives at a treatment facility responds to the staff at the facility in much the same way that he or she would respond to family members. Therefore, if the patient's relations with his or her family can be changed by psychosocial interventions, it would be appropriate to attempt changes in the patient's relations with staff members by these same techniques.

Much of the family intervention research is not strictly embedded in theoretical models as to why the interventions have the effects that they do on patients' relapse rates. As Yank et al. (1993) have pointed out, placing these interventions into a theoretical perspective gives us a better understanding of the reasons for their effects. Models such as the dynamic vulnerability perspective (Nicholson & Neufeld, 1992) enables us to predict the effects of these treatments (cf. Neufeld & Nicholson, 1991). For example, if an intervention is aimed at teaching coping skills, is there a change in coping skills and relapse, as well as concomitant changes in appraisal and stress? The intervention could be then assessed to determine why its effects occur (e.g., stress reduction, coping mechanism alterations, changes in appraisal techniques).

Finally, one possible area of treatment that has not been widely investigated has been the use of respite care for the families of schizophrenic patients. Geiser, Hoche, and King (1988) studied the effects of respite care on 14 patients with serious mental disorders, 12 of whom were schizophrenics. The patients were allowed brief admissions, 2–7 days in length, at intervals of approximately 6–8 weeks. With each patient serving as his or her own control, it was found that there was a drop from a prerespite program level of 1,240 days in the hospital to 615 days afterwards (380 planned respite days and 235 crisis/unplanned days). The mean number of hospital days dropped significantly, from 88.6 days per patient to 43.9 days. The number of days dropped for 13 of the 14 patients. Only 6 of the 14 patients had crisis/unplanned hospitalizations while in the program. Subjective family data showed that family members were pleased with the program and the rest it allowed them and the patients. In addition to giving the families and the patients time away from one another, the program was also found to increase the integration of the patients' families with the staff and to increase the staff's positive, supportive relationship with the families. The potential benefits of this type of program for families and patients, as well as the effects on relapse, support increased investigation of respite care.

CONCLUSION

This chapter has attempted to define schizophrenia and to outline the relation between the disorder and the patient's family. The psychodynamic theories have not stood the test of time, unlike theories based on more modern stress research, which are now more common. Research now supports the model that many families react to patients with schizophrenia and the symptoms they display in a manner that exacerbates the disorder (high EE). Many forms of family psychosocial interventions have been developed since this discovery, and they have repeatedly shown effectiveness in lowering the relapse rates for this chronic disorder. Although both the high-EE model and the family intervention research have been criticized for various reasons, the general findings are consistently obtained across studies. Future research in several areas may help to clarify these findings and to overcome these criticisms.

REFERENCES

Alanen, Y. O. (1994). An attempt to integrate the individual-psychological and interactional concepts of the origins of schizophrenia. *British Journal of Psychiatry, 164*(Suppl. 23), 56–61.
American Psychiatric Association. (1980). *Diagnostic and statistical manual of mental disorders* (3rd ed.). Washington, DC: Author.
American Psychiatric Association. (1994). *Diagnostic and statistical manual of mental disorders* (4th ed.). Washington, DC: Author.
Anderson, C. M., Reiss, D. J., & Hogarty, G. E. (1986). *Schizophrenia and the*

family: A practitioner's guide to psychoeducation and management. New York: Guilford Press.

Andreasen, N. C. (1989). The American concept of schizophrenia. *Schizophrenia Bulletin, 15,* 519–531.

Anonymous. (1994). First person account: Life with a mentally ill spouse. *Schizophrenia Bulletin, 20,* 227–229.

Arieti, S. (1957). The two aspects of schizophrenia. *Psychiatric Quarterly, 31,* 403–416.

Backer, T. E., & Richardson, D. (1989). Building bridges: Psychologists and families of the mentally ill. *American Psychologist, 44,* 546–550.

Ball, R. A., Moore, E., & Kuipers, L. (1992). EE in community care facilities: A comparison of patient outcome in a 9 month follow-up of two residential hostels. *Social Psychiatry and Psychiatric Epidemiology, 27,* 35–39.

Barlow, D. H. (Ed.). (1991). Diagnosis, dimensions, and DSM-IV: The science of classification [Special issue]. *Journal of Abnormal Psychology, 100,* 243–412.

Bebbington, P., & Kuipers, L. (1994a). The clinical utility of expressed emotion in schizophrenia. *Acta Psychiatrica Scandinavica, 89*(Suppl. 382), 46–53.

Bebbington, P., & Kuipers, L. (1994b). The predictive utility of expressed emotion in schizophrenia: An aggregate analysis. *Psychological Medicine, 24,* 707–718.

Bellack, A. S., & Mueser, K. T. (1993). Psychosocial treatment for schizophrenia. *Schizophrenia Bulletin, 19,* 317–326.

Birchwood, M. J., & Smith, J. (1987). Expressed emotion and first episodes of schizophrenia. *British Journal of Psychiatry, 152,* 859–860.

Blashfield, R. K., & Livesley, W. J. (1991). Metaphorical analysis of psychiatric classification as a psychological test. *Journal of Abnormal Psychology, 100,* 262–270.

Bleuler, E. (1950). *Dementia praecox or the group of schizophrenias* (J. Zinker, Trans.). New York: International Universities Press. (Original work published 1911)

Breslin, N. A. (1992). Treatment of schizophrenia: Current practice and future promise. *Hospital and Community Psychiatry, 43,* 877–886.

Brown, G. P. (1996). First person account: Paranoid schizophrenia—A sibling's story. *Schizophrenia Bulletin, 22,* 557–561.

Brown, G. W., Birley, J. L. T., & Wing, J. K. (1972). Influence of family life on the course of schizophrenic disorders: A replication. *British Journal of Psychiatry, 121,* 241–258.

Ciompi, L. (1989). The dynamics of complex biological-psychosocial systems: Four fundamental psychobiological mediators in the long-term evolution of schizophrenia. *British Journal of Psychiatry, 155*(Suppl. 5), 15–21.

Cole, J. D., & Kazarian, S. S. (1988). The Level of Expressed Emotion Scale: A new measure of expressed emotion. *Journal of Clinical Psychology, 44,* 392–397.

Cole, J. D., & Kazarian, S. S. (1993). Predictive validity of the Level of Expressed Emotion (LEE) Scale: Readmission follow-up data for 1, 2, and 5-year periods. *Journal of Clinical Psychology, 49,* 216–218.

Cozolino, L. J., Goldstein, M. J., Nuechterlein, K. H., West, K. L., & Snyder, K. S. (1988). The impact of education about schizophrenia on relatives varying in expressed emotion. *Schizophrenia Bulletin, 14,* 675–687.

Cromwell, R. L. (1975). Assessment of schizophrenia. *Annual Review of Psychology, 26,* 593–619.

Crow, T. J. (1980). Molecular pathology: More than one disease process? *British Medical Journal, 280,* 66–68.

Davis, J. A., Goldstein, M. J., & Nuechterlein, K. H. (1996). Gender differences in family attitudes about schizophrenia. *Psychological Medicine, 26,* 689–696.

Dixon, L. B., & Lehman, A. F. (1995). Family interventions for schizophrenia. *Schizophrenia Bulletin, 21,* 631–643.

Doane, J. A., Falloon, I. R. H., Goldstein, M. J., & Mintz, J. (1985). Parental affective style and the treatment of schizophrenia. *Archives of General Psychiatry, 42,* 34–42.

Dobson, D. J. G., & Neufeld, R. W. J. (1987). Association of social competence with episodic vs. remitted status in paranoid and nonparanoid schizophrenics. *Canadian Journal of Behavioural Science, 19,* 67–73.

Doran, A. R., Brier, A., & Roy, A. (1986). Differential diagnosis and diagnostic systems in schizophrenia. *Psychiatric Clinics of North America, 9,* 17–33.

Falloon, I. R. H. (1988). Expressed emotion: Current status. *Psychological Medicine, 18,* 269–274.

Falloon, I. R. H. (1992). Psychotherapy of schizophrenia. *British Journal of Hospital Medicine, 48,* 164–170.

Falloon, I. R. H., Boyd, J. L., & McGill, C. W. (1984). *Family care of schizophrenia: A problem-solving approach to the treatment of mental illness.* New York: Guilford Press.

Falloon, I. R. H., Boyd, J. L., McGill, C. W., Razani, J., Moss, H. B., & Gilderman, A. M. (1982). Family management in the prevention of exacerbations of schizophrenia: A controlled study. *New England Journal of Medicine, 306,* 1437–1440.

Falloon, I. R. H., & Pederson, J. (1985). Family management in the prevention of morbidity of schizophrenia: The adjustment of the family unit. *British Journal of Psychiatry, 147,* 156–163.

Feighner, J. P. . & Herbstein, J. (1987). Diagnostic validity. In C. G. Last & M. Hersen (Eds.), *Issues in diagnostic research* (pp. 121–140). New York: Plenum Press.

Fein, R. (1958). *Economics of mental illness.* New York: Basic Books.

Flanagan, D. A., & Wagner, H. L. (1991). Expressed emotion and panic–fear in the prediction of diet treatment compliance. *British Journal of Clinical Psychology, 30,* 231–240.

Fowles, D. C. (1992). Schizophrenia: Diathesis-stress revisited. *Annual Review of Psychology, 43,* 303–336.

Frances, A. J. (1982). Categorical and dimensional systems of personality diagnosis: A comparison. *Comprehensive Psychiatry, 23,* 516–527.

Fromm-Reichmann, F. (1948). Notes on the development of treatment of schizophrenics by psychoanalytic psychotherapy. *Psychiatry, 11,* 263–273.

Geiser, R., Hoche, L., & King, J. (1988). Respite care for mentally ill patients and their families. *Hospital and Community Psychiatry, 39,* 291–295.

Glynn, S. M., Randolph, E. T., Eth, S., Paz, G. G., Leong, G. B., Shaner, A. L., & Strachan, A. (1990). Patient psychopathology and expressed emotion in schizophrenia. *British Journal of Psychiatry, 157,* 877–880.

Goldman, C. R., & Quinn, F. L. (1988). Effects of a patient education program in the treatment of schizophrenia. *Hospital and Community Psychiatry, 39,* 282–286.

Goldstein, J. M., Miklowitz, D. J., Strachan, A. M., Doane, J. A., Nuechterlein, K. H., & Feingold, D. (1989). Patterns of expressed emotion and patient coping styles that characterise the families of recent onset schizophrenics. *British Journal of Psychiatry, 155*(Suppl. 5), 107–111.

Goldstein, J. M., Rodnick, E. H., Evans, J. R., May, P. R. A., & Steinberg, M. R. (1978). Drug and family therapy in aftercare of acute schizophrenics. *Archives of General Psychiatry, 35,* 1169–1177.

Goldstein, J. M., Santangelo, S. L., Simpson, J. C., & Tsuang, M. T. (1990). The role of gender in identifying subtypes of schizophrenia: A latent class analytic approach. *Schizophrenia Bulletin, 16,* 263–275.

Greedharry, D. (1987). Expressed emotion in the families of the mentally handicapped: A pilot study. *British Journal of Psychiatry, 150,* 400–402.

Greenley, J. R. (1986). Social control and expressed emotion. *Journal of Nervous and Mental Disease, 174,* 24–30.

Hans, S., & Marcus, J. (1987). A process model for the development of schizophrenia. *Psychiatry, 50,* 361–370.

Harrison, C. A., & Dadds, M. R. (1992). Attributions of symptomatology: An exploration of family factors associated with expressed emotion. *Australian and New Zealand Journal of Psychiatry, 26,* 408–416.

Hartmann, H. (1953). Contributions to the metapsychology of schizophrenia. *Psychoanalytic Study of the Child, 8,* 177–198.

Harvey, P. D., & Walker, E. E. (1987). *Positive and negative symptoms in psychosis: Description, research, and future directions.* Hillsdale, NJ: Erlbaum.

Hatfield, A. B., Spanoil, L., & Zipple, A. M. (1987). Expressed emotion: A family perspective. *Schizophrenia Bulletin, 13,* 221–226.

Heinrichs, R. W. (1993). Schizophrenia and the brain: Conditions for a neuropsychology of madness. *American Psychologist, 48,* 221–233.

Higson, M., & Kavanagh, D. J. (1988). A hostel-based psychoeducational intervention for schizophrenia: Programme development and preliminary findings. *Behaviour Change, 5,* 85–89.

Hogarty, G. E. (1985). Expressed emotion and schizophrenia relapse: Implications from the Pittsburgh study. In M. Alpert (Ed.), *Controversies in schizophrenia* (pp. 354–365). New York: Guilford Press.

Hogarty, G. E., Anderson, C. M., Reiss, D. J., Kornblith, S. J., Greenwald, D. P., Javna, C. D., Madonia, M. J., & the Environmental/Personal Indicators in the Course of Schizophrenia Research Group. (1986). Family psychoeducation, social skills training, and maintenance chemotherapy in the aftercare treatment of schizophrenia: I. One-year effects of a controlled study on relapse and expressed emotion. *Archives of General Psychiatry, 43,* 633–642.

Hogarty, G. E., Anderson, C. M., Reiss, D. J., Kornblith, S. J., Greenwald, D. P., Ulrich, R. F., Carter, M., & the Environmental/Personal Indicators in the Course of Schizophrenia Research Group. (1991). Family psychoeducation, social skills training, and maintenance chemotherapy in the aftercare treatment of schizophrenia: II. Two-year effects of a controlled study on relapse and adjustment. *Archives of General Psychiatry, 48,* 340–347.

Holden, D. F., & Levine, R. R. J. (1982). How families evaluate mental health professionals, resources, and effects of illness. *Schizophrenia Bulletin, 8,* 626–633.

Hooley, J. M., Orley, J., & Teasdale, J. (1986). Levels of expressed emotion and relapse in depressed patients. *British Journal of Psychiatry, 148,* 642–647.

Ivanovic, M., Vuletic, Z., & Bebbington, P. (1994). Expressed emotion in the families of patients with schizophrenia and its influence on the course of illness. *Social Psychiatry and Psychiatric Epidemiology, 29,* 61–65.

Jackson, H. J., Smith, N., & McGorry, P. (1990). Relationship between expressed emotion and family burden in psychotic disorders: An exploratory study. *Acta Psychiatrica Scandinavica, 82,* 243–249.

Jenkins, J. H., & Karno, M. (1992). The meaning of expressed emotion: Theoretical issues raised by cross-cultural research. *American Journal of Psychiatry, 149,* 9–21.

Johnson, D. L. (1989). Schizophrenia as a brain disease: Implications for psychologists and families. *American Psychologist, 44,* 553–555.

Kagigebi, A. (1995). First person account: Living in a nightmare. *Schizophrenia Bulletin, 21,* 155–159.

Kanter, J., Lamb, H. R., & Loeper, C. (1987). Expressed emotion in families: A critical review. *Hospital and Community Psychiatry, 38,* 374–380.

Kavanagh, D. J. (1992). Recent developments in expressed emotion and schizophrenia. *British Journal of Psychiatry, 160,* 601–620.

Kazarian, S. S. (1992). The measurement of expressed emotion: A review. *Canadian Journal of Psychiatry, 37,* 51–56.

Kazarian, S. S., Malla, A. K., Cole, J. D., & Baker, B. (1990). Comparisons of two expressed emotion scales with the Camberwell Family Interview. *Journal of Clinical Psychology, 46,* 306–309.

Kazarian, S. S., & Vanderheyden, D. A. (1992). Family education of relatives of people with psychiatric disabilities: A review. *Psychosocial Rehabilitation Journal, 15,* 67–83.

Kershner, J. G., Cohen, N. J., & Coyne, J. C. (1996). Expressed emotion in families of clinically referred and nonreferred children: Toward a further understanding of the expressed emotion index. *Journal of Family Psychology, 10,* 97–106.

Klein, M. (1948). *Contributions to psycho-analysis: 1921–1945.* London: Hogarth Press.

King, S., & Dixon, M. J. (1996). The influence of expressed emotion, family dynamics, and symptom type on the social adjustment of schizophrenic young adults. *Archives of General Psychiatry, 53,* 1098–1104.

Klerman, G. L. (1983). The significance of DSM-III in American psychiatry. In R. L. Spitzer, J. B. W. Williams, & A. E. Skodol (Eds.), *International perspectives on DSM-III* (pp. 3–25). Washington, DC: American Psychiatric Press.

Klerman, G. L. (1989). Psychiatric diagnostic categories: Issues of validity and measurement. *Journal of Health and Social Behavior, 30,* 26–32.

Koenigsberg, H. W., & Handley, R. (1986). Expressed emotion: From predictive index to clinical construct. *American Journal of Psychiatry, 143,* 1361–1373.

Köttgen, C., Sonnichsen, I., Mollenhauser, K., & Jurth, R. (1984). Group therapy with families of schizophrenia: III. Results of the Hamburg–Camberwell family intervention study. *International Journal of Family Psychiatry, 5,* 84–94.

Kraepelin, E. (1919). *Dementia praecox and paraphrenia* (R. M. Barklay, Trans.). Huntington, NY: Robert E. Krieger. (Original work published 1913)

Kuipers, L. (1992). Expressed emotion research in Europe. *British Journal of Clinical Psychology, 31,* 429–443.

Kuipers, L., & Bebbington, P. (1988). Expressed emotion research in schizophrenia: Theoretical and clinical implications. *Psychological Medicine, 18*, 893–909.

Lam, D. H. (1991). Psychosocial family intervention in schizophrenia. *Psychological Medicine, 21*, 423–441.

Lamb, H. R. (Ed.). (1984). *The homeless mentally ill: A task force report of the American Psychological Association.* Washington, DC: American Psychological Association.

Leff, J. (1994a). Stress reduction in the social environment of schizophrenic patients. *Acta Psychiatrica Scandinavica, 90*(Suppl. 384), 133–139.

Leff, J. (1994b). Working with the families of schizophrenic patients. *British Journal of Psychiatry, 164*(Suppl. 23), 71–76.

Leff, J., Berkowitz, R., Shavit, N., Strachan, A., Glass, I., & Vaughn, C. (1990). A trial of family therapy versus a relatives' group for schizophrenia: Two-year follow-up. *British Journal of Psychiatry, 157*, 571–577.

Leff, J. P., Wig, N., Ghosh, A., Bedi, H., Menon, D. K., Kuipers, L., Korten, A., Ernberg, G., Day, R., Sartorius, N., & Jablensky, A. (1987). Influence of relatives' expressed emotion on the course of schizophrenia in Chandigarh. *British Journal of Psychiatry, 151*, 166–173.

Lefley, H. P. (1989). Family burden and family stigma in major mental illness. *American Psychologist, 44*, 556–560.

Lefley, H. P. (1992). Expressed emotion: Conceptual, clinical, and social policy issues. *Hospital and Community Psychiatry, 43*, 591–598.

Liberman, R. P. (1994). Psychosocial treatments for schizophrenia. *Psychiatry, 57*, 104–114.

Lidz, T., Cornelison, A., Fleck, S., & Terry, D. (1957). The intrafamilial environment of schizophrenic patients: II. Marital schism and marital skew. *American Journal of Psychiatry, 114*, 241–248.

Linszen, D. H., Dingemans, P. M., Nugter, M. A., Van der Does, A. J. W., Scholte, W. F., & Lenoir, M. A. (1997). Patient attributes and expressed emotion as risk factors for psychotic relapse. *Schizophrenia Bulletin, 23*, 119–130.

Linszen, D. H., Dingemans, P. M., Van der Does, J. W., Nugter, M. A., Scholte, W. F., Lenoir, R., Goldstein, M. J. (1996). Treatment, expressed emotion and relapse in recent onset schizophrenic disorders. *Psychological Medicine, 26*, 333–342.

Lorr, M. (1986). Classifying psychotics: Dimensional and categorical approaches. In T. Millon & G. L. Klerman (Eds.), *Contemporary directions in psychopathology: Toward the DSM-IV* (pp. 331–345). New York: Guilford Press.

Magana, A. B., Goldstein, M. J., Karno, M., Miklowitz, D. J., Jenkins, J., & Falloon, I. R. H. (1986). A brief method for assessing expressed emotion in relatives of psychiatric patients. *Psychiatry Research, 17*, 203–212.

Mari, J. D. J., & Streiner, D. L. (1994). An overview of family interventions and relapse on schizophrenia. *Psychological Medicine, 24*, 565–578.

Malla, A. K., Kazarian, S. S., Barnes, S., & Cole, J. D. (1991). Validation of the Five Minute Speech Sample in measuring expressed emotion. *Canadian Journal of Psychiatry, 36*, 297–299.

Mavreas, V. G., Tomaras, V., Karydi, V., Economou, M., & Stefanis, C. N. (1992). Expressed emotion in families of chronic schizophrenics and its association with clinical measures. *Social Psychiatry and Psychiatric Epidemiology, 27*, 4–9.

McFarlane, W. R. (1994). Multiple-family groups and psychoeducation in the treatment of schizophrenia. *New Directions in Mental Health Services, 62,* 13–22.

McFarlane, W. R., Lukens, E., Link, B., Dushay, R., Deakins, S. A., Newmark, M., Dunne, E. J., Horen, B., & Toran, J. (1995). Multiple family group and psychoeducation in the treatment of schizophrenia. *Archives of General Psychiatry, 52,* 679–687.

McGlashan, T. H., & Fenton, W. S. (1991). Classical subtypes for schizophrenia: Literature review for DSM-IV. *Schizophrenia Bulletin, 17,* 609–632.

McGuire, T. G. (1991). Measuring the economic costs of schizophrenia. *Schizophrenia Bulletin, 17,* 375–388.

McReadie, R. G., & Robinson, A. D. T. (1987). The Nithsdale schizophrenia survey: 6. Relatives' expressed emotion: Prevalence, patterns, and clinical assessment. *British Journal of Psychiatry, 150,* 640–644.

Meehl, P. E. (1962). Schizotaxia, schizotypy, schizophrenia. *American Psychologist, 17,* 827–838.

Meehl, P. E., & Golden, R. R. (1982). Taxometric methods. In J. M. Butcher & P. C. Kendall (Eds.), *The handbook of research methods in clinical psychology* (pp. 127–181). New York: Wiley.

Miklowitz, D. J. (1994). Family risk indicators in schizophrenia. *Schizophrenia Bulletin, 20,* 137–149.

Mills, P. D., & Hansen, J. C. (1991). Short-term group interventions for mentally ill young adults living in a community residence and their families. *Hospital and Community Psychiatry, 42,* 1144–1150.

Mino, Y., Inoue, S., Tanaka, S., & Tsuda, T. (1997). Expressed emotion among families and course of schizophrenia in Japan: A 2-year cohort study. *Schizophrenia Research, 24,* 333–339.

Mintz, L. M., Liberman, R. P., Miklowitz, D. J., & Mintz, J. (1987). Expressed emotion: A call for partnership among relatives, patients, and professionals. *Schizophrenia Bulletin, 13,* 227–235.

Neufeld, R. W. J., & Nicholson, I. R. (1991). *Differential and other equations essential to a servocybernetic (systems) approach to stress–schizophrenia relations* (Research Bulletin No. 698). London, Ontario, Canada: Department of Psychology, University of Western Ontario.

Nicholson, I. R., & Neufeld, R. W. J. (1989). Forms and mechanisms of susceptibility to stress in schizophrenia. In R. W. J. Neufeld (Ed.), *Advances in the investigation of psychological stress* (pp. 392–420). New York: Wiley.

Nicholson, I. R., & Neufeld, R. W. J. (1992). Dynamic vulnerability perspective on stress and schizophrenia. *American Journal of Orthopsychiatry, 62,* 117–130.

Nicholson, I. R., & Neufeld, R. W. J. (1993). Classification of the schizophrenias according to symptomatology: A two-factor model. *Journal of Abnormal Psychology, 102,* 259–270.

Noh, S., & Turner, R. J. (1987). Living with psychiatric patients: Implications for the mental health of family members. *Social Science and Medicine, 25,* 263–271.

Nuechterlein, K. H. (1987). Vulnerability models for schizophrenia: State of the art. In H. Hafner, W. F. Gattaz, & W. Janzarik (Eds.), *Search for the causes of schizophrenia* (pp. 297–316). Berlin: Springer-Verlag.

Parker, G., Johnston, P., & Hayward, L. (1988). Parental expressed emotion as a predictor of schizophrenic relapse. *Archives of General Psychiatry, 45,* 806–813.

Penn, D. L., & Mueser, K. T. (1996). Research update on the psychosocial treatment of schizophrenia. *American Journal of Psychiatry, 153,* 607–617.

Perris, C. (1989). *Cognitive therapy with schizophrenic patients.* New York: Guilford Press.

Priebe, S., Wildgrube, C., & Muller-Oerlinghausen, B. (1989). Lithium prophylaxis and expressed emotion. *British Journal of Psychiatry, 154,* 396–399.

Randolph, E. A., Eth, S., Glynn, S. M., Paz, G. G., Leong, G. B., Shaner, A. L., Strachan, A., Van Vort, W., Escobar, J. I., & Liberman, R. P. (1994). Behavioral family management in schizophrenia: Outcome of a clinic-based intervention. *British Journal of Psychiatry, 164,* 501–506.

Rosenfarb, I. S., Goldstein, M. J., Mintz, J., & Nuechterlein, K. H. (1995). Expressed emotion and subclinical psychopathology observable within the transactions between schizophrenic patients and their family members. *Journal of Abnormal Psychology, 104,* 259–267.

Rupp, A., & Keith, S. J. (1993). The costs of schizophrenia: Assessing the burden. *Psychiatric Clinics of North America, 16,* 413–423.

Scazufca, M., & Kuipers, E. (1996). Link between expressed emotion and burden of care in relatives of patients with schizophrenia. *British Journal of Psychiatry, 168,* 580–587.

Schooler, N. R., Keith, S. J., Severe, J. B., & Matthews, S. M. (1995). Maintenance treatment of schizophrenia: A review of dose reduction and family treatment strategies. *Psychiatric Quarterly, 66,* 279–292.

Simpson, J. A., & Weiner, E. S. C. (Eds.). (1989). *The Oxford English dictionary* (2nd ed.). Oxford: Clarendon Press.

Smith, J., & Birchwood, M. (1990). Relatives and patients as partners in the management of schizophrenia: The development of a service model. *British Journal of Psychiatry, 156,* 654–660.

Snyder, K. S., Wallace, C. J., Moe, K., & Liberman, R. P. (1994). Expressed emotion by residential care operators and residents' symptoms and quality of life. *Hospital and Community Psychiatry, 45,* 1141–1143.

Solomon, P., Draine, J., Mannion, E., & Meisel, M. (1996). Impact of brief family psychoeducation on self-efficacy. *Schizophrenia Bulletin, 22,* 41–50.

Stengel, E. (1959). Classification of mental disorders. *Bulletin of the World Health Organization, 21,* 601–663.

Stirling, J., Tantam, D., Thomas, P., Newby, D., Montague, L., Ring, N., & Rowe, S. (1991). Expressed emotion and early onset schizophrenia: A one-year follow-up. *Psychological Medicine, 21,* 675–685.

Sturgeon, D., Turpin, G., Kuipers, L., Berkowitz, R., & Leff, J. (1984). Psychophysiological responses of schizophrenic patients to high and low expressed emotion relatives. *British Journal of Psychiatry, 145,* 62–69.

Sullivan, H. S. (1929). *The interpersonal theory of psychiatry.* Washington, DC: William Allanson White.

Szmukler, G. I., Eisler, I., Russell, G. F. M., & Dare, C. (1985). Anorexia nervosa, parental EE, and dropping out of treatment. *British Journal of Psychiatry, 147,* 265–271.

Tarrier, N. (1991a). Changes in the electrodermal activity of schizophrenic patients and the association with change in the expressed emotion status of their relatives. *Psychopathology, 24*, 203–208.

Tarrier, N. (1991b). Some aspects of family interventions in schizophrenia: I. Adherence to intervention programmes. *British Journal of Psychiatry, 159*, 475–480.

Tarrier, N., & Barrowclough, C. (1989). Electrodermal activity as a predictor of schizophrenic relapse. *Psychopathology, 22*, 320–324.

Tarrier, N., Barrowclough, C., Porceddu, K., & Fitzpatrick, E. (1994). The Salford Family Intervention Project: Relapse rates of schizophrenia at five and eight years. *British Journal of Psychiatry, 165*, 829–832.

Tarrier, N., Lownson, K., & Barrowclough, C. (1991). Some aspects of family interventions in schizophrenia: II. Financial considerations. *British Journal of Psychiatry, 159*, 481–484.

Tarrier, N., & Turpin, G. (1992). Psychosocial factors, arousal, and schizophrenic relapse: The psychophysiological data. *British Journal of Psychiatry, 161*, 3–11.

Tarrier, N., Vaughn, C., Lader, M., & Leff, J. (1979). Bodily reactions to people and events in schizophrenia. *Archives of General Psychiatry, 36*, 311–315.

Tompson, M. C., Goldstein, M. J., Lebell, M. B., Mintz, L. I., Marder, S. R., & Mintz, J. (1995). Schizophrenic patients' perceptions of their relatives' attitudes. *Psychiatry Research, 57*, 155–167.

Vaccaro, J. V., Young, A. S., & Glynn, S. (1993). Community-based care of individuals with schizophrenia: Combining psychosocial and pharmacologic therapies. *Psychiatric Clinics of North America, 16*, 387–399.

Vaughan, K., Doyle, M., McConaghy, N., Blaszczynski, A., Fox, A., & Tarrier, N. (1992). The Sydney intervention trial: A controlled trial of relatives' counselling to reduce schizophrenic relapse. *Social Psychiatry and Psychiatric Epidemiology, 27*, 16–21.

Vaughn, C. E. (1989). Expressed emotion in family relationships. *Journal of Child Psychology and Psychiatry, 30*, 13–22.

Vaughn, C. E., & Leff, J. P. (1976a). The influence of family and social factors on the course of psychiatric illness. *British Journal of Psychiatry, 129*, 125–137.

Vaughn, C. E., & Leff, J. P. (1976b). The measurement of expressed emotion in the families of psychiatric patients. *British Journal of Social and Clinical Psychology, 15*, 157–165.

Vaughn, C. E., & Leff, J. P. (1981). Patterns of emotional response in relatives of schizophrenic patients. *Schizophrenia Bulletin, 7*, 43–44.

Wilkinson, G. (1987). Commentary on *Dementia praecox and paraphrenia* (1919) and *Introduction lectures on clinical psychiatry* (1906) III Dementia Praecox by E. Kraepelin. In C. Thompson (Ed.), *The origins of modern psychiatry* (pp. 239–243). New York: Wiley.

William, P., Williams, A., Sommer, R., & Sommer, B. (1986). A survey of the California Alliance for the Mentally Ill. *Hospital and Community Psychiatry, 37*, 253–255.

Woo, S. M., Goldstein, M. J., & Neuchterlein, K. H. (1997). Relatives' expressed emotion and non-verbal signs of subclinical psychopathology in schizophrenic patients. *British Journal of Psychiatry, 170*, 58–61.

Wyatt, R. J., Henter, I., Leary, M. C., & Taylor, E. (1995). An economic evaluation of schizophrenia—1991. *Social Psychiatry and Psychiatric Epidemiology, 30,* 196–205.

Wynne, L. I., & Singer, M. T. (1963). Thought disorder and family relations of schizophrenics: I. A research strategy. *Archives of General Psychiatry, 9,* 191–198.

Yank, G. R., Bentley, K. J., & Hargrove, D. S. (1993). The vulnerability–stress model of schizophrenia: Advances in psychosocial treatment. *American Journal of Orthopsychiatry, 63,* 55–69.

Zilboorg, G. (1941). *A history of medical psychology.* New York: Norton.

Zubin, J., & Spring, B. (1977). Vulnerability: A new view of schizophrenia. *Journal of Abnormal Psychology, 86,* 103–126.

CHAPTER 13

Psychosomatic Illness and the Family

MANFRED CIERPKA
GÜNTER REICH
ACHIM KRAUL

"Patients have families," wrote Richardson (1948), calling attention in the English-language literature to the importance of family background in the development, course and prognosis of illness. In the German literature, Richter's (1970) book *Patient Familie* (*The Patient Family*) gave voice to the viewpoint that the psychic and physical suffering of the patient must also always be regarded as the suffering of the family. The influence of couple and family relationships on an individual's health and illness is now no longer disputed (see Figure 13.1). This recognition is based not only on clinical experience, but also on the relevant findings of empirical studies in quite different fields during the last 15 years:

1. The "salutogenetic" point of view (Antonowsky, 1979) emphasizes the resources derived from couples and families. A supportive couple relationship (Doherty, Schrott, Metcalf, & Iassiello-Vailas, 1983; Bunzel & Wollenek, 1994) and a supportive family system (Cohen & Syme, 1985) exercise a positive influence on health.

2. Many empirical studies (for reviews, see Campbell, 1986; Doherty & Campbell, 1988; Turk & Kerns, 1985; McDaniel, Campbell, & Seaburn, 1989) confirm that processes of interaction exist between family dysfunction on the one hand, and the etiology, pathogenesis, and course of an illness, the results of treatment, and the prognosis on the other. Psychosocial factors such as family stress and relationship conflicts within the family can be regarded as significant factors (Cohen, 1981). Further important factors,

such as the death of a relative, may exercise a negative influence on the morbidity or mortality of patients (Schleifer, Keller, & Stein, 1989). In complex experimental studies, there is a relationship between the health- or illness-related physiological processes of children and the quality of their parents' relationship (e.g., Gottman & Katz, 1989).

3. Better treatment results are obtained when the families of individuals with psychosomatic illnesses are included in treatment (Lask & Matthew, 1979; Clark et al., 1981; Gustaffson, Kjellman, & Cederblad, 1986; Onnis et al., 1993).

Research on the connection between psychosomatic illness and the family takes two directions. The first question is this: How does the family influence a patient's illness or symptoms? In this chapter, we concentrate on answering this question.

In the last 10 years, another question has received more attention— namely, to what extent do the patient's illness and symptoms influence the family? The constructive aspect of answering this question in an individual case is that it can facilitate the provision of help for a couple or family when a patient with a sometimes severe or fatal somatic illness is cared for in the couple or family context. In such cases, family medicine places great value on cooperation among the patient, the spouse/partner and family, the doctor, and other members of the health care system.

Family medicine, the theory of which is based on the biopsychosocial model (Engel, 1977; see below), views the family as a valuable resource and help in dealing with illness (Doherty & Baird, 1983; Sperling, 1983; McDaniel, Hepworth, & Doherty, 1992). How well a family is able to cope

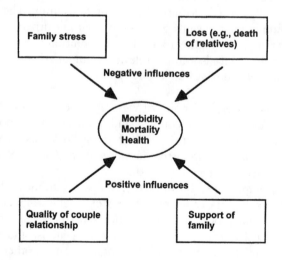

FIGURE 13.1. Couple and family influence on health or illness.

with a chronic illness depends on its functionality. By "functionality" we mean a family's ability to deal with crises; its ability to question existing patterns of coping, if necessary; and its ability to adapt to new ways of solving problems and reducing tension. Sometimes these resources are not forthcoming from a family—for example, when adaptation to the patient's physical symptoms maintains the family in balance, and changes are not desired. The following case example illustrates such a family.

CASE EXAMPLE

Mr. S is 27 years old and an industrial office assistant by profession. Since puberty he has had attacks of diarrhea once or twice a month, which are preceded by severe cramps and pain. During the last year, the symptoms of diarrhea have been occurring an average of three times a week. Mr. S suffers bouts of diarrhea before any kind of undertaking—for example, before tests, before going to lectures, before holidays, and on weekends—and increasingly in recent times without any external provocation at all. Only during the last year did he finally visit his family doctor, who, having failed to diagnose the problem or to treat it successfully with medication, referred Mr. S to the University Outpatient Clinic for further examination.

According to diagnostic criteria that distinguish 11 different functional gastrointestinal disturbances (Drossman, 1994), Mr. S has irritable bowel syndrome (IBS). In the psychological models most frequently applied to patients with IBS, such patients are characterized by psychopathological abnormalities, personality traits, and stressful events in their life histories. For example, IBS patients more frequently recall distressing events in their lives, such as the death of relatives, family conflicts, or professional changes, and experience these as more stressful than healthy people do (Arun, Kanwal, Vyas, & Sushil, 1993). Moreover, they report fewer positive experiences in life than IBS sufferers who are not receiving medical care do (Drossman, 1994).

Compared to control groups, IBS patients have more psychiatric diagnoses, higher rates of anxiety and depression, and more physical complaints, as well as additional psychovegetative problems (Lynn & Friedman, 1993; Lydiard, 1992; Kröger, 1986). How a person experiences pain correlates with his or her psychic state, and especially with the extent of depressive symptoms. Also indicative of the significance of perception processes is the fact that IBS patients with diagnosed depression do not describe themselves as depressive, unlike depressive patients without IBS (Toner et al., 1990).

To return to Mr. S, he gives the impression during his first interview of a pleasant, amiable young man, who answers questions briefly and precisely but without emotional involvement, and then stops to wait cautiously for further inquiries. He often remains vague, forcing the therapist into an active questioning role. In addition to his gastrointestinal complaint, he reports an occasional feeling of pressure "up to the throat," as well as persistent fatigue, lack of concentration, and tension, which are sometimes accompanied by nausea and dizziness.

Mr. S has had a girlfriend for about 2 years. She is much like him and is studying in a nearby city. "We have never had an argument," he reports. The two of them live together on the weekends, seeing each other less often during the week. Parting at the end of the weekend is hard for both of them. Mr. S often has diarrhea then and is very dejected, and his girlfriend tries to cheer him up. Because of problems at work, he has also recently begun a course of study in the evenings. He was promised a promotion a year ago, which was later abruptly withdrawn. As always, he did not protest. His colleagues occasionally refuse to do things, and to his disgust do only what is absolutely required. Then, when a backlog of work does build up, Mr. S feels ready to explode. He curses under his breath at work, but does not speak to any of his colleagues directly. They stay out of his way when this happens, and after a while Mr. S regrets the "incident," fearing that this time he's "let too much slip out."

The family interview reveals the following picture: The patient's parents have a small business. He has two older sisters, one of whom is married and has two children—"a very motherly type." The other sister has no partner or family and lives in another city. The patient's father takes care to present as unobtrusive and perfect a facade as possible, and "lives for his business." His mother appears somewhat more open, friendly, and conciliatory. Of the siblings, Mr. S has the best relationship with his parents, living in a separate apartment in his parents' house. The family regards itself as being divided into two groups: On one side are the patient and the parents, who solve their own problems and do not reveal anything to outsiders; on the other side are the sisters, who "let everything out, with no consideration for others." Everyone can do what he or she likes within the family—there are no clear and definite rules. It is typical also that it is left to the patient alone to decide whether he will undertake anything toward treating his illness. Each family member is allowed a high degree of autonomy, and the members do not "interfere" with one another.

Mr. S's grandparents, to whom he felt very attached, died 1½ and 3 years ago. Each family member dealt with the resulting grief alone and in his or her own way, except that once, when the family sat down together for dinner, the father suddenly began to cry and ran out of the room. The others, not knowing what they could do, did not say anything.

Other than a few back problems, the parents are healthy. But one sister also has digestion problems in the form of sudden attacks of diarrhea; the grandmother who died had similar troubles.

In the biography of Mr. S at the time of his increase in symptoms, we discover several unsettling new experiences in his life: the loss of his grandparents, his having been passed over for promotion at work, and the beginning of a relationship with his girlfriend based on harmony and equality. The S family has, on the one hand, a very strong tendency to avoid conflict and seek harmony. On the other, it is divided into two opposing camps. Mr. S and the parents place value on maintaining a perfect outer facade, whereas the sisters, on the contrary, do not control their emotions. The control of aggressive affects is for Mr. S and his parents a matter of the first priority, and is linked with fears that something might just "slip out." As in the family business, people are regarded as customers upon whom the family is dependent. At his own job as well, Mr. S must deal with the complaints of customers, must try to appease them, and must make an effort to present his company as running as smoothly and flawlessly as possible. Communication and the acceptance of affective relationships are subject to strict control not only in the workplace, but also within the family; the expression of emotions—for example, grief for the deceased grandparents—is avoided. If an outbreak of feeling does occur, the family regards it with helplessness and shame. Adaptability to inner or outer change and conflict is extremely limited.

The S family displays a relationship pattern typically described for the families of psychosomatic patients. It has few resources available, especially those needed for dealing with conflicts. The family members respond to change (e.g., the loss of a close relative) by distancing themselves from the outside world with increasing anxiety. The family climate is characterized by helplessness and depressive-like avoidance behavior. The expression of emotions is strictly discouraged; in particular, socially unusual and aggressive responses must be avoided. The patient's marked anxiety is based on a fear of uncontrolled, explosive outbreaks, which are also symbolically manifested in the patient's symptoms. Unlike his sisters, Mr. S has avoided taking developmental steps toward individuation, and he continues the habitual relationship style of his parents with regard to his own profession and partnership.

MINUCHIN'S CONCEPT OF THE PSYCHOSOMATIC FAMILY

Minuchin's theory of the "psychosomatic family" is one of the most influential and frequently cited theories in family therapy (Forman, 1986). In their 1978 book, the child psychiatrist Minuchin, the psychologist Rosman, and the psychiatrist Baker developed their experiences in treating children—using a case of diabetes mellitus, one of bronchial asthma, and later one of anorexia nervosa—into an explanatory model of dysfunctionality in a family with a psychosomatically ill adolescent. Based on their clinical experience, Minuchin et al. (1978) described the following modes of interaction in "anorexic families":

1. *Enmeshment.* Family relationships are marked by an extremely close and intense form of interaction, which is described as "enmeshment" or "fusion." There appears to be only weakly defined boundaries between the family system and the parent's families of origin.

2. *Overprotection.* Overprotection is expressed in the family members' excessive degree of care and concern for one another, which is not restricted to the patient or the illness. Nurturing and protective functions are kept constantly aroused and available.

3. *Rigidity.* These families are characterized by a rigid maintenance of the existing status quo. They experience phases of change and growth, such as adolescence, as a severe threat. Any need for change is denied.

4. *Lack of conflict resolution.* Arguing out or resolving conflict is avoided, or reaching a solution is hindered through constant interruption and distraction.

5. *Triangulation or parent–child coalitions.* In "triangulation," the parents use a child's behavior (e.g., the ill adolescent's symptoms) to avoid addressing areas of disagreement between themselves; in a parent–child "coalition," one parent aligns himself or herself directly with the child against the other parent. In either case, the boundary between generations is overstepped.

Many researchers came to similar conclusions for quite different syndromes, which were examined with different methods:

Anorexia nervosa (e.g., Selvini Palazzoli, 1963/1974; Minuchin et al., 1978; Kog & Vandereycken, 1989; Cierpka & Reich, 1997).

Atopic reactions (e.g., Pinkerton, 1970; Overbeck, 1985; Mrazek, Klinnert, Mrazek, & Macey, 1991).

Ulcerated colitis and Crohn's disease (e.g., Jackson & Yalom, 1966; Overbeck, 1985; Wirsching & Stierlin, 1982; Wirsching, 1984).

Juvenile diabetes (e.g., Cierpka, 1982; Hauser, Di Placido, & Jacobson, 1993).

Malignant diseases (e.g., Louhivuori, Huupponen, Riita, & Sormunen, 1976; Stierlin et al., 1983).

Kidney disease requiring hemodialysis (e.g., Engel, 1978).

Chronic pain (e.g., Roy, 1982; Flor & Fydrich, 1990; Joraschky, 1993).

The results of this research tended to be unsatisfactory, however, for various reasons (problems of methodology, retrospective designs, no differentiation observed between the ill individual and healthy family members; see Cierpka, 1989). Because of the differences in results, families with a psychosomatically ill member came to be described in review articles under even more general family dynamic headings, such as "rigid development standstill," "harmonizing conflict avoidance," and "fused boundaries" (Wirsching, 1996)—terms that apply to many families in crisis situations.

Confronted with change (e.g., life crises, threshold situations, or illness), the almost inevitable response is further avoidance of conflict, a tighter closing of ranks, and an increase in clinging to the status quo.

CRITICISM OF THE PSYCHOSOMATIC FAMILY MODEL

The influence of disturbed couple and family relationships on the development of psychosomatic illnesses has been the subject of controversial discussion since the publication of *Psychosomatic Families* (Minuchin et al., 1978). The debate has been marked in particular by the argument over *specific* familial dysfunctions that are said to characterize so-called "psychosomatic" families—that is, the postulation of a close causal link between certain clearly defined family interactions or configurations and a clearly defined syndrome in the patient.

The term "specificity" derives from the field of medicine. Infection with a "specific" pathogen (e.g., the tubercle bacillus) leads to certain morphological changes in tissue (i.e., the formation of tubercles). Even if we assume that other conditions must be present for an infection to develop, the tubercle bacillus can be regarded as the specific cause. In examining the development of psychic diseases, Freud (1962/1895) pointed out that one can only speak of a specific cause if in none of the cases the cause is lacking. A specificity hypothesis for psychosomatic illnesses was formulated by Alexander, French, and Pollock (1968). They postulated that in each of seven illnesses they examined at the time (bronchial asthma, rheumatoid arthritis, ulcerated colitis, essential hypertonia, hyperthyroidism, stomach ulcers, and neurodermititis), in addition to the predispositional, somatic "X factor" and the subjectively significant, "triggering" situation in the subject's life, the existence of a specific psychodynamic configuration that developed in childhood (together with the accompanying defensive processes) can be assumed. This hypothesis gave rise to a fierce argument regarding specificity versus nonspecificity in psychosomatic illness, which continues to the present day.

Furthermore, therapists have criticized Minuchin's approach because of the danger that parents could be blamed for the illness of their children. Indeed, some therapists working within the psychosomatic family model do tend to ignore the biological aspect of such illnesses as diabetes and asthma; a few even take the viewpoint that the family dynamics "cause" certain illnesses.

Another criticism is that the model lacks a sufficiently empirical basis (Coyne & Anderson, 1988, but see also the reply by Rosman & Baker, 1988). Vandereycken, Kog, and Vanderlinden (1989) pursued the question of whether evidence of this postulated specific family structure in psychosomatic families could be found in all families with eating disorders. A classification based on self-reports was used to determine a number of clinically useful subtypes; only some of these matched Minuchin et al.'s description, however. In the German literature, Wirsching and Stierlin (1982) studied a random sample of 55 families in which an adolescent had a severe, chronic psychosomatic illness. They found interaction patterns essentially in keeping with those of Minuchin et al. (1978) in only about half of the families. A linear causal relationship between an illness syndrome in one family member and an interaction disturbance in the family therefore does not exist.

To prevent an oversimplified application of Minuchin et al.'s concept, Beatrice Wood and her coworkers actualized the original model of the psychosomatic family with great theoretical finesse and better research methods (Wood et al., 1989). They studied the ways in which familial processes contributed to three different abdominal illnesses in children: Crohn's disease, ulcerated colitis, and recurrent functional abdominal pain. The families were assessed on the basis of standardized and videotaped interaction tasks during lunch and during an interview. For comparative values, the authors used the number of blood platelets and the volume of hematocrit and albumin in the blood. They discovered a connection between the activity of the illness on the one hand, and triangulation, parental dysfunctionality, and the overall psychosomatic values of the family on the other. There were two further important findings relevant to the psychosomatic family model: (1) The three illnesses differed from one another in how the family pattern related to the activity of the illness (Crohn's disease corresponded to the highest values for a "psychosomatic family"); and (2) parental dysfunctionality and triangulation proved to be more important than enmeshment, excessive care, rigidity, conflict avoidance, and poor conflict resolution.

In conclusive theoretical articles, Wood (1991, 1994) placed the psychosomatic family model within a wider frame—the "biopsychosocial development model"—in which the division between psyche and body in the original "psychosomatic" sense is included. The model is less disease-oriented; it includes relevant individual developmental factors and other social context variables (e.g., school). All of these factors influence the well-being of the child and the family through interaction processes.

Wood et al. (1989) emphasized that Minuchin et al. (1978) actually did start out from a vulnerability–stress model. That is, Minuchin et al. did postulate that in addition to the dysfunctionality of the family, factors such as physiological, endocrinal, and biochemical intermediate mechanisms play a role in triggering symptoms in an already genetically predisposed, "vulnerable" child. Thus, these authors described feedback mechanisms that are considered significantly more important from today's cognitive theory viewpoint. Family therapy can help interrupt these feedback processes at any given point. Thus Minuchin et al.'s model takes into consideration today's modern biopsychosocial views of psychosomatic diseases (Vandereycken et al., 1989).

ENGEL'S BIOPSYCHOSOCIAL MODEL

Complex processes in the development of illness or the maintenance of health are postulated in the biopsychosocial model developed by G. L. Engel (1977). In this model, a person is part of many broader systems and is also a system with many subsystems. The diagnostic concepts and the therapeutic approaches based on the model are correspondingly multifactored and connected to one another in an integrative approach.

The biopsychosocial model is formally designed according to general systems theory, as laid down by Ludwig von Bertalanffy (1956, 1962). This theory states that isomorphs can be identified over various levels of organization, ranging from the molecular level to that of institutional and social structures. All organizational levels are linked to sub-and suprasystems in hierarchical relationships. General principles can be established for the individual levels and the relationships between them. Hierarchical systems are dependent on one another, because changes at one organizational level can produce changes at higher or lower levels in the hierarchy.

Living systems are characterized by gradual or sudden change brought about by rhythm functions, feedback mechanisms, and nonlinear processes, in the course of which the system constantly seeks to recover its "autopoietic stability." It is a characteristic of nonlinear systems that a small change in one variable—particularly at a beginning stage—can have a disproportional and unpredictable effect on the other variables in the way they change over time. Moreover, nonlinear systems come about through the interactions of variables. These interactions can amplify the functions of the original variables or cancel them (or both).

Through the application of systems theory, we see the family as being organized by interpersonal structures and processes. A family member's symptom is part of this family context. The family dynamics can influence the pathogenesis, and the course of the symptom, like family dynamics, is influenced by that symptom. For many medical problems the relational context is important to assessment and treatment.

A THREE-STEP MODEL FOR PSYCHOSOMATIC ILLNESS AND FAMILY PROCESS

How do psychic and physical processes influence one another in psychosomatic illness? This problem has still not been satisfactorily resolved—perhaps because there is no *one* solution. What we regard as "psychosomatic illness" is a collection of very different, individual illness entities. Actual psychosomatic illnesses include an organic deficiency that must be distinguished from the somatic disorder of somatopsychic illnesses. In the case of somatization disorders, conversion neuroses are distinguished from functional disorders. These illnesses are due to quite different etiopathogenetic factors, with psychic and somatic factors of varying significance causing the development of the illness. Not remarkably, we find in the psychosomatic literature highly different explanatory approaches: concepts based on learning theory; the vulnerability–stress model; psychodynamically oriented conflict models (Alexander, 1950; Alexander et al., 1968); "desomatization" and "resomatization" models (Schur, 1955); the so-called "alexithymia" model (Marty, de M'Uzan, & David, 1963); and psychoneuroimmunological concepts (see Borysenko, 1989).

For each psychosomatic illness, therefore, we need a developmental model of the disturbance that must include quite different dysfunctional processes. Clinicians who ascribe to the biopsychosocial model usually define the borders of these related systems at the biomedical, the psychological, and the social levels. When dysfunctions reinforce one another at these different levels, causing disturbances or illness to develop or to be maintained, these are known as "coevolutionary processes." However, only those components that fit together like a key and a keyhole are codetermined to contribute to coevolutionary processes; in this sense, we speak of "key concepts" (see below). The patterns that evolve through the interaction of dysfunctional components and coevolutionary processes alter the structure of the system, which can be observed, for example, in the transition from an acute to a chronic illness. Through time and repetition, the new biopsychosocial pattern takes on another meaning, which contributes to its stabilization.

Our hypothesis for the relationship between psychosomatic illness and family psychopathology focuses on a three-step model for identifying and describing dysfunctions and resources:

1. Every level of the system must be assessed on its own. The view through the different diagnostic windows (Cierpka, 1996) is usually colored by the theoretical "spectacles" being used.
2. It must be determined which feedback processes between the levels lead to weakening or strengthening the dysfunctional processes on one level.
3. For each syndrome and each patient and family, special "key concepts" must identify and describe the interfaces between biological and psychological factors—but also among individual, familial, and social factors.

The coevolutionary feedback processes can be illustrated by the example described earlier in this chapter. Mr. S suffers from IBS, which can be explained by dysfunctions at different system levels. At the individual level, Mr. S shows—in addition to a somatic predisposition—strong inhibition of aggression, combined with highly controlled affects. The psychoanalytic literature describes a splitting of the feelings and experience areas from the ego, which can also be described as a basic psychosomatic disturbance in the sense of a pathology of the self (Gaddini, 1977). This can frequently be found in patients with psychosomatic illnesses. It is clinically striking in such patients that they appear to have little access to their affects and emotion-laden fantasies, which is explained by very early processes of disintegration between soma and psyche and their defenses. In empirical studies, Krause and Merten (1996) found a severe reduction in affectivity in ulcerated colitis patients' facial expressions.

Mr. S's family is characterized by an avoidance of conflict, unclear rules, and a striving for harmony. Interactive processes act to intensify individual and familial dysfunctionalities. In principle, the individual's inner psychic structure is developed through internalizing mechanisms such as identification or the introjection of object relations that develop primarily in the sphere of the family. Intrafamilial relationships that are characterized by "harmonizing conflict avoidance" and "fused boundaries" (Wirsching, 1996) contribute toward the forming of defenses against strong affects and hinder individuation processes, so that development-appropriate, affect-responsive, fantasized or real object relations are not available for individual internalization. This means that a complex world of self-representation and object representation, in the context of affective interactions, cannot be internalized. Fundamentally, Mr. S himself, by splitting off affect and experience areas, contributes to low-emotion family interactions—with which he himself in turn identifies. Viewed longitudinally, these feedback processes between intrapsychic and interpersonal object relations lead to a family interaction structure that can be summarized as "rigidity."

KEY CONCEPTS

As noted above, special "key concepts" are needed for each type of psychosomatic illness and each patient and family to describe the feedback processes at the interfaces among individual, familial, and social factors, as well as between biological and psychological factors. In this section, we discuss several key concepts concerning the interplay of individual, familial, and (to a certain extent) social factors in eating disorders; more briefly, we discuss key concepts concerning the interplay of biological and psychological factors in atopic dermatitis. Of course, all of these types of factors must be considered together in any particular situation.

Key Concepts in Eating Disorders: The Interplay among Individual, Familial, and Social Factors

Psychoanalytic object relations theory offers a starting point for understanding the interaction of developmental processes between the individual and the family. Identification processes with the psychosocial formulation of compromise in the family determine what the individual internalizes as the "inner family." The child may be born into a family, but he or she assimilates the concept of the family gradually over time. During their entire development, children impose change upon their parents, who must adjust to new developmental tasks and accept appropriate roles. A child's active relationship-inducing role means for the family that the child does not simply identify with the functions and processes of the family; he or she contributes toward the development of these functions. Interaction patterns, as family representatives, are internalized; however, the child himself or herself has helped to create these.

In what follows the identification processes and the coevolution of individual, familial, and social factors are shown for the etiology and pathogenesis of eating disorders. We emphasize a longitudinal view of the development of eating disorders. In the continuum of causal factors, the family plays a very important role, but not the only one. Hereditary factors, such as temperament and affectivity (Strober, 1991), social factors, such as the slimness ideal and sex role issues of women (who are overwhelmingly more at risk for these disorders); developmental factors, especially the transitions of adolescence and early adulthood; and the self-reinforcing dysfunctional eating behavior itself also play important roles.

Adolescent development requires reorganization both in the individual and in the family system. For the individual, adolescence is a crucial phase for self-development, for the development of sex role identity, and for the integration of familial and cultural role expectations. The body and the outer appearance change, often dramatically, with high increase of fat cells for girls. Bodily self-esteem seems to decrease or to fluctuate considerably. Comparison with social standards, either imagined or real, intensifies. The cultural thinness schema—linking slimness to attractiveness, social, and professional success, and thus to self-esteem—becomes very important. An adolescent girl's risk for frank eating disorders increases the more her self-esteem is connected with the thinness schema or the "superwoman-complex," the more her sense of achievement is felt to be threatened, and the more her self-definition emphasizes "success in multiple roles in order to secure an identity through external approval" (Smolak & Levine, 1994, p. 51). Family interaction preforms the way the slimness schema is adopted and internalized, as well as the way conflicts of self-esteem are experienced and handled. Eating disorders are often correlated with dysfunctional family processes (Cierpka & Reich, 1997; Humphrey, 1989a; Waller & Rachel, 1994). There are several paths of influence:

1. A strong relationship between disturbed parental attitudes toward eating and parental preoccupation with dieting and slimness on the one hand, and children's attitudes toward eating, dieting, and slimness and the corresponding behaviors and eating disorders on the other (as well as a negative body image, especially in girls), has been shown in several studies (see Cierpka & Reich, 1997). So the family has a very direct impact on pathological eating attitudes and behaviors.

2. There is empirical evidence for linking separation–individuation difficulties and eating disorders (Cierpka & Reich, 1997; Friedlander & Siegel, 1990; Vandereycken et al., 1989). In particular, anorexics seem to have tight bonds to their families of origin (Smolak & Levine, 1993). In families with permeable interpersonal and intergenerational boundaries and a high degree of interpersonal control, both factors also manifest themselves in eating behaviors and rituals. Often the boundaries between these family and the outside world are closed. These family systems do not give enough room and encouragement to the adolescent striving for autonomy, and eating becomes the secret or open battlefield for this striving.

3. In family systems where basic needs for affective responsiveness, consolation, recognition, and emotional support are not met, these needs are warded off. They tend to manifest themselves in more global dysphoric affect states, which an adolescent has difficulty in differentiating and in handling in subtly diversified ways. The intake or the refusal of food can become a primary method for the regulation of affects. Empirical evidence shows that families of bulimics in particular can be characterized by more open conflict, less cohesion, and affective attunement than those of anorexics or of normal control subjects (see Cierpka & Reich, 1997; Humphrey, 1989a; Kog & Vandereycken, 1989; Reich, 1997). In families of "classic anorexics," the expression of affection is often combined with attempts at control and negation of the adolescents' separate needs (Humphrey, 1989b).

4. In family systems where achievement orientation and striving for reputation contrast with impulsivity and/or an inclination to addictive behavior or substance misuse, similar conflicts are likely to be experienced by the adolescent offspring through identification processes. Eating disorders, misuse of alcohol and other substances, and depressive illnesses were found more often in families of bulimic patients than in those of anorexics or normal controls. Family members of bulimics show more problems with impulse control, and the general functioning of these families seems to be more disturbed than in the other groups mentioned (Cierpka & Reich, 1997). Empirical evidence shows more differences between normal families and families with bulimic or bulimic–anorexic members than between anorexic and normal groups (Cierpka & Reich, 1997; Humphrey, 1989a).

Systems with permeable intrafamiliar boundaries, closed family–environment boundaries, and high interpersonal control are likely to promote individual tendencies of high harm avoidance, low novelty seeking, and high reward dependence, as Strober (1991) describes for anorexic individuals. The protection and control of the self–other boundary and of self-esteem is then likely to be displaced to the intake of food and thinness, both inside and outside the family, and to lead to anorexia nervosa (Reich, 1997). In addition to these self-reinforcing interactional vicious circles, anorexia leads into physiological vicious circles, which further reinforce the maladaptive intrapsychic and interactional patterns. Starvation leads to disturbances of hormonal balance and a drop in serotonin, which increases the likelihood of depressive mood states. There is also a drop in leptin, and the consequences of this (e.g., a reduction in feelings of hunger) also often have a maladaptive impact on family interaction.

Whereas many anorexic patients try to arrest their progress into the turmoil of adolescence by turning the thinness schema into an ascetic ideal, bulimic patients are in the throes of this turmoil. They are often very "field-dependent" and try to fulfill the superwoman stereotype. Thus they tend to adopt the thinness schema in pursuing the conventional ideal of a young woman more than normal age-mates do (Habermas, 1990). They often seem to feel a wide gap between their ideal and their actual selves (Reich, 1992, 1997; Silberstein, Striegel-Moore, & Rodin, 1987; Teusch, 1988). This leads to intense feelings of shame.

As the regulation of unwanted affects and of affects in general is a central issue in understanding the links between family process and psychosomatic illnesses, there are several important links between eating disorders and shame. Shame is a holistic, global, and often undifferentiated affect, close to intense body sensations. Bulimics have considerable problems in differentiating their affects (Léon, Fulkerson, Perry, & Cudeck, 1993). This can be understood as a consequence of the disturbed affective attunement in their families of origin. As all experiences are filtered through the bulimic slimness schema, dieting becomes a means of reducing shame. Feelings of emotional isolation and shame often precipitate weight and food problems in the bulimic person (Teusch, 1988). The binge–purge cycle serves as an anesthetic against any intense feeling, and hence against shame. Many bulimics are ashamed of intense feelings of affection or dependence; some are ashamed of feelings of anger or revenge; some are ashamed of all feelings. Family systems that exhibit two groups of characteristics—high rates of conflict, low cohesion, low affective responsiveness, high impulsivity, and an inclination to alcohol or substance misuse on the one hand, and a tendency to high achievement standards, a strong striving for reputation, and a strong emphasis on outer appearance on the other—have a high probability of developing these conflicts and reinforcing them (Cierpka & Reich, 1997; Reich, 1996; Reich & Cierpka, 1998; Roberto, 1986).

The physiological consequences of bulimic symptoms are often not as drastic as in anorexia nervosa. Restricted eating alternating with binges impairs the regulation of hunger–satiety. The restriction of certain "forbidden" foods (e.g., foods containing chocolate, sugar, or carbohydrates) may produce a "craving" for these substances, which are devoured during the binges. This is often similar to addictive behavior.

We want to illustrate these remarks now with a case example of bulimia nervosa. The A family came for family therapy because of Maureen, an 18-year-old college student, who had binge–purge cycles three to four times a day. Periods of overeating and vomiting were followed by periods of dieting. At this time she was slightly but not extremely over-weight. Her menstruation was irregular. The family dynamics can be described as follows: Mr. A used to drink large quantities of alcohol. He had lost his driver's license twice because of driving while intoxicated, and had consequently lost his job. The mother was a regular user of tranquil-izers. There were severe conflicts between the parents, exploding into noisy fights at night, when the father became violent. Maureen and her sister, clinging together in their beds, were involuntary witnesses to these fights. The next morning everything was back to normal, like a bad dream vanishing with the dawn.

The father's family of origin was very respected in the family's home town and participated actively and prominently in its social life. Although Mr. A's father had died as a result of his excessive use of alcohol and tobacco, this did not keep his mother from looking down upon other families and thinking of her family as something special. Mrs. A's mother suffered from severe depression as a result of unresolved trauma, for which she was treated only medically. "Let us not dwell on these matters," was the motto in Mrs. A's family of origin, and this left the children with a strange feeling. Likewise, nothing about the mother's depression was allowed to become public knowledge. Mrs. A responded to her upbringing by developing an outwardly directed orientation. Concerned about order, appearance, and clothing, she often went on diets. Expressing strong emotions or having familial conflicts was not "done," because it could damage the family's smooth facade or the illusion of it. Both families of origin were strongly motivated to hide their various problems, although this was nearly impossible in a small town such as that in which they lived.

Between Maureen and her father was a feeling of attachment and similarity, which also had eroticized features. Again and again, however, this would be suddenly disrupted, as the father reacted coldly when she showed tender feelings. The feeling of attachment was also disrupted by the impulsive actions of Mr. A; these frightened Maureen, but she admired them at a deeper level because her father did not care about rules, especially those set up by the mother. On the other side, there were deep conflicts and rivalry between Maureen and Mrs. A, who often found fault with Maureen. While growing up, Maureen had the constant feeling that "I am wrong." Her mother frequently gave her new clothes to try on, but because Maureen was very thin before the onset of puberty, the clothes were too wide. With the beginning of puberty, she quickly became plump, and the clothes her mother gave her were now often too tight. She always felt she came off badly in this comparison: "My body was never the right one." Her mother now called her "Fatty." On the other hand, the family emphasized the significance of eating and the importance of all members' having a good appetite. Maureen's sister went on numerous diets.

During her high school years, Maureen became intimate with a man 5 years her senior, who praised her fantastic appearance. When she started taking birth control pills, she quickly gained weight. "That was a drastic experience. Not only my body was put out of joint; I myself grew totally insecure." Then the man left her. "The relationship was my point of orientation and stabilized me. Because I'd been dropped, I was worthless. I blamed my weight gain. I hated my body, and started dieting and forcing my good looks by vomiting. The better I look, the more I am worth. The thinner I am, the better I look." She constantly compared herself with other women and avoided looking in the mirror, fearing she was growing fat, ugly, and unpopular. In her binges she devoured "forbidden" foods such as chocolate, cake, cookies, and bread, which she "craved" after some days of restriction.

Key Concepts in Atopic Dermatitis: The Interplay between Psychological and Biological Factors

The interplay between psychological and biological factors can, with the aid of general systems theory, be understood as a series of feedback processes between the family system and the immunological and endocrinological parameters of a human being. The influence of family dynamics on an individual's immune status can be seen in the effects of stressful events on the cellular immune reaction, the consequences being higher rates of infectious illnesses and neoplasms (Ramsey, 1989). In the endocrine feedback cycles, family dynamics act as a stimulant in processing information through the brain to the endocrinologically influenced organs, which are ultimately affected. For example, family conflicts work as stressors to influence metabolism, growth, and reproductive processes.

The example of atopic dermatitis in small children illustrates how psychological parameters influence biological factors. Because a high percentage of atopic dermatitis manifests itself in infancy, the family must cope with considerable problems at the beginning of the familial life cycle—problems that then interfere with the causes of the child's symptoms. Carrying out treatment measures requires a relatively large amount of care and attention from the primary caregiver. Medication must be taken as prescribed; lotions must be applied regularly; dietary measures must often be adhered to; and/or the child must be kept away from allergenic substances. For parents who are sometimes still quite young, this means a high degree of responsibility. It is likely that functional, or otherwise less stressed, families manage the medical treatment better.

Studies have verified that emotional strain and family stress lead to increased scratching in children with atopic dermatitis, which in turn can exacerbate the illness (Jordan & Whitlock, 1972; Faulstich, Williamson, Duchmann, Conerly, & Brantley, 1985; Faulstich & Williamson, 1985). For example, a change in the autonomic level of excitement leads to disturbances in the vascular microcirculation, which in turn affect the itching and scratching. The child's chronic illness and increasing manifestation of symptoms become a burden to the family; through the above-mentioned influence of the family, a vicious circle develops.

CONCLUSIONS

To understand the dysfunctional conditions that contribute to or help maintain psychosomatic illnesses, narrower, "correlative" conditions for the examined connections must be given to specify in detail the conditions for possible occurrence (Luhmann, 1984, p. 84). In this chapter, we have described factors in the biopsychosocial model that can be regarded as dysfunctional for maintaining an individual's health. In our three-step model, we first identify at different system levels (e.g., the individual and the family) separate dysfunctional processes and possible resources, with the aid of different theories. In the second step, we look at the question of whether the individual disposition of the patient is reinforced or weakened by familial factors. Family diagnosis must include not only dysfunctional factors that contribute toward intensifying the individual's symptoms, but also the resources that promise a solution. Only in the third step do we examine the bridges between the individual and the familial factors, via key concepts.

Our three-step model contains several points that are relevant to assessing the different factors in the development or maintenance of psychosomatic illness:

1. The individual psychological and/or biological factors can occupy the foreground, while the familial dimensions, from a clinical point of view, should be taken into account but not emphasized. With regard to the development of illness, we must observe a hierarchy and differentiation of sufficient and necessary factors, whereby the pivotal factors in many "psychosomatic illnesses" (but especially in somatopsychic illnesses) are most probably not family interaction disturbances but somatic dispositions. In these cases, the family helps the individual in overcoming and dealing with illness. The resource-oriented strategy of family medicine builds on the method of supporting the individual to overcome pathology, in that the family provides or makes possible new solutions for the patient.

2. Individual and familial factors can interactively amplify each other, which may lead to escalation processes. In many cases, these interaction processes are accompanied by conflict denial. Many patients and many families thus feel "completely normal." In such cases, insight into dynamic processes and motivation for psychological change must first be developed.

3. Further interactive processes and key concepts are required for some interfaces with the social context—for example, with the health services and health insurance.

It should also be emphasized here that only the combination of different variables contributes to a higher probability that a psychosomatic illness will be manifested. Research clearly indicates that parents who (1) can be described as "warm-hearted" (i.e., tend to be emotionally positive, respond sensitively to the needs of the child, accept the child's individuality, and are open to communication with the child), and (2) exercise a moderate degree of influence and control on the child, contribute significantly to affectively balanced relationships in the family. The personality and temperament of the child, however, also have a considerable influence on the development of the relationship. Finally, in addition to these parent and child factors, the interaction effects play a major role in determining whether a family will develop as functional or dysfunctional.

Although we know a great deal about the different types of variables connected with certain psychosomatic illnesses, we still lack fundamental knowledge as to interactive processes and interactive effects between and among the variables. Research in this area should concentrate on the interfaces among individual, familial, and social factors, and between biological and psychological factors. We need to develop more key concepts concerning the particular factors and interactions that lead to maladaptive coevolutionary processes in a patient and family. Accordingly, studies must be designed to ensure that these various factors can be examined simultaneously, in order for us to arrive at a better understanding of the interaction between family dysfunctionalities and the etiology, course, and prognosis of psychosomatic illnesses.

REFERENCES

Alexander, F. (1950). *Psychosomatic medicine: Its principles and application.* London: Allen & Unwin.

Alexander, F., French, T., & Pollock, G. (1968). *Psychosomatic specificity.* Chicago: University of Chicago Press.

Antonowsky, A. (1979). *Health, stress, and coping: New perspectives on mental and physical well-being.* San Francisco: Jossey-Bass.

Arun, P., Kanwal, K., Vyas, J. N., & Sushil, C. S. (1993). Life events and irritable bowel syndrome. *Indian Journal of Clinical Psychology, 20,* 108–112.

Borysenko, J. (1989). Psychoneuroimmunology. In C. N. Ramsey (Ed.), *Family systems in medicine* (pp. 243–256). New York: Guilford Press.

Bunzel, B., & Wollenek, G. (1994). Heart transplantation: Are there psychosocial predictors for clinical success of surgery? *The Thoracic and Cardiovascular Surgeon, 42,* 103–107.

Campbell, T. (1986). Family's impact on health: A critical review and annotated bibliography. *Family Systems Medicine, 4,* 135–328.

Cierpka, M. (1982). Der juvenile Diabetiker und seine Familie. *Zeitschrift für Psychosomatische Medizin und Psychoanalyse, 28,* 363–384.

Cierpka, M. (1989). Das Problem der Spezifität in der Familientheorie. *System Familie, 2,* 197–216.

Cierpka, M. (1996). *Handbuch der Familiendiagnostik.* Heidelberg: Springer-Verlag.

Cierpka, M., & Reich, G. (1997). Die familientherapeutische Behandlung von Patientinnen mit Essstörungen. In G. Reich & M. Cierpka (Eds.), *Die Psychotherapie der Essstörungen* (pp.127–150). Stuttgart: Thieme.

Clark, N. M., Feldman, C. H., Evans, D., Millman, E. J., Wailewski, Y., & Valle, I. (1981). The effectiveness of education for family management of asthma in children: A preliminary report. *Health Education Quarterly, 8,* 166–174.

Cohen, F. (1981). Stress and bodily illness. *Psychiatric Clinics of North America, 4* 269–285.

Cohen, F., Syme, S. L. (Eds.). (1985). *Social support and health.* Orlando, FL: Academic Press.

Coyne, J. C., & Anderson, B. J. (1988). The "psychosomatic family" reconsidered: Diabetes in context. *Journal of Marital and Family Therapy, 14,* 113–123.

Doherty, W. J., & Baird, M. A. (1983). *Family therapy and family medicine.* New York: Guilford Press.

Doherty, W. J., & Campbell, T. (1988). *Families and health.* Newbury Park, CA: Sage.

Doherty, W. J., Schrott, H. G., Metcalf, L., & Iassiello-Vailas, L. (1983). Effect of spouse support and health beliefs on medication adherence. *Journal of Family Practice, 17,* 837–841.

Drossman, D. A. (1994). Irritable bowel syndrome: The role of psychosocial factors. *Stress Medicine, 10,* 45–55.

Engel, G. L. (1977). The need for a new medical model: A challenge for biomedicine. *Science, 196,* 129–136.

Engel, K. (1978). Testing cooperation in parents with children destined for home dialysis. *Psychotherapy amd Psychosomatics, 30,* 78–87.

Faulstich, M. E., & Williamson, D. A. (1985). An overview of atopic dermatitis: Towards a biobehavioral integration. *Journal of Psychosomatic Research, 29,* 647–654.

Faulstich, M. E., Williamson, D. A., Duchmann, E. G., Conerly, S. C., & Brantley, P. J. (1985). Psychophysiological analysis of atopic dermatitis. *Journal of Psychosomatic Research, 29,* 415–417.

Flor, H., & Fydrich, T. (1990). Die Rolle der Familie beim chronischen Schmerz. In H. D. Basler, C. Franz, B. Kroener-Herwig, H. P. Rehfisch, & H. P. Seemann (Eds.), *Psychologische Schmerztherapie* (pp. 135–142). Berlin: Springer-Verlag.

Forman, B. D. (1986). Citation classics in family therapy. *Journal of Marital and Family Therapy, 12,* 97–100.

Freud, S. (1962). A reply to criticisms of my paper on anxiety neurosis. In J. Strachey (Ed. and Trans.), *The standard edition of the complete psychological works of Sigmund Freud* (pp. 119–139). London: Hogarth Press. (Original work published 1895)

Friedlander, M. L., & Siegel, S. M. (1990). Separation–individuation difficulties and cognitive-behavioral indicators of eating disorders among college women. *Journal of Counseling Psychology, 37,* 74–78.

Gaddini, R. (1977). The pathology of the self as a basis of psychosomatic disorders. *Psychotherapy and Psychosomatics, 28,* 260–271.

Gottman, J. M., & Katz, L. F. (1989). Effects of marital discord on young children's peer interaction and health. *Developmental Psychology, 25,* 373–381.

Gustaffson, P. A., Kjellman, N. I., & Cederblad, M. (1986). Family therapy in the treatment of severe childhood asthma. *Journal of Psychosomatic Research, 30,* 369–374.

Habermas, T. (1990). *Heisshunger: Historische Entstehungsbedingungen der Bulimia Nervosa.* Frankfurt: Fischer.

Hauser, S. T., DiPlacido, J., & Jacobson, A. M. (1993). The family and the onset of its youngster's insulin-dependent diabetes: Ways of coping. In R. Cole & D. Reiss (Eds.), *How do families cope with chronic illness?* (pp. 25–55). Hillsdale, NJ: Erlbaum.

Humphrey, L. L. (1989a). Is there a causal link between disturbed family process and eating disorders? *Advances in Eating Disorders, 2,* 119–136.

Humphrey, L. L. (1989b). Observed family interactions among subtypes of eating disorders using Structural Analysis of Social Behavior. *Journal of Consulting and Clinical Psychology, 57,* 206–214.

Jackson, D. D., & Yalom, J. (1966). Family research on the problem of ulcerative colitis. *Archives of General Psychiatry, 15,* 410–415.

Joraschky, P. (1993). Familiendynamische und systemische Ansätze zum Schmerzverständnis. In U. Egle & S. O. Hoffmann (Eds.), *Der Schmerzkranke* (pp. 120–129). Stuttgart: Schattauer-Verlag.

Jordan J. M., & Whitlock, F. A. (1972). Emotions and the skin: The conditioning of scratch responses in cases of atopic dermatitis. *British Journal of Dermatology, 86,* 574–585.

Kog, E., & Vandereycken, W. (1989). Family interaction in eating disorder patients and normal controls. *International Journal of Eating Disorders, 8,* 11–23.

Krause, R., & Merten, J. (1996). Affekte, Beziehungsregulierung, Übertragung und Gegenübertragung. *Zeitschrift für Psychosomatische Medizin und Psychoanalyse, 42,* 261–280.

Kröger, C. (1986). *Funktionelle Darmstörungen.* Frankfurt: Verlag Peter Lang.

Lask, B., & Matthew, D. (1979). Childhood asthma: A controlled trial of family psychotherapy. *Archives of Disease in Childhood, 54,* 116–119.

Léon, G. R., Fulkerson, J. A., Perry, C. L., & Cudeck, R. (1993). Personal and behavioral vulnerabilities associated with risk status for eating disorders in adolescent girls. *Journal of Abnormal Psychology, 102,* 438–444.

Louhivuori, K., Huupponen, T., Riita, T., & Sormunen, E. (1976). Leukemic children and their families. *Psychiatria Fennica, 8,* 113–117.

Luhmann, N. (1984). *Soziale Systeme.* Frankfurt: Suhrkamp.

Lydiard, R. B. (1992). Anxiety and the irritable bowel syndrome. *Psychiatric Annals, 22,* 612–618.

Lynn, R. B., & Friedman L. S. (1993). Irritable bowel syndrome. *New England Journal of Medicine, 329,* 1940–1945.

Marty, P., de M'Uzan, M., & David, C. (1963). *L'investigation psychosomatique.* Paris: Presses Universitaires de France.

McDaniel, S., Campbell, T. L., & Seaburn, D. B. (1989). *Family-oriented primary care.* New York: Springer-Verlag.

McDaniel, S., Hepworth, J., & Doherty, W. (1992). *Medical family therapy.* New York: Basic Books.

Minuchin, S., Rosman, B., & Baker, L. (1978). *Psychosomatic families: Anorexia nervosa in context.* Cambridge, MA: Harvard University Press.

Mrazek, D. A., Klinnert, M. D., Mrazek, P., & Macey, T. (1991). Early asthma onset: Consideration of parenting issues. *Journal of the American Academy of Child and Adolescent Psychiatry, 30,* 277–282.

Onnis, L., di Gennaro, A., Cespa, G., Agostini, B., et al. (1993). Rapproche systémique et prévention de la chronicité. *Thérapie Familiale, 14,* 201–216.

Overbeck, G. (1985). *Familien mit psychosomatisch kranken Kindern: Familiendynamische Untersuchung zu Asthma bronchiale und zur Colitis ulcerosa.* Göttingen, Germany: Vandenhoeck & Ruprecht.

Pinkerton, P. (1970). The influence of sociopathology in childhood asthma. *Psychotherapy and Psychosomatics, 18,* 231–245.

Ramsey, C. N. (1989). The science of family medicine. In C. N. Ramsey (Ed.), *Family systems in medicine* (pp. 3–17). New York: Guilford Press.

Reich, G. (1992). Identitätskonflikte bulimischer Patientinnen: Klinische Beobachtungen zur inter- und intrapersonellen Dynamik. *Forum der Psychoanalyse, 8,* 121–133.

Reich, G. (1996). Familiendynamische Muster bei Magersucht und Bulimie. *Wege zum Menschen, 48,* 375–397.

Reich, G. (1997). Psychodynamische Aspekte der Bulimie und Anorexie. In G. Reich & M. Cierpka (Eds.), *Die Psychotherapie der Esstörungen* (pp. 44–60). Stuttgart: Thieme.

Reich, G., & Cierpka, M. (1998). Bulimia nervosa: Identity conflicts and psychoanalytic treatment. *Psychoanalytic Inquiry, 18,* 383–402.

Richardson, H. B. (1948). *Patients have families.* New York: Commonwealth Foundation.

Richter, H. E. (1970). *Patient Familie: Entstehung, Struktur und Therapie von Konflikten in Ehe und Familie.* Reinbek, Germany: Rowohlt.

Roberto, L. G. (1986). Bulimia: The transgenerational view. *Journal of Marital and Family Therapy, 12,* 231–240.

Rosman, B. L., & Baker, L. (1988). The "psychosomatic family" reconsidered: Diabetes in context—a reply. *Journal of Marital and Family Therapy, 14,* 125–132.

Roy, R. (1982). Marital and family issues in patients with chronic pain. *Psychotherapy and Psychosomatics, 37,* 1–12.

Schleifer, S. J., Keller, S. E., & Stein, M. (1989). Bereavement and immune function. In C. N. Ramsey (Ed.), *Family systems in medicine* (pp. 257–262). New York: Guilford Press.

Schur, M. (1955). Comments on the metapsychology of somatization. *Psychoanalytic Study of the Child, 10,* 119–164.

Selvini Palazzoli, M. (1974). *Self-starvation: From the intrapsychic to the transpersonal approach to anorexia nervosa* (A. Pomerans, Trans.). London: Chaucer. (Original work published 1963)

Silberstein, L. R., Striegel-Moore, R. H., & Rodin, J. (1987). Feeling fat: A woman's shame. In H. B. Lewis (Ed.), *The role of shame in symptom formation* (pp. 89–108). Hillsdale, NJ: Erlbaum.

Smolak, L., & Levine, M. P. (1993). Separation–individuation difficulties and the distinction between bulimia nervosa and anorexia nervosa in college women. *Internal Journal of Eating Disorders, 14,* 33–41.

Smolak, L., & Levine, M. P. (1994). Critical issues in the developmental psychopathology of eating disorders. In L. A. Alexander-Mott & B. D. Lumsden (Eds.), *Understanding eating disorders* (pp. 37–60). London: Taylor & Francis.

Sperling, E. (1983). Beobachtungen in Familien mit chronischem Leiden. *Familiendynamik, 8*, 32–47.

Stierlin, H., Wirsching, M., Haas, B., Hoffmann, F., Schmidt, G., Weber, G., & Wirsching, B. (1983). Familienmedizin mit Krebskranken. *Familiendynamik, 8*, 48–68.

Strober, M. (1991). Disorders of self in anorexia nervosa: An organismic–developmental paradigm. In C. L. Johnson (Ed.), *Psychodynamic treatment of anorexia nervosa and bulimia* (pp. 354–373). New York: Guilford Press.

Teusch, R. (1988). Levels of ego development and bulimics' conceptualizations of their disorder. *International Journal of Eating Disorders, 7*, 607–615.

Toner, B. B., Garfinkel, P. E., Jeejeebhoy, K. N., Scher, H., et al. (1990). Self-schema in irritable bowel syndrome and depression. *Psychosomatic Medicine, 52*, 149–155.

Turk, D. C., & Kerns, R. D. (1985). *Health, illness, and families: A life-span perspective.* New York: Wiley.

Vandereycken, W., Kog, E., & Vanderlinden, E. (Eds.). (1989). *The family approach to eating disorders.* New York: PMA.

von Bertalanffy, L. (1956). General systems theory. In *General systems yearbook* (Vol. 1). New York: George Braziller.

von Bertalanffy, L. (1962). General systems theory: A critical review. In *General systems yearbook* (Vol. 7). New York: George Braziller.

Waller, G., & Rachel, C. (1994). Parenting and family factors in eating problems. In L. A. Alexander-Mott & B. D. Lumsden (Eds.), *Understanding eating disorders* (pp. 61–76). London: Taylor & Francis.

Wirsching, M. (1984). Familientherapeutische Aspekte bei Colitis ulcerosa und Morbus Crohn. *Zeitschrift für Psychosomatische Medizin und Psychoanalyse, 30*, 238–246.

Wirsching, M. (1996). Familiendynamik und Familientherapie. In T. Uexkuell (Ed.), *Psychosomatische Medizin* (pp. 441–449). Munich: Urban & Schwarzenberg.

Wirsching, M., & Stierlin, H. (1982). *Krankheit und Familie.* Stuttgart: Klett.

Wood, B. (1991). Beyond the "psychosomatic family": A biobehavioral family model of pediatric illness. *Family Process, 32*, 261–278.

Wood, B. (1994). One articulation of the structural family therapy model: A biobehavioral family model of chronic illness in children. *Journal of Family Therapy, 16*, 53–72.

Wood, B., Watkins, J. B., Boyle, J. T., Nogueira, J., Zimand, E., & Carroll, L. (1989). The "psychosomatic family" model: An empirical and theoretical analysis. *Family Process, 28*, 399–417.

CHAPTER 14

The Family Roots of Aggression and Violence: A Life Span Perspective

KAREN H. ROSEN

This chapter provides a life span perspective on one of society's most pernicious problems—violence. Violent crime is a serious public health crisis, as well as a criminal justice problem (Campbell, 1995). The economic cost to victims is estimated at $100 billion per year; perhaps even worse, violent crime depresses the human spirit, wastes lives, and erodes confidence in our social system (Earls & Reiss, 1994). Unfortunately, for all too many people the home itself is not a "safe haven." In recent years, family violence, which was previously ignored as "private," has been recognized as a serious societal problem. Every day women are assaulted by spouses, children are assaulted by parents, and the elderly are assaulted by spouses or adult children within the confines of home. Many argue that understanding the developmental origins of violence is critical to diminishing its occurrence. Scholarly research plays a vital role in this effort. This chapter is an extensive review of research since the mid-1980s investigating the family roots of aggression and violence—both street violence and family violence—over the life span.

Violence has been studied from a multitude of theoretical perspectives. Macrotheories suggest that broad cultural forces (e.g., cultural acceptance, patriarchy, other social-structural factors) promote or allow violence to occur (Barnett, Miller-Perrin, & Perrin, 1997). Microtheories attempt to explain violent behavior by means of social learning, intrapersonal (e.g., psychopathological, psychological, and biological), interpersonal (e.g., dyadic stress, attachment problems, social exchange), or multidimensional (e.g., biopsychological, developmental–ecological) theories. The intergenerational transmission process, positing that violent behavior is passed from violent parents to children via social learning, is perhaps the most widely accepted explanation for the development of violent behavior (Widom, 1989a). However, although there is evidence that the intergenerational transmission of violence is a significant factor in the development of violent behavior, some have questioned its predictive strength (Kaufman & Zigler, 1993). Indeed, many theoretical perspectives are useful to an understanding of how violent behavior develops. However, few would argue with the notion that the family is a critical determinant of an individual's level of violence—whether it be via social learning or another avenue. The emphasis in this chapter is on the family roots of aggression. What is happening or has happened in an individual's family that seems to influence his or her tendency to be violent? Although the intergenerational transmission perspective is evident in many of the studies reviewed, the chapter considers a broad range of family dynamics and mechanisms of transmission. Genetic inheritance, another important aspect of a familial explanation (DiLalla & Gottesman, 1991), is addressed only to the extent that it is a component of multidimensional studies (i.e., studies that address both nature and nurture).

There is a lack of consensus regarding the definition and measurement of "violence," "aggression," or "violent crime," and this impedes the consolidation of research findings (Arias & Pape, 1994). For the purposes of this chapter, "violent acts" are defined as acts that are carried out with an actual or perceived intent to harm another person. The focus here is on the commission of physically violent acts. Although certainly psychological or sexual assault constitute violence, I have not included the extensive body of research investigating the family roots of these kinds of violence, because of space limitations.

I have tried to select studies that are methodologically robust. However, in general, studies of the development of aggression and violence have serious methodological shortcomings (Mash & Wolfe, 1991; Widom, 1989b). One problem lies in the lack of specificity and continuity in defining predictor and outcome variables. What constitutes child abuse, physical abuse, and delinquent behavior, and how these variables are measured, vary from one study to the next. Research in this area also often fails to use adequate control groups or to consider statistical base rates. Another problem is the use of weak sampling techniques involving convenience rather than representative samples, and thus detracting from the generalizability of the findings. Furthermore, studies are often retrospective or based on secondhand information rather than direct observation; this leaves them open to a number of potential biases and results in little predictive power. For many of the studies reviewed, I highlight methodological strengths, such as the use of control groups, representative sampling, or prospective designs.

AGGRESSIVE CHILDREN

From 14% to 73% of preschoolers have mild to severe behavioral problems, many of which include aggressive acting-out behaviors (Landy & Peters, 1992). Children's aggressive behavior is manifested both in the home toward parents or siblings and outside the home toward peers or authority figures. It has long been recognized that the family, where children are nurtured and socialized, plays an important role in their development and functioning. This section focuses on studies that investigate the relationship between children's aggressive behavior on the one hand, and parental child-rearing practices, both witnessing and receiving abuse, and broad family relationship factors on the other.

Parental Child-Rearing Practices

Harsh or abusive parental discipline is a parental child-rearing practice often linked to children's aggressive behavior. Being abused or neglected as a child increases one's risk of developing aggressive behavior. In a longitudinal study of 172 at-risk mother–child dyads, Egeland (1991) found a relationship between the early development of aggressive behavior in children and different patterns of maltreatment by mothers. Children whose mothers were physically abusive or psychologically unavailable were significantly more aggressive than children of mothers in other groups (verbally abusive and "good caretakers"), even when socioeconomic status (SES), life stress, school quality, and selected child characteristics were controlled for.

However, the relationship between physical punishment and children's aggressive behavior appears to be mediated by positive parent–child interaction. For example, in a large, nationally representative sample of parents and children, the relationship between physical punishment and children's aggressive behavior toward parents and siblings was mediated by parental discussion (Larzelere, 1986). The combination of frequent spanking and minimal discussion was highly associated with aggression toward parents. Similarly, in a more recent study, the relationship between children's maladjustment (including aggressive behavior) and their parents' harsh discipline was mediated by children's perception of their caretakers' acceptance (Rohner, Bourque, & Elordi, 1996).

Deviant or dysfunctional social information processing (SIP)—that is, the likelihood of attributing hostile intent in ambiguous situations and of not developing competent solutions to interpersonal problems—is a mechanism that links children's early socializing experiences and their aggressive behavior. Physical abuse received at home was predictive of both later child aggression and the development of dysfunctional SIP patterns in three prospective studies (Dodge, Bates, & Pettit, 1990; Dodge, Pettit, Bates, & Valente, 1995; Weiss, Dodge, Bates, & Pettit, 1992). As children became more deviant in their SIP patterns in response to early harsh discipline, they became more aggressive toward peers. In each of these three studies, a variety of contextual factors (e.g., SES, family structure, family life stressors, parent–parent conflict) and child factors (e.g., child temperament, medical problems) were controlled for. Interestingly, parental coercion and intrusiveness were also positively related to children's aggressive behavior and deviant SIP (Pettit, Harriest, Bates, & Dodge, 1991).

Dodge and his colleagues have associated the degree of physical punishment experienced at home and children's deviant SIP for subgroups of aggressive children. One subgroup of aggressive boys, labeled "reactively aggressive," tended to be hypervigilant to threat and to attribute hostile intentions to peers, whom they attacked at the slightest provocation (Dodge, 1991). Another group, labeled "proactively aggressive," tended to have deficits in the decision-making phase of SIP and to evaluate the outcomes of aggression positively. In a longitudinal study of a diverse group of preschoolers, children who were punished very harshly by their mothers had higher rates of both reactive and proactive (bullying) aggression than children who were just spanked (Strassberg, Dodge, Pettit, & Bates, 1994). However, boys spanked by fathers displayed the highest rates of bullying aggression. Apparently, paternal spanking has an additional meaning for boys—that of gender-based physical dominance.

Patterson (1986) proposed a process model to explain the development of aggression in children. According to the model, ineffective, coercive parental discipline that does not appropriately manage children's aggressive behavior inadvertently contributes to the increase of this behavior, often across contexts. One context is the home through fighting with siblings, who in effect provide in the home "training" for aggressive behavior. This theory was supported by several studies conducted by Patterson and colleagues (cited in Patterson, 1986). It was also supported by a nationwide study in which physically abused children were found to be more likely to attack a sibling than nonabused children; this suggests a vicious cycle in which children who are spanked because they aggress against siblings become even more aggressive toward siblings, and so on (Straus, 1994).

Witnessing Interparental Violence and Receiving Parental Abuse

Although witnessing interparental violence alone is related to children's aggression (Jaffe, Wolfe, Wilson, & Zak, 1986), there is probably a cumulative effect of receiving a "double whammy"—that is, both witnessing and receiving parental abuse—on children's aggressive behavior. In a small sample of at-risk children, witnesses of interparental violence who were also abused had more externalizing behavior problems (aggression, hostility, noncompliance) than children in the comparison groups (witnesses only and a no-witnessing, no-abuse control group) (Sternberg et al., 1993).

In another study, the more frequent and severe the marital violence witnessed and mother-to-child aggression experienced, the more aggressive the children, even when the effects of child age, race, and SES were controlled for (O'Keefe, 1994).

Cummings, Hennessy, Rabideau, and Cicchetti (1994) developed a process-based understanding of the relationship among parental abuse, interparental conflict, and children's aggression. In their experimental study of 12 abused boys and a matched sample of 12 nonabused boys (all witnesses to interparental aggression), abused boys were more reactive than comparison boys to interadult anger. That is, observing anger directed toward their mothers under experimental conditions triggered abused boys' impulsive, aggressive responses to a greater degree than those of the control group. Conflicts between adults may be more threatening for physically abused boys because they foster their hypervigilance, angry arousal, and aggression.

Familial Relationship Factors

The family roots of aggression in children are not limited to harsh discipline or interparental violence. Several different family relationship factors have been associated with the development of aggression in children. In a longitudinal study, eight factors in preschool children's familial and social context (i.e., harsh discipline, lack of maternal warmth, exposure to aggressive adult models, maternal aggressive values, family life stressors, lack of maternal support, lack of maternal cognitive stimulation, and peer group instability) significantly predicted teacher-rated and peer-rated aggression in kindergarten through third grade (Dodge, Pettit, & Bates, 1994). In another longitudinal study, although fathers' harsh discipline was the strongest predictor of preschool boys' initial clinic referral (for aggression among other behavior problems), fathers' life stress and levels of positive involvement with sons were most closely associated with the stability of behavior problems a year later (DeKlyen, Biernbaum, Speltz, & Greenberg, 1998).

Other researchers have identified mother–child interaction quality as an important factor in the development of externalizing behavior in young children. For a large sample of first-grade children, the effects of maternal depression on child externalizing behavior problems were partially mediated by the quality of mother–child interaction, even when the effect of SES was controlled for (Harnish, Dodge, & Valente, 1995). In another study, the quality of mother–child interaction mediated the effects of overt marital conflict on older siblings' tendency to behave aggressively toward younger siblings (Erel, Margolin, & John, 1998). Furthermore, in a longitudinal study, a broad measure of the quality of the parent–child relationship (including parental depression, attachment to child, restriction caused by parenting role, social isolation, and relationship to spouse) was related to children's aggressive behavior (Dubow & Reid, 1994).

Various family relationship factors were found to be relevant to the development of bullying behavior in the school setting. For a sample of 20 bullies, 20 victims, 20 children who were both bullies and victims, and 20 controls, the bullies were more likely than the other groups to lack a father figure, to express a concern for power, to perceive a lack of family cohesion, and to have negative relationships with siblings (Bowers, Smith, & Binney, 1994). In addition, the bully/victims rated their parents highest on overprotection and neglect, and lowest on accurate monitoring.

The results of a meta-analysis of parental caregiving and children's externalizing behavior suggest that parental caregiving variables are interrelated and are in fact aspects of a broader construct, acceptance/responsiveness (Rothbaum & Weisz, 1994). Apparently, parents who are accepting of and responsive to their children tend to have children who learn to seek control in appropriate ways. On the other hand, parents who are rejecting and unresponsive increase their children's learning of and motivation to use inappropriate, aggressive behavior.

AGGRESSIVE ADOLESCENTS AND YOUNG ADULTS

A small but significant minority of adolescents commit violent crimes. In a national sample of high school seniors, 22.2% had participated in a group fight, 17.7% had been involved in a serious fight at school or work, 13.4% had hurt someone badly enough to cause that person to need medical care, 4.6% had used a weapon against someone, and 3.6% had hit an instructor or supervisor (U.S. Department of Justice, 1993). Approximately 10% of adolescents attack a parent each year, 3.5% doing so severely. Two-thirds of U.S. adolescents assault a sibling at least once during the course of a year, one-third doing so severely (Straus & Gelles, 1990). The disturbing prevalence of adolescent violence has inspired a number of empirical studies investigating the familial roots of adolescent aggression.

Violent Delinquents

Research evidence consistently points to a relationship between aggressive juvenile delinquency and witnessing or experiencing violence in the family context. For example, when family backgrounds and psychoneurological evaluations of juvenile murderers, violent delinquents, and nonviolent delinquents were compared, both violent groups were much more likely than the nonviolent delinquent group to have a history of physical abuse and other family violence (Lewis et al., 1988). They also tended to be more impulsive, emotionally reactive, and cognitively impaired, suggesting that a "combination of serious vulnerabilities in the context of an abusive or violent environment" (Lewis et al., 1988, p. 587) is involved in the development of adolescent aggression.

In a large prospective study of abused and a matched sample of nonabused individuals, being abused and neglected significantly increased the risk of violent offending, particularly for males and blacks (Rivera & Widom, 1990). Furthermore, the abused and neglected subjects tended to begin their delinquent careers earlier than the nonabused. In fact, being abused or neglected as a child increased the likelihood of arrest as a juvenile by 53% and of arrest for a violent crime by 35% (Widom, 1992).

Delinquent behavior has also been linked to being spanked by parents. In a survey of 385 college students, participants who were punished physically (not necessarily abused) by their parents were more likely than those who did not experience corporal punishment to be involved in both violent crime and property crime (Straus, 1994). Corporal punishment was also related to delinquency in a national sample, even when interparental violence was controlled for, although the "double whammy" of both witnessing and experiencing aggression in the family context did increase the likelihood of delinquency.

However, Simons, Johnson, and Conger (1994) contend that it is not corporal punishment per se that fosters adolescents' maladjustment, but related dimensions of parenting. These researchers examined the impact of harsh corporal punishment and quality of parental involvement on adolescent aggressiveness, delinquency, and psychological well-being in a longitudinal study of 332 families. The quality of parental involvement was related to all three adolescent outcomes, whereas corporal punishment was not, once the effect of parental involvement was removed.

Patterson and his colleagues have developed an "early-starter" model for predicting juvenile delinquency that extends the process model discussed in the previous section on aggressive children (Patterson & Yoerger, 1993). According to the early-starter model, ineffective, coercive parent–child interaction patterns reinforce and solidify aggressive behavior in children, leading to early rejection by normal peers and failure in the school setting. This chain of events sets these young persons on a path toward the early onset of delinquency. Patterson and his colleagues found partial support for this model in the preliminary analyses of a 7-year longitudinal study of high-risk boys (Patterson, Capaldi, & Bank, 1991; Patterson, Crosby, & Vuchinich, 1992). Delinquency measured in early adolescence was predicted by lack of parental monitoring, association with deviant peers, and antisocial behaviors measured in the fourth grade. Although Patterson's group's work has employed samples of white males, ineffective parental supervision has also been related to violent crime in adolescent black males (Kruttschnitt & Dornfeld, 1991).

A series of prospective studies also lends credence to Patterson's model. In these studies, early influences on becoming delinquent were economic deprivation, family criminality, parental mishandling, and school failure; later influences were truancy, delinquent friends, antiestablishment attitudes, and unstable job records (Farrington, 1986, 1991, 1994). Delinquent youth were identified as troublesome, daring, dishonest, and aggressive by teachers, peers, and parents at an early age.

Aggressive Nondelinquents

Two recent studies of college students found a link between family conflict or violence and aggression in adolescents or young adults not labeled delinquent. For the males in a study of 300 college students, violence expressed toward sisters, observing interparental violence, and the severity of interparental violence were related to use of violence with peers (Mangold & Koski, 1990). For females, only being violent with brothers and witnessing mother-to-father violence were related to their being aggressive with peers. In another sample, violence expressed toward peers was predicted by a history of interparental violence (Cantrell, MacIntyre, Sharkey, & Thompson, 1995). Fathers appeared to be more powerful models of violent behavior, since father-to-mother violence predicted all combinations of peer violence for both men and women, whereas mother-to-father violence demonstrated a less consistent predictive pattern.

Forehand and his colleagues investigated the relationship between adolescent externalizing behavior and several family stressors, including family conflict, divorce, and maternal functioning. Marital conflict (nonviolent conflict) occurring in front of the child, general family conflict, and divorce were related to externalizing behavior problems, particularly for adolescent boys (David, Steels, Forehand, & Armistead, 1996; Tannenbaum, Neighbors, & Forehand, 1992). Poor maternal functioning (e.g., depression) and poor parenting skills were mechanisms through which parental divorce was associated with adolescent dysfunction (Forehand, Thomas, Wierson, Brody, & Fauber, 1990). However, in a prospective study, increased levels of maternal depression (regardless of marital status) led to increased levels of later adolescent aggression (Thomas, Forehand, & Neighbors, 1995). Apparently, a stressor like divorce or marital conflict may make parents more irritable and depressed, and less likely to be positive and responsive to their children's behavior problems. However, the negative impact of poor maternal functioning on adolescent functioning was buffered by a positive adolescent–father relationship (Tannenbaum & Forehand, 1994).

Dating Violence

A number of recent studies using college student samples examined the link between witnessing interparental violence and battering in premarital relationships. In one sample of 408 students, this was true for both males and females, but the effect was stronger for men if their mothers had been violent toward their fathers (Breslin, Riggs, O'Leary, & Arias, 1990). In another study of 289 students, witnessing more severe forms of interparental aggression was related to males' use of aggression, but not females' (Gwartney-Gibbs, Stockard, & Bohmer, 1987). In contrast, DeMaris (1990) found that only the females and black males in a sample of 536 tended to behave aggressively toward their partners when they had witnessed interparental violence.

However, several studies found no direct relationship between witnessing interparental violence and perpetrating violence in a dating relationship, for either men or women (Carlson, 1990; Follette & Alexander, 1992; Marshall & Rose, 1990; Tontodonato & Crew, 1992). Alexander, Moore, and Alexander (1991) offer a partial explanation for this contradictory evidence. In their study, the relationship between witnessing interparental violence and using aggression was mediated by men's and women's gender role attitudes. The men who witnessed marital violence tended to have more conservative attitudes toward women, whereas the female witnesses of interparental aggression had more liberal attitudes. Interestingly, women with liberal attitudes were more likely to be abused if their boyfriends had more conservative attitudes about women. Other mediating variables are SES, exposure to community or school violence, acceptance of violence in dating relationships, poor school performance, experiencing child abuse, and low self-esteem, according to a study of high school students who witnessed interparental violence (O'Keefe, 1998).

The relationship between sustaining violence in the family of origin and using aggression toward one's premarital partner has also been investigated. In two studies, receiving abuse or harsh discipline as a child was related to perpetuating abuse for men, but not for women (Alexander et al., 1991; Marshall & Rose, 1988). These gender differences were reversed in two other studies (Follette & Alexander, 1992; Marshall & Rose, 1990). In two additional studies, women's experience of parent-to-child aggression and their expression of aggression toward boyfriends were significantly correlated. However, in neither study were these variables significant when they were subjected to multivariate analyses that included other contextual variables (Tontodonato & Crew, 1992; Riggs, O'Leary, & Breslin, 1990).

In recent work (Rosen, Bartle-Haring, & Stith, 1996), we attempted to clarify these inconsistent findings. We found evidence to support the notion that in addition to family-of-origin violence, individual and family differentiation levels (boundary maintenance; Bowen, 1978) are intergenerational processes that relate to dating violence. Using structural equation modeling, we found that couple differentiation, which was influenced by both family-of-origin violence and individual differentiation levels, was the best predictor of current violence. Although being hit by one's parents also had direct effects on perpetrating violence, its effect was partially mediated by couple differentiation.

Parental divorce also seems to relate to the use of aggression by young adults in premarital relationships. In one study, the men who had experienced their parents' divorce were more likely both to be violent toward and to receive violence from their partners (Billingham & Gilbert, 1990). No gender effects were found in a second study, where both males and females from divorced families were more violent toward and received more violence from their partners than students from intact families (Billingham & Notebaert, 1993). These researchers concluded that coming from a divorced family may affect later relationships, either through ineffective conflict resolution skills or through the type of person selected as a partner.

Aggression Expressed toward Family Members

Hotaling, Straus, and Lincoln (1990) hypothesize not only that family assault trains children to be violent, but that some of that violent behavior is directed toward parents. In a large, representative sample of families, these researchers found heightened child assaults against parents in "mulltiassaultive" families (families where children both were assaulted by parents and observed assaults between parents). The rate of child violence against parents was 18 times higher in the multiassaultive families than in families where only one form of assault occurred. Furthermore, in a recent study of 469 college students, childhood experiences of parental violence were highly predictive of using aggressive tactics with parents, whereas maltreatment by people outside the family had almost no effect on respondents' behavior (Browne & Hamilton, 1998). In another study, the severity of adolescent-to-parent violence was directly related to the severity of violence adolescents experienced and witnessed within their families (Gelles & Cornell, 1987). Both sons and daughters were more likely to use severe violence toward mothers who were abused by their husbands, but were unlikely to aggress against their fathers. regardless of variations in family structure, SES, or stress levels.

In contrast, two studies found little support for the theory that adolescent-to-parent violence is related to violence witnessed or experienced within the family of origin. In a sample of at-risk adolescents, males who observed interparental violence were only somewhat more likely to hit their mothers than those who did not observe interparental violence. Instead, they were significantly more likely to run away or to have suicidal thoughts (Carlson, 1990). For females, family-of-origin violence was unrelated to either their behavior or their emotional well-being. Indeed, the effect of growing up in violent homes seems to be partially mediated by other factors such as connectedness to patents, especially for females (DeVet, 1997). In a national sample, adolescents who assaulted their parents were more likely to be white, to approve of violence, to believe that official consequences for their behavior were unlikely, to have friends who assaulted parents, and to be weakly attached to their parents (Agnew & Huguley, 1989). Thus, the family roots of these adolescents' aggression were indirect (approval of violence, lack of attachment toward parents, and lack of respect for authority) rather than direct (family-of-origin violence).

AGGRESSIVE ADULTS

Adults commit violent crimes against strangers and against family members of all ages at all stages of the family life cycle. Crimes of assault, homicide, armed robbery, and rape are committed by adults daily in the public sector. However, perhaps the most common form of violence is that committed by adults against their own family members. Approximately 90% of 3 to 4-year-olds are physically punished by their parents (Wauchope & Straus, 1990), with 1.5 million children being seriously assaulted each year in the United States (Gelles & Straus, 1990). Spouse abuse also occurs at alarming rates. Approximately 8.7 million couples experience at least one assault each year (Straus & Gelles, 1990). Of these violent experiences, 3.4 million are incidents that have a high risk of causing injury. Couple violence is not limited to heterosexual couples: The frequency of physical abuse in lesbian relationships varies from 25% to 47% (Renzetti, 1995), while an estimated 500,000 gay men are victims of abuse each year (Island & Letellier, 1991). Finally, elder abuse has generated significant public concern in the last decade (Gelles & Cornell, 1990). Approximately 3.2% of the elderly experience some form of abuse or neglect each year, with 2% experiencing physical abuse, most of which is perpetrated by spouses or adult children (Pillemer & Finkelhor, 1988).

Violent Criminals

Two prospective studies have linked experiencing abuse in the family of origin with adult criminal behavior. McCord (1988) compared the criminal records of at-risk boys who grew up in aggressive, nonaggressive, and punitive intact families. Families were comparable in terms of type of neighborhood, parental affection, and supervision. By middle age, almost 48% of the men raised in aggressive homes (homes where parents were frequently in conflict with each other, and at least one parent was generally aggressive) had been convicted of a violent crime, as compared to 27% of those reared in punitive homes (homes where at least one parent used physical punishment, but parents were not generally aggressive or in conflict with each other) and 13% from nonaggressive homes—a significant difference. Similarly, Widom (1989a) compared the adult criminal records of abused and neglected children and matched controls. The abused or neglected subjects were significantly more likely to have a criminal record at age 32 (28%) than the control group (21%). Furthermore, males who were abused as children had a significantly higher rate of arrests for violent crime (15.6%) than control group males (10.2%).

Similar results were obtained in a retrospective study of a large, nationally representative sample of adults (Straus, 1994). Adults who were hit (not necessarily abused) as teens were more likely to have physically assaulted someone outside the family, even when SES was controlled for.

For both men and women in the sample, as the frequency of physical punishment increased, the incidents of assault outside the family increased. Witnessing violence between one's parents was also associated with assaultive behavior toward nonfamily members and with increased arrest rates (Straus, 1992). However, this relationship was stronger for men than for women. Assaultive behavior outside the family was two or three times greater among men who witnessed interparental violence than among those who did not witness interparental violence.

In a large-scale longitudinal study, the best predictor of adult aggression was early aggression (Eron, Huesmann, & Zelli, 1991). Although the effects of parental rejection, punishment for aggression, and the degree of parental identification (measured at age 8) were related to children's aggression, early child-rearing styles were not predictive of aggression at age 30, once early aggression was accounted for. Based on these and prior results, Eron and colleagues argued that the tendency to be aggressive develops at a very young age (prior to age 6), in part from parental behavior and attitudes, and becomes very resistant to change as children grow older.

Three studies have examined the effects of biological factors, character traits, and family environmental precursors of adult criminal behavior. All three kinds of factors were implicated in a longitudinal study of boys from working-class families. The best independent predictors of convictions for violent criminal behavior at age 32 were restlessness at 12–14 years of age, parents with authoritarian child-rearing attitudes at 12, an unemployed father at 14, daring behavior at ages 8–10, and low parental interest in education at age 8 (Farrington, 1994).

In a follow-up study of 95 formerly incarcerated delinquents, the combination of intrinsic vulnerabilities (cognitive, psychiatric, and neurological) and history of family violence led to increased risk and severity of adult violent criminality (Lewis, Lovely, Yeager, & Femina, 1989). Lewis and colleagues contend that children who are neuropsychiatrically and cognitively intact are better equipped than those who are multiply handicapped to resist family models of aggressive behavior, to choose among alternative styles, and to make rational judgments regarding appropriate behavior. Furthermore, abuse may engender a kind of rage that neuropsychiatrically and cognitively impaired children find difficult to control. Severe abuse may even create psychiatric, neurological, and cognitive vulnerability; moreover, ironically, impaired children may invite further abuse.

McCord (1994) conducted a longitudinal study of two generations of 149 families to investigate genetic and environmental factors involved in the intergenerational transmission of criminality. Although McCord found no direct genetic link to criminal behavior, criminal fathers apparently tended to create the social environment conducive to developing aggressive behavior in sons, primarily through parental conflict. However, McCord asserts that "whatever genetic makeup has been passed from father to son ought to be viewed as providing susceptibilities or potentialities which require social condition for their expression in terms of crime" (1994, p. 248).

Child Abusers

Several recent studies provide evidence supporting the intergenerational transmission of child abuse. In a national sample, there was a significant relationship between experiencing corporal punishment as a teenager and abusing one's children (Straus & Kantor, 1994). The more corporal punishment subjects experienced, the greater the risk of their physically abusing their children. In fact, when corporal punishment was entered into the regression equation, parental SES, gender, age, and alcohol misuse were not significantly related to child abuse. Furthermore, parents who witnessed interparental violence were also more likely to abuse their own children, and the likelihood increased if both parents were violent toward each other (Straus, 1992). Similar results were obtained by taking a different methodological approach. For a sample of college students, childhood history of physical abuse was related to adult physical abuse potential (Milner, Robertson, & Rogers, 1990). Individuals who experienced physical abuse before puberty had higher abuse potential scores than those who experienced physical abuse after puberty. Increases in abuse severity also tended to be associated with increases in abuse potential. Not surprisingly, individuals who both observed and received abuse had the greatest abuse potential.

In a prospective study of 267 economically disadvantaged mothers, there was a 40% transmission rate of maltreatment across generations (Egeland, 1993). That is, 40% of the mothers who were abused as children were maltreating their own children. Although the history of abuse was a major risk factor, Egeland noted that it did not guarantee that abuse would occur in the next generation. A history of being maltreated as a child, the experience of life stress, lack of support, and the tendency to form dysfunctional interpersonal relationships were all part of the context of child maltreatment (Pianta, Egeland, & Erickson, 1989).

Several other studies have examined the broader family contexts of abusive families. In a sample of 888 intact child-rearing families, wife abuse was related to child abuse, and both were related to mothers' negative family-of-origin experiences (Cappell & Heiner, 1990). Women who had witnessed and experienced aggression in their families of origin were both more vulnerable to being hit by their husbands and more likely to hit their children. Similarly, in maritally violent homes, the frequency and severity of marital violence and the level of marital satisfaction were related to the incidence of child abuse (O'Keefe, 1995), as was parental disagreement about child-rearing practices (Trickett & Susman, 1989). Low SES, conflict, controlling/punitive discipline, and a negative emotional climate described the ecology of abusive homes (Trickett, Aber, Carlson, & Cicchetti, 1991).

The mechanisms of intergenerational transmission of child abuse have also been investigated. Straus (1991) suggested that approval of violence may link experiencing or witnessing violence as a child with becoming violent toward one's children as an adult. This hypothesis was supported by a path analysis in which corporal punishment received as a teenager was linked to the approval of interpersonal violence and then to harshly punishing one's own children (Straus, 1994). In fact, parents who approved of slapping a teenager who talks back reported hitting their teenagers about four times more often than parents who did not approve of such behavior (Straus, 1991). Similarly, in a study of abusive, intact families and matched controls, attitudes and values about child rearing, particularly as these related to harsh discipline, were related to child abuse (Trickett & Susman, 1989).

In contrast, in a large sample of low-risk rural families, there was only weak support for the contention that harsh parenting teaches a parenting philosophy that fosters the use of harsh discipline (Simons, Whitbeck, Conger, & Chyi-In, 1991). Instead, direct modeling (i.e., the idea that parenting practices are learned and reflexive) was the strongest explanation of the intergenerational transmission of harsh discipline. In another study, neither violence received as a child nor perceptions of the fairness of parents' punishment were associated with parental approval of corporal punishment as an adult (Ringwalt, Browne, Rosenbloom, Evans, & Kotch, 1989). Rather, mothers who saw themselves as having been poorly nurtured by their own mothers tended to express greater approval of corporal punishment.

In addition to familial risk factors associated with abusive parenting, protective factors have been identified. Childhood experience of a caring adult (Milner et al., 1990), and parental or sibling support (Caliso & Milner, 1994) apparently mediate the influence of childhood abuse on adult abuse potential. The intergenerational transmission process also appears to vary as a function of marital quality. In a study of middle- and working-class mothers, both mothers who had positive childhood experiences and those who had negative experiences had positive maternal affect toward their children when marital quality was high (Belsky, Youngblade, & Pensky, 1990).

Spouse Abusers

Much of the recent research on the family roots of spouse abuse investigate the relationship of witnessing or experiencing abuse as a child to perpetrating abuse as an adult. Like the research on dating violence, the research on the connection between witnessing violence in the family of origin and marital battering is compelling but inconsistent. Several recent studies found that males who observed interparental violence were more likely to behave aggressively toward their spouses (Choice, Lamke, & Pittman, 1995; Howell & Publiesi, 1988; Straus, 1992, 1994). In one study, the effect of witnessing abuse was stronger for men if their mothers had been violent toward their fathers (Straus, 1994). Females who witness interparental aggression are also more likely to aggress against their partners (Straus, 1992).

In contrast, Cappell and Heiner (1990) did not find a relationship between witnessing interparental violence and battering. For a national random sample of 2,143 couples, witnessing interparental violence predicted vulnerability to receiving aggression rather than perpetrating aggression, for both males and females. Several other studies found little support for the intergenerational transmission of violence via witnessing interparental abuse (Williams, 1989; MacEwen & Barling, 1988; Russell & Hulson, 1992).

In a nationally representative sample, wife beating was significantly related to receiving corporal punishment (not necessarily abuse) as an adolescent even when low SES, age, and alcohol misuse were controlled for (Straus, 1994; Straus & Kantor, 1994). Furthermore, ordinary corporal punishment and witnessing interparental violence had an additive affect for those men who had experienced both in their family of origin. In contrast, several studies found no relationship between experiencing violence as a child and expressing violence toward one's spouse, for either men or women (Cappell & Heiner, 1990; MacEwen & Barling, 1988; Russell & Hulson, 1992).

Several studies shed light on some of the differential effects that family-of-origin violence may have on men. In a study comparing maritally violent men with nonviolent control groups, all witnessing interparental violence, nonviolent men were less likely than violent men to view their mothers as victims in the fights they witnessed between their parents (Caesar, 1988). They also had a more balanced view of parental shortcomings, were less protective of violent parents, and had better coping mechanisms. In contrast, batterers appeared to ally with one parent or the other, and some had unrealized rescue fantasies. In another study, men who witnessed interparental violence were more likely to use ineffective conflict resolution strategies, leading to greater marital stress and wife battering (Choice et al., 1995). Observation of interparental violence also seems to have a negative effect on men's self-esteem, which increases the likelihood of marital distress, alcoholism, and the approval of violence (Stith & Farley, 1993). For both men and women, experiencing corporal punishment was also associated with depression, approval of hitting one's spouse, heightened levels of marital conflict, and physically assaulting one's spouse (Straus & Yodanis, 1996). Thus, individuals who have observed or experienced violence in their families of origin may have an increased likelihood of being violent toward their spouses, through psychological as well as social learning processes.

The results of other studies also suggest that the effects of abusive family-of-origin experiences may go beyond modeling abusive behavior. In a sample of court-referred and self-referred wife assaulters, shame-proneness was related to anger arousal and a tendency to blame others for one's own behavior (Dutton, van Ginkel, & Starzomski, 1995). Apparently significant childhood shame experiences lead to disturbances in self-identity and a sense of rage, while parental physical abuse experiences provide the modeling that determines how these disturbances are expressed. Similarly, in a study of wife assaulters and matched controls, parental rejection and abuse predicted the development of an abusive personality syndrome characterized by fearful attachment and identity diffusion (Dutton, Starzomski, & Ryan, 1996). These men were susceptible to self-generated rage related to perceptions of abandonment. Excessive dependency, fear of abandonment, relationship-dependent self-esteem, and jealousy have been related to marital violence in other studies as well (Barnett, Martinez, & Bluestein, 1995; Murphy, Meyer, & O'Leary, 1994).

Aggressive Homosexual Partners

Violence among gay and lesbian couples has largely been ignored by family violence researchers (Lockhart, White, Causby, & Isaac, 1994). However, the research that has been conducted seems to indicate that some of the same risk factors for abuse in heterosexual couples are also predictors of lesbian battering, such as substance misuse, conflict centering around attachment and power imbalances, and violence in the family of origin (Lockhart et al., 1994; Renzetti, 1992). Relatively little is known about the dynamics of abuse in gay relationships.

As is the case with research on heterosexual couples, research linking gay and lesbian violence to family-of-origin violence is inconclusive. In a study of lesbians, both the intergenerational transmission of aggression and the "double whammy" were supported (Lie, Schlitt, Bush, Montagne, & Reyes, 1991). Lesbians who experienced abuse as children were more likely to be both perpetrators and victims of abuse within their intimate relationships. This relationship was even stronger for lesbians who had both witnessed and experienced abuse in their families of origin. Similarly, in a study of gay and lesbian perpetrators of abuse, the majority of the men (93%) and women (88%) had experienced physical abuse in their families of origin (Farley, 1996). However, other research found no relationship between violence in the family of origin and subsequent abuse toward homosexual partners (Coleman, 1990; Renzetti, 1992).

Elder Abusers

Although abuse of the elderly has been a long-lived feature of the American family, there is a dearth of scholarly research on this form of family violence

(Barnett, Miller-Perrin, & Perrin, 1997). What little research evidence we do have indicates that elder abuse is a complex phenomenon that is difficult to study, in part because of the debate about what constitutes elder abuse. Several theoretical frameworks have been used to explain the occurrence of elder abuse: psychopathology, social exchange, stress, and intergenerational transmission (Boudreau, 1993).

The scanty research that has been conducted to test the intergenerational transmission theory is inconsistent. In a study of 15 adult children who were perpetrators of elder abuse, there was no support for intergenerational transmission, but abuse by adult offspring could be traced to pathological personality characteristics and current contextual factors such as stress and isolation (Pillemer, 1986). However, in a study comparing the family backgrounds of 21 child-abusing parents and 23 elder-abusing offspring, the rate of abuse experienced during childhood was high for both groups, although there were no significant differences between the groups (Korbin, Anetzberger, & Austin, 1995). Ninety-one percent of the child abusers and 65% of the elder abusers reported experiencing violence in their families of origin.

Although spouses are responsible for a significant portion of elder abuse, even less is known about this phenomenon. Recent decline in physical health (Wolf & Pillemer, 1989), abuser deviance, and high levels of spousal conflict (Pillemer & Finkelhor, 1989) are risk factors associated with elderly abuse perpetrated by spouses. It is not known whether spousal abuse of the elderly is a continuation of a long-term pattern or a late-onset phenomenon. Thus, although the intergenerational transmission theory provides an explanation for other types of violence, it appears to be less effective in predicting elder abuse.

SUMMARY AND DISCUSSION

This overview of research investigating the family roots of aggression connects the study of childhood and adult aggression by surveying familial determinants of aggression across the life span. Clearly, violence is a problem rooted in childhood. Aggression tends to be stable over the life span, with childhood aggression being a strong predictor of adolescent aggression, and so on. Although the intergenerational transmission of violence via social learning was supported across the life span in many studies, aggression was also related to a number of other forms of breakdown in the parent–child relationship (e.g., disturbed parent–child attachment, poor parental supervision). Furthermore, mechanisms of transmission encompass a broad range of social learning, psychological, biological, and interpersonal factors rooted in the family. The suggestion by Rothbaum and Weisz (1994) that the breakdown in the parent–child relationship should be viewed broadly as an oppositional familial environment, where parents fail to motivate and teach children to develop socially acceptable coping behaviors, seems reasonable.

Inconsistencies in research findings can be partially explained through methodological variations across studies, such as variations in how outcome and predictor variables are defined and measured, how samples and data are collected, and how data are analyzed. However, there are also large variations in individuals' responses to adversity and stress. Differences in individuals' responses to adversity and stress are due to variations in biological vulnerability, the impact of positive experiences, or a myriad of other factors (such as race, gender, or changes in the familial environment over the life span). Not all who grow up in oppositional familial environments become aggressive individuals.

Mechanisms of transmission, moderator variables (e.g., gender), and protective factors (e.g., parental warmth, supportive marital relationship) warrant further investigation. Now that we understand some of the direct effects of a few specific variables rooted in the family context, future investigations, rather than comparing the effect of one construct with another, can build on this knowledge base by developing and testing models predicting the causal pathways that lead to either vulnerability or resilience in individuals reared in oppositional familial environments. We also need integrated, developmentally focused research on individuals who are violent in different contexts and life cycle stages, as well as research that considers different types of aggressive behavior. Research designs need to be sophisticated enough to bring our understanding of the family roots of aggression to a higher level. We need comprehensive, longitudinal investigations where mothers, fathers, and children are assessed at various points in time. Experimental designs are also needed to unravel the reciprocal influences of parents and children and to enable us to make valid judgments about causality. Indeed, much has yet to be learned about the family roots of aggressive behavior.

REFERENCES

Agnew, R., & Huguley, S. (1989). Adolescent violence toward parents. *Journal of Marriage and the Family, 51,* 699–711.

Alexander, P. C., Moore, S., & Alexander, E. R. I. (1991). What is transmitted in the intergenerational transmission of violence? *Journal of Marriage and the Family, 53,* 657–668.

Arias, I., & Pape, K. T. (1994). Physical abuse. In L. L'Abate (Ed.), *Handbook of developmental family psychology and psychopathology* (pp. 284–308). New York: Wiley.

Barnett, O. W., Martinez, T. E., & Bluestein, B. W. (1995). Jealousy and romantic attachment in maritally violent and nonviolent men. *Journal of Interpersonal Violence, 10,* 473–486.

Barnett, O. W., Miller-Perrin, C. L., & Perrin, R. D. (1997). *Family violence across the lifespan: An introduction.* Thousand Oaks, CA: Sage.

Belsky, J., Youngblade, L., & Pensky, E. (1990). Childrearing history, marital quality, and maternal affect: Intergenerational transmission in a low-risk sample. *Development and Psychopathology, 1,* 291–304.

Billingham, R. E., & Gilbert, K. R. (1990). Parental divorce during childhood and use of violence in dating relationships. *Psychological Reports, 66,* 1003–1009.

Billingham, R. E., & Notebaert, N. L (1993). Divorce and dating violence revisited: Multivariate analyses using Straus's Conflict Tactics subscores. *Psychological Reports, 73,* 679–684.

Boudreau, F. A. (1993). Elder abuse. In R. L. Hampton, T. P. Gullotta, G. R. Adams, E. H. Potter, & R. P. Weissberg (Eds.), *Family violence: Prevention and treatment* (Vol. 1, pp. 142–158). Newbury Park, CA: Sage.

Bowen, M. (1978). *Family therapy in clinical practice.* New York: Jason Aronson.

Bowers, L., Smith, P. K., & Binney, V. (1994). Perceived family relationships of bullies, victims and bully/victims in middle childhood. *Journal of Social and Personal Relationships, 11,* 215–232.

Breslin, F. C., Riggs, D. S., O'Leary, K. D., & Arias, I. (1990). Family precursors: Expected and actual consequences of dating aggression. *Journal of Interpersonal Violence, 5,* 247–258.

Browne, K. D., & Hamilton, C. E. (1998). Physical violence between young adults and their parents: Associations with a history of child maltreatment. *Journal of Family Violence, 13,* 59–79.

Caesar, P. L. (1988). Exposure to violence in the families-of-origin among wife-abusers and maritally nonviolent men. *Violence and Victims, 3,* 49–63.

Caliso, J. A., & Milner, J. S. (1994). Childhood physical abuse, childhood social support, and adult child abuse potential. *Journal of Interpersonal Violence, 9,* 27–44.

Campbell, J. C. (1995). Violence research: An overview. *Scholarly Inquiry for Nursing Practice: An International Journal, 9,* 105–126.

Cantrell, P. J., MacIntyre, D. I., Sharkey, K. J., & Thompson, V. (1995). Violence in the marital dyad as a predictor of violence in the peer relationships of older adolescents/young adults. *Violence and Victims, 10,* 35–41.

Cappell, C., & Heiner, R. B. (1990). The intergenerational transmission of family aggression. *Journal of Family Violence, 5,* 135–152.

Carlson, B. E. (1990). Adolescent observers of marital violence. *Journal of Family Violence, 5,* 285–299.

Choice, P., Lamke, L. K., & Pittman, J. F. (1995). Conflict resolution strategies and marital distress as mediating factors in the link between witnessing interparental violence and wife battering. *Violence and Victims, 10,* 107–131.

Coleman, V. E. (1990). Violence in lesbian couples: A between groups comparison (Doctoral dissertation, California School of Professional Psychology, 1990). *Dissertation Abstracts International, 51-11B,* 5634.

Cummings, E. M., Hennessy, K. D., Rabideau, G. J., & Cicchetti, D. (1994). Responses of physically abused boys to interadult anger involving mothers. *Development and Psychopathology, 6,* 31–41.

David, C., Steels, R., Forehand, R., & Armistead, L. (1996). The role of family conflict and marital conflict in adolescent functioning. *Journal of Family Violence, 11,* 81–91.

DeKlyen, M., Biernbaum, M. A., Speltz, M. L., & Greenberg, M. T. (1998). Fathers and preschool behavior problems. *Developmental Psychology, 34,* 264–275.

DeMaris, A. (1990).The dynamics of generational transfer in courtship violence: A biracial exploration. *Journal of Marriage and the Family, 52,* 219–231.

DeVet, K. A. (1997). Parent–adolescent relationships, physical disciplinary history, and adjustment in adolescents. *Family Process, 36,* 311–322.

DiLalla, L. F., & Gottesman, I. I. (1991). Biological and genetic contributors to violence: Widom's untold tale. *Psychological Bulletin, 109,* 125–129.

Dodge, K. A. (1991). The structure and function of reactive and proactive aggression. In D. J. Peplar & K. H. Rubin (Eds.), *The development and treatment of childhood aggression* (pp. 201–218). Hillsdale, NJ: Erlbaum.

Dodge, K. A., Bates, J. E., & Pettit, G. S. (1990). Mechanisms in the cycle of violence. *Science, 250,* 1678–1683.

Dodge, K. A., Pettit, G. S., & Bates, J. E. (1994). Socialization mediators of the relation between socioeconomic status and child conduct problems. *Child Development, 65,* 649–665.

Dodge, K. A., Pettit, G. S., Bates, J. E., & Valente, E. (1995). Social information-processing patterns partially mediate the effect of early physical abuse on later conduct problems. *Journal of Abnormal Psychology, 104,* 632–643.

Dubow, E. F., & Reid, G. J. (1994). Risk and resource variables in children's aggressive behavior: A two-year longitudinal study. In L. R. Huesmann (Ed.), *Aggressive behavior: Current perspectives* (pp. 187–211). New York: Plenum Press.

Dutton, D. G., Starzomski, A., & Ryan, L. (1996). Antecedents of abusive personality and abusive behavior in wife assaulters. *Journal of Family Violence, 11,* 113–132.

Dutton, D. G., van Ginkel, C., & Starzomski, A. (1995). The role of shame and guilt in the intergenerational transmission of abusiveness. *Violence and Victims, 10,* 121–131.

Earls, F. J., & Reiss, A. J. (1994). *Breaking the cycle* (National Institute of Justice Research Report). Chicago: National Institute of Justice.

Egeland, B. (1991). A longitudinal study of high-risk families: Issues and findings. In R. H. Starr & D. A. Wolfe (Eds.), *The effects of child abuse and neglect* (pp. 33–56). New York: Guilford Press.

Egeland, B. (1993). A history of abuse is a major risk factor for abusing the next generation. In R. J. Gelles & D. R. Loseke (Eds.), *Current controversies on family violence* (pp. 197–208). Newbury Park, CA: Sage.

Erel, O., Margolin, G., & John, R. S. (1998). Observed sibling interaction: Links with the marital and the mother–child relationship. *Developmental Psychology, 34,* 288–298.

Eron, L. D., Huesmann, L. R., & Zelli, A. (1991). The role of parental variables in the learning of aggression. In D. J. Pepler & K. H. Rubin (Eds.), *The development and treatment of childhood aggression* (pp. 169–188). Hillsdale, NJ: Erlbaum.

Farley, N. (1996). A survey of factors contributing to gay and lesbian domestic violence. *Journal of Gay and Lesbian Social Services, 4,* 35–44.

Farrington, D. P. (1986). Stepping stones to adult criminal careers. In D. Olweus,

J. Block, & M. Radke-Yarrow (Eds.), *Development of antisocial and prosocial behavior: Research, theories, and issues* (pp. 359–384). Orlando, FL: Academic Press.

Farrington, D. P. (1991). Childhood aggression and adult violence: Early precursors and later life outcomes. In D. J. Pepler & K. H. Rubin (Eds.), *The development and treatment of childhood aggression* (pp. 5–30). Hillsdale, NJ: Erlbaum.

Farrington, D. P. (1994). Childhood, adolescent, and adult features of violent males. In L. R. Huesmann (Ed.), *Aggressive behavior: Current perspectives* (pp. 215–240). New York: Plenum Press.

Follette, V. M., & Alexander, P. C. (1992). Dating violence: Current and historical correlates. *Behavioral Assessment, 14,* 39–52.

Forehand, R., Thomas, A. M., Wierson, M., Brody, G., & Fauber, R. (1990). Role of maternal functioning and parenting skills in adolescent functioning following parental divorce. *Journal of Abnormal Psychology, 99,* 278–283.

Gelles, R. J., & Cornell, C. P. (1987). Adolescent-to-parent violence. In R. J. Gelles (Ed.), *Family violence* (pp. 153–167). Newbury Park, CA: Sage.

Gelles, R. J., & Cornell, C. P. (1990). *Intimate violence in families* (2nd ed.). Newbury Park, CA: Sage.

Gelles, R. J., & Straus, M. A. (1990). The medical and psychological costs of family violence. In M. A. Straus & R. J. Gelles (Eds.), *Physical violence in American families: Risk factors and adaptations to violence in 8,145 families* (pp. 425–430). New Brunswick, NJ: Transaction.

Gwartney-Gibbs, P. A., Stockard, J., & Bohmer, S. (1987). Learning courtship aggression: The influence of parents, peers, and personal experiences. *Family Relations, 38,* 276–282.

Harnish, J. D., Dodge, K. A., & Valente, E. (1995). Mother–child interactions quality as a partial mediator of the roles of maternal depressive symptomatology and socioeconomic status in the development of child behavior problems. *Child Development, 66,* 739–753.

Hotaling, G. T., Straus, M. S., & Lincoln, A. J. (1990). Intrafamily violence and crime and violence outside the family. In M. A. Straus & R. J. Gelles (Eds.), *Physical violence in American families: Risk factors and adaptations to violence in 8,145 families* (pp. 431–470). New Brunswick, NJ: Transaction.

Howell, M. J., & Publiesi, K. L. (1988). Husbands who harm: Predicting spousal violence by men. *Journal of Family Violence, 3,* 15–27.

Island, D., & Letellier, P. (1991). *Men who beat the men who love them: Battered gay men and domestic violence.* New York: Haworth Press.

Jaffe, P., Wolfe, D., Wilson, S., & Zak, L. (1986). Similarities in behavioral and social maladjustment among child victims and witnesses to family violence. *American Journal of Orthopsychiatry, 56,* 142–146.

Kaufman, J., & Zigler, E. (1993). The intergenerational transmission of abuse is overstated. In R. J. Gelles & D. R. Loseke (Eds.), *Current controversies on family violence* (pp. 209–221). Newbury Park, CA: Sage.

Korbin, J. E., Anetzberger, G., & Austin, C. (1995). The intergenerational cycle of violence in child and elder abuse. *Journal of Elder Abuse and Neglect, 7,* 1–15.

Kruttschnitt, C., & Dornfeld, M. (1991). Childhood victimization, race, and violent crime. *Criminal Justice and Behavior, 18,* 448–463.

Landy, S., & Peters, R. D. (1992). Toward an understanding of a developmental paradigm for aggressive conduct problems during the preschool years. In R.

354   INDIVIDUAL AND FAMILY PSYCHOPATHOLOGY

D. Peters, R. J. McMahon, & V. L. Quinsey (Eds.), *Aggression and violence throughout the life span* (pp. 1–30). Newbury Park, CA: Sage.

Larzelere, R. E. (1986). Moderate spanking: Model or deterrent of children's aggression in the family? *Journal of Family Violence, 1,* 27–36.

Lewis, D. O., Lovely, R., Yeager, C., & Femina, D. D. (1989). Toward a theory of the genesis of violence: A follow-up study of delinquents. *Journal of the American Academy of Child and Adolescent Psychiatry, 28,* 431–436.

Lewis, D. O., Lovely, R., Yeager, C., Ferguson, G., Friedman, M., Sloane, G., Friedman, H., & Pincus, J. H. (1988). Intrinsic and environmental characteristics of juvenile murderers. *Journal of the American Academy of Childhood and Adolescent Psychiatry, 27,* 582–587.

Lie, G., Schlitt, R., Bush, J., Montagne, M., & Reyes, L. (1991). Lesbians in currently aggressive relationships: How frequently do they report aggressive past relationships? *Violence and Victims, 6,* 121–135.

Lockhart, L. L., White, B. W., Causby, V., & Isaac, A. (1994). Letting out the secret: Violence in lesbian relationships. *Journal of Interpersonal Violence, 9,* 469–492.

MacEwen, K. E., & Barling, J. (1988). Multiple stressors, violence in the family of origin, and marital aggression: A longitudinal investigation. *Journal of Family Violence, 3,* 73–87.

Mangold, W. D., & Koski, P. R. (1990). Gender comparisons in the relationship between parental and sibling violence and nonfamily violence. *Journal of Family Violence, 5,* 225–235.

Marshall, L. L., & Rose, P. (1988). Family of origin violence and courtship abuse. *Journal of Counseling and Development, 66,* 414–418.

Marshall, L. L., & Rose, P. (1990). Premarital violence: The impact of family of origin violence, stress, and reciprocity. *Violence and Victims, 5,* 51–64.

Mash, E. J., & Wolfe, D. A. (1991). Methodological issues in research on physical child abuse. *Criminal Justice and Behavior, 18,* 8–29.

McCord, J. (1988). Parental aggressiveness and physical punishment in long-term perspective. In G. T. Hotaling, D. Finkelhor, J. T. Kirkpatrick, & M. A. Straus (Eds.), *Family abuse and its consequences* (pp. 91–98). Newbury Park, CA: Sage.

McCord, J. (1994). Aggression in two generations. In L. R. Huesmann (Ed.), *Aggressive behavior: Current perspectives* (pp. 241–251). New York: Plenum Press.

Milner, J. S., Robertson, K. R., & Rogers, D. L. (1990). Childhood history of abuse and adult child abuse potential. *Journal of Family Violence, 5,* 15–34.

Murphy, C. M., Meyer, S. L., & O'Leary, K. D. (1994). Dependency characteristics of partner assaultive men. *Journal of Abnormal Psychology, 103,* 729–735.

O'Keefe, M. (1994). Linking marital violence, mother–child/father–child aggression, and child behavior problems. *Journal of Family Violence, 9,* 63–78.

O'Keefe, M. (1995). Predictors of child abuse in maritally violent families. *Journal of Interpersonal Violence, 10,* 3–25.

O'Keefe, M. (1998). Factors mediating the link between witnessing interparental violence and dating violence. *Journal of Family Violence, 13,* 39–57.

Patterson, G. R. (1986). The contribution of siblings to training for fighting: A microsocial analysis. In D. Olweus, J. Block, & M. Radke-Yarrow (Eds.),

Development of antisocial and prosocial behavior: Research, theories, and issues (pp. 235–262). Orlando, FL: Academic Press.

Patterson, G. R., Capaldi, D., & Bank, L. (1991) An early starter model for predicting delinquency. In D. J. Pepler & K. H. Rubin (Eds.), *The development and treatment of childhood aggression* (139–168). Hillsdale, NJ: Erlbaum.

Patterson, G. R., Crosby, L., & Vuchinich, S. (1992). Predicting risk for early police arrest. *Journal of Quantitative Criminology, 8,* 335–355.

Patterson, G. R., & Yoerger, K. (1993). Developmental models for delinquent behavior. In S. Hodgins (Ed.), *Mental disorder and crime* (pp. 140–172). Newbury Park, CA: Sage.

Pettit, G. S., Harriest, A. W., Bates, J. E., & Dodge, K. A. (1991). Family interaction, social cognition and children's subsequent relations with peers at kindergarten. *Journal of Social and Personal Relationships, 8,* 383–402.

Pianta, R., Egeland, B., & Erickson, M. F. (1989). The antecedents of maltreatment: Results of the Mother–Child Interaction Research Project. In D. Cicchetti & V. Carlson (Eds.), *Child maltreatment: Theory and research on the causes and consequences of child abuse and neglect* (pp. 203–253). New York: Cambridge University Press.

Pillemer, K. A. (1986). Risk factors in elder abuse: Results from a case–control study. In K. A. Pillemer & R. S. Wolf (Eds.), *Elder abuse: Conflict in the family* (pp. 239–263). Dover, MA: Auburn House.

Pillemer, K. A., & Finkelhor, D. (1988). The prevalence of elder abuse: A random sample survey. *The Gerontologist, 28,* 51–57.

Pillemer, K. A., & Finkelhor, D. (1989). Causes of elder abuse: Caregiver stress versus problem relatives. *American Journal of Orthopsychiatry, 59,* 179–187.

Renzetti, C. M. (1992). *Violent betrayal: Partner abuse in lesbian relationships.* Newbury Park, CA: Sage.

Renzetti, C. M. (1995). Building a second closet: Third party responses to victims of lesbian partner violence. In S. M. Stith & M. A. Straus (Eds.), *Understanding partner violence: Prevalence, causes, consequences, and solutions* (pp. 58–66). Minneapolis: National Council on Family Relations.

Riggs, D. S., O'Leary, K. D., & Breslin, F. C. (1990). Multiple correlates of physical aggression in dating couples. *Journal of Interpersonal Violence, 5,* 61–73.

Ringwalt, C. L., Browne, D. C., Rosenbloom, L. B., Evans, G. A., & Kotch, J. B. (1989). Predicting adult approval of corporal punishment from childhood parenting experiences. *Journal of Family Violence, 4,* 339–351.

Rivera, B., & Widom, C. S. (1990). Childhood victimization and violent offending. *Violence and Victims, 5,* 19–35.

Rohner, R. P., Bourque, S. L., & Elordi, C. A. (1996). Children's perceptions of corporal punishment, caretaker acceptance, and psychological adjustment in a poor, biracial southern community. *Journal of Marriage and the Family, 58,* 842–852.

Rosen, K. H., Bartle-Haring, S. B., & Stith, S. M. (1996, November). *The relationship among partner violence, family of origin violence, and differentiation of self.* Paper presented at the annual meeting of the National Council on Family Relations, Kansas City, KS.

Rothbaum, F., & Weisz, J. R. (1994). Parental caregiving and child externalizing behavior in nonclinical samples: A meta-analysis. *Psychological Bulletin, 116,* 55–74.

Russell, R. J. H., & Hulson, B. (1992). Physical and psychological abuse of heterosexual partners. *Personality and Individual Differences, 13,* 457–473.

Simons, R. L., Johnson, C., & Conger, R. D. (1994). Harsh corporal punishment versus quality of parental involvement as an explanation of adolescent maladjustment. *Journal of Marriage and the Family, 56,* 591–607.

Simons, R. L., Whitbeck, L. B., Conger, R. D., & Chyi-In, W. (1991). Intergenerational transmission of harsh parenting. *Developmental Psychology, 27,* 159–171.

Sternberg, K. J., Lamb, M. E., Greenbaum, C., Cicchetti, D., Dawud, S., Cortes, R. M., Krispin, O., & Lorey, F. (1993). Effects of domestic violence on children's behavior problems and depression. *Developmental Psychology, 29,* 44–52.

Stith, S. M., & Farley, S. C. (1993). A predictive model of male spousal violence. *Journal of Family Violence, 8*(2), 183–201.

Strassberg, Z., Dodge, K. A., Pettit, G. S., & Bates, J. E. (1994). Spanking in the home and children's subsequent aggression toward kindergarten peers. *Development and Psychopathology, 6,* 445–461.

Straus, M. A. (1991). Discipline and deviance: Physical punishment of children and violence and other crime in adulthood. *Social Problems, 38,* 133–154.

Straus, M. A. (1992). Children as witnesses to marital violence: A risk factor for lifelong problems among a nationally representative sample of American men and women. In D. F. Schwarz (Ed.), *Children and violence* (pp. 98–109). Columbus, OH: Ross Laboratories.

Straus, M. A. (1994). *Beating the devil out of them: Corporal punishment in American families.* New York: Lexington Books.

Straus, M. A., & Gelles, R. J. (1990). How violent are American families?: Estimates from the National Family Violence Resurvey and other studies. In M. A. Straus & R. J. Gelles (Eds.), *Physical violence in American families: Risk factors and adaptations to violence in 8,145 families* (pp. 95–132). New Brunswick, NJ: Transaction.

Straus, M. A., & Kantor, G. K. (1994). Corporal punishment of adolescents by parents: A risk factor in the epidemiology of depression, suicide, alcohol abuse, child abuse, and wife beating. *Adolescence, 29,* 543–561.

Straus, M. A., & Yodanis, C. L. (1996). Corporal punishment in adolescence and physical assaults on spouses in later life: What accounts for the link? *Journal of Marriage and the Family, 58,* 825–841.

Tannenbaum, L., & Forehand, R. (1994). Maternal depressive mood: The role of the father in preventing adolescent problem behaviours. *Behaviour Research and Therapy, 32,* 321–325.

Tannenbaum, L., Neighbors, B., & Forehand, R. (1992). The unique contribution of four maternal stressors to adolescent functioning. *Journal of Early Adolescence, 12,* 314–325.

Thomas, A. M., Forehand, R., & Neighbors, B. (1995). Change in maternal depressive mood: Unique contributions to adolescent functioning over time. *Adolescence, 30*(117), 43–52.

Tontodonato, P., & Crew, B. K. (1992). Dating violence, social learning theory, and gender: A multivariate analysis. *Violence and Victims, 7,* 3–14.

Trickett, P. K., Aber, J. L., Carlson, V., & Cicchetti, D. (1991). Relationship of socioeconomic status to the etiology and developmental sequelae of physical child abuse. *Developmental Psychology, 27,* 148–158.

Trickett, P. K., & Susman, E. J. (1989). Perceived similarities and disagreements about childrearing practices in abusive and nonabusive families: Intergenerational and concurrent family processes. In D. Cicchetti & V. Carlson (Eds.), *Child maltreatment: Theory and research on the causes and consequences of child abuse and neglect* (pp. 280–301). New York: Cambridge University Press.

U.S. Department of Justice. (1993). *Sourcebook of criminal justice statistics—1993.* Rockville, MD: Author.

Wauchope, B. A., & Straus, M. A. (1990). Physical punishment and physical abuse of American children: Incidence rates by age, gender, and occupational status. In M. A. Straus & R. J. Gelles (Eds.), *Physical violence in American families: Risk factors and adaptations to violence in 8,145 families* (pp. 133–148). New Brunswick, NJ: Transaction.

Weiss, B., Dodge, K. A., Bates, J. E., & Pettit, G. S. (1992). Some consequences of early harsh discipline: Child aggression and a maladaptive social information processing style. *Child Development, 63,* 1321–1335.

Widom, C. S. (1989a). Child abuse, neglect, and adult behavior: Research design and findings on criminality, violence, and child abuse. *American Journal of Orthopsychiatry, 59,* 355–367.

Widom, C. S. (1989b). The intergenerational transmission of violence. In N. A. Weiner & M. E. Wolfgang (Eds.), *Pathways to criminal violence* (pp. 137–201). Newbury Park: CA: Sage.

Widom, C. S. (1992). *The cycle of violence* (Research in Brief, NCJ No. 136607). Washington, DC: U. S. Department of Justice.

Williams, O. (1989). Spouse abuse: Social learning, attribution and interventions. *Journal of Health and Social Policy, 1,* 91–107.

Wolf, R. S., & Pillemer, K. A. (1989). *Helping elderly victims: The reality of elder abuse.* New York: Columbia University Press.

CHAPTER 15

⇒➤◆◆⇐

Substance Abuse and Dependence

TERRY S. TREPPER
MARY E. DANKOSKI

Mental health researchers and practitioners have been called upon in ever-increasing numbers to provide information, prevention strategies, and treatment programs to handle the monumental problem of substance abuse and dependence. A number of useful models have emerged over the years to describe and treat substance use disorders—most notably the disease, compulsive behavior, and addictive personality disorder models (Williams, 1996). A new direction is that of looking at substance misuse as family psychopathology. O'Farrell (1993) has called for an identified research and clinical area focused on "families and addictions." This area would include the role of the family in the causes, treatment, and prevention of substance abuse and dependence.

This chapter examines the research on substance abuse and dependence as family psychopathology. We examine not only the specific research on the role of substance misuse in and its impact upon the family, but the research on other systemic factors that can affect the development of substance misuse in the family.

SYSTEMIC FACTORS CONTRIBUTING TO SUBSTANCE MISUSE VULNERABILITY

Although the addiction literature has traditionally been concerned with the individual, research on the *vulnerability* to substance use disorders seeks to broaden this focus to address the influences of multiple systems on substance use and misuse. Based on the general vulnerability model (e.g., Gottschalk, 1983; Zubin & Spring, 1977) and the diathesis–stress model (e.g., Rosenthal, 1971) common in abnormal psychology, this theoretical framework suggests that everyone is endowed with a certain degree of vulnerability to substance misuse. What determines the degree of vulnerability depends upon the person's genetic predisposition (which is not discussed in this chapter), the number and magnitude of specific factors, the likelihood of precipitating events, and the degree to which common coping mechanisms are lacking. Within this framework, the mere presence of a vulnerability factor does *not* mean that a person will develop a substance use disorder. In fact, one of the benefits of this model is that it avoids the unidimensional focus of many causal theories of and stereotypes surrounding substance misuse.

In this section, we focus on those specific nonbiological systemic factors that appear to make people more vulnerable to substance abuse or dependence. Although the primary focus of this chapter is on the family dynamics of substance misuse, the dynamics within the multisystemic context in which families exist must be examined if their complexity is to be fully understood. We have divided the vulnerability factors into socioenvironmental, family systemic, and intraindividual factors.

Socioenvironmental Factors

"Socioenvironmental factors" are the cultural, gender, socioeconomic, and community factors that exert influence upon families and individuals. Again it must be emphasized that possessing one of these factors makes an individual more vulnerable to substance abuse/dependence, but of course does not mean that he or she will develop a substance use disorder.

Culture

Many ethnicity comparison studies of alcohol and drug use patterns consistently show that European Americans are more likely than African Americans, Hispanics, Asians, or West Indians to use substances. For example, white college students are likely to be heavier drinkers than blacks (Barnes & Welte, 1983), and as adolescents, blacks have been found to have higher abstinence rates and lower rates of treatment for alcohol misuse than white teens (Barnes, Farrell, & Banerjee, 1994). European Americans have also been found to have higher lifetime prevalence rates of substance use than Hispanics (Schinke et al., 1992). In a study of high school students, European Americans and Native Americans had higher rates of heavy drinking than either Hispanics or African Americans, as well as West Indians and Asians (Barnes & Welte, 1986). Compared to those of European Americans, the overall drinking rates of Asians and Asian

Americans are low (Kitano & Chi, 1986–1987, cited in Zucker, Fitzgerald, & Moses, 1995).

The culture issue is more complex, however. For example, the Native American population is also characterized by high levels of heavy drinking and drug use; however, there is much variation among the many tribes and groups making up this population, and many tribes/groups have high rates of abstinence (Lex, 1987). The same holds true for the many different groups encompassed under the umbrella term "Hispanic" (Caetano, 1991). Variation of use in the Hispanic population may also be accounted for by differences in acculturation levels. Caetano (1986–1987) and Black and Markides (1993) found a positive relationship between acculturation level and increased rates of drunkenness among Hispanics, and Vega, Gil, and Zimmerman (1993) found greater acculturation levels to be related to earlier use of alcohol.

Gender

Another consistent finding in research studies is a clear gender difference in substance use. Almost unequivocally, males have higher rates of alcohol and drug use, abuse, and dependence than females (e.g., Barnes & Welte, 1990; Kandel, Simcha-Fagan, & Davies, 1986; O'Hare, 1995; Zucker et. al., 1995). There are also specific gender differences in substance use patterns, which are examined in various sections below.

Socioeconomic Status

An interesting finding for both males and females is that although African American and Hispanic youth have lower rates of drinking than European American adolescents, minority youth often experience more alcohol-related problems per ounce of alcohol consumed than European Americans do (Welte & Barnes, 1987). The difference in socioeconomic status between the majority and minorities groups is one hypothesis for why this trend occurs. Low-income families have been found to experience more lifetime alcohol problems than high-income families (Fitzgerald & Zucker, 1995).

Community Context

In addition to cultural influences, gender differences, and socioeconomic correlates, the community context of the alcohol/drug user is important in predicting patterns of use. Among adolescents, many studies have examined the relationship of school functioning and peer relations to substance use. The heavily using teenager can be characterized by frequent school misconduct and poor grades (Barnes & Welte, 1986), low satisfaction with school (McBride, Joe, & Simpson, 1991), and lack of receptiveness to traditional education programs (Babst, Miran, & Koval, 1976). Those who drop out of high school are over six times more likely to develop alcohol abuse or dependence as adults than are those with a college degree (Crum, Helzer, & Anthony, 1993). Furthermore, adolescent substance use is related to having a large number of friends who use substances on a weekly basis (Barnes & Welte, 1986), associations with deviant peers (Levine & Singer, 1988; McBride et al., 1991), high susceptibility to peer pressure, and peer approval of substance use (Dielman, Butchart, & Shope, 1993). In older adolescents and young adult college students, this susceptibility to peer pressure may account for the association between increased drinking and drug use rates and living in a residence hall (Barnes, Welte, & Dintcheff, 1992), a fraternity, or a sorority (Baer, Kivlahan, & Marlatt, 1995).

Another factor in the community context of the user is the level of religious involvement. Lack of participation in religious activities (Clapper, Buka, Goldfield, Lipsitt, & Tsuang, 1995) and not being strongly attached to a particular faith (Perkins, 1987) have been found to predict alcohol misuse. Indeed, a high level of religiousness may be a coping mechanism that protects an individual against drug use (Coombs & Paulson, 1988; Hays, Stacy, Widaman, DiMatteo, & Downey, 1986; Jessor & Jessor, 1977).

Family Systemic Factors

A growing body of research has recognized that family dynamics play a highly significant role in predicting drug and alcohol use, abuse, and dependence. Much of the research on adolescent use has focused on the current functioning of a teen's family, whereas much of the research on adult use has focused on an individual's family of origin. More recently, research has been conducted on the dynamics of current relationships of adult users. Each of these three areas is discussed below.

Current Family Dynamics of Adolescent Substance Users

Several studies that examine the impact of family structural variations (e.g., single-parent families) on adolescent substance use have been completed. Some studies have shown that adolescents in single-parent and stepfamilies use more alcohol and drugs than teens in intact families do (Barnes & Windle, 1987; Burnside, Baer, McLaughlin, & Pokorny, 1986). Yet in another study examining teen substance use in these different types of families, Selnow (1987) included a measure of the quality of the parent–child relationship and found that a better relationship between the teen and his or her parent(s) decreased substance use in single-parent families and stepfamilies, as well as in intact families. Indeed, research shows that the more interactional components of family functioning and parenting skills seem to be more predictive of adolescent substance use than are family structural components.

For example, Piercy, Volk, Trepper, Sprenkle, and Lewis (1991) found that the relational family factors of cohesion and open communication between the mother and teen were linked with the type, amount, and frequency of drugs used by teens, whereas family structural components were not. Similarly, high levels of parental support and positive parent–child communication have been determined to be important preventive predictors for adolescents (Barnes et al., 1994). Lower perceived parental love was also correlated with substance use involvement for teens (Pandina & Schuele, 1983). Compared to substance-using teens, nonusers were significantly more likely to feel "extremely or quite close" to their fathers (72% for nonusers vs. 47% for users) in a study of adolescent use conducted by Coombs and Paulson (1988). In the same study, nonusers also felt more trusted by their mothers and reported receiving more parental praise, especially from their fathers, than users did (Coombs & Paulson, 1988).

One way in which a teenager can gauge parental love is through his or her parents' discipline practices. Studies show that less parental monitoring of adolescents (Barnes et al., 1994; Dishion & Loeber, 1985), less parental discipline (Dishion & Loeber, 1985; Piercy et al., 1991), and poor child-rearing practices (Denoff, 1988) are related to increased alcohol and drug consumption in teens. Barnes and Windle (1987) found that the more specific rules parents had for their adolescents' behavior, the lower the reported number of adolescent alcohol-related problems, incidents of illicit drug use, and deviant acts.

Family members of adolescents may also model behaviors and attitudes that make an adolescent more vulnerable to substance use. Adolescent alcohol use has been found to correlate with parental alcohol use (Burnside et al., 1986). Stephenson, Henry, and Robinson (1996) found that teenagers' perceptions of their mothers' substance use was predictive of their own use. Barnes and Welte (1986) found that those teens who could be characterized as heavy drinkers were more likely to have parental approval of drinking. Thus, these teens may be receiving direct or indirect messages from their parents encouraging their use.

In addition to actual and perceived parental substance use, perceived and actual use by siblings influences teen substance use (Coombs & Paulson, 1988). Having an older brother who uses marijuana has been determined to be significantly related to adolescent substance use (Brook, Whiteman, Gordan, & Brendan, 1983), as have a younger teen's perceptions of his or her older sibling's drug use (Clayton & Lacy, 1982). In an all-female adolescent sample, not only sibling substance use but sibling conflict was significantly related to alcohol and marijuana use within the year prior to the testing, and sibling rivalry was significantly correlated with a life history of "hard drug" use (Hall, Henggeler, Ferreira, & East, 1992). Older siblings have also been found to be frequent suppliers of drugs and companions in use with their younger siblings (Needle et al., 1986).

For adolescents, then, family factors—such as the quality of the parent–child relationship, parental discipline, and parental and sibling substance use—are clearly related to risk for alcohol and other substance use, in addition to socioenvironmental predictors. For adult alcohol and drug users, a comprehensive examination of vulnerabilities must include an examination of the marital or committed relationship, as well as family functioning as a whole.

Current Family Dynamics of Adult Substance Users

On conventional measures of marital satisfaction, the marriages of alcoholics typically score in the conflicted or distressed range (Leonard, 1990; O'Farrell & Birchler, 1987), at least when the husbands are the alcoholic spouses (as was the case in these studies). Yet an alcoholic spouse and a nonalcoholic spouse may have differing views of their relationship. O'Farrell and Birchler (1987) found that alcoholic husbands tended to have positively biased views of their relationships, because of their self-reported increased levels of marital satisfaction and lowered awareness of their wives' desires for change, when they were compared to two nonalcoholic groups (maritally conflicted husbands and nonconflicted husbands). However, the drinking styles of alcoholics may influence these satisfaction levels. Leonard (1990) found that husbands who reported high levels of steady drinking (as opposed to episodic, or binge, drinkers) had wives who reported somewhat better marital functioning and decreased levels of depression. He concluded that the steadiness of the alcohol consumption in such relationships may have a stabilizing effect on the families (Leonard, 1990), while the alcoholics themselves may be in denial or have distorted cognitions about their relationships (O'Farrell & Birchler, 1987).

Further studies show gender differences in marital functioning and patterns of use among couples in which substance misuse is a problem for one spouse. For example, when male and female spouses were compared by Brown, Kokin, Seraganian, and Shields (1995), males were more likely to have symptoms of substance misuse, depression, and physical problems, and to have less frequent interaction with their children. In the same study, the researchers also found that support available to female substance misusers from their spouses was less than that available to male substance misusers (Brown et al., 1995). Similarly, Kingree (1995) found that women substance misusers reported less family support, and in turn lower self-esteem, more self-blame, and more blaming of their parents than male misusers did. Female substance misusers have also been shown to complain of more mental distress and family pathology than men, who may face more community problems and health concerns (O'Hare, 1995). Noel, McCrady, Stout, and Fisher-Nelson (1991) examined the marital functioning of alcoholics presenting for outpatient alcohol/marital therapy and found that spouses in couples with an alcoholic wife were more satisfied with each other and themselves in their role functioning than were couples with an alcoholic husband. Furthermore, in couples with an alcoholic wife, the frequency of sexual relations decreased as severity of alcohol problems increased, whereas this relationship was not found in were couples with an alcoholic husband. In a review of studies on the sexual functioning of male alcoholics, however, O'Farrell (1990) noted that alcoholic couples experience levels of sexual dissatisfaction similar to those of nonalcoholic/maritally conflicted couples; however, they experience less satisfaction with the frequency, privacy, and context of sex, and less overall sexual satisfaction for both partners, than do nonalcoholic/nonconflicted couples.

Gender differences have also been found in communication patterns of substance-misusing couples. Noel et al. (1991) found that alcoholic wives engaged in more positive communication with their husbands, while alcoholic husbands were more negative toward their wives. Leonard (1990) compared the marital functioning of steady and episodic male alcoholics in a laboratory setting and found that episodic alcoholic husbands decreased their problem solving and increased their negativity from a no-drinking to a drinking situation, whereas steady alcoholics increased their problem solving and both these husbands and wives increased in negativity. Thus the dynamics of the marital relations of couples in which one partner misuses alcohol or another substance may differ, depending on whether the user is male or female and is an episodic or a steady user.

An extreme form of marital dysfunction is spousal violence. Studies have shown that alcohol problems and spousal violence frequently go hand in hand (Kantor & Straus, 1989). O'Farrell and Choquette (1991) found that in the year prior to entering a behavioral marital therapy treatment program, alcoholic men and their wives had five to six times more occurrences of violent acts than the number reported by a 1985 U.S. national sample. In this study, the prevalence of violence by alcoholics remained significantly elevated compared to national norms in the year after treatment, being still more than twice as high as in the national sample.

To expand the focus from the marital relationship to the family as a whole, studies show that substance-using adults may struggle with parenthood, and that for women users in particular, children may actually be barriers to receiving treatment. Mutzell (1994) compared the families of adult men and women admitted to an inpatient facility for substance misuse treatment and found that the children of the female subjects had more contact with an educational welfare officer, psychologist, or physician than the children of the male alcoholics did. An investigation of barriers to treatment for substance-misusing African American women revealed that the most frequently identified barriers were responsibilities at home as a mother, wife, or partner; lack of insurance or money; needing alcohol/drugs to deal with the stress of daily life; and fear of losing their children and shame after admitting to a problem (Allen, 1995). Thus not only do women substance misusers seem to complain of more familial and relationship stressors as precipitants to using substances, but these same stressors may be barriers to treatment.

Family-of-Origin Dynamics of Adult Substance Users

It is well known within the field that children of alcoholics and other substance misusers are more likely to grow up to become alcoholics or substance misusers themselves than are the children of parents who do not misuse substances. Many studies show that a family history of substance abuse/dependence is a significant factor in prediction equations of the development of substance use disorders (e.g., Barnes & Welte, 1990; Dull, 1992; Neisen, 1993; Pullen, 1994; Stabenau, 1990). This family-of-origin transmission seems to be particularly strong from father to son (Barnes et al., 1992).

Not only is the existence of a family history of substance misuse a vulnerability factor in the development of such misuse, but histories of physical and other types of abuse tend to be fairly common in the histories of adult substance misusers. In a study of adults with both alcohol and drug addictions, one of the strongest predictors was the presence of traumatic events in childhood, such as physical abuse or violence in the home (Barr & Cohen, 1987). Bennett and Kemper (1994) found that in a sample of adult women, subjects who reported physical abuse were more likely to test positive for substance misuse, even after a family history of substance misuse was controlled for. Janikowski and Glover (1994) examined the history of incest among adult clients in substance use treatment. Of those reporting incest, 36% reported that they had used alcohol or drugs during at least one incestuous contact, and 53% reported that the relative was using substances during at least one such contact. About one-third reported that they believed the incest contributed to their substance misuse (Janikowski & Glover, 1994). Wallen and Berman (1992) also examined whether childhood sexual abuse was a possible indicator for substance misuse among clients in inpatient treatment by comparing subjects reporting a history of child sexual abuse with controls. Results showed that many of those with a history of sexual abuse were more likely to have fathers or mothers with an alcohol or drug problem. Few subjects reported positive relationships with their mothers, and many more reported that they were still troubled by their childhood experiences (Wallen & Berman, 1992). In a qualitative life history study of women substance misusers, Woodhouse (1992) reported that the following themes were common: sexual violence (rape and incest), physical abuse, male dominance, dependence, motherhood, and depression.

Therefore, physical or other abuse is a factor that may increase vulnerability to alcohol and drug use. Similarly, unfair, inconsistent, and harsh discipline by parents predicted alcohol and depressive disorders in a study by Holmes and Robins (1987). These researchers found that the frequency of being hit and/or punched with an object, and of being punished by parents in front of other people, differentiated alcoholics from controls. Downs, Miller, Testa, and Panek (1992) found that father–daughter verbal aggression was an especially important predictor of alcohol misuse in adult women.

Not only is aggression from parent to child a vulnerability factor, but conflict in one's parents' relationship is a family-of-origin vulnerability factor as well. Pardeck (1991) found that perceived conflict in college students' families of origin appeared to increase the students' potential for alcoholism; Klein, Forehand, Armistead, and Brody (1994) found that higher levels of parental conflict were consistently related to poorer quality of the mother–adolescent relationship, which has been found to be a predictor of substance misuse. Alcoholic families also tend to perceive the environments of their families of origin as less cohesive and expressive, and as more conflictual (Filstead, McElfresh, & Anderson, 1981).

In addition to the quality of relationships in substance-using families, structural factors and family environmental factors have been found to predict adult substance use. Parental absence and family size were found to influence the age of drug use onset among white and Chicano heroin addicts (McCarthy & Anglin, 1990). Fathers' absence during childhood also predicted heavy drinking in adults interviewed by Barnes and Welte (1990) about their current drinking, childhood family structure, and parental drinking patterns. As an example of family environmental issues, parental knowledge of their children's first drink significantly predicted the incidence of alcohol-related problems in a survey of college students who began drinking at an early age (Gonzalez, 1983). Bennett and Wolin (1990) examined the predictive quality of the stability of family rituals in the intergenerational transmission of alcoholism. Rituals were classified as either "distinctive" (alcohol use behavior remained distinct from the ritual itself) or "subsumptive" (alcohol use behavior subsumed the ritual). The researchers found that those families whose rituals were most completely subsumed by alcohol use behaviors had a greater incidence of intergenerational transmission of alcoholism in the grown children than did those whose families kept their rituals distinct. This study was then expanded to investigate the degree of deliberateness in establishing and maintaining family rituals in recently married couples. The investigators concluded that predictors of nontransmission were having a high degree of deliberateness in one's own family heritage, coming from a family with distinctive dinnertimes, marrying a spouse from a family with highly ritualized dinnertimes, and marrying a spouse from a nonalcoholic family (Bennett & Wolin, 1990).

Individual Factors

Psychopathology

Researchers are currently conducting a longitudinal study to examine the developmental pathways to alcoholism (Fitzgerald, Davies, Zucker, & Klinger, 1994; Fitzgerald et al., 1993; Zucker, Ellis, & Fitzgerald, 1994; Zucker, Ellis, Bingham, & Fitzgerald, 1996). Even at the age of 3, differences were found between the children in high-risk families and those in low-risk families: Sons of alcoholic fathers were found to be more impulsive, to exhibit high levels of hyperactivity, and to have more difficult temperaments than children of nonalcoholics (Zucker et al., 1996).

Antisocial personality disorder has been found to be comorbid with both alcoholism and misuse of other drugs, such as inhalants (Compton, Cottler, Dinwiddie, & Spitznagel, 1994), amphetamines, marijuana, and cocaine (Randolph & Yates, 1993). Other disorders are also frequently found in substance misusers. Barr and Cohen (1987) found that among a sample made up largely of heavy users of both alcohol and narcotics, histories of anxiety, depression, suicidality, and admissions to psychiatric hospitals were factors predicting severity of use. Pullen (1994) also found depression and state anxiety to be predictors of alcohol misuse. Among women, there is a higher prevalence of eating disorders among inpatient alcohol-dependent women than in community samples (Goebel, Scheibe, & Grahling, 1995). Also among women, posttraumatic stress disorder is sometimes present with substance misuse, especially when there is a history of physical or sexual abuse (Brady, Killeen, Saladin, & Dansky, 1994).

Personality Styles

On measures of personality differences between subjects who do not misuse substances, one factor that stands out is aggression. Adult aggression as measured in a laboratory setting was a significant predictor of abuse of or dependence on cigarettes, barbiturates, amphetamines, and marijuana in a study by Muntaner et al. (1990). Furthermore, a 10-year outcome study begun when subjects were in the first grade showed that aggressiveness predicted heavy drug, alcohol, and cigarette use in males (Kellam, Stevenson, & Rubin, 1982). In the personal histories of alcohol and drug users, an increased amount of fighting and arrests often predicts the severity of drug or alcohol use (Clapper et al., 1995; Holland & Griffin, 1984). Many misusers of alcohol and other substances show a history of difficult temperaments from a very early age, as noted in the discussion of psychopathology above (Fitzgerald et al., 1993; Zucker et al., 1996).

When children come from high-risk families, the lack of cognitive, social and emotional stimulation available to them (Noll, Zucker, Fitzgerald, & Curtis, 1992) may further impede their personality development as well as their coping skills. Cooper, Russell, and George (1988) found that subjects who drank alcohol to cope or had coping styles characterized by avoidance of emotion had the highest levels of heavy drinking, especially when they had a strong belief in alcohol's positive reinforcing properties (see below). Brennan, Moos, and Mertens (1994) also found that more avoidance coping strategies predicted poor outcomes in the adaptation of older problem drinkers (mean age = 61 years) to life stress.

Cognitions

Cognitive trends can also be seen as vulnerabilities predicting alcohol and other substance use. Denoff (1987) found that specific belief systems of adolescents predicted the frequency of drug use. These belief systems were characterized by a tendency toward catastrophizing, an irrational need for approval, and emphasis on blame and punishment. High risk-taking attitudes have also been found to predict drug and alcohol use in adolescents (Levine & Singer, 1988). Greater perceived benefits of drinking (Werner, Walker, & Greene, 1994), greater belief in alcohol's positive reinforcing qualities (Cooper et al., 1988), and expectations of positive effects from alcohol (Wood, Nagoshi, & Dennis, 1992) have all been found to predict alcohol consumption. Factual knowledge about alcohol and drugs alone does not always make a difference in mediating alcohol and drug use. In a study of undergraduates, knowledge of the risks of alcohol use did not predict reduced use or misuse patterns, nor did perceived risks of use (Smith & McCauley, 1991).

Age of Onset

A consistent predictor of alcohol and drug misuse is an early age of onset. Werner et al. (1994) found that younger age at first drinking significantly predicted more alcohol-related problems, and Clapper et al. (1995) found that the number of times a subject was intoxicated before his or her 16th birthday was a good indicator of adult alcohol abuse or dependence. Likewise, a survey of college students showed that students who began drinking during elementary and middle school had significantly higher levels of both the quantity and frequency of use and alcohol-related problems than did those who began drinking in high school or college (Gonzalez, 1983).

FAMILY-INVOLVED PREVENTION AND FAMILY PSYCHOTHERAPY

It would stand to reason that if family and other systemic factors contribute significantly to a family's vulnerability to substance abuse or dependence, family-systems-based prevention programs and psychotherapies should be effective in both reducing those vulnerabilities and ameliorating substance misuse. Although an extensive review of the literature on the family interventions for substance use disorders is beyond the scope of the chapter, there is strong evidence to support the efficacy of such interventions. Family therapy for adolescents, and couple therapy for adults, has been shown not only to improve overall substance use outcomes, but also to improve engagement and retention in therapy, to improve overall relationship and family functioning, and to bring about improvements in school/work performance and other types of social functioning (see Edwards & Steinglass, 1995; Liddle & Dakof, 1995; O'Farrell, 1993).

CONCLUSIONS

Some points emerge from the preceding review of factors that contribute to substance misuse vulnerability (for a summary of these factors, see Table 15.1). First, there are a great number of vulnerability factors from a number of dimensions. Since all of these factors have been empirically supported, it can be assumed that all have some degree of "truth" to them. It would be naïve, given this breadth of factors, to take a single-factor approach to the development of research designs or to clinical assessment. For example, having an alcoholic mother and father certainly increases a person's vulnerability, but it is probably not the "cause" of the person's substance misuse.

Second, the vulnerability factors are multisystemic. That is, to fully understand the complexity of substance abuse and dependence, both in choosing research designs and when developing treatment plans, one must examine the socioenvironmental, family systemic, and individual contributors. There is no evidence thus far that one dimension, such as the socioenvironmental or the family dimension, contributes a greater degree of vulnerability. Perhaps in the future, longitudinal, multivariate, and/or meta-analytic studies may be able to determine which dimension plays the greatest role in substance misuse vulnerability.

Third, though these factors are separate, they probably interact with one another systemically. Sometimes, in fact, it may be difficult or impossible ever to determine which causes which. For example, does alcohol misuse *cause* relationship dysfunction, or does a poor relationship lead to increased alcohol use? Certainly the reduction of one reduces the other. It is our view, having been involved both in substance misuse research and in treatment of couples where one partner is a substance misusers, that the two are inexorably and systemically linked.

Fourth, in the absence of a clear reason to do otherwise, treatment strategies should be designed to reduce individual and family vulnerabilities to substance abuse/dependence. The specific protocol that we use in our programs is quite simple: (1) assessing the vulnerability factors that play

TABLE 15.1. Factors Contributing to Substance Misuse Vulnerability

Socioenvironmental factors

European American ethnicity
Male gender
Low socioeconomic status
School problems
Unhealthy peer associations
Lack of or low levels of religiosity

Family systemic factors

Current family functioning of adolescent
    Poor parent–child relationship
    Lack of or poor discipline by parents
    Parental modeling of use or support of use
    Sibling use or sibling conflict

Current family functioning of adults
    Decreased support from spouses (for females)
    Increased mental distress and family pathology (for females)
    Increased community problems and health concerns (for males)
    Negative communication in marital relationship
    Poor problem solving in marital relationship
    Decreased marital satisfaction in general
    Sexual dissatisfaction
    Increased spousal violence
    Parenting problems

Family of origin of adults
    Family history of substance misuse
    History of childhood physical or sexual abuse
    Parental conflict
    Father or parental absence
    Alcohol-subsumed family rituals

Individual factors

Antisocial personality disorder
Increased comorbidity of other pathologies
Aggression
Poor coping skills
Belief systems supporting use
Increased risk-taking attitudes in adolescents
Early age of onset

the strongest roles for this particular substance misuser and/or family; (2) determining which of those are the most significant *and* that most accessible to therapeutic intervention (e.g., though poverty may be a vulnerability factor, it is not really accessible to intervention; on the other hand, a highly enmeshed family structure may be relatively easy to intervene with; and (3) planning direct interventions that reduce these significant and accessible vulnerability factors.

Substance misuse research and treatment is no longer in its childhood or even adolescence, but well into adulthood. We now know a great deal about the cause of and treatments for substance use disorders. It is our contention that the literature supports a multi-pronged approach to assessment and treatment, and that standard substance use treatment programs should include couple therapy and/or family systems therapy as one of the therapy components. Doing so will help assure that this major dimension is addressed, and should result in improved therapy outcomes.

REFERENCES

Allen, K. (1995). Barriers to treatment for addicted African American women. *Journal of the National Medical Association, 87*(10), 751–756.

Babst, D. V., Miran, M., & Koval, M. (1976). The relationship between friends' marijuana use, family cohesion, school interest, and drug abuse prevention. *Journal of Drug Education, 6*(1), 23–41.

Baer, J. S., Kivlahan, D. R., & Marlatt, G. A. (1995). High-risk drinking across the transition from high school to college. *Alcoholism: Clinical and Experimental Research, 19*(1), 54–61.

Barnes, G. M., Farrell, M. P., & Banerjee, S. (1994). Family influences on alcohol abuse and other problem behaviors among black and white adolescents in a general population sample. *Journal of Research on Adolescence, 4*(2), 183–201.

Barnes, G. M., & Welte, J. W. (1983). Predictors of alcohol use among college students in New York State. *Journal of American College Health, 31*(4), 150–157.

Barnes, G. M., & Welte, J. W. (1986). Patterns and predictors of alcohol use among 7th–12th grade students in New York State. *Journal of Studies on Alcohol, 47*(1), 53–62.

Barnes, G. M., & Welte, J. W. (1990). Prediction of adults' drinking patterns from the drinking of their parents. *Journal of Studies on Alcohol, 51*(6), 523–527.

Barnes, G. M., Welte, J. W., & Dintcheff, B. (1992). Alcohol misuse among college students and other young adults: Findings from a general population study in New York State. *International Journal of the Addictions, 27*(8), 917–934.

Barnes, G. M., & Windle, M. (1987). Family factors in adolescent alcohol and drug abuse. Pediatrician: International Journal of Child and Adolescent Health, 14, 13–18.

Barr, H. L., & Cohen, A. (1987). Abusers of alcohol and narcotics: Who are they? *International Journal of the Addictions, 22*(6), 525–541.

Bennett, E. M., & Kemper, K. J. (1994). Is abuse during childhood a risk factor for developing substance abuse problems as an adult? *Journal of Developmental and Behavioral Pediatrics, 15*(6), 426–429.

Bennett, L. A., & Wolin, S. J. (1990). Family culture and alcoholism transmission. In R. C. Collins, K. E. Leonard, & J. S. Searles (Eds.), *Alcohol and the family: Research and clinical perspectives* (pp. 194–219). New York: Guilford Press.

Black, S. A., & Markides, K. S. (1993). Acculturation and alcohol consumption in Puerto Rican, Cuban-American, and Mexican-American women in the United States. *American Journal of Public Health, 83*(6), 890–893.

Brady, K. T., Killeen, T., Saladin, M. E., & Dansky, B. (1994). Comorbid substance abuse and posttraumatic stress disorder: Characteristics of women in treatment. *American Journal on Addictions, 3*(2), 160–164.

Brennan, P. L., Moos, R. H., & Mertens, J. R. (1994). Personal and environmental risk factors as predictors of alcohol use, depression, and treatment seeking: A longitudinal analysis of late life problem drinkers. *Journal of Substance Abuse, 6*(2), 191–208.

Brook, J. S., Whiteman, M., Gordan, A. S., & Brendan, C. (1983). Older brothers' influence on younger siblings' drug use. *Journal of Psychology, 114,* 83–90.

Brown, T. G., Kokin, M., Seraganian, P., & Shields, N. (1995). The role of spouses of substance abusers in treatment: Gender differences. *Journal of Psychoactive Drugs, 27*(3), 223–229.

Burnside, M. A., Baer, P. E., McLaughlin, R. J., & Pokorny, A. D. (1986). Alcohol use by adolescents in disrupted families. *Alcoholism: Clinical and Experimental Research, 10,* 274–278.

Caetano, R. (1986–1987). Drinking and the Hispanic-American family life. *Alcohol Health and Research World, 11,* 26–34.

Caetano, R. (1991). Findings from the 1984 National Survey of alcohol use among United States Hispanics. In W. B. Clark & M. E. Hilton (Eds.), *Alcohol in America* (pp. 293–307). Albany: State University of New York Press.

Clapper, R. L., Buka, S. L., Goldfield, E. C., Lipsitt, L. P., & Tsuang, M. T. (1995). Adolescent problem behaviors as predictors of adult alcohol diagnoses. *International Journal of the Addictions, 30*(5), 507–523.

Clayton, R. R., & Lacy, W. B. (1982). Interpersonal influences on male drug use and drug use intentions. *International Journal of the Addictions, 17,* 655–666.

Compton, W. M., Cottler, L. B., Dinwiddie, S. H., & Spitznagel, E. L. (1994). Inhalant use: Characteristics and predictors. *American Journal on Addictions, 3*(3), 263–272.

Coombs, R. H., & Paulson, M. J. (1988). Contrasting family patterns of adolescent drug users and nonusers. In R. H. Coombs (Ed.), *The family context of adolescent drug use* (pp. 59–72). New York: Haworth Press.

Cooper, M. L., Russell, M., & George, W. H. (1988). Coping, expectancies, and alcohol abuse: A test of social learning formulations. *Journal of Abnormal Psychology, 97*(2), 218–230.

Crum, R. M., Helzer, J. E., & Anthony, J. C. (1993). Level of education and alcohol abuse and dependence in adulthood: A further inquiry. *American Journal of Public Health, 83*(6), 830–837.

Denoff, M. S. (1987). Irrational beliefs as predictors of adolescent drug abuse and running away. *Journal of Clinical Psychology, 43*(3), 412–423.

Denoff, M. S. (1988). An integrated analysis of the contribution made by irrational beliefs and parental interaction to adolescent drug abuse. *International Journal of the Addictions, 23*(7), 655–669.

Dielman, T. E., Butchart, A. T., & Shope, J. T. (1993). Structural equation model tests of patterns of family interaction, peer use, and intrapersonal predictors of adolescent alcohol use and misuse. *Journal of Drug Education, 23*(3), 273–316.

Dishion, T. J., & Loeber, R. (1985). Adolescent marijuana and alcohol use: The role of parents and peers revisited. *American Journal of Drug and Alcohol Abuse, 11,* 11–25.

Downs, W. R., Miller, B. A., Testa, M., & Panek, D. (1992). Long term effects of parent-to-child violence for women. *Journal of Interpersonal Violence, 7*(3), 365–382.

Dull, R. T. (1992). Correlates of alcohol and marijuana use within a college freshman population. *Journal of Alcohol and Drug Education, 38*(1), 1–10.

Edwards, M. E., & Steinglass, P. (1995). Family therapy treatment outcomes for alcoholism. *Journal of Marital and Family Therapy, 21*(4), 475–510.

Filstead, W. J., McElfresh, O., & Anderson, C. (1981). Comparing the family environments of alcoholic and "normal" families. *Journal of Alcohol and Drug Education, 26*, 24–31.

Fitzgerald, H. E., Davies, W. H., Zucker, R. A., & Klinger, M. (1994). Developmental systems theory and substance abuse: A conceptual and methodological framework for analyzing patterns of variation in families. In L. L'Abate (Ed.), *Handbook of developmental family psychology and psychopathology* (pp. 350–372). New York: Wiley.

Fitzgerald, H. E., Sullivan, L. A., Ham, H. P., Zucker, R. A., Bruckel, S., Schneider, A. M., & Noll, R. B. (1993). Predictors of behavior problems in three-year-old sons of alcoholics: Early evidence for the onset of risk. *Child Development, 64*, 110–123.

Fitzgerald, H. E., & Zucker, R. A. (1995). Socioeconomic status and alcoholism: The contextual structure of developmental pathways to addiction. In H. E. Fitzgerald, B. M. Lester, & B. Zuckerman (Eds.), *Children of poverty: Research, health care, and public policy issues* (pp. 1–12). New York: Garland Press.

Goebel, A. E., Scheibe, K. E., & Grahling, S. C. (1995). Disordered eating in female alcohol dependent inpatients: Prevalence and associated psychopathology. *Eating Disorders: The Journal of Treatment and Prevention, 3*(1), 37–46.

Gonzalez, G. M. (1983). Time and place of first drinking experience and parental knowledge as predictors of alcohol use and misuse in college. *Journal of Alcohol and Drug Education, 28*(3), 24–33.

Gottschalk, L. A. (1983). Vulnerability to stress. *American Journal of Psychotherapy, 37*, 5–23.

Hall, J. A., Henggeler, S. W., Ferreira, D. K., & East, P. L. (1992). Sibling relations and substance use in high-risk female adolescents. *Family Dynamics of Addiction Quarterly, 2*(1), 44–51.

Hays, R. D., Stacy, A. W., Widaman, K. F., DiMatteo, M. R., & Downey, R. (1986). Multistage path models of adolescent alcohol and drug use: A reanalysis. *Journal of Drug Issues, 16*(3), 357–369.

Holland, S., & Griffin, A. (1984). Adolescent and adult drug treatment clients: Patterns and consequences of use. *Journal of Psychoactive Drugs, 16*(1), 79–89.

Holmes, S. J., & Robins, L. N. (1987). The influence of childhood disciplinary experience on the development of alcoholism and depression. *Journal of Child Psychology and Psychiatry, 28*(3), 399–415.

Janikowski, T. P., & Glover, N. M. (1994). Incest and substance abuse: Implications for treatment professionals. *Journal of Substance Abuse Treatment, 11*(3), 177–183.

Jessor, R., & Jessor, S. L. (1977). *Problem behavior and psychosocial development: A longitudinal study of youth*. New York: Academic Press.

Kandel, D., Simcha-Fagan, O., & Davies, M. (1986). Risk factors for delinquency and illicit drug use from adolescence to young adulthood. *Journal of Drug Issues, 16*(1), 67–90.

Kantor, G. K., & Straus, M. A. (1989). Substance abuse as a precipitant of wife abuse victimizations. *American Journal of Drug and Alcohol Abuse, 15*(2), 173–189.

Kellam, S. G., Stevenson, D. L., & Rubin, B. R. (1982). How specific are the early predictors of teenage drug use? *NIDA Research Monograph Series, 43,* 329–334.

Kingree, J. B. (1995). Understanding gender differences in psychosocial functioning and treatment retention. *American Journal of Drug and Alcohol Abuse, 21*(2), 267–281.

Klein, K., Forehand, R., Armistead, L., & Brody, G. (1994). Adolescent family predictors of substance use during early adulthood: A theoretical model. *Advances in Behavior Research and Therapy, 16*(4), 217–252.

Leonard, K. E. (1990). Marital functioning among episodic and steady alcoholics. In R. L. Collins, K. E. Leonard, & J. S. Searles (Eds.), *Alcohol and the family: Research and clinical perspectives* (pp. 220–243). New York: Guilford Press.

Levine, M., & Singer, S. I. (1988). Delinquency, substance abuse, and risk taking in middle-class adolescents. *Behavioral Sciences and the Law, 6*(3), 385–400.

Lex, B. W. (1987). Review of alcohol problems in ethnic minority groups. *Journal of Consulting and Clinical Psychology, 55,* 293–300.

Liddle, H. A., & Dakof, G. A. (1995). Efficacy of family therapy for drug abuse: Promising but not definitive. *Journal of Marital and Family Therapy, 21*(4), 511–544.

McBride, A. A., Joe, G. W., & Simpson, D. D. (1991). Prediction of long-term alcohol use, drug use, and criminality among inhalant users. *Hispanic Journal of Behavioral Sciences, 13*(3), 315–323.

McCarthy, W. J., & Anglin, M. D. (1990). Narcotics addicts: Effect of family and parental risk factors on timing of emancipation, drug use onset, pre-addiction incarcerations and education achievement. *Journal of Drug Issues, 20*(1), 99–123.

Muntaner, C., Walter, D., Nagoshi, C., Fishbein, D., Haertzen, C. A., & Jaffe, J. H. (1990). Self-report vs. laboratory measures of aggression as predictors of substance abuse. *Drug and Alcohol Dependence, 25*(1), 1–11.

Mutzell, S. (1994). Alcoholism in women. *Early Child Development and Care, 101,* 71–80.

Needle, R., McCubbin, H., Wilson, M., Reineck, R., Lazar, A., & Mederer, H. (1986). Interpersonal influences in adolescent drug use: The role of older siblings, parents, and peers. *International Journal of the Addictions, 21,* 739–766.

Neisen, J. H. (1993). Parental substance abuse and divorce as predictors of injection drug use and high risk sexual behaviors known to transmit HIV. *Journal of Psychology and Human Sexuality, 6*(2), 29–49.

Noel, N. E., McCrady, B. S., Stout, R. L., & Fisher-Nelson, H. (1991). Gender differences in marital functioning of male and female alcoholics. *Family Dynamics of Addiction Quarterly, 1*(4), 31–38.

Noll, R. B., Zucker, R. A., Fitzgerald, H. E., & Curtis, W. J. (1992). Cognitive and motoric functioning of sons of alcoholic fathers and controls: The early childhood years. *Developmental Psychology, 28*(4), 665–675.

O'Farrell, T. J. (1990). Sexual functioning of male alcoholics. In R. L. Collins, K. E. Leonard, & J. S. Searles (Eds.), *Alcohol and the family: Research and clinical perspectives* (pp. 244–271). New York: Guilford Press.

O'Farrell, T. J. (1993). Conclusions and future direction in practice and research in marital and family therapy in alcoholism treatment. In T. J. O'Farrell (Ed.), *Treating alcohol problems: Marital and family interventions* (pp. 403–434). New York: Guilford Press.

O'Farrell, T. J., & Birchler, G. R. (1987). Marital relationships of alcoholic, conflicted, and nonconflicted couples. *Journal of Marital and Family Therapy, 13*(3), 259–274.

O'Farrell, T. J., & Choquette, K. (1991). Marital violence in the year before and after spouse-involved alcoholism treatment. *Family Dynamics of Addiction Quarterly, 1*(1), 32–40.

O'Hare, T. (1995). Mental health problems and alcohol abuse: Co-occurrence and gender differences. *Health and Social Work, 20*(3), 207–214.

Pandina, R. J., & Schuele, J. A. (1983). Psychosocial correlates of alcohol and drug use of adolescent students and adolescents in treatment. *Journal of Studies on Alcohol, 44*(6), 950–973.

Pardeck, J. T. (1991). A multiple regression analysis of family factors affecting the potential for alcoholism in college students. *Family Therapy, 18*(2), 115–121.

Perkins, H. W. (1987). Parental religion and alcohol use problems as intergenerational predictors of problem drinking among college youth. *Journal for the Scientific Study of Religion, 26*(3), 340–357.

Piercy, F. P., Volk, R. J., Trepper, T. S., Sprenkle, D. H., & Lewis, R. (1991). The relationship of family factors to patterns of adolescent substance abuse. *Family Dynamics of Addiction Quarterly, 1*(1), 41–54.

Pullen, L. M. (1994). The relationships among alcohol abuse in college students and selected psychological/demographic variables. *Journal of Alcohol and Drug Education, 40*(1), 36–50.

Randolph, M. J., & Yates, W. R. (1992). Antisocial personality in alcohol and drug dependent individuals: A study of gender effects. *American Journal on Addictions, 2*(1), 9–17.

Rosenthal, D. (1971). *Genetics of psychopathology.* New York: McGraw-Hill.

Schinke, S., Orlandi, M., Vaccaro, D., Espinoza, R., McAlister, A., & Botvin, G. (1992). Substance use among Hispanic and non-Hispanic adolescents. *Addictive Behaviors, 17*, 117–124.

Selnow, G. A. (1987). Parent–child relationships and single and two-parent families: Implications for substance usage. *Journal of Drug Education, 17*, 315–326.

Smith, R. H., & McCauley, C. R. (1991). Predictors of alcohol abuse behaviors of undergraduates. *Journal of Drug Education, 21*(2), 159–166.

Stabenau, J. R. (1990). Additive independent factors that predict risk for alcoholism. *Journal of Studies on Alcohol, 51*(2), 164–174.

Stephenson, A. L., Henry, C. S., & Robinson, L. C. (1996). Family characteristics and adolescent substance use. *Adolescence, 31*(121), 59–77.

Vega, W. A., Gil, A. G., & Zimmerman, R. S. (1993). Patterns of drug use among Cuban-American, African-American, and white non-Hispanic boys. *American Journal of Public Health, 83*(2), 257–259.

Wallen, J., & Berman, K. (1992). Possible indicators of childhood sexual abuse for individuals in substance abuse treatment. *Journal of Child Sexual Abuse, 1*(3), 63–74.

Welte, J. W., & Barnes, G. M. (1987). Alcohol use among adolescent minority groups. *Journal of Studies on Alcohol, 48,* 329–336.

Werner, M. J., Walker, L. S., & Greene, J. W. (1994). Screening for problem drinking among college freshmen. *Journal of Adolescent Health, 15*(4), 303–310.

Williams, T. G. (1996). Substance abuse and addictive personality disorders. In F. W. Kaslow (Ed.), *Handbook of relational diagnosis and dysfunctional family patterns* (pp. 448–462). New York: Wiley.

Wood, M. D., Nagoshi, C. T., & Dennis, D. A. (1992). Alcohol norms and expectations as predictors of alcohol use and problems in a college student sample. *American Journal of Drug and Alcohol Abuse, 18*(4), 461–476.

Woodhouse, L. D. (1992). Women with jagged edges: Voices from a culture of substance abuse. *Qualitative Health Research, 2*(3), 262–281.

Zubin, J., & Spring, B. (1977). Vulnerability: A new view of schizophrenia. *Journal of Abnormal Psychology, 86,* 103–126.

Zucker, R. A., Ellis, D. A., Bingham, C. R., & Fitzgerald, H. E. (1996). The development of alcoholic subtypes: Risk variation among alcoholic families during the early chilhood years. *Alcohol Health and Research World, 20*(1), 46–54.

Zucker, R. A., Ellis, D. A., & Fitzgerald, H. E. (1994). Developmental evidence for at least two alcoholisms: I. Biopsychosocial variation among pathways into symptomatic difficulty. *Annals of the New York Academy of Sciences, 708,* 134–145.

Zucker, R. A., Fitzgerald, H. E., & Moses, H. D. (1995). Emergence of alcohol problems and the several alcoholisms: A developmental perspective on etiologic theory and life course trajectory. In D. Cicchetti & D. J. Cohen (Eds.), *Developmental psychopathology: Vol. 2. Risk, disorder, and adaptation* (pp. 677–711). New York: Wiley.

SECTION IV

---◆---

HELPING FAMILIES AT RISK, IN NEED, AND IN CRISIS

CHAPTER 16

<=>•◊•<=>

Prevention Approaches
for Families

PATRICK H. TOLAN
ELENA QUINTANA
DEBORAH GORMAN-SMITH

Few people would challenge the importance of family units in shaping the lives of children, who will inherit the power to define our future. This suggests that prevention efforts focusing on families as agents of change should be highly valued. However, few prevention efforts to date have assisted families in an effort to change child behavior. This chapter is an examination of family participation in prevention efforts designed to cause long-term changes in children, and thereby to reduce the incidence of such social ills as violence, illiteracy, and substance use.

This chapter examines five aspects of prevention with families. First, theoretical and practical characteristics that differentiate prevention from treatment interventions are described, in order to provide a framework for family-focused prevention research. Second, a review of the current typology for distinguishing levels of prevention is presented, and the implications of this typology for intervention design and evaluation are explained. Third, different types of family-focused interventions that can be applied in prevention are reviewed, with examples of each type noted. Fourth, reasons for the underemphasis on family in child-oriented prevention research are discussed, together with a call for more inspired and careful efforts in the field of prevention with families. Finally, a suggested framework for integrating each area is presented, including benefits and limitations of family-focused prevention research, suggested research priorities, and related design considerations.

DIFFERENCES BETWEEN PREVENTION AND
TREATMENT RESEARCH AND PROGRAMMING

As part of the originating and initial promoting of preventive efforts for behavioral problems, some unfortunate rhetoric has described prevention as better than, undermined by, or antithetical to treatment and other "after-the-fact" interventions (Mrazek & Haggerty, 1994). As noted by the Institute of Medicine and the National Institute of Mental Health (NIMH) reviews (National Institute of Mental Health, 1990), prevention is a part of a continuum of useful interventions whose utility is dependent on etiological factors, intervention technology, and economic and other practical considerations. The differences in sampling, program design, and evaluation outlined do not address the oft-stated criticism that prevention designs, particularly "indicated" interventions (see below), are not distinct from treatment. This may be due to the fact that much of what is called "prevention" is, by these standards, treatment (which ameliorates symptoms or noxious effects of symptoms), and much of what is called "treatment" is actually intended to be prevention (whose impact is defined in terms of lessened risk in the future) (Cowen, 1973). However, differences in focus, design, and implementation distinguish family-oriented interventions that are treatments from those that are preventive in nature.

Differences in Focus

First, the focus of prevention is on populations, whereas treatment focuses on individuals. Individuals are of interest in prevention only as they are part of a population. Samples in prevention are valid to the extent that they include all those who are qualified or in need from a population with defined characteristics relating to risk and/or inclusion (Kellam, 1990).

In treatment, other than for purposes of symptom verification or problem definition (e.g., determining that someone is depressed), the sample is of interest as an aggregate of individuals. This has implications for how treatment efficacy or effectiveness is judged, how interventions are prescriptively adjusted to the needs of a family, and how case management is approached (Brown, 1993a).

Differences in Judging Efficacy or Effectiveness

An important distinction between prevention and other types of intervention research is in how efficacy or effectiveness is evaluated. In prevention research, the interest is not in evaluating immediate effects, but the long-term differences between the treatment and control groups. Also, the effects are interpreted differently. In treatment, the usual interest is in "means" comparisons between treated and untreated subjects from the same population, so that the average effect on a presumably homogeneous sample of recipients can be estimated. Also, the clinical interest is not, as it is in treatment, in reducing clinical levels of problems to normal levels (Kendall & Grove, 1988). Instead, prevention focuses on reduced rates of later occurrence of the "to-be-prevented" outcome, with the interest in immediate effects depending on the theoretical relation of proximal effects to the ultimate outcome (Kellam, 1990). Also, there is no presumption that all research participants are in equal need of an intervention, or are even receptive to it; heterogeneity is expected, as is meaningful variation in intervention impact (Brown, 1993b).

The currently prevailing approach is that preventive interventions for mental health problems are best conceptualized and analyzed as interactions with developmental trajectories, which are likely to be further modified by contextual constraints (Coie et al., 1993; Kellam, 1990). For example, it is not uncommon in prevention research to expect and find variations in the impact of an intervention depending on preintervention risk status, covarying characteristics, and/or timing and setting of the intervention (Brown, 1993a, 1993b; The Metropolitan Area Child Study, 1997). Thus, there is a primary focus on assessing outcome by the rate of problems' not occurring by some specified point in the future, rather than on using relative level on a scale to measure effects and focusing on variations in rates among epidemiologically meaningful subgroups. Also, a failure to find immediate differences between treated and untreated groups may be deceiving, as it is important to take into account the relation between proximal risk markers and eventual status (Tolan & Brown, 1997).

One important difference is the relationship between proximal or immediate postintervention effects and distal or later effects (Brown, 1993a, 1993b; Kellam, 1990). In most treatment programs, the most basic question is whether or not there are immediate effects, and, if so, whether or not they are maintained. The follow-up effects are often secondary to the immediate ones in indicating efficacy, and follow-up is undertaken to indicate maintenance of the initial impact.

In prevention, the immediate effects are of interest to the extent that they help explain distal effects. The immediate postintervention outcome may tell us little about the value of the intervention; this judgment may have to wait for a point in the future. For example, it appears that the age of about 25 is the point at which risk for initiating involvement in serious antisocial behavior is over for almost all individuals. Thus, any preventive efforts carried out in childhood cannot be fully judged until the population that has received these efforts reaches that age.

Differences in Measurement Emphasis

Differences between prevention and treatment in measurement emphasis affect more than outcome analysis. Measurement development may vary when individuals represent subgroups or constituents within a population (rather than interchangeable representatives of the population). For example, it may be appropriate to organize clusters of subjects who have pertinent characteristics, rather than to examine the linear combination of relative scores on such measures, to characterize how subjects with different characteristics fare (Tolan, Gorman-Smith, Henry, Chung, & Hunt, in press). Also, because of the inherently longitudinal nature of measurement of effects, developmental issues in measurement and the constructs of interest must be considered. Such issues often cause substantial complications in measuring effects; one must measure impact against a normative model of change informed by a longitudinal measurement model (Patterson & Bank, 1989). For example, changes in measurement reliability due to developmental changes may obscure intervention effects (Muthen & Curran, 1997).

Differences in Intervention Design

In treatment studies, the approach applied is usually tailored and structured to test a specific protocol; however, there is a general recognition that this is only a prototype that is to be modified when case characteristics indicate a need for modification, and certainly when the prototype is implemented by practitioners. In prevention research, variations in activities, accentuation, staff orientation, and staff members' prescriptive responsiveness to clients' needs are undesirable rather than optimal. Applied prevention research explicitly acknowledges that some participants may not benefit from such research. Clinically oriented staff members may need to be trained to rethink "case management": Instead of focusing more on the least responsive cases, they may need to redirect their efforts toward applying equal levels of involvement across cases, and to recognize that differential response is to be expected. In prevention design, the efficacy test rests on the understanding that other issues may arise, but that adherence to the protocol is critical to test the population effect. This difference is not absolute, but is present as a relative difference in weighing prescriptive response versus specific program application.

Difference in the Importance of the Relation of Proximal to Distal Effects

Prevention can also be differentiated from treatment in the importance of an articulated theory of the relations between proximal effects and distal status. In turn, during the intervention, this relation must be consistent with the type of prevention selected and the targets. It is uncommon for treatments to have an articulated theory, other than maintenance of effect. However, because prevention is focused on status at some point in the future, the selection of the type of prevention, inclusion criteria, and the methods to be used must be tied to that future status by a theoretical (and, ideally, empirically demonstrated) relationship among the risk factors identified, the targets of intervention, the intervention activities, the proximal outcomes, and the distal outcomes (Kellam, 1990; West, Aiken, & Todd, 1993). Thus, as in treatment, one needs to articulate a set of intervention activities based on a theory about how affecting risk factors will have immediate impact, but one must also specify how this immediate impact will lead to long-term effects (Lorion, Tolan, & Wahler, 1987; Lorion, Price, & Eaton, 1989). Inherently, this requires a developmental model of the psychopathology or problem, mapped onto a model of normal development (Coie et al., 1993). It is also increasingly recognized that the developmental model must be contextualized, so that the focus is on developmentally targeted intervention that is ecologically sound (Elliott & Tolan, in press; Tolan, Guerra, & Kendall, 1995).

Differences in Implementation

Participation in a preventive intervention is not decided primarily by those receiving the intervention. Although, of course, participation is usually voluntary to some degree (particularly among research participants), prevention is meant to be offered not by choice, but rather by need and benefit. In reality, there is a complicated and difficult process of getting clients, or those who act as gatekeepers for participation, to agree that the intervention has value or may keep a future problem from occurring (Tolan & McKay, 1996). In addition, if participation is based on some inclusion criteria in regard to relative risk, that risk must be reliably defined and must determine inclusion to a greater degree than motivation for help does. Not only does this add another wrinkle to evaluation of effects, but it adds considerable complexity to how programs are set up, where they should be located, how participation is solicited, and how participation rates affect validity (Tolan & Brown, 1997).

Prevention programs may need to be offered through venues other than traditional mental health and social service agencies, because these settings can connote an identified deficit. In most cases, it means soliciting people who have not been identified by themselves or others as having a need for intervention and who may not be experiencing specific distress. They may not accept or understand the conception of risk and its relation to later problems. This needs to be presented to them in such a way as to convince busy, serious people that they should devote limited time and other resources to such an activity. In prevention, in short, there is no client-identified problem that provides a clear contract of mutual activity between the intervention staff and the recipients. In fact, there may not even be an externally defined problem (e.g., a school or court referral). For example, in our Metropolitan Area Child Study and our SAFEChildren studies (Tolan & McKay, 1996), we engage families in 22-week interventions at a time when children are in elementary school, with the goal of decreasing risk for later behavioral and social problems. When the proximal mediators are better educated in social functioning and in greater compliance with parental management, families can be engaged in this immediate goal. However, it is our impression that some families come to a program because they see it as addressing immediate concerns about their children's behavior, whereas others come because they want to improve their child's chances in the future. Few engage in it simply as a "mental hygiene" exercise to prevent some problem that may occur 5–8 years later, or that may never occur.

Is Treatment a Special Case of the Prevention Approach?

These differences may seem to characterize prevention as a more complex and theoretically cumbersome intervention approach than treatment. However, it may also be that prevention research has required the articulation of issues that were latent in treatment studies and should be incorporated. For example, it can be argued that family therapy to reduce substance misuse among adolescents needs to consider the developmental issues of adolescents and the context in which the clients live to understand the intervention impact (Liddle & Dakof, 1995). In addition, follow-up or maintenance effects may have complex relations to proximal findings. It may be that much of what has been identified here as differentiating prevention from treatment represents features that are influential in treatment research but have not been recognized. Ideally, prevention research directly affects treatment research, casting light on important considerations such as the long-term effects of intervention over developmental transformations in various environmental contexts (Mrazek & Haggerty, 1994).

PREVENTION DESIGN BASED ON THE TYPE OF POPULATION FOCUS

The historical perspective on prevention has been that three levels can be differentiated: "primary," "secondary," and "tertiary" (Afifi & Breslow, 1994). In this public health schema, which was originally developed to combat biologically induced disease, all prevention is distinguished from treatment by two major features. First, the interest is in intervention before the disease, problem, or syndrome develops, rather than in ameliorating the ailment or minimizing its symptoms once it has occurred. Second, the interest is in populations rather than individuals (Coie et al., 1993). The goal is to decrease the rate (incidence or prevalence) of disease or disorder among the target *population*, rather than to cure or ease the ailment of specific patients (Caplan, 1964). The value of the intervention depends on changes in these rates, and primarily the rates of onset or new incidence of disorder subsequent to the intervention (Lorion et al., 1989).

This schema has been applied to psychopathology and social adaptation regularly, but during the history of such application students of the field and designers of preventive efforts have had difficulty in distinguishing the levels of prevention clearly; in distinguishing prevention from early treatment (e.g., a parenting program to lessen conduct disorder) and from maintenance of treatment benefits (e.g., a program to reduce relapse among schizophrenics); and in distinguishing among the different levels of treatment (e.g., is family therapy for first offenders secondary or tertiary prevention?). Despite extended discussions and complex definitions designed to adapt this biomedical model of the levels of prevention to behavioral areas, none seem to provide simple, clear distinctions (Cowen, 1983; Lorion et al., 1989; Price, Cowen, Lorion, & Ramos, 1989; Steinberg & Silverman, 1987).

A fairly recent development has been the adoption of a variation on the primary–secondary–tertiary distinction for prevention related to behavioral problems—a variation that brings to the fore the type of risk to the population of interest and the related intended impact (Lorion et al., 1989). This approach provides many advantages to behavioral prevention researchers, enabling them to design approaches based on the risk level of the target group. The differentiation was pioneered by Gordon (1983) and has been adopted by the Institute of Medicine (Mrazek & Haggerty, 1994) and the NIMH (Munoz et al., 1996). This approach distinguishes preventive interventions that target everyone in a given population, labeled "Universal" Prevention, from efforts that target a subpopulation for inclusion because it is judged to be at heightened risk, labeled "Selective" Prevention. Selective interventions often target subgroups because of some shared characteristic that may relate to risk (e.g., children from families with illiterate parents are selected for inclusion in a preventive effort during first grade to support acquisition of reading skills). This approach is distinguished from the third type, labeled "Indicated" Prevention, which targets only the portion of the sample with evidence of *specific* risk, usually due to individual differences. Thus, this approach makes a primary distinction about what portion of the population is targeted and the relative risk of that portion (Gordon, 1983). The distinction is not determined primarily by etiological formulations, which are supposed to be the basis for implementing primary, secondary, or tertiary prevention. However, there are implications about how risk is carried and which portion of the population is targeted.

It is important to note that Gordon's interest and this schema were predicated on the fact that prevention is not an intervention that is based on clients' consent. It is based on estimated risk or benefits, not on help seeking or other indications of interest from the clientele (Caplan, 1964). This difference reflects, as well as engenders, a different approach to determination of resource allocation and the type of social contract between the provider and the client (or the researcher and the participant, in prevention trials). For example, instead of engaging clients about a self-identified problem and engaging participants who are self-referred, the prevention researcher engages clients who are at risk or have some characteristic related to targeting (Tolan & McKay, 1996). A client may not understand that characteristic as denoting risk, may have difficulty understanding the certainty of risk, and may not agree with the implications. Also, the potential participants are approached apart from any specific initiation by them. Thus, the participation agreement can be less specific and may require different types of engagement activities (Tolan & McKay, 1996; Hanish, Tolan, McKay, & Dickey, in press). For example, the Metropolitan Area Child Study engaged families with children who were nominated by their peers and teachers as those at highest risk for a variety of undesirable characteristics; however, the program emphasized family strengths and concrete exercises for families, without explicitly stating the assumed risk status of the participants. Families were often willing to participate in a program that would help their children do their best in school, but they were wary of participating in a program that would label the children as potentially problematic within their larger community.

The differentiation of prevention types according to Gordon's (1983) schema implies differentiating several aspects of the design and understanding the nature of the prevention effort. Figure 16.1 provides a summary of the major differences among universal, selective, and indicated prevention efforts. This figure shows that these differences relate to the portion of the population targeted, the utility and importance of accurate discrimination procedures for selecting participants, the type of statistical measure or population effects of interest, and the criterion for "clinical significance" or substantial benefit. In addition, each type varies as to the intensity of intervention and the expected increment of benefit and risk for each participant (see Figure 16.1). These characteristics show that the differentiation of prevention types into universal, selective, and indicated types is more than nominal and should guide the design and application of family-focused prevention research.

Differentiating Universal, Selective, and Indicated Prevention

Universal interventions include participants regardless of possible differences in risk (Lorion et al., 1989). Most such programs have the intended purpose of preventing the incidence of disorder(s) at some later point, and thus of reducing the overall prevalence of the disorder(s) in the population. Such efforts often include attempts to increase resources, competencies, and skills to inoculate participants against the "pathogen" or to remediate circumstances or skills that create general risk (Kazdin, Bass, Ayers, & Rodgers, 1990). Family-focused examples include public education campaigns to alert parents to the importance of curfews; parenting classes that

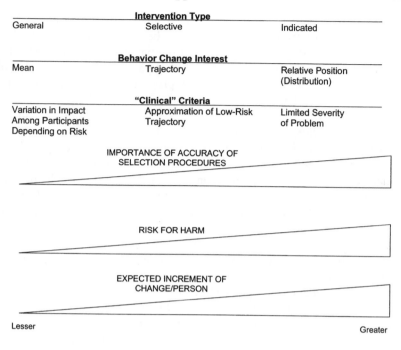

FIGURE 16.1. Prevention design characteristics.

coach parents in monitoring of their children's peers and other skills to reduce the children's involvement in antisocial behavior; and general prenatal classes in a health maintenance organization. In most cases, these interventions are mass-distributed and have low costs and intensity per person receiving the services. They may be meant to address a set of problems, and so are likely to have general rather than specific effects. For example, a universal program to improve parents' involvement in their children's academic achievement may address such issues as aiding children in learning to read, organizing a place for the children to do homework, and working with the children's teachers. Each of these specific skills may carry some risk for some persons, but all need addressing in a broad, mass-distributed universal prevention effort. Because universal interventions are mass-distributed, low in intensity, and minimally intrusive, they are likely to have a less dramatic impact on each participant. Their public health benefits, however, may be dramatic by reducing risk a small amount for large numbers of persons; similarly, they are generally likely to have a limited risk of harmful impact on those exposed.

An implicit assumption of such efforts is that risk is relatively evenly distributed within the population, that it is usually not carried by individuals, and that population characteristics are the main determinants of risk. Also there is an implicit assumption either that intervention effects may be equal across most persons receiving the benefits, or that there is some self-selection (with those in need reaping the benefit, without harm to those not in need). To return to the example of the parenting program for aiding academic achievement, the assumption is that parents who are already able in such areas will not be harmed by the program, but that they will also have children with less risk. In short, such programs hinge on the belief that what is provided probably can help everyone and cannot hurt anyone (Lorion et al., 1989).

Because universal interventions are intended to affect population incidence rates, the most direct measure of such an intervention's effect is change or difference in the population rates of those free from the problem at which the intervention is targeted. In general, the outcomes of interest are categorical, although in some instances the interest is in reducing the average (mean or median) on a scale representing the extent of a problem (e.g., favorable attitudes toward substance use). Because universal interventions are often large-scale and given to a whole population, comparison to a matched population in similar circumstances and historical context may be the optimal balance of control and external validity. Random assignment within a population may not be plausible, because of the mass distribution of the intervention and the likelihood of uncontrollable or unmeasurable "contamination" of control groups. When random assignment or comparison with a matched community is not possible, comparison with a prior cohort is necessary (Tolan & Brown, 1997).

Selected interventions differ from universal interventions by focusing on a subgroup or population that shares exposure to a particular risk factor (or set of factors). This approach is useful when the assumption is that risk is not distributed evenly and the risk is related to some group membership. For example, we are conducting a selective intervention for families of children entering first grade. We are providing tutoring for the children and a family support and skills group to aid in the children's adaptation to school and to academic achievement. Inclusion is based on families' residence in neighborhoods that are among the most destitute in Chicago. In this case, the risk factor for school failure and later behavior problems is seen as exposure to these neighborhood and school contexts, and the tutoring and family intervention are intended to inoculate children against the risk (Gorman-Smith, Henry, & Tolan, in press). Like indicated interventions, selective interventions usually focus on a theoretical model of development of risk and the empirically identified elements of risk. However, selective interventions focus more on a group's exposure to a risk factor, whereas indicated interventions focus on individual risk. For example, a selective intervention may focus on children exposed to parental divorce, because there is a relation between experiencing parental divorce and increases rates of internalizing disorders (Pillow, Sandler, Braver, Wolchik, & Gersten, 1991). An indicated program may focus on those children among those experiencing divorce who also show poor coping skills, because such individual differences mediate the divorce–internalization relationship (Pillow et al., 1991).

Because a subpopulation is targeted, selective interventions are usually more intensive than universal programs; therefore, they have a greater cost per person/family served and an accompanying increased risk of negative impact. Accurate identification of the risk group, and the extent to which its estimated level of risk is attributable to the shared characteristics, are important in determining the justification of selective interventions (Loeber, Dishion, & Patterson, 1984). If identification is reasonably accurate, a selective program may have a lower overall cost than an indiscriminately or inappropriately applied universal program may (Lorion et al., 1989).

Evaluation of selective programs differs from that of universal and indicated programs in how effects are measured. The statistical interest is in decreasing the rate of the problem's occurrence among the subgroup exposed to an intervention, but the clinical interest is in approximating the incidence of the problem among the low-risk portions of the population. From a developmental perspective, the interest is having the treated high-risk subgroup approximate the trajectory (or trajectories) of the low-risk group (Coie et al., 1993). Inclusion of those who are not really in need (false positives), as well as exclusion of those who actually are in need (false negatives), can increase error in the estimate of the intervention's impact. In a cross-sectional analysis or pre–post comparison, a reduction in the problem's occurrence rate among those with elevated risk is evidenced as reducing the proportion of the population with a problem at a given point. If linear measures of a characteristics are examined, an effective selected intervention is one that attenuates distribution among the overall population (Brown, 1993a, 1993b).

As noted above, indicated interventions focus on individual risk rather than subpopulation risk. Interventions of this third type are intended to lessen the seriousness, chronicity, or continuation of symptoms and disorders (Lorion et al., 1989). These interventions target those who may have relatively minor problems that could become more severe without intervention. Thus, those who are targeted may be asymptomatic for a specific condition, but appear to be predisposed to develop this condition because of the presence of less severe abnormalities (Gordon, 1983). In practice, such programs focus on serving individuals with early signs of problems or early manifestations of problems—for example, early aggression, which predicts later delinquency (Gordon, 1983). They are designed to curtail or eliminate the long-term consequences of a disorder (Caplan, 1964). Thus, the focus is on altering the natural course of the problem to lessen its harmful impact (Kellam, 1990).

Indicated programs, like selected programs, rely on epidemiology and screening to determine inclusion; however, because inclusion in indicated programs is usually based on the presence of specific symptoms or behaviors, accuracy of identification is more critical (Kellam, 1990). Their application is indicated when it is assumed that risk is carried by individuals and that individuals must be changed to reduce risk. Indicated programs should have a greater intensity, and may be expected to have a greater impact on each individual participating, than other prevention programs. Accordingly, they are usually more costly per person served than other prevention programs and have a greater probability of unintended harmful treatment effects. These concerns are balanced, however, by the high probability of worsening or continued serious problems without intervention, the greater costs of managing more serious and chronic forms of the problem, and the need for an immediate response. An indicated program may be the most cost-effective prevention when the population risk is concentrated among a small portion of the population and the risk carriers can be accurately identified (Lorion et al., 1989).

For indicated interventions, the logical outcomes of interest are control of the disorder, lessening of symptoms or undesired behaviors, and shorter duration or arrested development of a disorder. Evaluation of such efforts should focus on decreased seriousness and duration of problems in treated subjects, compared to untreated subjects with similar preintervention risk. For example, indicated interventions for antisocial behavior should lessen the seriousness and the duration of delinquency involvement. Borduin et al. (1995) reported on the use of a multisystemic family-focused intervention designed to prevent the recurrence of arrest and continuation of juvenile delinquent behavior into adult criminality. They showed that this program could reduce rates of violent behavior and rearrest.

Because the primary comparison in the evaluation of an indicated program is that between treated and untreated subjects in the risk group, random assignment is an appropriate design for such a study (Tolan & Brown, 1997). The interest may be either in reducing the extent of the problem (e.g., number of incidents of acute psychosis and relapse among subjects with a single prior psychotic episode) or in changing the relative position in the population distribution of those with the problem. At a population level, the interest is in changing the incidence rate of categorically defined problems and decreasing the total number of problems measured via extent of symptoms. The benefits of an indicated program can be quite misleading if it is assumed that the effect should create an approximation of the developmental trajectory of low-risk populations or a change in the group average.

Implications for Family-Focused Prevention

The differences noted above suggest that quite different methods of targeting, implementation, and evaluation criteria are appropriate, depending on the relation of risk factors to the outcome and on the distribution of such characteristics among the population of interest (Brown, 1993a). Family prevention efforts that are cognizant of such differences and incorporate their implications into program design are more likely to have the intended impact, to be adequately implemented, and to be appropriately evaluated. As in other areas of prevention, the question is not which type of prevention is best, but which is most useful and justified for a given goal to prevent a given problem. In addition to the differences among types of prevention, several important characteristics of family-focused prevention differ from those of family-focused treatment. However, these differences have not usually been specified and often impede the effects of prevention.

EXAMPLES OF FAMILY-FOCUSED PREVENTION

As indicated in the preceding section, family-focused prevention can take many forms and vary in the way in which families are viewed. A review of the literature suggests three primary types of family-focused prevention activities, particularly in regard to children (Pinsof & Wynne, 1995).

First and most common are activities that focus on the family, particularly parenting practices, as the direct causes of risk (Patterson, Reid, & Dishion, 1992). In such interventions, the family relationships and practices are the direct targets, and impact is thought to depend on the extent to which such family characteristics are changed (Tolan et al., 1995; Hanish et al., in press; Shadish et al., 1993). There are numerous examples of such programs (see Tolan & McKay, 1996). For example, Webster-Stratton and colleagues (Webster-Stratton, 1991; Webster-Stratton, Kolpacoff, & Hollinsworth, 1988) have carried out universal and selective interventions with parents of preschool children and early elementary-age children, in order to reduce the later incidence of oppositional defiant disorder and conduct disorder. They have shown reductions in rates of these disorders, positive long-term effects, and cost-effectiveness (Webster-Stratton et al., 1988).

Although there have been many family prevention programs targeted at disruptive behavior problems, there have been few such programs aimed at other types of child and adolescent psychopathology or at social problems (Chamberlain & Rosicky, 1995; Liddle & Dakof, 1995). In addition, many of the studies have not been focused on measuring family processes other than parenting practices (Tolan & Guerra, 1994; Tolan, Gorman-Smith, Zelli, & Huesmann, 1997). Even fewer have evaluated the process by which the effects were obtained. Those underway show promising results. For example, we have recently investigated the extent to which our Metropolitan Area Child Study family intervention (Tolan & McKay, 1996) affects change in child aggression by increasing parenting skills and child compliance with parental directives. Our results suggest that this is the path of effects and that changes in parenting practices are related to the alliance with the intervention provider (Tolan et al., in press). However, a second study suggests that there are different reactions to the intervention, depending on initial parenting skills, family systemic relations, and child aggression level (Hanish et al., in press).

A second type of family-focused prevention is most commonly provided for families with a physically ill child (Campbell & Peterson, 1995) and families with a schizophrenic member (Goldstein & Miklowitz, 1995). Although many such interventions focus on reducing pathogenic family processes, most focus on developing and supporting a family's capacity to maintain its ill member over time. Research suggests that multiple dimensions may merit targeting, but these types of family-focused prevention can be described as focusing on family processes and skills as moderators of risk. For example, Kliewer and Lewis (1995) found that more positive (active) coping among children with sickle cell anemia was related to family cohesion and parental coping. In such prevention efforts, the focus is usually on increasing family knowledge and resource utilization, as well as on providing technical support for managing the illness. For example, Sanders, Shepherd, Cleghorn, and Woolford (1994) applied a cognitive-behavioral intervention for families of children with abdominal pain, and found that it prevented relapses, increased the length of time between relapses, and resulted in lower rates of pain. Like the type of family-focused prevention emphasizing family processes as risk-inducing, this type of prevention has many problems that have not been investigated. In particular, it may be that family-focused health service delivery or psychoeducational and family support adjuncts to necessary health care may be as valuable as this type of prevention in reducing rates of full symptomatology or severity of acute episodes of chronic disorders. Also, there is a need for evaluation of universal prevention programs such as health promotion efforts that are family-focused.

The third major type of family-focused prevention focuses on the family not as a direct cause of problems or as a moderator of risk, but as a venue for enhancing receipt of and benefit from prevention services (Combrinck-Graham, 1989). For example, parental involvement to improve academic functioning can be undertaken to increase the likelihood that children will understand academic expectations or comply, without directly implicating family processes in risk or seeing change in parental behavior as important in determining the eventual outcome for the children. Similarly, child compliance with needed medical care can be increased by focusing on family involvement in treatment and incorporation of medical needs into family routines and plans (Kliewer, 1997). Although it has been less researched than other types of family-focused prevention, this third type of prevention may provide some of the most important information about the benefits of prevention, as its results tend to have implications for how service should be delivered, as well as how effective specific activities are. Thus, for example, one can test the impact of a family-based approach to reading practice versus a traditional individual-practice method for children with poor initial reading skills, to see which method is more effective and whether it has cost advantages as well (Combrinck-Graham, 1989).

There are probably several other areas of family prevention that could be distinguished, but the three types described above these represent the areas with the most research activity to date. However, even in these most active areas there has not been extensive research, and few of the studies that have been done have the sophistication suggested as necessary in the initial review of different types of prevention. A review of the literature suggests that research with increasing sophistication is beginning to be carried out, but much basic work is still needed. From Gordon's (1983) conceptualization of prevention types, the differentiation of prevention from treatment, the specific issues of family-focused prevention, and the examples of such work that we have listed here, it seems that some suggested directions for further work can be extracted.

THE UNDEREMPHASIS ON FAMILIES IN PREVENTION

To date there have been relatively few family-focused prevention efforts, particularly ones in which children's functioning is the outcome of interest. Most prevention has not focused on families as units of service or as the targets of change to reduce risk factors. The theoretical models of individual development and individual risk identification are far more advanced and have much more extensive empirical support than their counterparts regarding families (Coie et al., 1993; Tolan et al., 1997). The high cost of program delivery, and the difficulty in securing adequate rates of prevention for confidence in judging effects with families, may explain in part why individuals are more often the focus of prevention efforts. Much child-focused prevention has occurred within schools, because schools represent normative developmental settings that almost all children attend and in which prevention programs can be delivered with cost-efficiency. Thus, prevention has been provided through a venue and in a setting based on convenience. When one starts working with families, one confronts the multidimensionality of risk, as well as the variation in circumstances among children within a given group or school. Defining risk is much more complicated. There are many more covariates to consider in analyses (Tolan & McKay, 1996). Also, if a prevention program requires parental inclusion, one finds, not surprisingly, that the parents of the children most at risk are least able to participate or interested in participating (Tolan & McKay, 1996). In addition, parents may not participate for many other reasons. Economic demands, work schedules, disruptive family events, and other impediments can influence participation, just as more obvious impediments such as parental substance misuse, illiteracy, and psychopathology can (Tolan & McKay, 1996).

Family prevention, like other family intervention, introduces measurement complexities as well (Dakof, 1996; Tolan et al., 1997). Families can be conduits through which intervention effects are provided, can be seen as risk-inducing via problematic family processes, or may be viewed as intervention resources to develop and support skills and processes designed to prevent an undesirable outcome (Combrinck-Graham, 1989). Of course, these are not mutually exclusive perspectives, but they do represent different approaches, and they now show how defining a family's impact on the proximal and distal outcomes involves more than parallel analyses of individuals (Shadish et al., 1993) . Also, there are theoretical complications in interventions targeting families that do not arise in interventions aimed at individuals (Liddle & Dakof, 1995; Pinsof & Wynne, 1995). For example, how does one evaluate an intervention that makes mothers better able to monitor and discipline their sons, but does not affect fathers? Is it a failure, a partial success, or a full success if this is enough to reduce risk substantially among the population?

School-based and other institution-based preventions are also more common than family-focused prevention because the school provides ease of access to recipients. Schools and recreational centers have children present in large groups over adequate periods of time to permit delivery of the services. Scheduling can be simplified to accommodate efficient delivery. If one focuses on peers and school factors, prevention efforts can be applied to children without the nuisance of getting parents to come to meetings or making them welcome in schools. Parents are not bound to attend school or come to our prevention efforts. They cannot be included by coercion from principals, judges, or special education teams; rather, they must be persuaded to see the value of the intervention, beyond its removing the threats of gatekeepers. These limitations can be formidable, requiring substantial scientific work to be overcome. However, as this volume and other work attest, the extent and rate of development of family intervention science and its bases are increasing rapidly.

SOME SUGGESTIONS FOR FAMILY PREVENTION

Family-focused prevention holds great promise for providing a public good while enabling such work to be scientifically scrutinized (Cowen, 1983; Shadish et al., 1993). The emerging evidence is that family-focused prevention may be quite effective and may have cost advantages over treatment and other forms of prevention for children (Tolan & Guerra, 1994; Shadish et al., 1993). However, it is also a complex enterprise that has many theoretical and practical problems. Among the complexities is the need to locate intervention design and targeting within epidemiological, risk, and intervention technology research, as well as the ecological factors affecting service delivery and impact (Tolan & McKay, 1996; Tolan et al., 1995). The state of the science is one in which we can identify the limitations of present paradigms and borrowed methods. There is an urgent need to define the structure of prevention science and to develop more apt models and methods for family-focused prevention (Coie et al., 1993). A tradeoff must be made between exciting possibilities and simple, clear direction.

Within these qualifications and general conclusions, some guidelines merit consideration in the development, design, implementation, and evaluation of prevention efforts involving the family.

1. Clarifying the type of prevention is important, because, as we have shown in this chapter, this affects proper evaluation. Defining the type of population that should be included by the distribution of risk among the population, the expected costs and benefits of inclusion versus exclusion, and the likely population benefits of a given prevention approach constitutes an advance over the prior typology borrowed from biomedical epidemiology. Universal, selective, and indicated interventions differ not only in which portion of the population is included, but also in specific design and evaluation features. Failure to consider these adequately, or to follow the implications of each type for inclusion methods, program design, or evaluation, can lead to erroneous and perhaps misleading evaluation.

2. In prevention, base rates are critical for determining what type of intervention is warranted, what the likely risk markers are, and how much of a population effect can be expected. In concert with cost–benefit analyses, these statistics help guide the level of prevention that is advisable. This is different from a concrete application of risk models. For example, there is evidence that parental hostility relates to delinquency, so a prevention program may aim to reduce the relative level of hostility within a target population. However, even if the mean hostility in a population can be reduced substantially, this may have no effect on prevalence if the relationship is between extreme hostility and delinquency rather than the lower but more common levels of hostility.

3. It is critical in any prevention effort to articulate a relation between proximal and distal outcomes, and to do so within a developmental model that locates the intervention as an interaction with such development, with due attention to developmental timing effects and contextual influences. Without such specification, the rationale for intervention components is usually weak, and any relation to long-term effects may be indeterminable. Also, the nature of variations in effects on meaningful subgroups among participants will be hard to clarify.

4. Families probably represent the most optimal intervention target for many child and adult disorders and social problems. However, to date there has been less scientific development of needed construct assessment and developmental models to guide such prevention than there has been for individual-focused prevention. Also, family-focused prevention can entail more complex and unfamiliar service delivery issues than those involved in many preventions provided in schools and other institutional settings that focus on children only. Similarly, it is important to distinguish family prevention efforts that focus on family processes as risk factors,

efforts that focus on family processes and skills as moderators of risk–outcome links, and efforts that aim to increase prevention benefits by providing services in a family-friendly environment. All three areas merit investigation and can contribute to strengthening the field of family intervention science, as well as aiding in the cost-effective delivery of needed aid to families and children.

5. The evaluation of proximal and distal outcomes should depend on the type of intervention provided. If the family is merely a venue for prevention targeting an individual member (e.g., parents or other family members are present while cognitive-behavioral training is done with an impulsive child to prevent school failure), then it is important to measure the family's support of the program, but it may not be critical to assess systemic characteristics (Kumpfer, 1989). If family processes are implicated as causes of risk or as important protective factors in linking proximal effects to distal outcomes, then these must be measured in a manner that reflects family-level constructs, not merely a collection of individual measures (Tolan et al., 1997). If the family is the unit of intervention focus (e.g., the objective is to make family members less abusive with each other), then there is a need to show how change in the family will be measured.

CONCLUSION

Although family prevention efforts are often more costly and cumbersome than individual-level efforts to administer and evaluate, the continued belief that families have the power to effect long-term change fuels the ongoing development of prevention work with families (Tolan & McKay, 1996). It is insufficient merely to care about poor communities and the children and families living there. Even the most well-meaning efforts can fail if they are not conducted with precision and an accurate knowledge of appropriate implementation and evaluation strategies to use with families. It appears that the ingredients of inspired intervention include scrupulous scientific considerations; dedicated, approachable staff members who are motivated to find and engage highly mobile families with few resources; and the families themselves, whose members invest their time, effort, and faith that they can move a step in the right direction. Although many of us profess a yearning to leave the world a better place, it is vital for us to evaluate our efforts carefully along the way, to ensure that we are working toward what is truly a greater good.

ACKNOWLEDGMENTS

The development and writing of this chapter were conducted with support from NIMH Grants No. R1848034 and No. RO148248, NICHD Grant No. HS35415,

CDC Grant No. R49/CCR512739, SAMHSA/CSAP Grant No. CCR512379, and NSF Grant No. SPR-9601157; W.T. Grant Faculty Scholar Award to Deborah Gorman-Smith; and a University of Illinois at Chicago Great Cities Institute Faculty Scholar Award to Patrick H. Tolan. In addition, although we are responsible for all of the viewpoints presented, this work has benefited from collaborations with Drs. David Henry, Mary McKay, Nancy Guerra, and numerous others who have worked or currently work on the Metropolitan Area Child Study, the Chicago Youth Development Study, and the SAFEChildren project. Finally, the families, children, and community representatives who have aided our work are thanked for their belief in these studies and for their continuing patience.

REFERENCES

Afifi, A. A., & Breslow, L. (1994). The maturing paradigm of public health. *Annual Review of Public Health, 15,* 223–235.

Borduin, C. M., Mann, B. J., Cone, L. T., Henggeler, S. W., Fucci, D. R., Blaske, D. M., & Williams, J. R. (1995). Multisystemic treatment of serious juvenile offenders: Long-term prevention of criminality and violence. *Journal of Consulting and Clinical Psychology, 63,* 569–575.

Brown, C. H. (1993a). Statistical methods for preventive trials in mental health. *Statistics in Medicine, 12,* 289–300.

Brown, C. H. (1993b). Analyzing preventive trials with generalized additive models. *American Journal of Community Psychology, 21,* 635–664.

Campbell, T. L., & Peterson, J. (1995). The effectiveness of family interventions in the treatment of physical illness. *Journal of Marital and Family Therapy, 21,* 545–584.

Caplan, G. (1964). *Principles of preventive psychiatry.* New York: Basic Books.

Chamberlain, P., & Rosicky, J. G. (1995). The effectiveness of family therapy in the treatment of adolescents with conduct disorders and delinquency. *Journal of Marital and Family Therapy, 21,* 441–460.

Coie, J. D., Watt, N. F., West, S. G., Hawkins, J. D., Asarnow, J. R., Markham, H. J., Ramey, S. L., Shure, M. B., & Long, B. (1993). The science of prevention: A conceptual framework and some directions for a national research program. *American Psychologist, 48,* 1013–1022.

Combrinck-Graham, L. (Ed.). (1989). *Children in family contexts.* New York: Guilford Press.

Cowen, E.L. (1973). Baby-steps toward primary prevention. *American Journal of Community Psychology, 5,* 1–22.

Dakof, G. (1996). Meaning and measurement of family. *Journal of Family Psychology, 10,* 142–146.

Elliott, D., & Tolan, P. H. (in press). Overview of adolescent violence from a lifespan–ecological perspective. *Psychiatric Clinics of North America.*

Goldstein, M. J., & Miklowitz, D. J. (1995). The effectiveness of psychoeducational family therapy in the treatment of schizophrenic disorders. *Journal of Marital and Family Therapy, 21,* 361–377.

Gordon, R. (1983). An operational definition of prevention. *Public Health Reports, 98,* 107–109.

Gorman-Smith, D., Tolan, P. H., & Henry, D. (in press). The relation of community and family to risk among urban poor adolescents. In P. Cohen, L. Robins, & C. Slomkowski (Eds.), *Where and when: Influence of historical time and place on aspects of psychopathology.* Mahwah, NJ: Erlbaum.

Hanish, L. D., Tolan, P. H., McKay, M. M., & Dickey, M. H. (in press). Measuring process in child and family interventions: An example in prevention of aggression. *Journal of Family Psychology.*

Kazdin, A. E., Bass, D., Ayers, W. A., & Rodgers, A. (1990). Empirical and clinical focus of child and adolescent psychotherapy research. *Journal of Consulting and Clinical Psychology, 58*(6), 729–740.

Kellam, S. G. (1990). Developmental epidemiological framework for family research on depression and aggression. In G. R. Patterson (Ed.), *Depression and aggression in family interaction* (pp. 11–48). Hillsdale, NJ: Erlbaum.

Kendall, P. C., & Grove, W. (1988). Normative comparisons in therapy outcome. Special issue: Defining clinically significant change. *Behavioral Assessment, 10*(2), 147–158.

Kliewer, W. (1997). Children coping with chronic illness. In S. A. Wolchik & I. N. Sandler (Eds.), *Handbook of children's coping* (pp. 275–300). New York: Plenum Press.

Kliewer, W., & Lewis, H. (1995). Family influences on coping processes in children and adolescents with sickle cell disease. *Journal of Pediatric Psychology, 20,* 511–525.

Kumpfer, K. L. (1989). Prevention of alcohol and drug use: A critical review of risk factors and prevention. In D. Shaffer, I. Philips, N. B. Enzer, & M. M. Silverman (Eds.), *Prevention of mental disorders, alcohol, and other drug use in children and adolescents* (pp. 309–371). Rockville, MD: U.S. Department of Health and Human Services.

Liddle, H. A., & Dakof, G. A. (1995). Family therapy for drug abuse: Promising but not definitive efficacy evidence. *Journal of Marital and Family Therapy, 21,* 511–544.

Loeber, R., Dishion, T., & Patterson, G. R. (1984). Multiple-gating: A multistage assessment procedure for identifying youths at risk for delinquency. *Journal of Research in Crime and Delinquency, 21,* 7–32.

Lorion, R. P., Price, R. H., & Eaton, W. E., (1989). The prevention of child adolescent disorders: From theory to research. In D. Shaffer, I. Philips, N. B. Enzer, & M. M. Silverman (Eds.), *Prevention of mental disorders, alcohol, and other drug use in children and adolescents* (pp. 55–96). Rockville, MD: U.S. Department of Health and Human Services.

Lorion, R. P., Tolan, P. H., & Wahler, R. G. (1987). Prevention. In H. C. Quay (Ed.) *Handbook of juvenile delinquency* (pp. 383–416). New York: Wiley.

Metropolitan Area Child Study. (1997). *A cognitive–ecological approach to preventing aggression in urban and inner-city settings: Preliminary outcomes.* Manuscript submitted for publication.

Mrazek, P. J., & Haggerty, R. J. (1994). *Reducing risks for mental disorders: Frontiers for preventive intervention research.* Washington, DC: National Academy Press.

Munoz, R. F., Mrazek, P. J., & Haggerty, R. J. (1996). Institute of Medicine report on prevention of mental disorders: Summary and commentary. *American Psychologist, 51*(11), 1116–1122.

Muthen, B. O., & Curran, P. (1997). General longitudinal modeling of individual differences in experimental designs: A latent variable framework for analysis and power estimation. In M. I. Appelbaum & H. M. Sandler (Eds.), *Psychological Methods, 2*(4), 371–402.

National Institute of Mental Health. (1990). *National plan for research on child and adolescent mental disorders* (DHHS Publication No. ADM 90-1683). Washington, DC: U.S. Government Printing Office.

Patterson, G. R., & Bank, L. (1989). Some amplifying mechanisms for pathologic processes in families. In M. R. Gunnar & E. Thalen (Eds.), *Systems and development: The Minnesota Symposium on Child Psychology, 22,* 167–209.

Patterson, G. R., Reid, J. B., & Dishion, T. J. (1992). *Antisocial boys: A social interactional approach* (Vol. 4). Eugene, OR: Castalia.

Pillow, D. R., Sandler, I. N., Braver, S. L., Wolchik, S. A., & Gersten, J. C. (1991). Theory based screening for prevention: Focusing on mediating processes in children of divorce. *American Journal of Community Psychology, 19,* 809–836.

Pinsof, W. M., & Wynne, L. C. (1995). The effectiveness of marital and family therapy: An empirical overview, conclusions and recommendations. *Journal of Marital and Family Therapy, 21,* 585–613.

Price, R. H., Cowen, E. L., Lorion, R. P., & Ramos, M. J. (1989). The search for effective prevention programs: What we learned along the way. *American Journal of Orthopsychiatry, 59*(1), 49–58.

Sanders, M. R., Shepherd, R. W., Cleghorn, G., & Woolford, H. (1994). The treatment of recurrent abdominal pain in children: A controlled comparison of cognitive-behavioral family intervention and standard pediatric care. *Journal of Consulting and Clinical Psychology, 62,* 306–314.

Shadish, W. R., Montgomery, L. M., Wilson, P., Wilson, M. R., Bright, I., & Okumabua, T. (1993). The effects of family and marital psychotherapies: A meta-analysis. *Journal of Consulting and Clinical Psychology, 61,* 992–1002.

Steinberg, J. A., & Silverman, M. M. (Eds.). (1987). *Preventing mental disorders: A research persepctive.* Washington, DC: U.S. Government Printing Office.

Tolan, P. H., & Brown, C. H. (1997). Methods for evaluating intervention and prevention efforts. In. P. K. Trickett & C. Schellenbach (Eds.), *Violence against children in the family and the community* (pp. 439–464). Washington, DC: American Psychological Association.

Tolan, P. H., Gorman-Smith, D., Henry, D., Chung, K., & Hunt, M. (in press). The relation of patterns of coping of inner-city youth to social competence and psychopathology symptoms. *Journal of Personality and Social Psychology.*

Tolan, P. H., Gorman-Smith, D., Zelli, A., & Huesmann, L. R. (1997). Assessment of family relationship characteristics: A measure to explain risk for antisocial behavior and depression in youth. *Psychological Assessment, 9*(3), 212–223.

Tolan, P. H., & Guerra, N. G. (1994). *What works in reducing adolescent violence: An empirical review of the field* (Monograph prepared for the Center for the Study and Prevention of Youth Violence). Boulder: University of Colorado.

Tolan, P. H., Guerra, N. G., & Kendall, P. (1995). A developmental–ecological perspective on antisocial behavior in children and adolescents: Towards a unified risk and intervention framework. *Journal of Consulting and Clinical Psychology, 63,* 579–584.

Tolan, P. H., & McKay, M. (1996). Preventing serious antisocial behavior in inner-city children: An empirically based family prevention program. *Family Relations, 45,* 148–155.

Webster-Stratton, C. (1991). Annotation: Strategies for helping families with conduct disordered children. *Journal of Child Psychology and Psychiatry, 32,* 1047–1062.

Webster-Stratton, C., Kolpacoff, M., & Hollinsworth, T. (1988). Self-administered videotape therapy for families with conduct-problem children: Comparison with two cost-effective treatments and a control group. *Journal of Consulting and Clinical Psychology, 56,* 558–566.

West, S. G., Aiken, L. S., & Todd, M. (1993). Probing the effects of individual components in multiple component prevention programs. *American Journal of Community Psychology, 21,* 571–605.

CHAPTER 17

━━━▷◆◁━━━

From Parent Education to Family Empowerment Programs

JAN R. M. GERRIS
NICOLE M. C. VAN AS
PAUL M. A. WELS
JAN M. A. M. JANSSENS

In other chapters of this book, several authors have described their views of family psychopathology. Family psychopathology has been related to several family domains: It may be localized in the child, in the parent, in the parent–child relationship, and in the relationship between parents. In this chapter, we restrict ourselves to those aspects of family psychopathology that parent education programs try to change. Parent education can be defined as "a systematic and conceptually based program, intended to impart information, awareness, or skills to the participants on aspects of parenting" (Fine, 1980, p. 5). Programs are usually designed for use with relatively small groups of parents (about 8–15 parents; Alvy, 1994).

Generally parent education programs have several goals. These include providing information on child development and child-rearing strategies, developing parental self-awareness, teaching effective methods of discipline and problem solving, improving parent–child communication, and making family life more enjoyable (Dembo, Sweitzer, & Lauritzen, 1985; Fine, 1980; Fine & Henry, 1989). All types of parent education programs are based on the idea that parental and familial functioning are somehow related to children's functioning, and thus aim at improving the level of the former (Lamb & Lamb, 1978). Parent education may serve the goals of

401

early intervention and prevention of child behavior problems. Parent education is distinguished from parent or family therapy, in that therapists have a more personal, in-depth relationship with the family members, whereas parent education deals primarily with common child-rearing problems faced by many parents. Furthermore, parent education programs are limited to a fixed number of weekly sessions, whereas therapy usually has no predetermined number of sessions (Dembo et al., 1985; Fine, 1980).

To which types of family psychopathology are parent education programs addressed? With regard to child psychopathology, a distinction is usually made between "externalizing" and "internalizing" behavior (Achenbach, 1978; Achenbach & Edelbrock, 1979). A primary aim of most parent education programs is to reduce both kinds of child behavior problems. As far as parental psychopathology is concerned, many authors are interested in the dysfunctional child-rearing practices parents employ (e.g., Patterson & Forgatch, 1987). An important aim of most parent education programs is to teach parents a more functional child-rearing style, in order to improve their relationship with their children. Other authors (Abidin, 1976a, 1976b) refer to dysfunctional parental cognitions about child rearing. In this view, child-rearing problems occur if parents misinterpret their children's behavior, and the quality of child rearing will be enhanced if parental cognitions are changed. Still other authors are not so interested in cognitions of parents or in the specific child-rearing practices parents use, but emphasize the importance of a good parent–child relationship (Gordon, 1970, 1980); their purpose is the improvement of parent–child communication. With regard to the relationship between parents, parent education programs are aimed to create or to restore a family child-rearing system in which parents support each other in the child-rearing decisions they make.

In the first section of this chapter, we first give a review of relationships that have been found between child psychopathology on the one hand and psychopathology related to the parent, to the parent–child relationship, and to the relationship between parents on the other. Second, we examine five types of parent education programs: programs based on (1) the individual psychology of Adler, (2) humanistic psychology (client-centered therapy), (3) social learning theory (behavior modification approaches), (4) rational–emotive theory, and (5) combinations of these theoretical perspectives. We give a brief description of the theoretical assumptions of each type of program, and consider what aspects of parental functioning are addressed by each type. Third, we consider which techniques are used to change parental functioning. Fourth, we comment on the effectiveness of these types of parent education programs, based on the results of evaluation studies.

In contrast with parent education programs focusing on dimensions of parenting and parent–child interactions, in the next section we examine approaches and programs oriented toward family empowerment. This type of program is the result of a general movement from child-centered to family-centered service (Whittaker, 1996). The general goals of empowerment approaches are to let families work for their members by addressing and mobilizing forces within and/or around the families themselves.

In the discussion section of the chapter, we take the opportunity to review the rich diversity of perspectives on parent–family functioning that are found in prevailing parenting and family programs.

PARENT EDUCATION PROGRAMS
Child Pathology and Parental Functioning

In the literature (for reviews, see Maccoby & Martin, 1983; Rollins & Thomas, 1979), many relationships have been found between child psychopathology on the one hand and psychopathology related to the parents, to the parent–child relationship, and to the relationship between parents on the other. These relationships are usually interpreted unicausally: Dysfunctional child rearing, inappropriate communication between parent and child, and inappropriate communication between parents are assumed to cause or to reinforce child psychopathology. Based on the assumption that changing child-rearing practices and improving family communication patterns will diminish child psychopathology, many parent education programs are intended to change these practices or to improve these patterns.

Which child-rearing practices and communication patterns are considered to have harmful effects on child outcome? With regard to child-rearing practices, most authors point to the negative influence of a nonsupportive and an authoritarian child-rearing style; however, a lack of authoritative child rearing is also considered negative for a child's development (Maccoby & Martin, 1983; Rollins & Thomas, 1979). Therefore, most parent education programs are intended to change these dysfunctional child-rearing practices.

Some programs, however, do not emphasize parental practices that have to be changed, but parental cognitions. Parents may interpret their children's behavior irrationally (Abidin, 1976a, 1976b) and these misinterpretations may lead to intense emotional feelings about the children's behavior, which result in dysfunctional child-rearing behavior. Thus, the problem is thought to be localized in parents' cognitions, and it is assumed that changing these cognitions will change parents' child-rearing behavior.

Other authors emphasize that the problem has to be situated in the way parents and children communicate with each other (Gordon, 1970, 1980), and thus that parent education programs have to improve parent–child communication.

Finally, the relationship between parents may be an issue of intervention in parent education programs. If parents have different points of view about how to rear their child, a child is inclined to form a coalition with one parent against the other one, and to play the parents off against each other (Haley, 1971; Minuchin, 1974).

Types of Parent Education Programs

Programs Based on the Individual Psychology of Adler

Adlerian parenting programs are based on the ideas that Western society is based on the principles of democracy and social equality, and that parent–child interaction should reflect these values (Christensen & Thomas, 1980). There are four main Adlerian parent education techniques: teaching parents about the goals of children's misbehavior, the use of encouragement, the use of natural and logical consequences, and family meetings.

What are the "goals" of children's misbehavior? It is assumed in Adlerian parenting programs that a child's behavior always reflects a need to belong—that is, to feel accepted and useful. If children cannot meet their goals of belonging through constructive behavior, they may show destructive behavior. A child who does not feel accepted may try to belong by asking for undue attention, exerting power, aiming at revenge (hurting others as he or she feels hurt by others), or finally giving up in discouragement (Alvy, 1994; Christensen & Thomas, 1980; Dinkmeyer & McKay, 1976a, 1976b; Dreikurs & Blumenthal, 1976). Parents can help their children to show cooperative and desirable behavior by using encouragement, using natural and logical consequences, and holding family meetings. Encouragement consists of showing acceptance and appreciation of a child and his or her behavior, and is meant to develop self-confidence in children. Using natural and logical consequences involves allowing children to learn from the results of their behavior and to be responsible for their choices and decisions. "Natural" consequences are those that follow from the natural order of events (e.g., no gloves in winter means cold hands), whereas "logical" consequences are those that result from what is called the "reality of the social order" (e.g., not being dressed in time means being late for school). Finally, family meetings are regular meetings with all family members present, whose purposes are to plan for family chores and family fun, to resolve conflicts, and to make decisions (Alvy, 1994; Dinkmeyer & McKay, 1976a, 1976b).

Concerning child-rearing style, we have noted above that child behavior problems have been linked to nonsupportive parenting, to authoritarian parenting, and to a lack of authoritative parenting. In Adlerian parent education, parents are taught that supporting their children may contribute to building a positive relationship. An important aspect of support is the technique of encouragement. Furthermore, parents are taught to show respect for children's feelings, thoughts, and beliefs, which can be interpreted as parents' being responsive to their children's needs and wishes. Therefore, in Adlerian parent education parents are highly stimulated to support their children. In regard to the issue of parental control, individual independence and responsibility are promoted in Adlerian parent education. Natural and logical consequences are used to encourage children to make responsible decisions, without forcing their submission. In other words, parents are stimulated not to use *authoritarian* control techniques, but to use *authoritative* ones.

Programs Based on Humanistic Psychology and Client-Centered Therapy

Parent education programs based on humanistic psychology and on Carl Rogers's client-centered therapy aim at building warm, close, and democratic parent–child relationships. From this perspective, human relationships should be characterized by acceptance (being nonjudgmental toward each other), and genuineness (being honest in expressing one's feelings) (Alvy, 1994). It is assumed that people are able to find their own solutions to problems, once they recognize, express, and accept their feelings. Parent education programs based on this philosophy emphasize the expression of feelings between parents and children (Lamb & Lamb, 1978).

Gordon (1970, 1980) has developed a well-known parent education program called Parent Effectiveness Training (PET). The PET program aims at building a warm relationship between parents and children, based on mutual positive feelings and respect, by using Rogerian/client-centered communication skills. That is, parents learn to communicate respect and acceptance of their children's feelings, as well as their own feelings (Lamb & Lamb, 1978). Parents are taught that they can feel either accepting or unaccepting toward their children's behavior. If a child experiences a problem, and his or her behavior is acceptable to a parent, the parent can use the "language of acceptance" or "active listening"; this means that parent reflects back the feelings of the child, thus stimulating the child to find his or her own solutions to the problem. When the child's behavior is unacceptable to the parent because it interferes with the parent's needs and wishes, the parent can use (confrontative) "I-messages." Using I-messages, the parent nonblamefully describes the child's unacceptable behavior, the parent's feelings about the child's behavior, and the effect that the child's behavior is having on him or her. Thus, the child is stimulated to consider the parent's needs, without being forced to change behavior. The child is held responsible for his or her own behavior. When parent and child share a problem, they learn to reach agreement using a six-step problem-solving method: (1) identifying the conflicting needs, (2) generating possible alternative solutions, (3) evaluating the solutions, (4) deciding on the best acceptable solution, (5) working out ways of implementing the solution, and (6) evaluating the solution (Alvy, 1994, p. 79; Lamb & Lamb, 1978).

In short, in client-centered parent education, parents are taught to be supportive by listening actively and by showing respect and acceptance of children's feelings. This may help children to express their feelings, and to become independent and responsible for their feelings and behavior. When parents think their children's behavior is unacceptable, they send I-messages to stimulate the children to consider the parents' needs. This can be interpreted as a form of authoritative control, in that parents expect mature behavior of the children without forcing the children to comply. Again, parents are stimulated to be supportive and to use authoritative instead of authoritarian control techniques to influence their children's behavior.

Behavior Modification Approaches Based on Social Learning Theory

There are many different kinds of behavioral parent educations programs, all of which include basic behavioral concepts. Examples of such programs include Parents Are Teachers (Becker, 1971), Parents and Adolescents Living Together (Patterson & Forgatch, 1987), and Confident Parenting (Eimers & Aitchison, 1977). It is assumed in these approaches that human behavior is learned in social interaction. Thus, children's problem behaviors represent inadequate learning, and parents can be instructed to weaken undesirable and strengthen desirable child behavior. As behavior is assumed to be primarily a function of events that precede and follow the behavior, a lot of attention is given to these events. Parents learn to manipulate these factors in order to change children's behavior.

In behavioral parent education programs, parents are taught how to set up a behavior modification program consisting of four steps (Abidin, 1976a, 1976b; Alvy, 1994; Dembo et al., 1985; Fine, 1980; Lamb & Lamb, 1978; Patterson & Forgatch, 1987; Simpson, 1980):

1. *Selection of the target behavior that parents want to change.* The target behavior that parents want to increase or decrease must be observable and specifically defined.

2. *Observing and recording.* Parents measure the frequency, rate, duration, or intensity of the target behavior, in order to determine how serious the problem really is (and also whether any changes in the behavior occur after the consequences of the behavior are altered).

3. *Setting the consequences.* Parents are taught either to increase or to decrease the frequency of occurrence of the selected behavior, through systematic manipulation of the consequences of the behavior (Simpson, 1980). A positive consequence or reinforcer is an event that strengthens a behavior it follows (e.g., praise, compliments, a present). An aversive consequence, on the other hand, is an event that weakens the behavior it follows (e.g. time out, punishment).

4. *Evaluating the results.* After parents have set the consequences, they continue to measure whether the target behavior has indeed been weakened or strengthened.

In parent education programs based on social learning theory, the emphasis is on teaching parents to influence and control children's behavior by manipulating the consequences of that behavior. Compared to the parent education programs described above, behavior modification programs strongly emphasize parental control. However, a lot of attention is given to positively reinforcing children's desirable behavior. In particular, parents learn to use social reinforcers (e.g., hugs, praise, and compliments). Although social reinforcement is meant to increase desirable behavior, it also contributes to building a warm parent–child relationship and can be viewed as parental support. In behavioral parent education programs, parents also learn to set limits on their children's behaviors and to enforce those limits by using positive and negative consequences (Alvy, 1994). Although it seems that behavioral parent education relies somewhat more on techniques of punishment and the use of aversive consequences than Adlerian and client-centered parent education programs do, it can be said that in behavioral parent education too, parents are taught how to use authoritative control instead of authoritarian control. That is, the limits they set must be fair and reasonable; the emphasis is on using positive consequences; and if negative consequences are used, parents are taught to use only mild forms of punishment.

Programs Based on Rational–Emotive Theory

Rational–emotive parent education is based on the theory and therapy developed by Ellis (1962, 1973). According to this theory, emotional or psychological disturbances are largely a result of thinking illogically or irrationally. Ellis (1962, 1973) developed the "A-B-C" method to teach people to maximize rational and minimize irrational thinking. A represents the "Activating" event or situation; B stands for the individual's "beliefs" or "belief system" (the way in which the person thinks about situation A); and C stands for the "consequences" (the person's reactions and feelings in that situation). According to rational–emotive theory, negative feelings (C) are not caused by the situation or event (A), but by people's beliefs about the situation or event (B). These beliefs can be either rational or irrational. Rational beliefs assist people to achieve their goals, and relate to observable events that can be empirically validated. Irrational or illogical beliefs prevent people from meeting their goals, and relate to hypotheses that cannot be empirically verified (Ellis, 1973; Ellis & Harper, 1977). An example of a common irrational belief pertaining to child management is "Children can upset their parents" (rational alternative: "Parents upset themselves by what they say to themselves about their children") (Lamb & Lamb, 1978). Many irrational beliefs and thoughts contain absolutes, such as "must," "should (not)," or "ought (not)"; they are based on all-or-nothing, exaggerated thinking (Ellis & Harper, 1977). Parents can be challenged to dispute their irrational beliefs and to train themselves to think and behave more efficiently, and thus to manage and control their feelings and their reactions to their children (Abidin, 1976a, 1976b; Lamb & Lamb, 1978).

In rational–emotive parent education, the emphasis is not so much on parents' behavior toward their children as on parents' thoughts and beliefs (B in the A-B-C chain). Parents are taught that their own thoughts about their children's behavior are what determine their feelings and reactions to that behavior. This approach suggests that sometimes a child's behavior may not be the problem, but a parent's way of interpreting that behavior may be (at least part of) the problem. Child behavior problems may be easier to handle when parents view them more rationally. The focus in rational–emotive parent education is on examining parents' perceptions of children's behavior and situations and on teaching parents to think more rationally. This may lead to parents' reacting more adequately to children's behavior. Rational–emotive theory is mostly part of parent education programs that combine several theoretical perspectives, and in which parents' behavior toward their children is also a focus. Combined parent education programs are described next.

Programs That Combine Theoretical Approaches

Many parent education programs combine aspects of several of the theoretical approaches described above. Abidin (1976a, 1976b), for example, has developed a parenting program called Parenting Skills that teaches parents communication skills, behavior modification techniques, and rational–emotive techniques. Dinkmeyer and McKay (1976a, 1976b) have developed Systematic Training for Effective Parenting (STEP), an Adlerian parenting program that also includes communication skills from the client-centered approach. Patterson and Forgatch have developed a parent education program for parents of adolescents that consists of two parts: one based on behavior modification principles, and one based on conflict resolution techniques and communication skills (Forgatch & Patterson, 1989; Patterson & Forgatch, 1987).

According to Popkin (1989), many parent education books and programs are based on one or more of the theoretical perspectives mentioned before. For this reason, he has shifted attention from the content of parenting programs to the process (*how* can parents effectively and efficiently be instructed?) by developing the program Active Parenting, in which video is introduced to teach parents the skills of effective communication and behavior modification.

Techniques in Parent Education Programs

The question to be answered in this subsection is which methods or techniques are used by parent education programs to change parents' child-rearing style, parental cognitions, and communication patterns among family members.

A number of techniques have been developed to teach parents ways they can adequately support their children. Parents learn how to give attention to a child, how to react responsively to the child's needs, how to show affection, how to use humor effectively, how to initiate activities the child likes, and how to praise the child for doing well. In praising a child, the parent explains which child behavior he or she appreciates, and also points to the positive consequences this behavior has for the child himself or herself. Supporting a child also means that a parent listens to what the child tries to tell; a child has to experience the parent as responsive. Being responsive means that a parent asks for more information when the child is telling his or her story, or tries to put the child's feelings into words. As described above in connection with PET, this is known as "active listening" (Gordon, 1970, 1980). In parent education programs, these communication skills are explained and trained through role playing.

Role playing, is used to teach parents not only how to be supportive, but also how to control their children. Two basic mechanisms are used: reinforcement of desired behavior, and extinction of undesired behavior. Reinforcement of desired behavior is achieved by offering rewards if a child shows the behavior parents want. Several kinds of rewards may be used. First, material rewards may be applied; that is, the child is rewarded with candy, fruit, money, a book, a ticket for a baseball game, or the like if the child shows the behavior parents want. Second, besides or instead of material reinforcers, social reinforcers may be used—for example, praising the child, giving the child a kiss or a hug, or paying a compliment, as noted earlier.

Extinction of undesired behavior can be achieved by applying one or more of the following techniques. First, parents may be able to change the child's environment so that it is physically impossible for the child to behave in a way parents do not want (e.g., putting money under lock and key, if a child is inclined to steal money). Second, constructive criticism or I-messages may be used. A parent tells the child what behavior is unacceptable and why, by referring to the consequences this behavior has for both parent and child. The parent also tells the child which behavior is more appropriate than the behavior the child has shown. Third, a parent may decide that the child has to experience the natural consequences of the undesired behavior (e.g., a child who forgets to take a book to school will be punished by his or her teacher). Fourth, parents may clearly set limits to their child's behavior. Parents tell the child which behavior is not allowed and why. In parent education programs, it is emphasized that after a decision is made, parents have to resist the child's attempts to transgress the limits they have set. Fifth, parents may ignore a child's behavior they do not like. To do this effectively, parents must ignore the child's behavior directly, must not look at the child, and must not discuss the unacceptable behavior. In parent education programs, parents are advised to combine ignoring with reinforcement of desired behavior, because the child does not learn which behavior the parents desire if parents only ignore the child's undesired behavior.

A sixth method to decrease undesired behavior is to employ punishment. Baumrind (1996) has recently argued that punishment may fit in an authoritative child-rearing pattern, if the kind of punishment is contingent upon the child's transgression. Several kinds of punishment are mentioned in the literature. First, parents may decide to give a reprimand if the child transgresses a rule. Second, time out may be applied; the child is sent to his or her room or to another quiet place and receives no positive reinforcement for a short period. Third, parents may withdraw privileges. Fourth, they may decide that the child has to repair the damage he or she has caused. All these kinds of punishment are appropriate to be used contingently upon a child's transgression. Inappropriate forms of punishment include spanking and making the child ridiculous in the presence of other people. In most parent education programs, parents are taught to combine punishment with rewarding. If a parent only employs punishment, the child does not learn which behavior is desired. Rewarding desired behavior makes the child clear which behavior the parent expects.

A final technique parents may use is to set up a behavior modification program. It makes sense to apply such a program if an undesired behavior occurs very frequently and has become a persistent habit.

Thus far, we have focused on techniques parents may use to support or to control a child. As noted above, however, some parent education programs are intended to change parents' own cognitions. Parents are taught to think rationally about a child's behavior by applying the A-B-C method described before.

In other parent education programs, much attention is given to the ways parents and children may communicate more effectively. Parents are taught how they may solve child-rearing problems by employing a model of deliberation. This model usually consists of several steps. A first step is that a child and parents have to clarify the problem. To be successful at this step, parents have to learn two skills. First, they have to learn how they may introduce a problem in a constructive way. That is, they have to introduce the problem in behavioral terms—explaining with constructive criticism which behavior is unacceptable, rather than blaming the child as a person. A second skill to be learned is listening to the child's point of view. Parents are taught how they may actively listen to their child's wants and needs.

A second step is to generate possible solutions. Parents are taught various methods of generating solutions together with their child. The parents and child have to accept all the solutions that are proposed and are forbidden to criticize solutions generated in this step. In a third step, the parents and child have to discuss the pros and cons of all solutions generated in the second step. After that, all parties decide which solution is most acceptable.

Child-rearing problems may occur because parents disagree on how to rear a child. In parent educational programs, parents are taught to support each other after a decision has been made, and to avoid forming a coalition with the child against the other parent.

Evaluation of Parent Education Programs

Concerning Adlerian parent education programs, Dembo et al. (1985) evaluated 10 studies on the effects of such programs. According to these authors, Adlerian parent education resulted in positive changes in parents' child-rearing attitudes, although there was little evidence of resulting changes in children's behavior. According to Roberts (1994), considerable research has been conducted on the Adlerian parent education approach, and it generally supports this approach.

Concerning client-centered parent education programs, Dembo et al. (1985) reviewed 18 evaluation studies of PET. Most of these studies measured parental attitudes. Some positive changes were found in parental child-rearing attitudes, and in some studies children reported positive changes in parents' acceptance. However, Dembo et al. concluded that there was little evidence of changes in children's behavior; indeed, children's or parents' behavior was hardly studied. However, the results of a meta-analysis of 26 studies on the results of PET indicated that these studies did find changes in parental behavior, and also in child behavior (although, again, the main changes were in parental attitudes—e.g., more understanding of children) (Cedar & Levant, cited in Alvy, 1994). Regarding child outcomes, the results indicated that children improved on self-esteem.

Regarding behavioral parent education, Dembo et al. (1985) evaluated 15 studies, and Alvy (1994) evaluated 10 studies. Both reviews concluded that the majority of studies demonstrated some positive outcomes of behavioral parent training (e.g., positive changes in child behavior), although a few studies failed to demonstrate significant positive changes. Of the studies examining follow-up data, about three-fourths mentioned positive results (Dembo et al., 1985). Socioeconomic status appeared to be an important characteristic influencing the results: Less favorable outcomes were obtained with lower-income parents (Dembo et al., 1985).

Regarding combinations of parent education approaches, Alvy (1994) evaluated 31 studies of STEP, a parent education program based on a combination of client-centered and Adlerian principles. Of these 31 studies, only 20 used an adequate design with an experimental and control group. In 26 studies, children without severe disabilities participated. According to Alvy (1994), the STEP program resulted in changes in parental attitudes, but there was less evidence of changes in child attitudes and behavior or in parent–child interactions. Alvy also reported on some studies of Active

Parenting, a video-based approach in which client-centered, Adlerian, and behavioral principles are integrated. Combination parent education programs such as Active Parenting appear to have positive effects on parental attitudes and behaviors.

Dembo et al. (1985) reviewed five studies comparing of the effectiveness of different educational approaches. Four of these compared Adlerian with behavioral parent education, and one compared client-centered with Adlerian parent education. These studies failed to find differences in effectiveness between these types of programs. However, comparing different parent education programs is difficult, because different programs have different goals. Comparison studies should therefore use attitude measures as well as measures to assess behavior change.

Interestingly, the results of studies evaluating the client-centered and Adlerian approaches yielded more positive outcomes on parent attitude measures than on measures assessing parents' and children's behavior, whereas in studies of behavioral approaches, measures of parents' or children's behavior yielded more positive outcomes than parent attitude measures. According to Dembo et al. (1985), these findings are consistent with the goals of the different parent education approaches. Each type of program has different goals, and its effectiveness may depend on the specific needs of parents. Maybe the question "Which parent education program works best?" should be replaced by the question of "Which parent education program works best for which parents and which children?"

Medway (1989) used meta-analysis to review the results of 27 empirical studies on the effectiveness of parent education—12 studies of behavioral programs, 7 of Adlerian programs, 5 of client-centered programs, and 3 studies that compared behavioral approaches with other forms of parent education. The studies of behavioral parent education programs were most consistent in producing data on children's behavior. Results of the meta-analysis showed that on the whole, these studies yielded positive effects (62% greater improvement in treatment groups than in control groups), with about equally strong effects on parents and on children, and with about equally strong effects on attitudes and on behavior. According to Medway, the question whether one type of parent education is any better than any other could not be answered, because the studies differed in the outcome measures used. The three studies comparing a behavioral approach with another approach yielded stronger effects on child behavior measures for the behavioral model than for the client-centered or Adlerian model. However, these findings are tentative, because they are based on only three studies. Analysis of the studies with follow-up assessment (three studies of behavioral parent education) indicated promising long-term results. In summary, Medway (1989) found empirical support for all three of the models assessed. Parents' choice of a parent education program can be based on the effectiveness of the program in relationship to the parents' own goals.

FAMILY EMPOWERMENT PROGRAMS
The Concept of Empowerment

In this section of the chapter, we summarize and evaluate a contrasting approach in parenting programs—namely, programs based on a family systems orientation. This new approach deals with the issue of how parents can be involved in a more activate and therefore perhaps more effective manner in these programs. In the past 10 years, new forms of parenting programs have emerged that emphasize the responsibility of the family and the parents. Accordingly, there has been a shift from a problem-oriented approach to forms of empowerment-based care.

There are at least three different perspectives on family empowerment practice. The first perspective (Berger & Neuhaus, 1977) reflects the aspects of mediating structures in communities. The second perspective (Dunst, Trivette, & Deal, 1994) establishes the principles and premises of a contextual ecological perspective (Bronfenbrenner, 1977, 1979; Gerris, 1990). The third perspective focuses on the process of empowerment according to principles laid out by Solomon (1976, 1987) and represented by the Cornell Empowerment Group (Cochran, 1985).

In the framework of this chapter, we refer to two very important meanings of "empowerment": (1) empowerment as a philosophy and (2) empowerment as a paradigm. Empowerment as a *philosophy* encompasses three guiding principles as formulated by Rappoport (1984): (1) All people have existing strengths and capabilities, as well as the capacity to become more competent; (2) the failure of a person to display competence is not due to deficits within the person, but rather to a failure of social systems to provide or create opportunities for competence to be displayed or acquired; and (3) in situations where existing capabilities need to be strengthened or new skills need to be learned, they are best learned through experiences that lead people to make self-attributions about their capabilities to influence important life events. Empowerment as a *paradigm* is an intervention principle related to this philosophy, in which activating strengths, competence, and possibilities for change are assumed to exist in the person and in the social context.

Empowerment practice in family care, according to the Cornell Empowerment Group (1989; see also Cochran, 1985), encompasses a long-term and continuing process in several stages, involving mutual respect and critical reflection. "Mutual respect" needs some clarification. It includes the following (Warren & Hartless, 1995): (1) a focus on power (i.e., a desire to share it and devolve it); (2) an acknowledgment of people's adaptive capacity, and thus the need to identify and develop their strengths (see, e.g., Maluccio, Fein & Olmstead, 1986); (3) an emphasis on diversity, history, and culture; (4) the need for clients to play the primary role; and (5) the need for programs to be located at the local community level.

New Forms of Parenting Programs

We now describe three new forms of parenting programs in which the principles of empowerment have been explicitly incorporated within a home training format: Families First (FF), Home Start, and Video Home Training (VHT).

Families First

FF is a systematic support program for cases in which out-of-home placement of a child is being considered in order to solve a family crisis. The main objective of FF is to prevent such a placement by offering to the family a program of immediate, short-term, intensive help in the home situation, in which the involvement of all family members is sought. Practical as well as therapeutic help is available within 24 hours; duration is usually not longer than 1 month; and help is offered on a 24-hour standby basis (including holidays), with daily visits typically lasting several hours each. Practical help includes assisting in household chores and visits at local statutory care institutions (e.g., social services agencies). Therapeutic help is offered in the form of instruction in such skills as resolving conflicts, managing child behavior problems, or establishing contacts outside the family; the instruction is based on (cognitive) learning theoretical principles and is offered in the form of modeling or role playing. The program ends when the crisis is over and the threat of out-of-home placement of the child is no longer imminent. In many cases, of course, some sort of outpatient help is still needed to prevent further negative developments.

FF was originally based on the Homebuilders model (see Kinney, Haapala, & Booth, 1991) and was begun in 1974. It is based on five elements: (1) bringing about a calmer situation, (2) building a working relationship, (3) gathering information, (4) formulating goals, and (5) intervening through empowerment. The three relevant theoretical orientations of FF are a family systems approach, social learning theory, and the insight that a crisis creates opportunities for change. Program principles and features, as well as some scientific results, are described by Kinney et al. (1991).

In an evaluation study (Schuerman, Rzepnicky, & Little, 1994), 995 families that received the FF program were compared to 593 families that received some other traditional program. Families were randomly assigned to either the FF program or the other program. No differences in effect were found between FF and the traditional program, since the percentages of out-of-home placement prevention were more or less the same in the two groups. In a review article, Blythe, Patterson Salley, and Jayaratne (1994) reported that after 1 year 70% of the FF group children were still living at home, whereas in 77% of the traditional group out-of-home child placement was prevented. Thus, the FF program's results were not superior to those of a traditional approach.

Home Start

Home Start is an organization in which volunteers, who are usually parents themselves, complement the efforts of professional workers by offering regular support, friendship, and practical help to young families under stress in their own homes, thus helping to prevent family breakdown and emphasizing the pleasures of family life. The time that volunteers can spend in the families, their informal role, their friendship and spontaneity, and their common-sense approach are all focused on the family members themselves rather than on their problems. Through getting to know a family rather well, volunteers can encourage the family's strengths and its members' emotional well-being. Home Start therefore provides a breathing space for parents, as well as "elbow room" for many professional workers, who can refer any family with at least one child under school age to the scheme.

The program was initiated in Leicester, England, in 1973 and has now spread throughout the United Kingdom and to other countries as well. The program's trained volunteers are supported and guided by a multidisciplinary professional management committee; this ensures close links with other voluntary and statutory caring agencies working with young families in the community. The working format is home training, and the volunteers visit the families on a regular basis (typically once or twice a week) for a few months to a year or more. As an extension to the family visits, and because many parents and small children need experiences outside the home, most Home Start schemes hold weekly family groups for parents and their children, which offer opportunities for meeting others socially as well. Each Home Start scheme is firmly rooted in its community, operating with a committee of local representatives from relevant statutory agencies, such as social services, health, and education departments.

There are a few studies on the Home Start program indicating positive results (Van der Eyken, 1990; Shinman, 1996a, 1996b).

Video Home Training

VHT is a short, intensive parenting program in which a family is treated in its own home. The VHT method was conceived by workers in the field of residential and outpatient treatment of emotionally disturbed children. They were seeking an answer to the question of how to involve families in the children's treatment to a greater extent. Both the daily realities of treatment in a specific institution and research on the early communication process in young children, especially the work of Trevarthen (1979, 1989), served as useful resources in determining the features of the program. The originators of the program, Aarts, Biemans, and Van Rees, based their method on several principles derived from interactional theories, developmental psychology, and the ethological field (Dekker & Biemans, 1994). They started from the basic idea that parents and children want a good relationship and good communication with each other. When they do not know how to achieve these aims, a negative communication pattern will prevail (e.g., ignoring, turning down, aggression), and this in turn can lead to an increase all sorts of problem behavior on the children's part.

The program focuses on the communication behavior of family members. The method makes use of video as a therapeutically helpful medium and consists of three main elements: video recording of family interactions, interaction analysis, and feedback. After a diagnostic intake, an introduction section is scheduled for each family separately. This introduction consists of making the family's acquaintance in the home, showing an introductory video, and/or making a short video recording of a family interaction. A week later, the trainer replays this recording in a feedback session with the parents. Both the video recording and the feedback session are analyzed for the parents, in order to get an impression of the communication patterns in the family and of the way parents are able to learn from the trainer's feedback. The trainer typically films selectively and, on the basis of the video interaction analysis, shows to the parents a specific selection of these recordings. This selection preferably contains situations in which the interaction between parent and child is successful in terms of pleasant and effective communication and effective contact principles. In cases where negative communication patterns are visible, the trainer "invites" parents to devise a possible positive continuation of the interaction. In the training of basic communication behavior, a particular scheme containing elements of basic communication patterns is used in order to analyze the video recordings and to give feedback to the parents. This scheme contains various elements of successful communication behavior: being attentive, approving, conversing in a pleasant tone of voice, taking turns in a balanced manner, engaging in mutual consultation, being cooperative, resolving conflicts, guiding the communication, sending positive initiatives (e.g., looking at the person, smiling, nodding), and receiving these initiatives positively (e.g., eye contact, naming in approval).

After the introduction, a training plan is made, containing information in five areas: (1) basic family communication patterns, (2) daily family life organization, (3) development of the children, (4) development of the parents, and (5) the family's participation in society. According to this plan, a series of home sessions alternating between recording and feedback sessions is scheduled. The intensity and duration of the training program depend on the severity of the problems involved, on the presence or absence of protective and risk factors, and on the amount of experience of the trainer. The duration of the training can therefore vary from less than 3 months to more than a year. The ending of VHT depends on whether signs that the parents are able to cope in their daily child-rearing process are emerging, and on whether the aims set in the training plan are being achieved. Normally, a successful interaction between parents and children for one or several days, without any problems that the parents themselves cannot cope with, serves as a useful criterion. Improvements in schoolwork or the child's behavior at school, as well as a parent's getting a job or starting an education, are examples of improvements in the other areas of the training plan that can serve as indications for the ending of the training. After a period of about 6 months, the trainer usually makes a follow-up contact with the family to see how things are going. Sometimes a visit or a training session is necessary to stimulate things in a positive direction. A complete VHT process contains a schedule of further follow-up contacts after 1, 2, and 5 years.

Only a few scientific studies have been published on the effects of VHT. Weiner, Kuppermintz, and Guttmann (1994) published a study on the effects of the Orion program (comparable to the VHT program), which had been introduced shortly before in Israel. The study included a group of parents ($n = 52$) who received the Orion program and a control group ($n = 64$), and showed positive effects of the intervention. As expected, a reduction of negative interactions was found. A follow-up after 6 months revealed that significant differences between the Orion families and a control group still existed.

In The Netherlands, Vogelvang (1993) was the first researcher to perform a study on the effects of VHT in comparison with another family intervention program called Projekt aan Huis (Project at Home). Results were rather disappointing and inconclusive. On a number of family characteristics, almost no positive effects were found as a result of VHT. There were no improvements found in the children's behavioral problems, except in 2 children (in a group of 15). However, a study by Muris et al. (1994) reported positive effects of VHT in a group of 135 families. Results showed that 70% of the families involved benefited from VHT, and follow-up results after 1 year revealed improved family situations.

A few studies have reported changes in the communication behavior of parents as a result of VHT. Simpson, Forsyth, and Kennedy (1995) developed a category system in order to reveal these changes. In their analysis, they applied a reduced two-component coding system: "attuned" and "not attuned" or "discordant" responses. In a group of five families, they were able to show a significant increase (from a 35% to a 94% average) in "attuned" responses to the children's initiatives, and a decrease (from a 34% to a 4% average) in "not attuned" or "discordant" interactions. Moreover, they found a significant increase in turn-taking sequences and in positive responses to the children's initiatives.

Janssens and Kemper (1997) developed a detailed communication category system for written protocols based on videotaped interactions. These protocols contained all verbal and nonverbal behavior, recorded, for example, as information about "looking at the child," "intonation" (friendly or unfriendly), and who was addressing whom. Janssens and Kemper reported an increase in positive communication behavior and in parents' looking at the child as a result of VHT; they also found a decrease in negative communication behavior.

In another study (Jansen & Wels, in press), the effects of VHT in terms of positive changes in the communication behavior of parents could be ascertained.

Parent Education Programs and Family Empowerment Programs Compared

To illustrate the differences between traditional parent education programs and programs based on family empowerment, we compare the way in which parents are approached in traditional programs with the way they are approached in an empowerment program such as VHT. The parent education format seems to convey implicit messages such as the following:

- "You as parents have been indicated to possess inadequate or insufficient parenting abilities. We, as professionals in family care, are experts in this field. We therefore have both the knowledge and the resulting authority and attitude to suggest to you what adequate parenting behavior should be."
- "We are the teachers and you are the students, and what we suggest you should follow. We mean well. As a result of these positions, you should be glad to get this teaching and should be motivated to participate."
- "When you follow our instructions, the parenting situation should improve. If the situation does not improve, you as parents are not motivated enough, or things are more complicated than we thought. You may not blame the method or us for this."
- "We as trainers are in competition with you as parents in modeling good parenting behavior."

The VHT program does not convey these messages. The trainer makes suggestions only on the basis of the behavior of the parents themselves; the parents are usually their own models on the videotapes. The concept of self-imposed modeling applies here, as opposed to trainer-imposed modeling. In using VHT, the trainer has the advantage of not being a messenger or a judge of good or bad behavior. The well-known distinction in therapy between content and relational processes is relevant here. The video is a neutral medium, without reserve; it does not spare or flatter. In principle, video does not comment on the situation either positively nor negatively— which, by the way, does not imply that the medium will not evoke emotions in the viewer. Video may be seen as a nonhuman "messenger" that conveys the content of the message, as well as a relational process component in the message; that gives parents feedback on their parenting abilities; and that parents can get angry with or can value like a trainer. When a trainer or therapist observes and reports, he or she is automatically the judge of and the messenger concerning good or bad behavior. Therapists sometimes find this role annoying or are inclined to weaken it, as appears from a description by Farrelly and Brandsma (1985). These authors use the concept of "disowning the communication" for a particular communication strategy in which therapists sometimes give the messenger role to "another." In these cases, they use such phrases as "Research has shown that . . . " or "Some therapists think that. . . . " The responsibility for the message is given to another authority in a way that gives the therapist more room for other roles, especially the helping role of the care provider.

DISCUSSION

How effective are parent education programs? According to Alvy (1994, p. 230), it is not realistic to expect parent education programs to have "a profound impact on the behavior and functioning of all parents," because there are many other factors influencing parental functioning. Parental behavior is also influenced by the personality and health characteristics of both parents and children, by children's developmental stage, by the parents' marital relationship, by environmental aspects (e.g., neighborhood, financial stresses), and by the norms and values of the parents' cultural background. All these factors may play a role and may influence one another, which makes parental functioning a very complex matter. Parent education can be viewed as a short-term intervention that attempts to influence the "long-term and multidetermined" parenting process and parent–child interactions (Alvy, 1994, p. 232). During the parent education program, parents are stimulated to focus their attention on parenting. When the program has ended, it may be difficult for parents to remain focused on their style of parenting (Alvy, 1994).

Furthermore, just like parental behavior, child behavior is multidetermined. Although parental functioning is a major influence on the development of children, other factors influence child development as well, such as internal biological factors (personality, temperament, health characteristics) and external factors (siblings, peers, school, television) (Alvy, 1994).

In general, the intervention approaches of Adlerian, client-centered, behavioral, and rational–emotive parent education are based on a unidirectional model of influence: The parent is viewed as the change agent, and the child is viewed as the target of change. Probably the reality is more complex, and parent–child interaction is bidirectional rather than unidirectional (Patterson, Reid, & Dishion, 1992): Children influence the relationship with their parents, too. The complexity not only of the parent–child relationship, but also of relationships with other family members and of extrafamilial relationships, hardly receives any attention in parent education programs (Dembo et al., 1985; Roberts, 1994). It may be possible to include both parents and children as change agents in parent education programs. Thus, authors are increasingly arguing in favor of applying an interactive or systemic perspective in parent education approaches.

According to Roberts (1994), at present there are no parent education programs operating from a systemic perspective. When we look at differences in the "style" of intervention between traditional parent education programs and approaches based upon a family empowerment model (see above), it seems obvious that traditional approaches view families with problems as client systems asking for help. The family is in a "one-down" position in relation to the care system. In responding to these needs and in delivering care, the care provider puts himself or herself in a "one-up" position. That is, the professional assumes an image of superiority as an expert in family pathology. In the intake process, the family members give information, and the professional asks for information. His or her job is to analyze and assess the pathology and to offer a diagnosis of what the problem is; to explain by which mechanism or processes the difficulties have developed and continue to influence family interaction ;and, finally, to suggest a suitable treatment. The family listens to these messages, promises to be motivated to follow advice, and promises to comply in general with treatment suggestions, in order to be able to remedy the family weaknesses and to overcome the difficulties involved. During this intake process, the professional couches his or her observations in terms of shortcomings of family members, of the family interaction, or of the system that are in need of treatment. Clients are inclined to expect answers to the questions on family problems and pathology, thus in turn acknowledging the professional in his or her expert role. Clients often report disappointment and tend to show suspicion when professionals are vague in their answers. Instead of assuming a deficit in the family system, both the family–ecological perspective and the Cornell Empowerment Group's approach share a strong interest in bringing out the existing skills and strengths in parents, children, and families (Arcus, 1995; Cochran, 1985, 1987).

In the Family Matters program developed by Cochran and Woolever (1983), the following six goals are illustrative of the empowerment approach as a whole: (1) reducing isolation; (2) recognizing parents as experts; (3) reinforcing and encouraging parent–child activities; (4) sharing information about children, neighborhood, services, and work; (5) promoting the exchange of resources among neighboring families; and (6) promoting concerted action by participating parents on behalf of their children.

When we take the assumptions underlying an empowerment approach a step further, we may ask ourselves what implications for evaluation studies follow from the basic principle that parents and families should be respected and should set their own range of objectives and desired outcomes. And, of course, there are similar implications for family educators and family counselors. Looking at program evaluation studies and reflecting upon what should be the central question for program evaluation, several authors come to the conclusion that the traditional question— namely, "Do parenting programs work and why?"—should be reframed as "Which programs work best for which parents and which children, under which ecological conditions?" (Arcus, 1995). In this reframing, we can see growing acknowledgment of the intentions and conditions of parents as they are. The reframing also indicates that there is no such thing as a superior parenting program that is effective for all kind of parents and families in all kind of conditions. As a way to answer the question "Which program works best for which parents . . . ?", comparative evaluation studies do not make sense any more, because the objectives and intended outcomes of different parents or groups of parents may not be comparable. Forcing differing objectives and intentions of different parents into a comparative effect evaluation could lead to implicit value judgments that some parents' objectives are "better"—more child-oriented or better for preparing children for adaptation to societal standards, for instance.

Even when our evaluation efforts would meet criteria for a full process account of a program's effects, whether the program in question is a traditional parent education program or an empowering one, we would still be left with the problem of how to give a full account of parents' ways of conceptualizing their parenting in their context, their beliefs, their objectives, and their ways of striving to reach their short-term and/or long-term objectives (if they have any at all). This problem follows inevitably from the empowerment approach's emphasis on recognizing and respecting parents for their responsibility and their competence. But even when we eschew a deficit model with its implicit blaming of parents, we may ask ourselves whether it is possible even in the empowerment approach—working with the principles of making parents aware of their child-rearing practices, and, in VHT, of giving them insight through video sessions into their ongoing interactions with their children—to overcome implicit value judgments about the functionality of parenting practices. Does it make any sense to try to orient families and parents toward their surrounding environment, and to inform parents how they can mobilize and construct supporting networks of families in their neighborhood? On what grounds can we stipulate in our empowering strategies and programs that it might be better for isolated inner-city families to engage in supporting contacts, and that it is better for parents to be made aware of their existing abilities and to strengthen and elaborate their child-rearing skills?

As a matter of fact, there are hidden ethical, political, and philosophical problems behind different answers to these questions. The ethical problem is that the empowerment approach gives the impression of not involving expert value judgments; in fact, however, there always will be an external criterion saying that it is better for these parents to get insight into their (limited?) range of abilities, but that it is possible and effective to build upon those existing abilities, that it is the parents' own responsibility to make up their minds to pursue such a co-constructing approach. In the end, all parenting programs—however empowering they may be, and however they support parents in enhancing their parenting abilities themselves—will always be subjected to external value criteria because parenting is not a self-sufficient and self-sustaining act, but is inherently directed toward the well-being and functional behavioral development of a child. Children and their development toward personal and societal adulthood are the ultimate functional bases for conceptualizing and evaluating parenting programs. And in all societies, communities, authorities, and governments take position on the issue of whether and how far parents are to be held responsible and thus are "to blame for" their level of effective parenting and their way of arranging family life.

In the context of this chapter, we should emphasize that in our view, empowerment of parenting seems to be the better option—not only at the micro level of parent–child interactions, but also at the levels of community development (Henderson, 1997) and of family policy (Gerris, 1996, 1998; Warren, 1997). Both in empowerment programs and in more traditional parent education programs as well, parents are still viewed as the main vehicles for bringing about changes in their children and their family life. However, parents need to be made aware of the relevance of their surrounding environment and its potentials for support. They should be helped to mobilize their already existing social network and to use it on a sustainable basis of reciprocal exchange for the benefit of their children and themselves.

REFERENCES

Abidin, R. R. (1976a). *Parenting Skills: Trainer's manual*. New York: Human Sciences Press.
Abidin, R. R. (1976b). *Parenting Skills: Workbook*. New York: Human Sciences Press.
Achenbach, T. M. (1978). The Child Behavior Profile: I. Boys aged 6–11. *Journal of Consulting and Clinical Psychology, 46*, 478–488.
Achenbach, T. M., & Edelbrock, C. S. (1979). The Child Behavior Profile: II. Boys aged 12–16 and girls aged 6–11 and 12–16. *Journal of Consulting and Clinical Psychology, 47*, 223–233.
Alvy, K. T. (1994). *Parent training today: A social necessity*. Studio City, CA: Center for the Improvement of Child Caring.
Arcus, M. E. (1995). Advances in family life education: Past, present and future. *Family Relations, 44*, 336–344.
Baumrind, D. (1996). The discipline controversy revisited. *Family Relations, 45*, 405–414.

Becker, W. C. (1971). *Parents Are Teachers: A child management program.* Champaign, IL: Research Press.

Berger, P. L., & Neuhaus, R. J. (1977). *To empower people: The role of mediating structures in public policy.* Washington, DC: American Enterprise Institute for Public Policy Research.

Blythe, B. J., Patterson Salley, M., & Jayaratne, S. (1994). A review of intensive family preservation services research. *Social Work Research, 18,* 213–224.

Bronfenbrenner, U. (1977). Toward an experimental ecology of human development. *American Psychologist, 32,* 513–531.

Bronfenbrenner, U. (1979). *The ecology of human development: Experiments by nature and design.* Cambridge, MA: Harvard University Press.

Christensen, O. C., & Thomas, C. R. (1980). Dreikurs and the search for equality. In M. J. Fine (Ed.), *Handbook on parent education* (pp. 53–74). New York: Academic Press.

Cochran, M. (1985). The parental empowerment process: Building upon family strengths. In J. Harris (Ed.), *Child psychology in action: Linking research and practice* (pp. 12–33). London: Croom Helm.

Cochran, M. (1987). Empowering families: An alternative to the deficit model. In K. Hurrelmann & F. Kaufmann (Eds.), *The limits and potential of social interventions* (pp. 105–120). Berlin: De Gruyter.

Cochran, M., & Woolever, F. (1983). Beyond the deficit model. The empowerment of parents with information and informal support. In J. E. Sigel & L. M. Laoso (Eds.), *Changing families* (pp. 225–245). New York: Plenum Press.

Cornell Empowerment Group. (1989). Empowerment through family support. *Empowerment and Family Support, 1*(1), 2–12.

Dekker, J. M. & Biemans, H. (Eds.). (1994). *Video-hometraining in gezinnen* [*Video home training in families*]. Houten, The Netherlands: Bohn Stafleu Van Loghum.

Dembo, M. H., Sweitzer, M., & Lauritzen, P. (1985). An evaluation of group parent education: Behavioral, PET, and Adlerian programs. *Review of Educational Research, 55,* 155–200.

Dinkmeyer, D., & McKay, G. D. (1976a). *Systematic Training for Effective Parenting: Leader's manual.* Circle Pines, MN: American Guidance Service.

Dinkmeyer, D., & McKay, G. D. (1976b). *Systematic Training for Effective Parenting: Parents' handbook.* Circle Pines, MN: American Guidance Service.

Dreikurs, R., & Blumenthal, E. (1976). *Ouders en kinderen, vrienden of vijanden?* [*Parents and children, friends or enemies?*]. Amsterdam: Uitgeverij Contact.

Dunst, C., Trivette, C., & Deal, A. (Eds.). (1994). *Supporting and strengthening families.* Cambridge MA: Brookline Books.

Eimers, R., & Aitchison, R. (1977). *Effective parents—responsible children: A guide to confident parenting.* New York: McGraw-Hill.

Ellis, A. (1962). *Reason and emotion in psychotherapy.* New York: Lyle Stuart.

Ellis, A. (1973). *Humanistic psychotherapy. The rational–emotive approach.* New York: Julian Press.

Ellis, A., & Harper, R. A. (1977). *A new guide to rational living.* North Hollywood, CA: Wilshire.

Farrelly, F., & Brandsma, J. (1985). *Provocative therapy.* Cupertino, CA: Meta.

Fine, M. J. (Ed.). (1980). *Handbook of parent education.* New York: Academic Press.

Fine, M. J., & Henry, S. A. (1989). Professional issues in parent education. In M. J. Fine (Ed.), *The second handbook on parent education: Contemporary perspectives* (pp. 3–20). New York: Academic Press.

Forgatch, M., & Patterson, G. (1989). *Parents and adolescents living together: Part 2. Family problem solving.* Eugene, OR: Castalia.

Gerris, J. R. M. (1990). Research of parent–child interactions within a system-ecological process model of family research. In W. Koops & H. Soppe (Eds.), *Developmental psychology behind the dikes* (pp. 195–210). Delft, The Netherlands: Eburon.

Gerris, J. R. M. (1996). Gezinsbeleid: Nationale redding of nationale kwaal? [Family policy: National salvation or national disease?] *Tijdschrift voor Orthopedagogiek, 35*(1), 28–32.

Gerris, J. R. M. (1998). Gezin en gezinsopvoeding: Moreel fundament van de samenleving? [Family and familial child-rearing: Moral foundations for society?]. In G. W. Meijnen (Ed.), *Opvoeding, Onderwijs en Sociale Integratie [Child-rearing, Education and Social Integration]* (pp. 25–112). Groningen, The Netherlands: Wolters-Noordhoff.

Gordon, T. (1970). *Parent Effectiveness Training.* New York: Wyden.

Gordon, T. (1980). Parent Effectiveness Training: A preventive program and its effects on families. In M. J. Fine (Ed.), *Handbook on parent education* (pp. 101–121). New York: Academic Press.

Haley, J. (1971). Family therapy. *International Journal of Psychiatry, 9,* 233–248.

Henderson, P. (1997). Community development and children: A contemporary agenda. In C. Cannan & C. Warren (Eds.), *Social action with children and families* (pp. 23–42). London: Routledge.

Jansen, R. J. A. H., & Wels, P. M. A. (in press). Videohometraining: Pedagogische ondersteuning voor gezinnen met een hyperactief kind [Video home training: Paedagogical support for families with a hyperactive child]. In W. Hellinckx & B. van den Bruel (Eds.), *Pedagogische thuishulp in problematische opvoedingssituaties [Pedagogical home-based care in problematic child-rearing situations].* Leuven, Belgium: Garant.

Janssens, J. M. A. M., & Kemper, A. A. M. (1997). Effects of video hometraining on parental communication and a child's behavioral problems. *International Journal of Child and Family Welfare, 2,* 137–148.

Kinney, J., Haapala, D., & Booth, C. (1991). *Keeping families together: The Homebuilders model.* New York: Aldine de Gruyter.

Lamb, J., & Lamb, W. A. (1978). *Parent education and elementary counseling.* New York: Human Sciences Press.

Maccoby, E. E., & Martin, J. A. (1983). Socialization in the context of the family: Parent–child interaction. In P. H. Mussen (Series Ed.) & E. M. Hetherington (Vol. Ed.), *Handbook of child psychology: Vol. 4. Socialization, personality, and social development* (4th ed., pp. 1–101). New York: Wiley.

Maluccio, A., Fein, E., & Olmstead, K. A. (1986). *Permanency planning for children.* New York, London: Tavistock.

Medway, F. J. (1989). Measuring the effectiveness of parent education. In M. J. Fine (Ed.), *The second handbook on parent education: Contemporary perspectives* (pp. 237–255). New York: Academic Press.

Minuchin, S. (1974). *Families and family therapy.* Cambridge, MA: Harvard University Press.

Muris, P., Vernaus, A., Hooren, M. van, Merckelbach, H., Heldens, H., Hochsten-bach, P., Smeets, M., & Postema, C. (1994). Effecten van video-hometraining: Een pilot-onderzoek [Effects of video home training: A pilot study]. *Gedragstherapie, 27,* 51–62.

Patterson, G., & Forgatch, M. (1987). *Parents and Adolescents Living Together: Part 1. The basics.* Eugene, OR: Castalia.

Patterson, G. R., Reid, J. B., & Dishion, T. J. (1992). *Antisocial boys: A social interactional approach* (Vol. 4.). Eugene, OR: Castalia.

Popkin, M. H. (1989). Active Parenting: A video-based approach. In M. J. Fine (Ed.), *The second handbook on parent education: Contemporary perspectives* (pp. 77–98). New York: Academic Press.

Rappoport, J. (1984). Studies in empowerment. *Prevention in Human Services, 3,* 1–7.

Roberts, T. W. (1994). *A systems perspective of parenting: The individual, the family, and the social network.* Pacific Grove, CA: Brooks/Cole.

Rollins, B. C., & Thomas, D. L. (1979). Parental support, power and control techniques in the socialization of children. In W. R. Burr, R. Hill, F. I. Nye, & I. L. Reiss (Eds.), *Contemporary theories about the family* (Vol. 1, pp. 317–364). London: Free Press.

Schuerman, J. R., Rzepnicky, T. L., & Little, J. H. (1994). *Putting families first: An experiment in family preservation.* New York: Aldine de Gruyter.

Shinman, S. M. (1996a). *Needs and outcomes in families supported by Home Start.* Unpublished manuscript, Brunel University, Runnymede, England.

Shinman, S. M. (1996b). *Family Health and Home Start: Information for commissioners and purchasers of family support services* (Report). Runnymede, England: Brunel University.

Simpson, R. L. (1980). Behavior modification and child management. In M. J. Fine (Ed.), *Handbook on parent education* (pp. 153–178). New York: Academic Press.

Simpson, R., Forsyth, P., & Kennedy, H. (1995). An evaluation of video interaction analysis in families and teaching situations. In *Professional development initiatives 1993–1994,* (Paper No. 6, pp.129–154). SOED, Regional Psychological Services.

Solomon, B. (1976). *Black empowerment.* New York: Columbia University Press.

Solomon, B. (1987). Empowerment: Social work in oppressed communities. *Journal of Social Work Practice, 2*(4), 79–91.

Trevarthen, C. (1979). Communication and cooperation in early infancy. A description of primary intersubjectivity. In M. Bullowa (Ed.), *Before speech: The beginning of human communication* (pp. 321–347). London: Cambridge University Press.

Trevarthen, C. (1989). *Intuitive emotions: Their changing role in communication between mother and infant.* Edinburgh: Department of Psychology, University of Edinburgh.

Van der Eyken, W. (1990). *Home Start: A four-year evaluation.* Leicester, England: Home Start.

Vogelvang, B. O. (1993). *Video-hometraining "Plus" en het Projekt aan Huis: Verheldering van twee methodieken voor intensieve pedagogische thuisbehandeling* [Video home training "Plus" and the Project at Home: Clarification of two programs for intensive pedagogical treatments at home]. Unpublished doctoral dissertation, Free University of Amsterdam.

Warren, C. (1997). Family support and the journey to empowerment. In C. Cannan & C. Warren (Eds.), *Social action with children and families* (pp. 103–123). London: Routledge.

Warren, C., & Hartless, J. (1995, September). *Family support and the journey to empowerment.* Paper presented at the 4th European Scientific Association for Residential and Foster Care for Children and Adolescents (EUSARF) Congress, Leuven, Belgium.

Weiner, A., Kuppermintz, H., & Guttmann, D. (1994). Video home training (The orion project): A short-term preventive and treatment intervention for families with young children. *Family Process, 33,* 441–453.

Whittaker, J. K. (1996). Community based prevention programs: A selective North American perspective. *International Journal of Child and Family Welfare, 2,* 114–126.

CHAPTER 18

The Empirical Status of Psychological Interventions with Families of Children and Adolescents

MATTHEW R. SANDERS

The family provides the first and most important social, emotional, interpersonal, economic, and cultural context for human development; as a result, family relationships have a profound influence on mental health. Disturbed interpersonal relationships are generic risk factors, and positive interpersonal relationships are protective factors, related to a wide variety of mental health problems from infancy to old age. This chapter provides an overview of the empirical evidence examining the effectiveness of family interventions in treating and preventing mental health problems in children and adolescents. Space limitations preclude analysis of the growing literature on family and marital interventions with adults (see Baucom, Shoham, Mueser, Daiuto, & Stickle, 1998; Halford & Markman, 1997, for reviews of this literature), and the growing literature on the effects of parent training with children with autism and other developmental disabilities.

DEFINITION OF "FAMILY INTERVENTION"

In this chapter, "family intervention" is defined broadly as a therapeutic process that helps modify individuals' psychological distress by targeting their interpersonal relationships within the family. Family interventions typically aim to change aspects of family functioning that are related to the etiology, maintenance, relapse, or exacerbation of an individual's functioning. This may include attempts to alleviate the behavioral or emotional problems of individual family members, to change relationships between family members (marital partners, parent–child relationships, sibling relationships), or to alter relationships between the family and the broader community. The approach is broadly educative and emphasizes reciprocity among family members. Hence, this definition incorporates parent training interventions that aim to improve parent–child relationships and marital interventions that target the marital dyad, along with more traditional family therapies. The term "family intervention" is preferred to "family therapy," as it allows both prevention and treatment studies to be considered.

Hence, family intervention broadly emphasizes the importance of family relationships and interactions to psychological distress, rather than a single approach or therapeutic modality. Three main theoretical perspectives have dominated the family intervention literature: the psychoanalytic, systemic, and cognitive-behavioral or social learning perspectives. These different approaches share the assumption that the individual's behavior is functionally related to the family context and that causality is bidirectional and complex. However, the empirical evidence supporting the efficacy of these different approaches is very unevenly weighted. Several reviews of the family therapy literature have commented on the poor quality of much of the research (Bednar, Burlingame, & Masters, 1988; Dadds, 1995; Gurman, Kniskern, & Pinsof, 1986; Hazelrigg, Cooper, & Borduin, 1987). Many forms of family therapy (systemic, structural) have limited empirical support both on outcome with clearly defined client groups, and on the question of whether observed changes in clients is related to the theoretical mechanisms of family functioning postulated by these theories. Progress in establishing a credible scientific basis for family intervention methods has been made primarily within cognitive-behavioral, social learning, and family psychoeducational models.

EMERGING PERSPECTIVES IN FAMILY INTERVENTION RESEARCH

Several new themes are emerging in family intervention research, including an increasing emphasis on a public health perspective, which stresses the importance of developing cost-effective prevention initiatives targeting entire populations rather than individual families; the concept of levels of intervention, which argues for the idea that the strength of intervention should vary according to known risk and protective factors and to stage of therapy; and a developmental perspective, which seeks to identify key transition points in the family life cycle that may constitute periods of greater receptivity to intervention. These issues are elaborated below.

A Preventive Perspective in Family Mental Health

Raphael (1993) has argued that in contrast to the massive efforts put into the prevention of physical diseases in recent decades, the prevention of mental health problems has been neglected, despite increasing evidence that some forms of mental health problems can be prevented at a community level. Given the widespread nature of mental health problems in the community, and the critical shortage of qualified mental health professionals who are available in the community to provide treatment services, a public health perspective becomes increasingly important.

However, an effective prevention agenda in mental health needs to incorporate strategies that strengthen and promote the stability of family relationships as a central focus. According to the terminology recommended by the Committee on Prevention of Mental Disorders of the National Institute of Medicine (see also Tolan, Quintana, Gorman-Smith, Chapter 16, this volume), family interventions for mental disorders fall into three categories:

1. "Universal" preventive interventions are provided to entire populations. Two examples are prenatal care and programs designed to prevent distress and divorce in couples who are married or planning marriage and are not currently experiencing difficulties in their relationships.

2. "Selective" preventive interventions are targeted toward groups or individuals whose risk of developing mental disorders is significantly higher than average (e.g., home visitation for low-birthweight children).

3. "Indicated" preventive interventions target high-risk individuals who are identified as having minimal but detectable behavioral symptoms that could later develop into a full-blown mental disorder, or biological markers indicating predisposition for mental disorder (e.g., a parent–child interaction training program for preschool children who have been identified by their parents as displaying difficult behaviors).

These three categories of preventive family intervention are part of an intervention spectrum that also includes treatment and maintenance, which are equally important types of mental health interventions.

Levels of Family Intervention

It is increasingly being recognized that a variety of family intervention methods can be effective. These vary in complexity along a number of dimensions, including the strength, intensity, and scope of the intervention; the setting in which it takes place; the mode of delivery (self-directed, individual, group); the target population; the providers of the intervention; and the cost of delivery. To illustrate how different families may require interventions of varying strength, a multilevel parenting and family support strategy that my colleagues and I have developed at the University of Queensland is described below. This program, known as "Triple P" (Positive Parenting Program), consists of five levels of intervention.

Level 1 interventions essentially involve information-based strategies. Educational materials are a form of minimal, relatively low-cost intervention. Written or videotape materials can provide specific information on ways to manage identified problems (e.g., toilet training or sleep disturbances in a toddler), strategies for advocating for a child in the school system, or ways to ask a family doctor questions about the effects of medication. Alternatively, educational materials can be fairly comprehensive, dealing with a series of related problems. Detailed materials can be delivered as a program for family members to work through over a period of weeks (e.g., by correspondence). Elsewhere (Sanders, 1997), I have described a 12-episode television series called *Families,* on parenting and family survival skills; this series was shown at prime time on a commercial network in New Zealand in 1995.

A second level of intervention may combine the use of self-help materials with the provision of professional support to family members. At this level, professional contact is minimal. The self-help materials may be combined with telephone counseling or brief face-to-face contact. The professional role may be adequately filled by care providers who are not mental health specialists, such as general practitioners or community nurses (see Sanders & Markie-Dadds, 1997).

A third level of intervention is appropriate for family members who require more than information and support. Active skills training is used to complement the provision of information. Such an approach includes the extensive use of modeling, rehearsal (via role playing or *in vivo* practice), skills practice, feedback, and support, combined with the use of self-selected or therapist-assisted homework assignments or tasks. This active skills training approach has been shown to be effective with a variety of clinical problems. The focus of this level of intervention is relatively narrow (i.e., it targets specific skills to solve specific problems). Research illustrating this level of intervention includes studies examining the treatment of feeding problems (Turner, Sanders, & Wall, 1994) and recurrent abdominal pain (Sanders et al., 1989).

The fourth level of intervention is similar to the third level, except that the focus of the intervention is broader. The intervention targets a broad range of skills to solve a variety of problems of several family members. Examples of this work include research into the management of multiple behavior problems of oppositional and conduct problem children (Sanders & Glynn, 1981; Sanders & Christensen, 1985).

The fifth level of intervention provides intensive intervention and typically addresses family problems at a broader systemic level. The focus extends beyond individual dyads and target problems to address multiple problems within a family. Again, the key components are education, active skills training, and structured homework activities. An illustration of this approach comes from work within the Triple P model combining marital and parenting interventions for families with concurrent marital and child management problems (e.g., Dadds, Schwartz, & Sanders, 1987) or with concurrent parental depression and child management problems (McFarland & Sanders, 1998). Research on the treatment of child abuse and neglect (e.g., Lutzker, 1992) provides further examples.

A Life Span Perspective in Family Intervention

A life span perspective in family intervention involves a recognition that families are dynamic systems that continually change throughout each member's life, from infancy to old age. It also reflects the recognition that at different points in the life cycle, certain mental health and family problems are more common than at other points. As individuals move from one developmental stage to the next, the developmental tasks and challenges facing them change, as does the nature of the risk and protective factors influencing mental disorder. Problems can arise at any stage of development. If left untreated, they may multiply, intensify, and lead to even greater difficulties when an individual faces subsequent developmental tasks. Interventions targeting key life transitions have the potential to halt this "snowball" effect.

One possible advantage of scheduling interventions at developmental transition points is that families are often more amenable to change at these times. Developmentally sensitive interventions that equip families to deal with stressful life changes reduce risk factors for mental health problems. For example, programs aimed at reducing children's problem behaviors and promoting social skills, initiated during the preschool and early school years, may prevent severe conduct disorders during middle childhood and later delinquent behaviors during adolescence. Since psychopathology can develop at any point in a child's development, it is unlikely that any intervention at a single point in time can prevent mental health problems for a lifetime. A life span perspective is particularly helpful for planning mental health services focused on the prevention of mental disorders.

A developmentally sensitive intervention is one that takes into account the current developmental competencies and characteristics of the individual and his or her social network, and tailors the intervention to meet the cognitive capabilities, language proficiencies, activities, interests, preferences, and aspirations of the age group. Hence, a parenting intervention that is appropriate for a preschooler requires substantial modification if it is to be successful with families of teenagers. Family interventions involving adolescent children must involve the teenagers more in family decisions because of their increasing independence and autonomy, as well as their higher cognitive capabilities compared to younger children (Forehand & Wierson, 1993).

In sum, enhancing psychological well-being and preventing mental health problems require intervention efforts that take into account the changing needs of the individual and family over vulnerable life transitions. A developmental perspective highlights the importance of continuity and the integration of family intervention services across the entire life span.

FAMILY INTERVENTION WITH CHILDREN AND ADOLESCENTS

This section provides an overview of the evidence on the effectiveness of family intervention methods in treating or preventing problems in children of various ages and in adolescents.

Family Interventions with Infants and Toddlers

Family intervention research targeting infants and toddlers has primarily focused on supporting parents of vulnerable infants whose development is considered "at risk." There has been considerable debate regarding the continuity and stability of infant behavior as a predictor of later behavior difficulties in children (e.g., Greenberg, Speltz, & DeKlyen, 1993; Moffitt, 1993). Infant behavior is a better predictor of subsequent developmental and behavior problems when more than a single risk factor is present (e.g., developmental delay, low birthweight, insecure attachment, and difficult temperament). Given the dependence of infants on their parents, it is not surprising that family factors are important determinants of developmental outcome (Greenberg et al., 1993; Rutter, 1985). For example, infants who develop secure attachments to their parents are less likely to develop mental health problems later, are more sociable with other adults and children, achieve better at school, are more compliant, and have greater emotional self-regulation (Greenberg et al., 1993). Other evidence links parenting factors to behavior difficulties in infants. For example, parental anxiety and lack of developmentally appropriate knowledge are associated with excessive crying in young children (Carey, 1968; Pritchard, 1984). Blampied and France (1993) have developed a model of infant–caregiver interaction to explain the development of sleep disturbance in infants, and similar models have been proposed linking parenting to feeding difficulties (e.g., Douglas, 1989). Hart and Risley (1995) have shown that the amount and type of language stimulation children receive between the ages of 12 and 36 months are significant predictors of intellectual and language accomplishments at age 9–10 years.

Other family factors may be generic risk factors for a variety of adverse developmental outcomes. These factors include maternal smoking, maternal substance misuse, young maternal age, living in poverty or violent relationships, and parental psychopathology, particularly depression (Morriset, Barnard, Greenberg, & Booth, 1990; Batshaw & Perret, 1992; Cohn, Campbell, Matias, & Hopkins, 1990). Consequently, the effects of family factors are complex and do not operate independently of other risk variables. The prediction of adverse developmental outcomes for infants requires better understanding of the complex interaction among biological vulnerability factors (e.g., temperament), the broader social context of the family (e.g., poverty), parents' management practices, and the quality of their attachment relationship with their infants.

Promoting Children's Intellectual Development

Some studies seek to promote children's intellectual and social development through parent education programs, often through home visiting programs. For example, the Parents as Teachers program (Ehlers & Ruffin, 1990) is a universal early intervention for first-time parents that begins at birth and continues during the first 3 years of life. Families receive information on child development, periodic developmental and health screenings, monthly home visits by parent educators, and monthly meetings at neighborhood parent resource centers. Early evaluations of this program have been limited by the use of quasi-experimental designs and low participation by minority groups. Nevertheless, Pfannenstiel and Seltzer (1989) found that participating children were significantly more advanced than a comparison group on measures of children's language development, problem-solving skills, and intellectual abilities. Parents were also more knowledgeable about their children's development. However, the program's long-term effects are unclear, and its specific impact on measures of children's behavior and adjustment has yet to be clearly delineated.

Promoting Development in Low-Birthweight Infants

Several literature reviews have concluded that home visiting programs are effective in promoting better parenting. Olds and Kitzman (1990) concluded that home visiting during pregnancy reduced the risks of low birthweight and preterm delivery in a high-risk sample. Postnatal interventions with low-birthweight infants also show positive effects (see Sandall, 1992, for a review). Several studies show that home nursing visits, facilitation of access to pediatric care, and developmental activities can improve cognitive development and indices of growth maturity in these infants (Field, Widmayer, Stringer, & Ignatoff, 1980). These effects have been observed at 36 months (Infant Health and Development Program, 1990; Ramey et al., 1992) and at 9 years (Achenbach, Howell, Aoki, & Rauh, 1993). However, as home visiting parent education forms part of a multicomponent intervention, it is difficult to determine which components are essential.

Improving Attachment Relationships

Anisfeld, Casper, Nozyce, and Cunningham (1990) found that increased physical contact improved maternal responsiveness and ratings of attachment in low socioeconomic-status mother–infant dyads, compared to a control group. Booth, Barnard, Mitchell, and Spieker (1987) used a nursing intervention to improve mothers' social skills and found improvements in mother–child interactions for mothers who increased their social skills. Mothers who did not change had infants with insecure attachment. Erikson, Korfmacher, and Egeland (1992) found that mothers involved in a program to promote healthy parent–infant relationships had a better understanding of their children's needs and less depression and anxiety than control mothers did. Jacobson and Frye (1991) found that providing home visitor support prenatally and during the first year resulted in improved attachment. Lieberman, Weston, and Pawl (1991) carried out a controlled study providing therapy to insecurely attached infant–mother dyads. Their intervention group scored much better than their insecurely attached controls, and as well as their securely attached control group, on several measures of infant–mother interaction.

Preventing Child Abuse and Neglect

Several reviews of the home visiting literature (e.g., Roberts, Wasik, Casto, & Ramey, 1991; Wekerle & Wolfe, 1993) have concluded that intensive home visitation programs for 1- to 3-year-olds that provide parents with support and instruction in child management techniques are effective in changing parental attitudes and behavior, in improving mothers' adjustment, and in decreasing risk of child abuse and neglect. Olds, Henderson, Tatelbaum, and Chamberlin (1986) examined a home visitation program as a means of preventing child abuse and neglect. Nurse home care visitors provided parent education regarding fetal and infant development, and assisted families in gaining access to other health and human services. There was a trend for the visited group to have a lower rate (4% vs. 19%) of reported abuse, they were less likely to visit a physician for an injury or ingestion, and lived in homes with fewer safety hazards (Olds, 1997). Interventions for child abuse per se have been confined to older children. Home visits and education opportunities were provided for mothers in high-risk circumstances by Johnson (1990, 1991). At 36 months of age, the mothers showed better parenting behaviors than control mothers, but there were few differences in the children. When the children were 8 and 11 years, their teachers rated them as more prosocial and less acting out than control children, but there were no effects on their intellectual ability. More conclusive results were obtained by the Milwaukee Program for Prenatal Care (Heber & Garber, 1975). This program provided parents in high-risk circumstances with home visits, parent training, vocational training, facilitation of the use of social services, and a preschool program. At age 14, there was a 30-point difference in IQ between the experimental and control groups (Garber, 1988).

There is also evidence that interventions begun in infancy bring better results than interventions started later in the preschool years. Horacek, Ramey, Campbell, Hoffman, and Fletcher (1987) intervened with children from high-risk families. Day care, home visits, a toy library, and parent supports were provided from infancy for one group, and from kindergarten entry for another. Both groups received better grades in school, but the better outcome was for the children who received intervention from infancy; their results were nearly equal to those of the low-risk comparison group. Interventions in infancy also need to be sustained past infancy. Horacek et al. (1987) stopped intervening with one group at kindergarten entry, and these children lost many of their gains.

Managing Feeding and Sleep Difficulties

Sleep problems have responded well to interventions that involve training parents to modify how they provide attention to their infants when they cry after being put to bed (see France & Hudson, 1993, for a review). Excessive infant crying has responded to increased carrying in the early weeks (Hunziker & Barr, 1986). Training parents to understand the reasons behind different cries has also been effective (Kirkland, 1990; Pritchard, 1984; Taubman, 1984). Feeding problems in infancy include rumination and refusal of food, particularly food containing lumps. Rumination has traditionally been treated with aversive conditioning (Linscheid & Cunningham, 1977; Sajwaj, Libet, & Agras, 1974), but more recently Larson, Ayllon, and Barrett (1987) have described other techniques for decreasing maladaptive feeding in failure-to-thrive infants, which could be applied to specific infant feeding problems such as rumination and refusal of food. Palmer, Thompson, and Linscheid (1975) describe a case study where an infant's insistence on pureed food was treated by the gradual introduction of more solid foods. Douglas (1989) reported several approaches to managing feeding problems in infants and young children, but presented no evaluation of their efficacy.

Family Interventions with Preschool-Age Children

Risk factors for the development of behavior problems during the preschool period include (1) child characteristics, such as being perceived by parents as having a difficult temperament (Prior, Smart, Sanson, & Oberklaid, 1993), being oppositional, or having attentional problems; (2) ineffective parenting, which includes low involvement and harsh, irritable, and inconsistent discipline (McMahon, 1994); and (3) distal factors, including parental psychopathology (particularly maternal depression), parental divorce or conflict, parental antisocial behavior and substance misuse, and low socio-economic status (Sanders & Markie-Dadds, 1992). Children whose parents use harsh, coercive parenting methods, and children with insecure attachments, are at greater risk of developing disruptive behavior problems (Speltz, Greenberg, & DeKlyen, 1990; McMahon, 1994). However, it is important to note that the relationship between various risk factors is reciprocal. For example, a child with severe conduct problems is more likely to elicit negative parental responses (Dumas, 1989). Other known family risk factors, including poverty, marital discord, being raised in a single-parent home, parental psychiatric illness, alcohol misuse, and a history of criminal behavior, have their primary effects on children by modifying parenting and caregiving practices (Patterson, 1982; Reid, 1993; Sanders & Markie-Dadds, 1992).

There is also evidence showing that child abuse frequently occurs in the context of a disturbed parent–child relationship (Belsky, 1993). Parent characteristics that increase the risk of abuse include an absence of warmth and positive attention, a high level of negative attention (e.g., threats and disapproving comments), a lack of empathy, a negative bias in perceptions and attributions of their children's behavior, failure to discriminate accurately between positive and negative child behaviors, use of harsh styles of discipline, unrealistic expectations and standards, difficulty in handling daily stressors, and a general tendency to view normal, innocuous child behavior as aversive (see Frude, 1989, for a review). Child characteristics that increase the risk of abuse include developmental difficulties, as well as behavioral symptoms such as tantrums, enuresis, oppositional behavior, compulsivity, hypervigilance, and aggressive tendencies (Frude, 1989). Thus, relationships between abusing parents and their children are often chronically and seriously disturbed. In such an environment, the probability of serious disciplinary encounters increases, thereby increasing the chances of an escalation of anger and subsequent abuse.

Positive parent–child experiences during this period protect against the development of behavioral problems and the likelihood of abuse (Pettit & Bates, 1989). Protective factors relating to parenting include having warm, affectionate relationships with one's own parents, having realistic expectations about a child's developmental capabilities, actively teaching children necessary social skills, and using consistent discipline techniques. In non-clinic children, parental responsiveness is associated with lower levels of externalizing behavior problems (Rothbaum & Weisz, 1994). Longitudinal research reveals that levels of parental responsiveness during infancy predict subsequent child aggressiveness during preschool and at age 10 (Bradley, Caldwell, & Rock, 1988). Research with clinical samples shows that parents of problem children initiate fewer spontaneous interactions, make fewer contributions to keep the activity going, are less responsive to the children's questions and requests, use more imperative controlling actions, and show more negative affect than parents of nonproblem children do (Gardner, 1994).

A number of well-controlled trials have been conducted to evaluate the effectiveness of family intervention programs for preschool-age children who are considered at risk for later conduct and emotional problems. Many of these early interventions focus on improving parenting and enhancing the children's social and cognitive development in order to prevent later conduct or learning difficulties (Committee on the Prevention of Mental Disorders, 1994). In most successful prevention programs, parent training forms a central focus for the intervention (e.g., Johnson, 1991; Levenstein, 1992; Strayhorn & Weidman, 1991).

There is strong evidence that parent training interventions can be effective in reducing oppositional, aggressive, and disruptive behaviors in preschool children (Berrueta-Clement, Schweinhart, Barnett, & Weikart, 1987; Hawkins, VonCleve, & Catalano, 1991; Johnson & Walker, 1987; Webster-Stratton, 1990). This pattern of behavior is an early precursor of more severe forms of conduct disorder and delinquency. These programs typically involve training parents to use positive parenting methods, such as increasing positive attention and affection when a child behaves appropriately, providing age-appropriate activities, and using more effective discipline strategies (e.g., clear, calm instructions; use of backup consequences such as time out or removal of privileges). Several recent reviews of this literature show that parents can be trained to use more effective parenting skills, and that when this training occurs, there is often rapid improvement in the children's behavior and adjustment (Kendziora & O'Leary, 1993; Sanders, 1996; Webster-Stratton, 1994). Parents often show improvements in their attitudes toward their children, reductions in negativity and hostility, a greater sense of parenting competence, and reduced stress (Pisterman et al., 1992). The recipients of such programs generally report high levels of consumer satisfaction with the intervention (Webster-Stratton, 1994).

Parent training programs can also be relatively brief and largely self-administered. For example, Webster-Stratton, Kolpacoff, and Hollinsworth (1988) demonstrated that video modeling can be an effective medium for teaching parenting skills. They developed a series of parenting videotapes on child management techniques, which parents watched in groups without a therapist. Results at a 1-year follow-up showed that, compared to the control group, parents in the video modeling group reported highly significant improvements in their children's behavior (Webster-Stratton et al., 1989). However, Webster-Stratton (1990) found that of the parents who had participated in one of three different parent training programs, only parents who had received a video modeling program *and* a therapist-led group discussion maintained their gains. Parents receiving a self-directed videotape program did not maintain gains. Overall, the children who failed to maintain improvements came from more disadvantaged families (single parents; lower income; increased alcoholism, drug use, and depression in the immediate families). Thus, the challenge is to match families to the most appropriate, cost-effective level of intervention that will meet their needs.

My colleagues and I have shown that parent training is an effective intervention for young children with conduct problems. The Triple P (Positive Parenting Program), described earlier in this chapter, is a multilevel system of intervention for the families of young children at risk for developing severe conduct problems. The intervention methods used in Triple P have been subjected to a series of controlled evaluations, using both intrasubject replication designs and traditional randomized control group designs (see Sanders & Dadds, 1993, for a review). Early studies demonstrated that parents could be trained to implement behavior change and positive parenting strategies with their children in the home, and that the effects of intervention transferred to out-of-home situations in the community (Sanders & Glynn, 1981; Sanders & Dadds, 1982). Children receiving intervention showed significantly lower levels of disruptive and oppositional behavior following intervention. After training, parents showed increases in positive parent–child interaction and reduced levels of negativity. Later studies demonstrated that the same intervention methods were also effective with oppositional children who were mildly intellectually disabled (Sanders & Plant, 1989).

From this initial research, which established the viability of the intervention, a series of studies examined the effects of intervention when children's problems were complicated by marital discord. Marital conflict has been shown to be a significant risk factor for the development of antisocial behavior in children, particularly boys. It also predicts poor response to parent training interventions. We (Dadds et al., 1987) developed a brief marital communication intervention to complement parenting skills training. This intervention involved teaching parents of an oppositional child to support each other's parenting efforts, rather than undermining or criticizing each other. It also taught couples problem-solving skills to resolve disagreements about parenting. This adjunctive intervention significantly improved outcome on both child and parent observational measures for families with marital discord. There were no additional benefits for parents without marital discord.

Parent training can also be effective with clinically depressed parents of oppositional children. Another study (McFarland & Sanders, 1993) evaluated the effectiveness of behavioral family intervention (BFI) with 47 clinically depressed mothers who met diagnostic criteria for either major depression or dysthymia. The mothers were randomly assigned either to a standard BFI condition or to an enhanced condition. The enhanced condition provided additional treatment components that specifically targeted the mothers' depression, including mood monitoring, cognitive restructuring techniques, and coping skills training. Both the standard condition and the enhanced condition produced significant reductions in children's aversive behavior and in mothers' depression at a 6-month follow-up. These findings suggest that parent training can be an effective intervention for improving mothers' mood and reducing child disruptive behavior.

Preliminary data (Sanders & Markie-Dadds, 1994) have been presented from a large-scale community trial comparing three different versions of the Triple P intervention. The parents of 300 high-risk 3-year-olds were randomly assigned either to a self-help condition, to a standard BFI condition in which parents received 12 weeks of child-focused parent training, or to an enhanced BFI condition where parents received additional interventions focusing on marital communication, mood management, and stress coping skills training. Immediately after treatment, all three interventions were more effective than a waiting-list control, and the two therapy-assisted conditions showed greater treatment effects than the self-directed condition. The two therapy-assisted conditions were not significantly different from each other. Compared to the control group, families receiving intervention had lower levels of oppositional and aggressive behavior, lower levels of parental negativity (including much less reliance on physical punishment in disciplining children), and increases in parents' sense of competence. All three interventions had high levels of consumer satisfaction. These findings also revealed that after intervention, over 90% of children moved out of the clinically significant range on parent report measures of child conduct problems. At one year follow-up treatment effects were maintained or further improved for all three treatment conditions. These are encouraging findings, and if these intervention effects are maintained in the longer term, they will point to a powerful intervention technology for assisting parents with young behaviorally disturbed children.

An extension of Triple P with a sample of rural families has been recently reported (Connell, Sanders, & Markie-Dadds, 1997). Twenty-four families living in rural and remote areas were randomly assigned either to a self-directed intervention, which included brief telephone counseling, or to a waiting-list control condition. The telephone counseling intervention lasted 10 weeks, with once-weekly contact that lasted for an average of 20 minutes (range = 5–30 minutes). Telephone contacts were used to prompt parents to use the self-help materials, which included a copy of *Every Parent* (Sanders, 1992) and a workbook containing a series of weekly tasks to be completed by a parent in conjunction with the parenting text (Sanders, Lynch, & Markie-Dadds, 1994). Following intervention, treated families showed significant reductions in parental reports of child behavior problems; improvements in parenting skills; a greater sense of parenting competence; and reduced levels of parenting stress, anxiety, and depression. Parents completing the program were highly satisfied with the program, according to a consumer satisfaction survey. The waiting-list group either showed no change or deteriorated on measures of child adjustment. These findings show that a brief, largely self-directed version of Triple P can be effective with families that traditionally have had little access to mental health services.

Overall, Triple P is an example of a family intervention program derived from experimental clinical research that has clearly established the effectiveness of the intervention strategies for reducing oppositional behavior in a variety of populations, including children from maritally discordant homes, children of depressed parents, children in stepfamilies, developmentally disabled children, and children in rural and remote areas. Similar parent training methods have been used successfully with young children who have persistent feeding difficulties (Dadds, Sanders, & Bor, 1984; Turner et al., 1994; Werle, Murphy, & Budd, 1993). The family intervention methods have been evaluated with mildly and moderately intellectually disabled children (Harrold, Lutzker, Campbell, & Touchette, 1992; Huynen, Lutzker, Bigelow, Touchette, & Campbell, 1996). Parent training has also been used successfully with children with language impairments (Alpert & Kaiser, 1992) and sleep disturbance (Seymour, Brock, During, & Poole, 1989). There is some evidence that children from maritally discordant homes or from single-parent homes do less well in parent training programs than other children. However, outcomes for these children can be improved with the provision of marital counseling for parents, or by changing dysfunctional patterns of communication and problem solving within the family (e.g., Dadds et al., 1987).

Parent training programs focusing on child management have been combined with stress reduction procedures, with some success in reducing abusive parenting behaviors and reports of child behavior problems (e.g., Lutzker, 1992; Wolfe, Edwards, Manion, & Koverola, 1988). It is now generally accepted that a more comprehensive, ecobehavioral approach to treating and preventing child abuse is likely to result in better long-term maintenance of treatment gains than programs focused on parenting skills alone. An example of a large-scale project that assessed and treated cases of child abuse and neglect from a multifaceted perspective is Project 12-Ways (Lutzker, 1992). Families referred to Project 12-Ways underwent intensive behavioral assessment, followed by family-based treatment services. After participation in the project, some families clearly made dramatic changes—so dramatic that they were no longer considered to be at risk. More research is needed with large groups of at-risk families to determine the external validity of such broader approaches to the treatment of child abuse.

Several studies have shown that parent training programs can produce highly durable treatment effects. For example, a long-term follow-up of adolescents whose parents participated in a parent training program for young children found that on most measures of functioning, treated children were indistinguishable from nonclinic children (Forehand & Long, 1988). A further follow-up of these same children in late adolescence or early adulthood showed that they were similar to a matched community sample on measures of delinquency, emotional adjustment, academic progress, and relationships with parents (Long, Forehand, Wierson, & Morgan, 1994).

In summary, there is clear evidence that early intervention programs aimed at preventing conduct problems can be effective. These programs have shown large intervention effects and have been replicated by different groups in different countries. The strongest evidence for the value of family intervention with children of preschool age is based on the behavioral parent training model; parents can learn new parenting skills, and when they do, their children's psychological adjustment improves. There is a need to develop large-scale, multisite, preventively focused parenting skills interventions commencing when children reach age 3. A priority for such work is the development of systematic early intervention programs for parents of preschool-age children showing early signs of significant disruptive or oppositional behavior, as this behavior pattern seems to be readily modifiable. Mental health services for young children should be prevention-oriented if any significant impact on psychosocial morbidity is to be achieved.

Family Interventions with Elementary-School-Age Children

There is a paucity of well-controlled evaluations of child psychotherapy, compared to research with adults (Kazdin, Bass, Ayers, & Rodgers, 1990). This situation is beginning to change, and there is now increasing evidence that family intervention is the treatment of choice for a range of behavioral and emotional problems in children (Kazdin & Weisz, 1998; Sanders, 1996). There is now evidence showing that family intervention strategies can be effective in treating children with conduct and attention problems, anxiety disorders, recurrent pain syndromes, language problems and stuttering, obesity, sleep disorders, and habit disorders (e.g., thumbsucking); they can also be useful in teaching children personal safety skills and social skills (Sanders, 1996).

Interventions for Specific Problems

Conduct Problems. Treatment outcome studies support the role of family interaction patterns in the development of conduct problems in children. Behavioral intervention programs that teach parents to use effective discipline strategies, and that provide attention and rewards for prosocial behavior, result in reliable decreases in conduct problems in school-age children (Kazdin, 1997; Kazdin et al., 1990; Lochman, 1990). Interventions that modify parents' personal distress, marital discord, or problem-solving and communication skills have also produced reductions in conduct problems in children (Miller & Prinz, 1990). However, it should be noted that these parental factors have typically been modified in conjunction with training parents in child management skills. It is unlikely that modification of parental factors alone would lead to direct changes in a child's adjustment without the parallel change in child-rearing techniques.

Anxiety Disorders. Controlled treatment studies have shown that exposure to the fearful stimuli (often with associated cognitive therapy), and family interventions directly focused on how parents respond to children's anxious behavior, are effective in treating children's anxiety problems. Helping anxious children face the stimuli they are afraid of helps decrease their level of fear. Many of these studies also involve a cognitive component in which a child is taught to process information about threat in a more constructive way. Only one controlled treatment study has evaluated the role of family variables in the remediation of child anxiety. Barrett, Dadds, and Rapee (1993) treated a large group of anxious children who were randomly assigned to either a cognitive-behavioral treatment (CBT) or the same CBT model plus a family intervention that ran in parallel over a 14-week period. At the end of treatment, 88% of children in the combined group no longer met formal diagnostic criteria for an anxiety disorder, compared with 61% in the CBT-only treatment and fewer than 30% in the waiting-list control group. At a 12-month follow-up, the relative superiority of the CBT-plus-family condition was maintained. Thus, it appears that the modification of parental skills can have a significant effect on anxiety in children when combined with a CBT program for the children. However, it is not clear whether a change in parental skills on its own will result in an improvement in child behavior, and it is not clear which aspect of the parental intervention is associated with the extra improvement.

Somatic Complaints. Several studies have attempted to modify recurrent abdominal pain (RAP) in children by changing family interaction patterns. We (Sanders et al., 1989) assessed a BFI for children with RAP. The intervention produced significant decreases in the frequency of child pain behaviors, compared to a control condition in which matched RAP sufferers and their families received standard pediatric care. The majority of BFI children reported that they were no longer experiencing pain after the intervention. This finding was later replicated and extended (Sanders, Shepherd, Cleghorn, & Woolford, 1994). A cognitive BFI was again superior to standard pediatric care. Children receiving the BFI had higher rates of complete elimination of the pain, lower levels of relapse at 6- and 12-month follow-ups, and lower levels of interference with their activities as a result of pain; there were also higher levels of parent satisfaction with the BFI than with standard pediatric care.

Academic Underachievement. Poor academic achievement is a major contributor to children's dropping out of school, which in turn increases the risk of a variety of antisocial behavior problems (Loeber, 1990). Some evidence from controlled single-case studies supports the value of training a child's parents to employ remedial tutoring procedures. Glynn and associates have shown that parents can successfully employ Pause, Prompt, Praise, a remedial tutoring procedure, to assist their children with severe reading difficulties (McNaughton, Glynn, & Robinson, 1987). Parental involvement in children's education has been widely supported by educators as facilitating learning, particularly for children with learning difficulties. It should be noted that there is no evidence that parent training on its own is effective in the long run in overcoming the multiple problems of children with clearly documented learning difficulties. However, parent involvement can complement other approaches, and in many instances it is vital to ensure that the school's efforts are not undermined. Glynn, Fairweather, and Donald (1992) have argued that parental involvement in children's literacy (oral language, reading, writing) should be based on collaborative partnerships between parents and schools in which decision making is shared.

Comparisons of Different Family Therapies

Most of the empirical work on family intervention has employed BFI or family skills training models. There is much less evidence available concerning the effectiveness of other types of family therapy. Reviews of the family therapy literature have repeatedly pointed to the lack of research and the generally poor methodologies used in studies that are available. Although some evidence suggests that families receiving family therapy show greater improvement than waiting-list subjects, definitive conclusions have been difficult to draw (Gurman et al., 1986; Hazelrigg et al., 1987).

Hazelrigg et al. (1987) based their conclusions on 20 studies that met rigorous methodological standards. These outcome studies included a mixture of structural, strategic, and behavioral interventions (no studies of systemic family intervention met the inclusion criteria). Bednar et al. (1988) questioned whether systemic family interventions actually achieve change through the mechanisms proposed by the theory. Outcome studies typically do not measure the theoretical constructs hypothesized to be critical to change in the family. Bednar et al. (1988) argued that there is no evidence that these models of therapy actually modify the family system at all. Rather, when change occurs, it probably does so as a result of mechanisms that are common to all "good" psychotherapy—that is, a positive relationship with clients, opportunities for problem solving, ventilation of emotion, and formulation of plans for change. Bednar et al. argued that BFI is not subject to the same criticism. Evaluations of this mode of therapy generally take measures of family processes hypothesized to be important in maintaining a particular problem. Researchers have shown that changes in these family processes are associated with improvement in the related problem (Sanders & Dadds, 1993).

Only a handful of studies have directly compared different types of family therapy. Szykula, Morris, Sudweeks, and Saygar (1987) compared the effectiveness of strategic and behavioral family therapy for a sample of behaviorally and emotionally disturbed children and their families. Only self-report measures were used to evaluate outcome. The outcome was similar and positive for both therapy groups. However, an analysis of the outcome by severity of presenting problem showed that families with more severe problems responded more favorably to the behavioral intervention.

Wells and Egan (1988) compared behavioral family therapy with systems family therapy in the treatment of childhood oppositional disorder. The results showed no differences between the two therapies on measures of parental emotional and marital adjustment; parents in both groups had a decrease in depression and anxiety. Direct observations of the family, however, showed that the behavioral intervention was superior in producing improvements in positive parent attention and child compliance (the referral problem).

Evaluations of Commercially Available Parent Training Programs

A number of commercially available programs give parents advice on raising children and promoting successful family relationships. These programs include Parent Effectiveness Training (PET), based on the work of Gordon (1975), and Systematic Training for Effective Parenting (STEP), based on the work of Dinkmeyer and McKay (1976). The PET program makes use of the concepts and techniques of Carl Rogers (1951). The program emphasizes the use of active listening, "I-messages," and democratic problem-solving skills. The STEP program uses similar skills but also draws on the work of an Adlerian, Rudolf Dreikurs (Cedar & Levant, 1990; Schultz, 1981; Schultz & Khan, 1982). Although there is some evidence showing that the PET and STEP programs are viewed favorably by participants (Noller & Taylor, 1989), there is a paucity of adequately controlled studies using children with properly documented, clinically significant levels of behavioral disturbance. In many studies the diagnostic status of the children is not reported. In one of the few studies with adequate methodology, Schultz (1981) compared PET, STEP, and a behavioral parent training program. The study used placebo and nonattendant control conditions and had a 12-month follow-up. The main finding was that all treatments produced positive changes in parental attitudes and maternal ratings of household happiness, compared with the controls. However, it is not possible to conclude from these studies that the psychological functioning of children actually improved.

Consequently, although some data suggest that the PET and STEP programs are associated with some changes in parental attitudes, the clinical significance of these findings has not been adequately demonstrated. These programs cannot be recommended as treatments for children with significant mental health problems. Their effectiveness as preventive interventions for high-risk families is unknown at this time.

Evaluations of Parenting Books

A large number of books have been written on parenting and family relationships. Even though most of these books have been written for the North American market, there is little doubt that books on parenting are popular in many countries and are one of the main sources of information parents have about child rearing. It is unfortunate that so few of these books have been systematically evaluated, even though some of the ideas they contain may be based on research findings. It would be useful to know to what extent recommending that a parent read a particular book results in changes in a child's behavior or adjustment, or changes in parenting practices and family relationships. One of the few studies to examine this issue (Sanders & Markie-Dadds, 1994) evaluated a self-help program for parents of oppositional children that involved reading *Every Parent: A Positive Approach to Children's Behaviour* (Sanders, 1992). Compared to parents in a waiting-list control condition, parents in the self-help condition had significantly greater reductions in reports of behavior problems and positive changes in parenting practices. Other studies have also shown that written materials can be an effective intervention in teaching parents toilet training routines and ways of managing sleep problems (see Sanders, 1996). The work of Webster-Stratton (1990) has shown that parenting skills can be taught effectively through use of videotape modeling procedures. Clearly, however, further research is needed to determine who benefits from self-help parenting programs (perhaps programs combining written and video materials), as these constitute brief, low-cost, effective alternatives to more intensive programs.

Summary

The most thoroughly researched treatment intervention for elementary-school-age children has been BFI for childhood conduct problems. Research evaluating the use of BFI for child conduct problems has supported the efficacy of this approach, both in the short term and over follow-up periods up to 17 years after the termination of treatment (Forehand & Long, 1988; Long et al., 1994). There is increasing evidence to support the efficacy of BFI with anxiety disorders, recurrent pain syndromes, social skills deficits, language problems, and academic underachievement. There is less evidence to show that strategic and systemic approaches to family therapy are effective, although a small number of methodologically adequate studies have shown that these approaches have some positive effects. Much more concerning is the lack of scientific evidence that the improvements observed have anything to do with changes in the family system (Dadds, 1995). Other than BFI, commercially available parent training programs without a behavioral focus (e.g., PET, STEP) have not been adequately evaluated. Although some positive changes in parental attitudes have been shown (Schultz, 1981), there is little evidence of the clinical significance of these changes, the impact on children's psychological functioning, and the effectiveness of the programs as preventive interventions for high-risk families. While further research evaluating parenting books and videotapes is required, they have been shown to be an effective intervention tool (Sanders & Markie-Dadds, 1994; Sanders, 1996; Webster-Stratton, 1990).

Family Interventions with Adolescents

There is considerable evidence that family functioning has a pervasive effect on adolescents' psychological adjustment. Family conflict is a common source of psychological distress for both parents and adolescents. From a parenting perspective, the period of adolescence can be a difficult one. Many of the risk factors that predict psychopathology in younger children may continue in adolescence. Some adolescents with disruptive behavior disorders or attention-deficit/hyperactivity disorder experience further escalation of preexisting problem behaviors, as well as involvement in serious antisocial behavior and substance misuse. Until relatively recently, there were few well-controlled studies examining family interventions with adolescents. This situation has changed, and it is reasonable to conclude that family interventions are potentially effective with a variety of adolescent problems, including substance misuse (Liddle & Dakof, 1995; Alexander, Holtzworth-Munroe, & Jameson, 1994), antisocial behavior (Henggeler, Borduin, & Mann, 1993), and eating disorders (Le Grange, Eisler, Dare, & Russell, 1992).

Interventions for Substance Misuse

A promising form of family intervention known as multidimensional family therapy (MDFT) has been effective in reducing drug use in adolescents. Liddle and Dakof (1995) compared MDFT to either adolescent group therapy or a multifamily education intervention. The greatest and most consistent improvements occurred for the MDFT group, including better school grades. MDFT targets four areas of an adolescent's and family's functioning: the adolescent's intrapersonal and interpersonal functioning, parenting practices, parent–adolescent interactions, and family member's interactions with the community (e.g., welfare officers). In a subsequent study, Schmidt, Liddle, and Dakof (1996) showed that MDFT did indeed produce changes in parenting practices. Specifically, 29 parents and their drug-using adolescents completed a 16-session therapy program. Two-thirds of parents showed significant reductions in negative parenting (such as power-assertive discipline and negative monitoring), and increases in positive parenting (such as positive discipline and communication), as assessed through behavioral observation.

Interventions for Antisocial Behavior and Delinquency

The management of seriously conduct-disordered youth is a major mental health and social problem. Parent management training (PMT) has produced good results with preadolescent children. However, PMT has not been as successful with adolescents. This may be partly due to the need to include adolescents as partners in treatment, and partly due to the need to address peer relational and academic skills, which are outside parents' immediate control. Dishion and Andrews (1995) compared a group parent training intervention with an adolescent group intervention, a combined parent and adolescent group program, a self-directed intervention involving information but no face-to-face therapy contact, and a no-treatment control group. Results showed that although both the parent-focused and adolescent group programs produced greater short-term improvements in observed and reported family conflict, only the parent condition reduced subsequent tobacco use at follow-up, and long-term effects on problem behavior were minimal. An interesting finding was that the adolescent group program resulted in higher rates of tobacco use and problem behavior than the control condition; this suggests the possible dangers of peer interventions with high risk adolescent samples.

A more promising example of effective intervention that targets family relationships stems from work by Henggeler and colleagues. Multisystemic therapy (MST) is a comprehensive multisetting intervention for adolescent offenders. The approach uses present-focused, action-oriented, individually tailored strategies targeting intrapersonal (e.g., cognitive), family, peer, and school factors associated with antisocial behavior. Treatment is usually conducted in the adolescents' homes and in the local community (schools, recreation centers). The program has a strong emphasis on teaching parents skills so that they can independently tackle their concerns in raising adolescents. The results from this research have been impressive, given the severity of the conduct problems experienced by participating families. Borduin et al. (1995) compared MST and individual therapy in a study involving 176 juvenile offenders. Results showed that MST was more effective in preventing future offending and in reducing family correlates of disturbance (i.e., more cohesion, adaptability, and supportiveness, and less observed conflict and hostility, during family interactions).

A combination of PMT and family systems therapy has been shown to be successful with adolescent offenders (Alexander & Parsons, 1973). However, the results of this research were difficult to interpret because of methodological problems, and no replication has yet succeeded in producing similar results. Intensive PMT with adolescent chronic offenders by pairs of highly experienced therapists produced significant reductions in police-recorded offenses. Although the results persisted during a 3-year follow-up, offending gradually increased to the point where it was not significantly different from that of a control group (Bank, Marlowe, Reid, Patterson, & Weinrott, 1991). The high level of training and experience necessary to implement these procedures militate against their widespread adoption for handling community-level problems. Classroom-based interventions have also reduced antisocial behavior, but there has been no study that combines PMT with a systematic classroom management program.

Another significant finding with implications for family intervention is that improvements in prosocial behavior and reductions in delinquent behavior obtained via contingency management in a halfway house (Kirigin, Braukman, Atwater, & Wolf, 1982) were lost when the adolescents returned to their home settings (Jones, Weinrott, & Howard, 1981). However, the use of well-developed treatment foster care has shown good results (Chamberlain, 1990, 1996; Chamberlain, Moreland, & Reid, 1992; Chamberlain & Reid, 1991). This package includes PMT for the biological family, home contingency management by trained foster parents, a school program monitored by teachers and foster parents, and close monitoring and supervision of peer relationships. Other components for such problems as substance misuse are added as needed. Typical placement length is 6 months, after which adolescents return to their biological parents.

Robin (1981) compared "behavioral–systems" family therapy for parent–adolescent conflict with alternative treatments that included a mixture of systemic, eclectic, and psychodynamic family therapies. Both groups showed reductions in self-reported parent–adolescent conflict immediately after treatment. However, the behavioral–systems therapy showed superior outcome on measures of problem solving, communication, and self-reported satisfaction with therapy.

Although drug treatments have often had a positive effect on antisocial behavior, they appear to be most beneficial when combined with PMT. The interaction between physiological predisposition to conduct or attention problems and the social environment requires further systematic investigation.

Interventions for Attention-Deficit/Hyperactivity Disorder

There is little evidence examining the effects of family therapy with adolescents with attention-deficit/hyperactivity disorder, even though parent–adolescent conflict is a major problem in many of these families. In one of the few studies, Barkley, Guevremont, Anastopoulos, and Fletcher (1992) examined three different types of family therapy: behavioral parent training, based on Forehand's and Barkley's work; family problem solving and communication training, based on Patterson and colleagues' work; and structural family therapy, based on Minuchin's work. All three therapies reduced negative communication, anger during conflicts, maternal depression, and the number of internalizing and externalizing symptoms. All three therapies also improved ratings of school adjustment. Despite these improvements, most of the adolescents (70–95%) in each group showed no clinically significant change in the number or intensity of family conflicts. These authors emphasize the importance of long-term multimodal combined pharmacological–psychological interventions for adolescents with attention-deficit/hyperactivity disorder.

Interventions for Depression

Controlled group outcome studies have shown that cognitive-behavioral therapies can produce significant reductions in adolescent depression (Kahn, Kehle, Jenson, & Clark, 1990; Lewinsohn, Clarke, Hops, & Andrews, 1990). However, one-third to one-half of adolescents treated in these studies showed little improvement. Greater parental involvement in treatment has been shown to predict greater improvement during treatment (Clarke et al., 1992). Although these gains were maintained at follow-up in this study, adolescents who received the intervention without parental involvement continued to improve beyond the gains made by the parental involvement group. It is worth noting, however, that the parental group program was conducted separately from the adolescent group program.

Interventions for Eating Disorders

Although there have been numerous clinical descriptions of family therapy for adolescent eating disorders, based on Minuchin's work (Minuchin, Rosman, & Baker, 1978) in the treatment of anorexia nervosa, there are few well-controlled clinical trials evaluating the efficacy of any form of family therapy for these disorders. Indeed, skepticism about the value of such trials and the generalizability of findings to clinical practice has been expressed, and this skepticism has served to slow the development of a scientific understanding of who responds to treatment (Dare, Eisler, Russell, & Szmukler, 1990).

Although hospitalization is common for chronically underweight individuals, Fairburn and Cooper (1989) suggest that better research into outpatient treatment could prevent this in most cases, especially when parents and other family members could be involved. This involvement would include an educational component about the nature of the disorder, plus training in conflict resolution and management of food intake. Anorexia nervosa is currently a poorly understood disorder of low but increasing prevalence, with serious implications for mental and physical health.

Three studies have shown that family intervention strategies are effective in the treatment of adolescents with eating disorders (Russell, Szmukler, Dare, & Eisler, 1987; Le Grange et al., 1992; Robin, Siegel, Koepke, Moye, & Tice, 1994). Russell et al. (1987) compared the effects of family therapy and individual supportive psychotherapy after a period of inpatient treatment. For patients with an onset prior to 19 years of age and a duration of less than 3 years, family therapy was superior in terms of weight gain. A subsequent report from the same trial (Dare et al., 1990) revealed that engagement of families in therapy was a significant problem, with quite high levels of dropout in both family therapy (36%) and individual therapy (33%). More recently, Robin et al. (1994) found that behavioral–family systems therapy emphasizing parental influences over eating and weight gain, coupled with communication skills training and cognitive restructuring, was more effective than psychodynamically oriented individual therapy in changing measures of body mass index. The two programs were comparable on measures of psychopathology and eating-related family conflict. It is important to note that the individual therapy program involved some collateral parent sessions.

Interventions for Chronic Illness

Recently, the possibility of family intervention program's improving the clinical status and adjustment of medically ill adolescents has been examined. Satin, La Greca, Zigo, and Skyler (1995) evaluated the effects of a 6-week family-oriented group intervention for adolescents with insulin-dependent diabetes. The family therapy was provided either alone or in combination with a parent simulation exercise. This involved parents' experiencing a simulation of the regimen their adolescents were expected to follow (e.g., administering injections, monitoring urinary glucose and acetone, following a meal plan). Results showed that adolescents in families receiving the family intervention combined with the simulation exercise had better metabolic control following intervention, compared to adolescents in the control group. The results for the family-therapy-alone group were unclear.

Summary

Family interventions have the potential to contribute meaningfully to the management and prevention of substance misuse, conduct disorder, eating disorders, depression, and other disorders in adolescents. With respect to conduct disorder and substance misuse, there is increasing evidence that family interventions that engage parents of adolescents can be effective. Numerous studies show that adolescents with conduct problems are particularly resistant to treatment, and considerable effort and expertise are needed to make any impact on this problem; these findings emphasize the need to intervene earlier. The most promising procedures for problem youth seem to be MST and the foster care approach.

Programs such as the Adolescent Coping with Depression Course (Clarke, Lewinsohn, & Hops, 1990) need to examine whether more active parent participation enhances outcome in adolescent depression. This type of intervention should be carried out in a way that enhances communication between parents and adolescents. Research studies need to evaluate the various intervention components and the means for delivering them, with particular reference to family communication and problem solving. Prevention should focus on identifying children at or near puberty who are at significant risk of depression. Parents may need to be educated to recognize early warning signs and to seek early assistance. Examples include bereavement counseling in the event of the death or loss of a parent, and couple therapy (Markman, Renick, Floyd, Stanley, & Clements, 1993) for parents in distress. At this level, interventions by means of self-help manuals and/or audiotape–videotape delivery need to be developed and evaluated.

Although I have not discussed adolescent schizophrenia in this section, the potential genetic vulnerability of adolescents with a schizophrenic parent makes them a known risk group. However, the preferred treatment is likely to be similar to that described for depression (reducing stress and marital discord or breakdown) and substance misuse and conduct disorder (improving parenting skills), plus a specific educational component to explain the nature of the disorder and its associated risks. Given the high cost to the community of schizophrenia and the trend toward deinstitutionalization, the development, dissemination, and evaluation of community-delivered interventions should be a high priority.

To turn to methodological concerns, parents' and/or adolescents' resistance to treatment and the demonstration of treatment integrity are crucial issues that require attention in future research. Research has demonstrated that the number of parental resistance statements early in treatment is highly predictive of treatment completion and dropout (Chamberlain, Patterson, Reid, Forgatch, & Kavanagh, 1984). Training therapists to identify and respond appropriately to this behavior is extremely important. Similarly, results from outcome studies that do not satisfactorily demonstrate treatment integrity in delivering the variables under investigation may be misleading (e.g., Botvin, Baker, Filazzola, & Botvin, 1990). Research studies that do not include stringent tests that therapists are delivering the treatment in the desired manner should not be funded. However, this must be balanced against the development and implementation of highly complex protocols that are unlikely to be used by a wide range of practitioners. Prevention or early intervention must be available to large numbers of people, and delivery cannot be restricted to a small number of highly trained personnel.

In addition, valid and reliable measures of interpersonal communication and problem solving are required that are robust enough to be widely accepted and used to demonstrate change. These changes must then be shown to be associated with significant and socially valuable improvements in functioning that are maintained over time. More attention needs to be given to reaching agreement on what indicators of functioning should be used to provide this information. Attempts must also be made to compute the savings achieved (through the prevention of health care expenditures, imprisonment, welfare or social security payments, unemployment, and lost productivity) as a result of such improvements.

General Summary

There is strong evidence supporting the effectiveness of family intervention methods in the treatment of preschool, child, and (to a lesser extent) adolescent psychopathology. Most of the scientific evidence has focused on BFI approaches, specifically parent training and functional family therapy. There is little evidence concerning the effectiveness of other approaches to family intervention, such as the PET or STEP programs, even though such programs are widely used and have strong advocates. Studies evaluating these two programs have generally employed weak methodologies (e.g., reliance on questionnaire measures of outcome, lack of appropriate control conditions, lack of measures of hypothesized family mechanisms, and inadequate descriptions of the clinical status of the children involved). Also, the clinical significance of the treatment effects has not been adequately reported (e.g., Wood & Davidson, 1993).

Consequently, it is essential that all mental health services for children and adolescents have expertise available in the treatment modalities with the strongest empirical support. It is of concern that some of the most widely used forms of family therapy are those with the weakest scientific support (e.g., strategic and systemic approaches to family therapy). If these approaches continue to be employed in mental health services proper scientific evaluation of them must be undertaken. It is important that forms of family intervention with demonstrated effectiveness be more widely used, that proper training be available, and that staff members using these methods receive adequate supervision.

Although family intervention is a powerful intervention, it is not a panacea. Many forms of child psychopathology involve significant comorbidity, and family factors are one of several groups of etiological factors (albeit an important one) influencing children's adjustment. As children move through the school system, peers and academic learning failure increasingly affect their children's adjustment. As they move toward adolescence, many forms of behavioral disturbance become more firmly established. Consequently, a preventive emphasis on early childhood and the early years of primary schooling is likely to have the greatest yield in terms of impact on child psychopathology.

A major challenge in delivering better treatment services to children and families is the need to develop more effective ways of reaching the many high-risk families who at present receive no treatment services at all. Graziano (1977) argued that parent training has revolutionized clinical services for children, and it is now widely used in many clinical settings. Although techniques of behavior change constitute the therapeutic centerpiece of the approach, the consultation process strongly influences the acceptability of treatment to families and therefore has an important role in the overall strategy (Sanders & Lawton, 1993).

TOWARD A MODEL OF EFFECTIVE FAMILY CONSULTATION

Reports of clinical trials documenting the effects of family intervention programs often mask the complexity of the therapeutic process issues involved in successful family intervention. In addition to relevant theoretical and conceptual knowledge of psychopathology, family relationships, life-long human development, principles and techniques of behavior, and attitude and cognitive change, practitioners must be interpersonally skilled. They require well-developed communication skills, with advanced-level training in the theory and principles of family intervention. In this section, several principles that optimize the effectiveness of family intervention work are proposed.

1. *Family intervention should empower families.* Interventions should aim to enhance individual's competence and the family's ability as a whole to solve problems for itself. In most (but not all) instances, families will have a lesser need for support over time. Family interventions that promote dependence are destructive.

2. *Family interventions should build on existing strengths.* Successful interventions build on the existing skills and abilities of family members. It is assumed that individuals are capable of becoming active problem solvers, even though their previous attempts to resolve problems may not have been successful. This may be due to lack of necessary knowledge, skills, or motivation.

3. *The therapeutic relationship is an important part of effective family intervention.* Regardless of theoretical orientation, most family intervention experts agree that the therapeutic relationship between the clinician and relevant family members is critical to successful long-term outcome (Patterson & Chamberlain, 1994; Sanders & Lawton, 1993). Clinical skills such as rapport building, effective interviewing and communication skills, session structuring, and the development of empathic, caring relationships with family members are important to all forms of family intervention. Such skills are particularly important in face-to-face programs,

but they are also important in models of counseling that involve brief or minimal contact, including telephone counseling or correspondence programs. Consequently, mental health professionals undertaking family intervention work need advanced-level training and supervision in both the science and the clinical practice of family intervention.

4. *The goals of intervention should address known risk variables.* Family interventions vary according to the focus or goals of the intervention. Interventions that have proven most successful address variables that are known to increase the risk of individual psychopathology. Some interventions focus heavily on behavioral change (e.g., Forehand & McMahon, 1981), whereas others concentrate on cognitive, affective, and attitude change as well (e.g., Webster-Stratton, 1994; Sanders & Dadds, 1993). The focus of the intervention depends greatly on the theoretical underpinnings and assumptions of the approach. However, common goals in most effective forms of family intervention are to improve family communication, problem solving, conflict resolution, and parenting skills.

5. *Intervention services should be designed to facilitate access.* It is essential that interventions be delivered in ways that increase, rather than restrict, access to services. Professional practices can sometimes restrict access to services. For example, inflexible clinic hours from 9 A.M. to 5 P.M. may be a barrier to working parents' participation in family intervention programs. Family intervention consultations may take place in many different settings, such as clinics or hospitals, family homes, kindergartens, preschools, schools, and worksites. The type of setting selected should vary, depending on the goals of the intervention and the needs of the target group. Practitioners must become more flexible to allow better tailoring of services.

6. *Family intervention programs should be developmentally timed to optimize impact.* "Developmentally timing" an intervention means taking the age and developmental level of the target group into consideration. Family intervention methods have been used across the life span, including prebirth, infancy, toddlerhood, middle childhood, adolescence, early adulthood, middle adulthood, and late adulthood. A developmentally well-timed family intervention for a particular problem may have a greater impact than the same sort of intervention delivered at another time in the life cycle. For example, premarital counseling may be more effective in reducing subsequent relationship breakdown than a marriage enrichment program delivered after marital distress has already developed.

7. *Family interventions can complement and enhance other interventions.* Family interventions can be effective interventions in their own right for a variety of clinical problems. However, for other problems such as schizophrenia, bipolar disorder, depression, and learning difficulties, family interventions can be successfully combined with other interventions, such as drug therapy, individual therapy, social and community

survival skills training, classroom management, and academic instruction. Family intervention can complement other interventions for individuals by increasing compliance with medication, and by ensuring the cooperation and support of family members. Family interventions should be an integral component of comprehensive mental health services for all disorders.

8. *Family interventions should be gender-sensitive.* Family interventions have the potential to promote more equitable gender relationships within the family. Intervention programs may directly or indirectly promote inequitable relationships between marital partners by inadvertently promoting traditional gender stereotypes and power relationships that increase women's dependence on men and restrict their choices. Consequently, family intervention programs should promote gender equality.

9. *Theories underlying family interventions should be scientifically validated.* Family interventions should be based on coherent and explicit theoretical principles that allow key assumptions to be tested. This extends beyond demonstrating that an intervention works, although that may be an important first step. It involves showing that the mechanisms purported to underlie improvement (specific family interaction processes) actually change and are responsible for the observed improvement, rather than other, nonspecific factors.

10. *Family interventions should be culturally appropriate.* Family intervention programs should be tailored in such a way as to respect and not to undermine the cultural values, aspirations, traditions, and needs of different ethnic groups. There is much to learn about how to achieve this objective. However, there is increasing evidence that sensitively tailored family interventions can be effective with minority cultures (Myers et al., 1992).

CONCLUSION

This chapter attests to the critical importance of family relationships throughout the life span, and shows how families can be meaningfully involved in both the prevention and treatment of mental health problems. There is clear evidence that family intervention is a powerful intervention technology for a wide range of mental health problems. However, many unresolved problems must be addressed before the field makes a significant impact on community mental health. First, research is clearly needed to examine the dissemination process. Too few practitioners have had adequate training in the delivery of family intervention programs. The knowledge domain should be an integral part of the training of all mental health practitioners. Second, despite the repeated calls for empirical research into other forms of family therapy, the weight of the evidence clearly shows that cognitive-behavioral and social learning approaches to working with families have the most empirical support. Training programs should give priority to training practitioners in empirically validated forms of family intervention. Finally, much more research is required to examine how treatment strength can be better tailored to family characteristics, preferences, and needs. Empirically based decision rules are needed to guide practitioners in determining which type of approach (e.g., self-directed, group, brief, intensive) is needed at different points of the developmental trajectory for different constellations of problems.

REFERENCES

Achenbach, T., Howell, C., Aoki, M., & Rauh, V. (1993). Nine-year outcome of the Vermont Intervention Program for low birthweight infants. *Pediatrics, 91,* 45–55.

Alexander, J. F., Holtzworth-Munroe, A., & Jameson, P. B. (1994). The process and outcome of marital and family therapy: Research review and evaluation. In A. E. Bergin & S. L. Garfield (Eds.), *Handbook of psychotherapy and behavior change* (4th ed., pp. 595–630). New York: Wiley.

Alexander, J. F., & Parsons, B. V. (1973). Short-term behavioral intervention with delinquent families: Impact on family process and recidivism. *Journal of Abnormal Child Psychology, 81,* 219–225.

Alpert, C. L., & Kaiser, A. P. C. (1992). Training parents as milieu language teachers. *Journal of Early Intervention, 16,* 31–52.

Anisfeld, E., Casper, V., Nozyce, M., & Cunningham, N. (1990). Does infant crying promote attachment?: An experimental study of the effects of increased physical contact on the development of attachment. *Child Development, 61,* 1617–1627.

Bank, L., Marlowe, J. H., Reid, J. B., Patterson, G. R., & Weinrott, M. R. (1991). A comparative evaluation of parent training for families of chronic delinquents. *Journal of Abnormal Child Psychology, 19,* 15–35.

Barkley, R. A., Guevremont, D. C., Anastopoulos, A. D., & Fletcher, K. E. (1992). A comparison of three family therapy programs for treating family conflicts in adolescents with attention-deficit hyperactivity disorder. *Journal of Consulting and Clinical Psychology, 60*(3), 450–462.

Barrett, P. M., Dadds, M. R., & Rapee, R. M. (1993, November). *Family intervention for childhood anxiety disorders: A controlled trial.* Paper presented at the 27th Annual Convention of the Association for Advancement of Behavior Therapy, Atlanta, GA.

Batshaw, M. L., & Perret, Y. M. (1992). *Children with disabilities: A medical primer* (3rd ed.). York, PA: Maple Press.

Baucom, D. H., Shoham, V., Mueser, K. T., Daiuto, A. D., & Stickle, T. R. (1998). Empirically supported couple and family interventions for marital distress and adult mental health problems. *Journal of Consulting and Clinical Psychology, 66,* 53–88.

Bednar, R. L., Burlingame, G. M., & Masters, K. S. (1988). Systems of family treatment: Substance or semantics? *Annual Review of Psychology, 39,* 401–434.

Belsky, J. (1993). Etiology of child maltreatment: A developmental–ecological analysis. *Psychological Bulletin, 114*(3), 413–434

Berrueta-Clement, J. R., Schweinhart, L. J., Barnett, W. S., & Weikart, D. P. (1987). The effects of early educational intervention on crime and delinquency in adolescence and early adulthood. In J. D. Burchard & S. N. Burchard (Eds.), *Prevention of delinquent behaviour* (pp. 220–240). London: Sage.

Blampied, N. M., & France, K. G. (1993). A behavioral model of infant sleep disturbance. *Journal of Applied Behavior Analysis, 26,* 477–492.

Booth, C. L., Barnard, K. E., Mitchell, S. K., & Spieker, S. J. (1987). Successful intervention with multi-problem mothers: Effects on the mother–infant relationship. *Infant Mental Health Journal, 8,* 288–306.

Borduin, C. M., Mann, B. J., Cone, L. T., Henggeler, S. W., Fucci, D., Blaske, D. M., & Williams, J. R. (1995). Multisystemic treatment of serious juvenile offenders: Long-term prevention of criminality and violence. *Journal of Consulting and Clinical Psychology, 63*(4), 569–575.

Botvin, G. J., Baker, E., Filazzola, A. D., & Botvin, E. M. (1990). A cognitive-behavioral approach to substance abuse prevention: One-year follow-up. *Addictive Behaviors, 15,* 47–63.

Bradley, R. H., Caldwell, B. M., & Rock, S. L. (1988). Home environment and school performance: A ten-year follow-up and examination of three models of environmental action. *Child Development, 59,* 852–867.

Carey, W. B. (1968). Maternal anxiety and infant colic: Is there a relationship? *Clinical Pediatrics, 7,* 590–595.

Cedar, B., & Levant, R. F. (1990). A meta-analysis of the effects of parent effectiveness training. *American Journal of Family Therapy, 18*(4), 373–384.

Chamberlain, P. (1990). Comparative evaluation of specialized foster care for seriously delinquent youths: A first step. *Community Alternatives: International Journal of Family Care, 2*(2), 21–36.

Chamberlain, P. (1996). Community-based residential treatment for adolescents with conduct disorder. In T. H. Ollendick & R. J. Prinz (Eds.), *Advances in clinical child psychology* (Vol. 18, pp. 63–90). New York: Plenum Press.

Chamberlain, P., Moreland, S., & Reid, K. (1992). Enhanced services and stipends for foster parents: Effects on retention rates and outcomes for children. *Child Welfare, 71*(5), 387–401.

Chamberlain, P., Patterson, G. R., Reid, J. B., Forgatch, M. S., & Kavanagh, K. (1984). Observation of client resistance. *Behavior Therapy, 15,* 144–155.

Chamberlain, P., & Reid, J. B. (1991). Using a specialized foster care treatment model for children and adolescents leaving the state mental hospital. *Journal of Community Psychology, 19,* 266–276.

Clarke, G., Hops, H., Lewinsohn, P. M., Andrews, J., Seeley, J. R., & Williams, J. (1992). Cognitive-behavioral group treatment of adolescent depression: Prediction of outcome. *Behavior Therapy, 23,* 341–354.

Clarke, G., Lewinsohn, P. M., & Hops, H. (1990). *The Adolescent Coping with Depression Course.* Eugene, OR: Castalia.

Cohn, J. F., Campbell, S. B., Matias, R., & Hopkins, J. (1990). Face-to-face interactions of postpartum depressed and nondepressed mother–infant pairs at 2 months. *Developmental Psychology, 26,* 15–23.

Committee on the Prevention of Mental Disorders. (1994). *Reducing risks for mental disorders: Frontiers for preventive intervention research.* Washington DC: National Academy Press.

Connell, S., Sanders, M. R., & Markie-Dadds, C. (1997). Self-directed behavioral family intervention for parents of oppositional children in rural and remote areas. *Behavior Modification, 21*(4), 379–408.

Dadds, M. R. (1995). *Families, children and the development of dysfunction.* New York: Sage.

Dadds, M. R., Sanders, M. R., & Bor, W. (1984). Training children to eat independently: Evaluation of mealtime management training for parents. *Behavioral Psychotherapy, 12,* 356–366.

Dadds, M. R., Schwartz, S., & Sanders, M. R. (1987). Marital discord and treatment outcome in the treatment of child conduct disorders. *Journal of Consulting and Clinical Psychology, 55,* 396–403.

Dare, C., Eisler, I., Russell, G. F. M., & Szmukler, G. I. (1990). The clinical and theoretical impact of a controlled trial of family therapy in anorexia nervosa. *Journal of Marital and Family Therapy, 16,* 39–57.

Dinkmeyer, D., & McKay, G. D. (1976). *Systematic Training for Effective Parenting: Parent's Handbook.* Circle Pines, MN: American Guidance Service.

Dishion, T. J., & Andrews, D. W. (1995). Preventing escalation in problem behavior with high-risk young adolescents: Immediate and 1-year outcomes. *Journal of Consulting and Clinical Psychology, 63,* 538–548.

Douglas, J. (1989). *Behavior problems in young children: Assessment and management.* London: Tavistock/Routledge.

Dumas, J. E. (1989). Treating antisocial behavior in children: Child and family approaches. *Clinical Psychology Review, 9,* 197–222.

Ehlers, V. L., & Ruffin, M. (1990). The Missouri Project: Parents as Teachers. *Focus on Exceptional Children, 23*(2), 1–14.

Erikson, M. F., Korfmacher, J., & Egeland, B. R. (1992). Attachments past and present: Implications for therapeutic intervention with mother–infant dyads. *Development and Psychopathology, 4,* 495–507.

Fairburn, C. G., & Cooper, P. J. (1989). Eating disorders. In K. Hawton, P. M. Salkovskis, J. Kirk, & D. M. Clark (Eds.), *Cognitive behaviour therapy for psychiatric problems: A practical guide* (pp. 277–314). Oxford: Oxford University Press.

Field, T. M., Widmayer, S. M., Stringer, S., & Ignatoff, E. (1980). Teenage, lower-class, black mothers and their preterm infants: An intervention and developmental follow-up. *Child Development, 51,* 426–436.

Forehand, R. L., & Long, N. (1988). Outpatient treatment of the acting out child: Procedures, long term follow-up data, and clinical problems. *Advances in Behavior Research and Therapy, 10,* 129–177.

Forehand, R. L., & McMahon, R. J. (1981). *Helping the noncompliant child: A clinician's guide to parent training.* New York: Guilford Press.

Forehand, R. L., & Wierson, M. (1993). The role of developmental factors in planning behavioral interventions for children: Disruptive behavior as an example. *Behavior Therapy, 24,* 117–141.

France, K. G., & Hudson, S. M. (1993). Management of infant sleep disturbance: A review. *Clinical Psychology Review, 13,* 635–647.

Frude, N. (1989). The physical abuse of children. In K. Howells & C. R. Hollin (Eds.), *Clinical approaches to violence* (pp. 155–181). New York: Wiley.

Garber, H. (1988). *The Milwaukee Project: Preventing mental retardation in children at risk.* Washington, DC: American Association on Mental Retardation.

Gardner, F. E. M. (1994). The quality of joint activity between mothers and their children with behavior problems. *Journal of Child Psychology and Allied Disciplines, 35*(5), 935–948.

Glynn, T., Fairweather, R., & Donald, S. (1992). Involving parents in improving children's learning at school: Policy issues for behavioural research. *Behaviour Change, 9*(3), 178–185.

Gordon, T. (1975). *Parent Effectiveness Training.* New York: Plume.

Graziano, A. M. (1977). Parents as behavior therapists. In M. Herson, R. M. Eisler, & P. M. Miller (Eds.), *Progress in behavior modification* (Vol. 4, pp. 251–298). New York: Academic Press.

Greenberg, M. T., Speltz, M. L., & DeKlyen, M. (1993). The role of attachment in the early development of disruptive behavior problems. *Development and Psychopathology, 5,* 191–213.

Gurman, A. S., Kniskern, D. P., & Pinsof, W. M. (1986). Research on the process and outcome of marital and family therapy. In S. L. Garfield & A. E. Bergin (Eds.), *Handbook of psychotherapy and behavior change* (3rd ed., pp. 565–624). New York: Wiley.

Halford, W. K., & Markman, H. J. (Eds.). (1997). *Clinical handbook of marriage and couples interventions.* Chichester, England: Wiley.

Hart, B., & Risley, T. R. (1995). *Meaningful differences in everyday experiences of young American children.* Baltimore: Paul H. Brookes.

Harrold, M., Lutzker, J. R., Campbell, R. V., & Touchette, P. E. (1992). Improving parent–child interactions for families with developmental disabilities. *Journal of Behavior Therapy and Experimental Psychiatry, 23,* 89–100.

Hawkins, J. D., VonCleve, E., & Catalano, R. F. (1991). Reducing early childhood aggression: Results of a primary prevention program. *Journal of the American Academy of Child and Adolescent Psychiatry, 30,* 208–217.

Hazelrigg, M. D., Cooper, H. M., & Borduin, C. M. (1987). Evaluating the effectiveness of family therapies: An integrative review and analysis. *Psychological Review, 101,* 428–442.

Heber, R., & Garber, H. (1975). The Milwaukee Project: A study of the use of family intervention to prevent cultural–familial mental retardation. In B. Z. Friedlander, G. Sterritt, & G. Kirk (Eds.), *Exceptional infant: Assessment and intervention* (Vol. 3, pp. 399–433). New York: Brunner/Mazel.

Henggeler, S. W., Borduin, C. M., & Mann, B. J. (1993). Advances in family therapy: Empirical foundations. In T. H. Ollendick & R. H. Prinz (Eds.), *Advances in clinical child psychology* (Vol. 15, pp. 207–241). New York: Plenum Press.

Horacek, H. J., Ramey, C. T., Campbell, F. A., Hoffman, K. P., & Fletcher, M. D. (1987). Predicting school failure and assessing early intervention with high risk children. *Journal of the American Academy of Child and Adolescent Psychiatry, 26,* 758–763.

Hunziker, U. A., & Barr, R. G. (1986). Increased carrying reduces infant crying: A randomized control trial. *Pediatrics, 77,* 641–648.

Huynen, K. B., Lutzker, J. R., Bigelow, K. M., Touchette, P. E., & Campbell, R. V. (1996). Planned activities training for mothers of children with developmental disabilities. *Behavior Modification, 4,* 406–427.

Infant Health and Development Program. (1990). Enhancing the outcomes of low birthweight, premature infants: A multi-site randomized trial. *Journal of the American Medical Association, 263,* 3035–3042.

Jacobson, S. W., & Frye, K. F. (1991). Effect of maternal social support on attachment: Experimental evidence. *Child Development, 62,* 572–582.

Johnson, D. L. (1990). The Houston Parent–Child Development Center Project: Disseminating a viable program for enhancing at-risk families. *Prevention in Human Services, 7,* 89–108.

Johnson, D. L. (1991). Primary prevention of problem behaviors in young children: The Houston Parent–Child Development Center. In R. Price, E. L. Cowen, R. P. Lorian, & J. Ramos-McKay (Eds.), *Fourteen ounces of prevention: A casebook for practitioners* (pp. 44–52). Washington, DC: American Psychological Association.

Johnson, D. L., & Walker, T. (1987). Primary prevention of behavior problems in Mexican-American children. *American Journal of Community Psychology, 15,* 375–385.

Jones, R. C., Weinrott, M. R., & Howard, J. R. (1981). *The national evaluation of the Teaching Family Model.* Final report to the Center for Studies of Antisocial and Violent Behavior, National Institute of Mental Health, Bethesda, MD. (Available from the Oregon Social Learning Center, 207 E. 5th Ave., Suite 202, Eugene, OR 97401)

Kahn, J. S., Kehle, T. J., Jenson, W. R., & Clark, E. (1990). Comparison or cognitive-behavioral relaxation, and self- monitoring interventions for depression among middle-school students. *School Psychology Review, 19,* 196–210.

Kazdin, A. E. (1997). Parent management training: Evidence outcomes and issues. *Journal of the Academy of Child and Adolescent Psychiatry, 36,* 1349–1356.

Kazdin, A. E., Bass, D., Ayers, W. A., & Rodgers, A. (1990). Empirical and clinical focus of child and adolescent psychotherapy research. *Journal of Consulting and Clinical Psychology, 58*(6), 729–740.

Kazdin, A. E., & Weisz, J. R. (1998). Identifying and developing empirically supported child and adolescent treatments. *Journal of Consulting and Clinical Psychology, 66,* 19–36.

Kendziora, K. T., & O'Leary, S. G. (1993). Dysfunctional parenting as a focus for prevention and treatment of child behavior problems. In T. H. Ollendick & R. J. Prinz (Eds.), *Advances in clinical child psychology* (Vol. 15, pp. 175–206). New York: Plenum Press.

Kirigin, K. A., Braukmann, C. J., Atwater, J. D., & Wolf, M. M. (1982). An evaluation of Teaching Family (Achievement Place) group homes for juvenile offenders. *Journal of Applied Behavior Analysis, 15,* 1–16.

Kirkland, J. (1990). Adults' perceptual shifts between infant fussing and crying: A proposition. *Early Child Development and Care, 65,* 77–82.

Larson, K. L., Ayllon, T., & Barrett, D. H. (1987). A behavioural feeding program for failure-to-thrive infants. *Behaviour Research and Therapy, 25,* 39–47.

Le Grange, D., Eisler, I., Dare, C., & Russell, G. F. M. (1992). Evaluation of family treatments in adolescent anorexia nervosa: A pilot study. *International Journal of Eating Disorders, 12,* 347–357.

Lewinsohn, P. M., Clarke, G. N., Hops, H., & Andrews, J. (1990). Cognitive-behavioral treatment for depressed adolescents. *Behavior Therapy, 21,* 385–401.

Liddle, H. A., & Dakof, G. A. (1995). Efficacy of family therapy for drug abuse: Promising but not definitive. *Journal of Marital and Family Therapy, 21*(4), 511–543.

Lieberman, A. F., Weston, D. R., & Pawl, J. H. (1991). Preventive intervention and outcome with anxiously attached dyads. *Child Development, 62,* 199–209.

Linscheid, T. R., & Cunningham, C. E. (1977). A controlled demonstration of the effectiveness of shock in eliminating chronic infant rumination. *Journal of Applied Behavior Analysis, 10,* 500–521.

Levenstein, P. (1992). The mother–child home program: Research methodology and the real world. In J. McCord & R. E. Tremblay (Eds.), *Preventing antisocial behavior: Interventions from birth through adolescence* (pp. 43–66). New York: Guilford Press.

Lochman, J. E. (1990). Modification of childhood aggression. In M. Hersen, R. M. Eisler, & P. M. Miller (Eds.), *Progress in behavior modification* (Vol. 25, pp. 47–85). New York: Academic Press.

Loeber, R. (1990). Development and risk factors of juvenile antisocial behavior and delinquency. *Clinical Psychology Review, 10,* 1–41.

Long, P., Forehand, R., Wierson, M., & Morgan, A. (1994). Does parent training with young noncompliant children have long-term effects? *Behaviour Research and Therapy, 32,* 101–107.

Lutzker, J. R. (1992). Developmental disabilities and child abuse and neglect: The ecobehavioural imperative. *Behaviour Change, 9*(3), 149–156.

Markman, H. J., Renick, M. J., Floyd, F., Stanley, S., M., & Clements, M. (1993). Preventing marital distress through effective communication and conflict management: A 4- and 5-year follow-up. *Journal of Consulting and Clinical Psychology, 61*(1), 70–77.

McFarland, M., & Sanders, M. R. (1993, November). *A comparison of behavioral and cognitive-behavioral family intervention with maternally depressed families of disruptive children.* Paper presented at the 27th Annual Convention of the Association for Advancement of Behavior Therapy, Atlanta, GA.

McFarland, M., & Sanders, M. R. (1998). *The treatment of parental depression: A comparison of standard behavioral family intervention and cognitive behavioral family intervention.* Manuscript submitted for publication.

McMahon, R. J. (1994). Diagnosis, assessment and treatment of externalizing problems in children: The role of longitudinal data. *Journal of Consulting and Clinical Psychology, 62,* 901–917.

McNaughton, S. Glynn, T., & Robinson, V. M. J. (1987). *Parents as remedial tutors: Issues for home and school.* Wellington: New Zealand Council for Educational Research.

Miller, G. E., & Prinz, R. J. (1990). Enhancement of social learning family interventions for child conduct disorder. *Psychological Bulletin, 108,* 291–307.

Minuchin, S., Rosman, B. L., & Baker, L. (1978). *Psychosomatic families: Anorexia nervosa in context.* Cambridge, MA: Harvard University Press.

Moffitt, T. E. (1993). Adolescence-limited and life-course-persistent antisocial behavior: A developmental taxonomy. *Psychological Review, 100,* 674–701.

Morriset, C. E., Barnard, K. E., Greenberg, M. T., & Booth, C. L. (1990). Environmental influences on early language development: The context of social risk. *Development and Psychopathology, 2,* 127–149.

Myers, H. F., Alvy, K. T., Arrington, A., Richardson, M. A., Marigna, M., Huff,

R., Main, M., & Newcomb, M. D. (1992). The impact of a parent training program on inner-city African-American families. *Journal of Community Psychology, 20,* 132–147.

Noller, P., & Taylor, R. (1989). Parent education and family relations. *Family Relations, 38,* 196–200.

Olds, D. L. (1997). The Prenatal Early Infancy Project: Preventing child abuse and neglect in the context of promoting maternal and child health. In D. A. Wolfe, R. J. McMahon, & R. D. Peters (Eds.), *Child abuse: New directions in prevention and treatment across the life span* (pp. 130–154). Thousand Oaks, CA: Sage.

Olds, D. L., & Kitzman, H. (1990). Can home visitation improve the health of women and children at environmental risk? *Pediatrics, 86,* 108–116.

Olds, D. S., Henderson, C., Tatelbaum, R., & Chamberlin, R. (1986). Preventing child abuse and neglect: A randomized trial of home visitation. *Pediatrics, 78,* 65–78.

Palmer, S., Thompson, R. J., & Linscheid, T. R. (1975). Applied behavioural analysis in the treatment of childhood feeding problems. *Developmental Medicine and Child Neurology, 17,* 333–339.

Patterson, G. R. (1982). *Coercive family process.* Eugene, OR: Castalia.

Patterson, G., & Chamberlain, P. (1994). A functional analysis of resistance during parent training therapy. *Clinical Psychology: Science and Practice, 1,* 53–70.

Pettit, G. S., & Bates, J. E. (1989). Family interaction patterns and children's behavior problems from infancy to 4 years. *Developmental Psychology, 25,* 413–420.

Pfannenstiel, J. C., & Seltzer, D. A. (1989). New parents as teachers: Evaluation of an early parent education program. *Early Childhood Research Quarterly, 4,* 1–18.

Pisterman, S., Firestone, P., McGrath, P., Goodman, J. T., Webster, I., Mallory, R., & Goffin, B. (1992). The effects of parent training on parenting stress and sense of competence. *Canadian Journal of Behavioural Science, 24,* 41–58.

Prior, M., Smart, D., Sanson, A., & Oberklaid, F. (1993). Sex differences in psychological adjustment from infancy to 8 years. *Journal of the American Academy of Child and Adolescent Psychiatry, 32*(2), 291–304.

Pritchard, P. (1984). An infant crying clinic. *Health Visitor, 59,* 375–377.

Ramey, C., Bryant, D., Wasik, B., Sparling, J., Fendt, K., & La Vange, L. (1992). Infant health and development program for low birthweight, premature infants: Program elements, family participation, and child intelligence. *Pediatrics, 89,* 454–465.

Raphael, B. (1993). *Scope for prevention in mental health.* Report prepared for the National Health and Medical Research Council (NHMRC).

Reid, J. B. (1993). Prevention of conduct disorder before and after school entry: Relating interventions to developmental findings. *Development and Psychopathology, 5,* 243–262.

Roberts, R. N., Wasik, B. H., Casto, G., & Ramey, C. T. (1991). Family support in the home: Programs, policy and social change. *American Psychologist, 46,* 131–137.

Robin, A. L. (1981). A controlled evaluation of problem solving communication training with parent–adolescent conflict. *Behavior Therapy, 12,* 593–609.

Robin, A. L., Siegel, P. T., Koepke, T., Moye, A. W., & Tice, S. (1994). Family therapy versus individual therapy for adolescent females with anorexia nervosa. *Journal of Developmental and Behavioral Pediatrics, 15*(2), 111–116.

Rogers, C. R. (1951). *Client-centered therapy.* Boston: Houghton Mifflin.

Rothbaum, F., & Weisz, J. R. (1994). Parental caregiving and child externalizing behaviour in nonclinical samples: A meta-analysis. *Psychological Bulletin, 116,* 55–74.

Russell, G. F. M., Szmukler, G. I., Dare, C., & Eisler, I. (1987). An evaluation of family therapy in anorexia nervosa and bulimia nervosa. *Archives of General Psychiatry, 44,* 1047–1056.

Rutter, M. (1985). Family and school influences on behavioural development. *Journal of Child Psychology and Psychiatry, 26,* 349–368.

Sajwaj, T., Libet, J., & Agras, S. (1974). Lemon juice therapy: The control of life threatening rumination in a six month old infant. *Journal of Applied Behavior Analysis, 7*(4), 557–563.

Sandall, S. (1992). Developmental interventions for biologically at-risk infants at home. *Topics in Early Childhood Special Education, 10,* 1–13.

Sanders, M. R. (1992). *Every parent: A positive approach to children's behaviour.* Sydney: Addison-Wesley.

Sanders, M. R. (1996). New directions in behavioral family intervention with children. In T. H. Ollendick & R. J. Prinz (Eds.), *Advances in clinical child psychology* (Vol. 18, pp. 283–330). New York: Plenum Press.

Sanders, M. R. (1997). Media, parenting and children's mental health. *Bulletin of the Faculty of Child and Adolescent Psychiatry, 1,* 10.

Sanders, M. R., & Christensen, A. P. (1985). A comparison of the effects of child management and planned activities training across five parenting environments. *Journal of Abnormal Child Psychology, 13,* 101–117.

Sanders, M. R., & Dadds, M. R. (1982). The effects of planned activities and child management training: An analysis of setting generality. *Behavior Therapy, 13,* 1–11.

Sanders, M. R., & Dadds, M. R. (1993). *Behavioral family intervention.* Needham Heights, MA: Allyn & Bacon.

Sanders, M. R., & Glynn, T. (1981). Training parents in behavioral self management: An analysis of generalization and maintenance. *Journal of Applied Behavior Analysis, 14,* 223–237.

Sanders, M. R., & Lawton, J. M. (1993). Discussing assessment findings with families: A guided participation model for information transfer. *Child and Family Behavior Therapy, 15,* 5–35.

Sanders, M. R., Lynch, M. E., & Markie-Dadds, C. (1994). *Every parent's workbook: A practical guide to positive parenting.* Brisbane: Australian Academic Press.

Sanders, M. R., & Markie-Dadds, C. (1992). Toward a technology of prevention of disruptive behaviour disorders: The role of behavioural family intervention. *Behaviour Change, 9,* 186–200.

Sanders, M. R., & Markie-Dadds, C. (Chairs). (1994, November). *Triple P (Positive Parenting of Preschoolers) program: A controlled evaluation of an early intervention program for children with disruptive behavior problems.* Symposium conducted at the 28th Annual Convention of the Association for Advancement of Behavior Therapy, San Diego, CA.

Sanders, M. R., & Markie-Dadds, C. (1997). Managing common childhood behavior problems. In M. R. Sanders, C. Mitchell, & G. J. A. Byrne (Eds.), *Medical consultation skills: Behavioral and interpersonal dimension of health care.* Melbourne: Addison Wesley Longman.

Sanders, M. R., & Plant, K. (1989). Programming for generalization to high and low risk parenting situations in families with oppositional developmentally disabled preschoolers. *Behavior Modification, 13,* 283–305.

Sanders, M. R., Rebgetz, M., Morrison, M., Bor, W., Gordon, A., Dadds, M. R., & Shepherd, R. (1989). Cognitive-behavioral treatment of recurrent nonspecific abdominal pain in children: An analysis of generalization, maintenance and side effects. *Journal of Consulting and Clinical Psychology, 57*(2), 294–300.

Sanders, M. R., Shepherd, R. W., Cleghorn, G., & Woolford, H. (1994). The treatment of recurrent abdominal pain in children: A controlled comparison of cognitive-behavioral family intervention and standard pediatric care. *Journal of Consulting and Clinical Psychology, 62,* 306–314.

Satin, W., La Greca, A. M., Zigo, M. A., & Skyler, J. S. (1995). Diabetes in adolescence: Effects of multifamily group intervention and parent simulation of diabetes. *Journal of Pediatric Psychology, 14*(2), 259–275.

Schmidt, S. E., Liddle, H. A., & Dakof, G. A. (1996). Changes in parenting practices and adolescent drug abuse during multidimensional family therapy. *Journal of Family Psychology, 10,* 12–27.

Schultz, C. (1981). Family and parent effectiveness training. *Australian Journal of Sex, Marriage, and the Family, 2,* 135–142.

Schultz, C., & Khan, J. A. (1982). Mother–child interaction behaviour and parent effectiveness training, *Australian Journal of Sex, Marriage, and the Family, 3,* 133–138.

Seymour, F. W., Brock, P., During, M., & Poole, G. (1989). Reducing sleep disruptions in young children: Evaluation of therapist-guided and written information approaches. A brief report. *Journal of Child Psychology and Psychiatry, 30,* 913–918.

Speltz, M. L., Greenberg, M. T., & DeKlyen, M. (1990). Attachment in preschoolers with disruptive behaviour: A comparison of clinic-referred and non-problem children. *Development and Psychopathology, 2,* 31–46.

Strayhorn, J. M., & Weidman, C. S. (1991). Follow-up one year after parent–child interaction training: Effects on behavior of preschool children. *Journal of the American Academy of Child and Adolescent Psychiatry, 30,* 138–143.

Szykula, S. A., Morris, S. B., Sudweeks, C., & Saygar, T. V. (1987). Child focussed behavior and strategic therapy: Outcome comparison. *Psychotherapy, 35,* 546–551.

Taubman, B. (1984). Clinical trial of the treatment of colic by modification of parent–infant interaction. *Pediatrics, 74,* 998–1003.

Turner, K. M. T., Sanders, M. R., & Wall, C. (1994). A comparison of behavioural parent training and dietary education in the treatment of children with persistent feeding difficulties. *Behaviour Change, 4,* 242–258.

Webster-Stratton, C. (1990). Long-term follow-up of families with young conduct problem children: From preschool to grade school. *Journal of Clinical Child Psychology, 19,* 144–149.

Webster-Stratton, C. (1994). Advancing videotape parent training: A comparison study. *Journal of Consulting and Clinical Psychology, 62,* 583–593.

Webster-Stratton, C., Kolpacoff, M., & Hollinsworth, T. (1988). Self-administered videotape therapy for families with conduct-problem children: Comparison with two cost-effective treatments and a control group. *Journal of Consulting and Clinical Psychology, 56*(4), 558–566.

Wekerle, C., & Wolfe, D. A. (1993). Prevention of child abuse and neglect: Promising new directions. *Clinical Psychology Review, 13,* 501–540.

Wells, K. C., & Egan, J. (1988). Social learning and systems family therapy for childhood oppositional disorder: Comparative treatment outcome. *Comprehensive Psychiatry, 29*(2), 138–145.

Werle, M. A., Murphy, T. B., & Budd, K. S. (1993). Treating chronic food refusal in young children. *Journal of Applied Behavior Analysis, 26,* 421–433.

Wolfe, D. A., Edwards, B., Manion, I., & Koverola, C. (1988). Early intervention for parents at risk of child abuse and neglect: A preliminary investigation. *Journal of Consulting and Clinical Psychology, 56,* 40–47.

Wood, C., & Davidson, J. (1993). Conflict resolution in the family: A PET evaluation study. *Australian Psychologist, 28*(2), 100–104.

SECTION V

RESEARCH ISSUES

CHAPTER 19

<=>◆<=>

Methodological Problems in Studying Family Psychopathology

WOLFGANG TSCHACHER

This chapter examines various types of methodological problems in studying family psychopathology. First, the traditional criteria for clinical research are summarized. In this first section, reliability, validity, hypothesis testing, and objectivity are introduced and discussed. The next section focuses on how method depends on theory. Several theoretical approaches to family psychopathology are distinguished: the transactional approach, the constructivist approach, and the dynamic systems approach. The last of these is chosen as a comprehensive framework for the study of family psychopathology. An empirical case study is then described. It is argued that the methods of the dynamic systems view are capable of integrating longitudinal with cross-sectional research. Other dichotomies in clinical psychological research, such as experiments versus field studies and the nomothetic approach versus the idiographic approach, may also be resolved within a dynamic framework.

THE PROBLEMS OF STUDYING PSYCHOPATHOLOGY: CRITERIA FOR CLINICAL RESEARCH

This chapter begins with an indication of what questions are *not* addressed in it. In particular, the following theoretical and conceptual topics are not addressed:

- How should the distinction between normal development and abnormal, pathological development be made? Is there a qualitative difference, or are these the extremes of a continuum?
- Is psychopathology a state or a trait?
- Is psychopathology based on a personality attribute or on an individual's environment?

These and numerous other polarities represent major points of discussion in the field of family psychology (L'Abate & Baggett, 1997) and are dealt with in other chapters of this handbook. They are not, however, relevant to this chapter on methodological problems—or are they?

In attempting to characterize and classify methodological issues in family psychopathology, I am nonetheless obliged to acknowledge that the conceptualization of psychopathology plays an important part in the selection of the methods used to study its empirical realization. For instance, if psychopathology lies on a continuum, methods of data acquisition and analysis must differ in the scaling properties they support from the methods developed for nominal or ordinal data. Furthermore, if psychopathology is seen as a trait, it makes sense to look at cross-sections in order to find out about the covariance of psychopathology with other variables. But if psychopathology has the characteristics of a state, there may be nontrivial change with time, so that the analysis of averages and distributions of samples may be entirely misleading.

Thus, beginning with a well-known caveat in psychological scale construction seems justified: Namely, the method of measurement changes that which is being measured (Dawis, 1987). Theoretical conceptualization cannot be isolated from the methods that are used to operationalize and measure the elements of the theory.

Cursorily, I now turn to the classical methodological criteria for the study of psychopathology, and for clinical research more generally (Kazdin, 1992). These consist of reliability, validity, objectivity, and hypothesis testing.

Reliability

The basic requirement of good measurement is obviously correctness and precision—that is, reliability. The concept of reliability in classical test theory is derived from the notion that an observed value can be split up into the sum of "true score" and "measurement error." Any measure of reliability estimates the degree of overlap of observed values with true values. "Reliability" is accordingly defined as the ratio of true-score variance and observed-score variance.

Different methods are used to assess reliability. First, test–retest reliability employs the same test (or measurement) after some period of time. The correlation of both is then taken as a measure of reliability. Second, for a number of test instruments parallel versions exist, so that the overlap between parallel tests can be used as a measure of reliability. A variant (interrater reliability) is commonly used in clinical and psychiatric research to detect the quality of psychopathology rating scales and coding schemes. Third, split-half methods compare different parts of a homogeneous test (e.g., odd- and even-numbered items) with each other.

All of these methods have their specific problems. To name only a few, different sources of error are assessed in the various methods to establish reliability. If, for example, a measure is used repeatedly, deviations in measurements can be due to measurement error and to the natural fluctuation of the variable measured—which is especially obvious from a dynamic perspective on psychopathology (see below). There is also a connection between reliability and validity, in that optimizing the reliability of a measure or an instrument may affect its validity in a negative way (Tukey, 1979). Thus, achieving poor measurement of the right entity is preferable to having an exact measure of the wrong thing.

Let me illustrate the principles and problems of reliability with two examples. First, in a study on the course of systemic couple therapy (Tschacher & Scheier, 1995; Brunner, Tschacher, Ruff, & Quast, 1997), time series were generated by two observers, based on the videotaped recordings of therapy sessions. The value of each of nine variables (e.g., empathy of therapist) was rated in 3-minute intervals. To optimize reliability, the raters were trained extensively, using videotaped material from other therapies. The rating experience was also discussed, and a rating manual was written. Then the interrater correlation was computed repeatedly until a .90 criterion was reached. The ratings of the target videotapes showed a mean .91 agreement over all variables (i.e., very good reliability).

Second, in an investigation of daily symptoms shown by psychotic patients (Tschacher, Scheier, & Hashimoto, 1997), observations were made by milieu therapists. The philosophy of treatment at the therapeutic community where the study was conducted (the Soteria in Bern, Switzerland) derives from close and continuous interaction of one staff member with a patient during the acute phase, while all external stimulation is shielded off. In this situation, it was difficult to measure reliability. Parallel observations were ruled out by the therapeutic approach, and retesting would yield uninterpretable results because of the dynamics of the variables (autocorrelation is not reliability). Rater training and good documentation of the rating instrument were the remaining possibilities to achieve satisfying reliability.

Validity

"Validity" refers to the meaning of a test or measure. For example, to assess the validity of a paper-and-pencil measure of family psychopathology, one may compute the correlation of this measure with independent ratings of the same families done by experts. A high correlation between the measure and the experts' judgment would point to high validity; that is, the measure expresses what it is supposed to measure. Campbell and Stanley (1967) and other authors discriminate among several kinds of validity (internal and external validity, construct validity, statistical conclusion validity). I do not intend to go into detail about these different types here, as these are common topics in psychological methodology.

Many problems arise when one tries to specify how valid a statement is. Validity depends crucially on reliability: If a test or measure is not reliable (i.e., does not correlate with itself), it cannot be valid (i.e., cannot correlate with an outside criterion). In many cases, the criteria are less reliable than the tests they are intended to validate (Green, 1981). Therefore, it generally remains unclear which of the two (a criterion or a test) should be trusted more. Moreover, there are many possible ways to assess validity, and this makes quantification and comparison across tests difficult. Validity serves rather as a constant admonition to control for variables that could jeopardize valid explanations (e.g., internal validity is maintained by ruling out alternative explanations, randomizing subjects in a study, keeping the number of dropouts low, etc.).

For example, in a descriptive study of psychosocial crises (Tschacher, 1996), all patients admitted to a crisis unit were asked to complete diary self-ratings on mood, tension, and activity. Some patients did not consent to participate in the study; others consented but later dropped out. The diagnoses and demographic attributes of these patients had to be compared to those of participating patients in order to assess internal validity. If the nonparticipants and dropouts differed from the patients who completed the study, this selectivity would reduce validity.

Hypothesis Testing

Empirical psychology is based to a great extent on statistical tests of null hypotheses, according to the Fisherian tradition in statistics. That is, instead of attempting to prove that some specific hypothesis is correct, the usual procedure is to try to falsify the corresponding null hypothesis (i.e., that there is no effect that can be attributed to experimental variation). In scientific practice in psychology, it often seems that progress is achieved by repeated hypothesis testing in a yes-or-no manner, using the "magic" .05 probability (p) level; the contribution of the Neyman–Pearson approach is often neglected (Cohen, 1990). Yet in evaluations of studies, more than just the p of rejecting the null hypothesis is relevant. Many authors claim, as Neyman and Pearson did, that the power details of tests have to be considered—not only the α risk of falsely rejecting the null hypothesis, but also the β risk of falsely adopting the null hypothesis ($1 - \beta$ defines the power of the test), the clinically significant effect size, and the sample size (n). As the first three of these measures can be conveniently chosen, the optimal n needed in a study follows directly (Bortz, 1993). With this procedure, common problems of interpretation can be avoided, such as the occurrence of significant differences that turn out to be of quite marginal effect size (as the null hypothesis is almost never "correct" and can be rejected in any study, provided that n is large enough).

The related issue of clinical significance (Jacobson & Truax, 1991) has consequently raised increasing concerns in clinical research. The prerequisite of properly choosing effect sizes and statistical power should be observed in any quantitative research that uses psychopathology data. The following is a cautionary example: Sedlmeier and Gigerenzer (1989) reviewed the entire 1984 volume of the *Journal of Abnormal Psychology* in order to assess how much attention was paid to test power. They found that the median power of experimental tests was below .50, given a medium effect size and $\alpha = .05$. In other words, there was generally less than the 50% or "coin toss" chance that existing differences were actually detected in these experiments.

Objectivity

The "objectivity" of a scientific method or measure can be defined as the degree of intersubjective agreement that can be reached. An "objective" method, therefore, is considered to minimize the "subjective" distortion and error that result from the very process of observation. In psychology, the following rank order of methods according to their objectivity is commonly presupposed: introspective self-reports of one's own cognitions (low objectivity), self-reports of one's own behaviors, observation of behaviors, and observation of biological markers (high objectivity). In psychological testing, objective tests are those that do not reveal the intentions and hypotheses of the author of the test (Cattell & Warburton, 1967). The less obtrusive the observations are, the more objective observational methods are.

Where psychopathology is concerned, it is obviously of some importance which data are used in analysis, because data may have different degrees of objectivity. For example, heart rate may be an objective test for "anxiety" (but it must be considered that it may have low validity, as "joy" can also lead to an increase in heart rate).

The concept of objectivity points to questions of philosophical interest, eventually leading to the so-called "subject–object problem" of ontology and epistemology. Because such questions have recently been addressed in family psychology and are important issues in clinical settings, I feel that some pertinent remarks are appropriate at this point. The context of observation includes two entities: the observer and the system under study. Spontaneously, we might define "observation" as the relationship, "observer ← system," where the arrow symbolizes some flow of information. The observer receives information but remains totally outside the system;

this idealized information uptake of a deistic observer may be called "Einstein measurement" (Crutchfield, 1994).

But in our world of irreversibility and time, the premise of deistic observation does not hold. We have to face "Heisenberg measurement," or the relationship "observer ↔ system." If we apply test A to system X, we will never again be able to apply test B to the same system, all other things being equal. But tests B, C, and so on may be necessary to investigate the system objectively. Thus, for a complete description of the system, the testing procedure and hence the observer must be included. (Heisenberg's name has been proposed in this respect because of the congruence with his uncertainty principle: In quantum theory, measurement of the impact of a particle precludes exact measurement of its locus, and vice versa.)

The Heisenberg observer inescapably participates in the system he or she observes, thereby creating a self-referential constellation. Whenever a cognitive system models its environment, this endeavor always carries "self-modeling" with it (Tschacher, 1997). Observation is observation from within ("endo"-observation; cf. Rössler, 1996). This may sound familiar to the therapist observing and diagnosing a client or family. Observing a client in therapy means observing behavior that is modulated by the therapeutic relationship, and therefore means using endo-observation.

How may we account for the problem of endo-observation? First of all, I propose that it need not lead to postmodern relativism and defiance of scientific methodology. Second, in the context of clinical psychology, such endo-systems may not be problems at all; rather, they may have some interesting and even beneficial side effects.

The first answer to the objectivity problem is statistics. The self-referentiality of observation cannot be avoided, but its general impact can be assessed in cross-sections, using the criteria of reliability and validity mentioned above. Thus, we may apply tests A and B in different order to a random sample of copies or variants of system X. This procedure is in no way perfect, but the fact that it deals directly with the problem of endo-observation or self-reference is often overlooked in the systemic literature.

The second answer to the problem of endo-observation is to study systematically how it influences the system under study. To my knowledge, there has been no such investigation except in hermeneutical approaches. From studying exemplary systems with high degrees of self-modeling (e.g., evolutionary biological systems, market systems, psychotherapy systems), one may derive the working hypothesis that such systems generically show increasing complexity. It is interesting to examine self-modeling systems (i.e., systems that increase their complexity) that are also self-organizing (i.e., systems that reduce their complexity). These systems have two vectors of complexity with opposing directions. An approach to determine complexity has been discussed in theoretical biology (Banerjee, Sibbald, & Maze, 1990). In psychotherapy systems one usually finds increasing levels of order, whereas potential complexity is also increasing (Tschacher, Scheier, & Grawe, 1998).

To summarize, this first section has focused on the more conventional methodological problems that must be taken into consideration in studying psychopathology: reliability, validity, hypothesis testing, and objectivity. To obtain acceptable results, a tradeoff is needed in most cases. In the next section, I discuss methodological concerns regarding specific research in *family* psychopathology.

PROBLEMS IN STUDYING *FAMILY* PSYCHOPATHOLOGY

As we have seen, the study of psychopathology unavoidably means encounters with various general problems. Yet the concept of *family* psychopathology has an extra, systemic quality to it, making the difficulties in its study even more severe. Let us therefore first look at the systemic nature of family psychopathology.

Dependence of Method on Theory

Psychopathology is pathology of the psyche. This straightforward definition immediately gives rise to the question of whose psyche we are referring to when we address the concept of family psychopathology. Are we dealing with the sum of all family members' pathologies, with the pathology of a "family psyche" yet to be defined, or with the pathology of the identified patient's psyche? The answers to these seemingly simple questions have been the subject of heated debates throughout the history of family psychology and therapy, and have varied considerably in accordance with developments in these fields.

The Transactional Approach

Initially, the key element in the definition of "family therapy" was the notion that pathology (or, to paraphrase the term, dysfunction) rested in the relationships among family members, rather than in their individual personality attributes. Consequently, the prescribed concepts were those of communication and information theory (Watzlawick, Beavin, & Jackson, 1967). Minuchin's group used the concept of "patterns of transaction," defined as recurring sequences of interpersonal actions (Minuchin, Rosman, & Baker, 1978). In the practice of most schools of family therapy, "psychopathology" per se was no longer referred to. An individual's maladaptive behavior was seen from a different angle, as an epiphenomenal symptom of the family system's functioning.

One possible approach to dealing with symptoms of this sort was changing the point of view—rephrasing pathology into the newly emerging systemic code of communications and transactions (i.e., reframing the problem). Doubtless this novel perspective of systems theory in psychology had its merits: The onus of blame could be lifted from the individual person, whether this was the symptomatic family member behavior therapy would concentrate on, or the "pathogenic mother" of early psychoanalytic thinking. This development allowed the problem of pathology to be opened up to familial and therapeutic negotiations. For the field of social psychiatry, however, more problems resulted, because the blame in a way had merely been shifted to another agent—the "schizophrenogenic system" (i.e., the family).

Constructivist Theory

In the 1980s, the field of systems-oriented psychology underwent a somewhat unexpected change (Maturana & Varela, 1980). Constructivist theory elaborated upon the idea of the observer's influence on observation in quite a fundamental way. Reframing the "linear" thinking of individual family members about the origin of problems was also considered to be beneficial, just as in the transactional approach; however, there was no longer one valid "systemic perspective" that would have the potential to resolve the conflicting individual views (von Schlippe & Schweitzer, 1996). Reality was constructed in much the same manner within each of the individual stances, and in principle none of the individual constructions (including the therapist's) could be superior or closer to reality, to the world of facts. Indeed, this world did not "exist" in any ontological sense, but owed its "existence" to individual constructions.

Thus, the individual was once again in charge, so that the field of systemic therapy and psychology in part returned to a person-centered view resurrected under the auspices of constructivism. The "system" of the original perspective was reintegrated into cognition in a way that did not deviate much from the thinking of the psychological and psychotherapeutic mainstream, except for its epistemological underpinnings.

The Dynamic Systems View

A third line of thought in psychology has made a connection to the interdisciplinary field of dynamic systems theory, especially to the branches of self-organization theory (Nicolis & Prigogine, 1977) or "synergetics" (Haken, 1983, 1996) and of chaos theory (Abraham & Shaw, 1992). In this view, the family is conceptualized as a complex system. Family behavior patterns—both functional and dysfunctional—emerge from this system by spontaneous self-organization. The focus is on the attribute of stability in these patterns ("attractors" in terms of dynamic systems theory). Therefore, treatment of family psychopathology means perturbating and destabilizing these attractors through therapeutic interventions (Hayes & Strauss, in press); reframing may be one item in a list of such interventions, but it need not have the philosophical implications that it has in the constructivist view. I share this dynamic systems view of psychopathology. Recently, I have outlined the integration of dynamic systems theory and self-organization research in psychology, using the concept of "processual Gestalts" (Tschacher, 1997).

In medicine and biology, an approach similar to the dynamic systems view—the concept of "dynamic diseases"—has provided valuable contributions to the understanding of disorders (an der Heiden, 1992; Bélair, Glass, an der Heiden, & Milton, 1995). This concept implies that the processing of a dynamic system (which is often nonlinear) underlies the symptoms of an individual. Accordingly, psychopathology is equivalent to a significant change within a system's dynamic regime, in that pathological behavior evolves out of healthy behavior by way of a bifurcation (a transition between two different dynamic regimes). In psychiatry, bipolar depression and schizophrenia are the primary disorders that have been analyzed from this angle (Gottschalk, Bauer, & Whybrow, 1995; Pezard et al., 1996; Tschacher et al., 1997).

In short, consensus on a working definition of family psychopathology must be reached to afford a platform for our analyses and to facilitate discussion of related methodological problems. If we choose the transactional view of strategic family therapy and similar approaches, little can be said without accounting for the interactional behavior in a family. Communicational variables must be recorded. The constructivist approach has relied mostly on qualitative and hermeneutical methods. The dynamic systems approach focuses on the quantification of processes that are modeled in order to describe and predict the dynamics of a system. This approach does not stipulate any specific type of data, as long as the data can be collected repeatedly to yield one or several time series. Variables may be on the macro level of a complex system (e.g., global family atmosphere) or on the mesoscopic or microscopic levels of the system (e.g., intensity of irritated mood in one specific family member).

At this juncture, I shall restrict the discussion to problems of the dynamic systems approach. Most of the quantitative research considerations of the transactional approach are included as they are covered by the methods of the dynamic systems approach as well. A minor difference may be the transactional approach's greater reliance on content-analytical methods (Brunner & Tschacher, 1995, 1996) and generally on the observation of nominal data (e.g., qualitative sequential analysis; Revenstorf & Vogel, 1989; Gottman & Roy, 1990). "Symbolic dynamics" may be called for here instead—a fledgling field in dynamic systems methodology, which may in the future afford better insight into the behavior of sequences of qualitative data (e.g., Rapp, Jiménez-Montano, Langs, Thomson, & Mees, 1991). Furthermore, I will not pursue the methodological issues of the constructivist view. As the objectivity of quantitative data receives little credit in constructivist theory, strict methods can only be of minor importance in this view. Why bother much with operationalization and data recording if all reality is constructed?

From the viewpoint of dynamic systems theory, the methodological problems that must be dealt with in family psychopathology research can be grouped as follows. First, there is the pivotal topic of how to analyze a dynamic characteristic of a family, such as its psychological state, its psychopathology, or its well-being (see "Analysis of Dynamics," below). Second, and as a result, we are confronted with the question of how to generalize the findings of dynamic analysis (see "Single-System Approach or Multiple-Systems Approach?," below).

Analysis of Dynamics

The Static and Dynamic Principles

In contemporary psychology and psychiatry, there are two opposing principles: the static and the dynamic principles (Table 19.1). These two principles can be differentiated on the basis of the respective phenomenological entities selected for investigation.

The static principle singles out those measures that are assumed to be

TABLE 19.1. Comparison of the Static and the Dynamic Principles in Empirical Psychological Research

	Static principle	Dynamic principle
Philosophical background	Eleatics Platonic philosophy	Heraclitus Hegelian philosophy
Target variables	Traits, constants describing an individual or social system	Momentary states $x(t)$ of an individual or social system
Single-system measurement variance is . . .	Error	Dynamics plus error
Goal of investigation	Relations between true scores in a population (nomothetic approach)	1. Modeling the dynamic system 2. Predicting its behavior 3. Classifying dynamic invariants
Invariant	True score (single system) or mean of true scores (sample/population)	Dynamic invariant—that is, attractor (single system) or class of attractors (population)

inert in terms of time and situation. An example of a static measure is a personality trait—a hypothetical constant that underlies an individual's behavior, such as "verbal intelligence" or "psychoticism." The variance of this measure due to time and situation is regarded as error. As I have pointed out in the first section of this chapter, a retest of a static measure is considered to be just another measurement of the same virtual "true score." The variance resulting from retests does not indicate real change, but endangers the reliability of measurements. One may identify the Eleatic and Platonic origins of this principle: The static view is concerned with the unchanging idea that characterizes the system under study. Change is illusion.

The dynamic principle proceeds in quite another (Heraclitean and Hegelian) fashion. Change is considered as real and generic; for this reason, the dynamics of the system under study become the subject of measurement. The dynamic principle selects observables that span the phase space of the system (e.g., an individual or a family). A constant state—temporal variation is absent—will give a point in phase space. Yet this is not a common finding. Generally, the system describes a curve ("trajectory") into phase space that can be analyzed for its geometrical and topological characteristics. The trajectory may approach certain patterns ("attractors" or "processual Gestalts"). These patterns are the invariants of the dynamic approach. A geometric introduction to this theoretical framework can be found in Abraham and Shaw (1992). Kaplan and Glass (1995) present an accessible treatment of nonlinear dynamics. Psychological applications are given in Tschacher, Schiepek, and Brunner (1992) and Tschacher (1997).

Mainstream psychology and psychiatry are based largely on the static approach. The typical methods related to it are cross-sectional: Variables are measured in samples drawn from a population. The samples differ from one another only with respect to the experimental factor(s) induced by the investigator and with respect to stochastic differences. The scheme of analysis of variance can thus separate the variance of the experimental factor(s) from unaccountable error variance. Surveys of the published literature have shown that psychology and psychiatry rely almost exclusively on static methodology. Even in subdisciplines that are intrinsically dynamic in nature (e.g., developmental psychology or clinical psychology), the use of longitudinal methods is dramatically underrepresented. Thus, a serious gap ensues between research and application: Practitioners are confronted with changing and developing systems, whereas research does not address change but some hypothetical structure underlying it.

The dynamic principle therefore advocates various methods of time series analysis. As it is not within the scope of this chapter to give an introduction to time series methods, it may suffice to present a classification

TABLE 19.2. Overview of Linear Time Series Methods

	Autoregressive moving average (ARMA) models	State space approach	Factor analysis	Spectral analysis
Description	Temporal correlation as linear regression (AR) and/or weighed stochastic input (MA)	(Multivariate) Analysis of canonical correlations in time series	Correlational analysis of items × time matrix (O technique and T technique)	Time series = sum of sine and cosine components (Fourier transformation)
Characteristics	Univariate, stochastic	Multivariate, stochastic	Multivariate	Univariate, deterministic
Goals	Prediction, description	Multivariate prediction, description; interaction between time series	Data reduction and description; linear dimensionality	Description, detection of periodicity
Reference	Box & Jenkins (1976)	Chatfield (1989)	Cattell (1966)	Bloomfield (1976)

and overview of these methods in Tables 19.2 and 19.3. Table 19.2 covers linear analysis, whereas Table 19.3 covers nonlinear methods.

The Goals of Investigation

Given the premise that family psychopathology may be investigated like any other dynamic characteristic of families, the goals of investigation can be formulated as follows:

1. The dynamics of psychopathology are analyzed in a certain family that has been observed (the single-system approach). In terms of dynamics, we formulate a model of the dynamics.

2. The influences of various variables on the dynamics are studied. This analysis may be intrasystemic, yielding the interaction among different variables of a multivariate system. If environmental variables have been recorded, the interaction between the system and its environment can be modeled in much the same way.

3. The results of analysis can be utilized in several ways. Obviously, the results may themselves stand for a dynamic description of the system we are interested in. In addition, we may use the dynamic model to generate predictions of what may be expected from the future evolution of the system or what the system's response to intervention will be. Finally, several possibilities exist for generalizing from the single-system results; these possibilities are discussed later.

TABLE 19.3. Overview of Nonlinear Time Series Methods

	Lyapounov exponents	Dimension analysis	Nonlinear forecasting
Description	Divergence of neighboring trajectories	Scaling laws in embedding spaces	Prediction of future values using the known dynamics of nearest neighbors
Result	Estimation of the largest exponent (indicator of chaos)	(Fractal) Dimension of an attractor	Predictability within time series
Reference	Wolf, Swift, Swinney, & Vastano (1985)	Theiler (1990)	Sugihara & May (1990)

Case Example

The prerequisites and problems of time series modeling may be best illustrated by means of a case example. Fred and Gina, pseudonyms for a young married couple, volunteered to participate in a study that required them to record various aspects of their moods/feelings on an hourly basis during 30 days of vacation at home.

Goal of Study. The goal of this study in the context of this chapter was to provide an example of a dynamic model of a dyad. This study may serve as an analogy to explorations of family psychopathology (e.g., Tschacher & Scheier, 1995).

Method. The data were collected by means of small pocket computers (cf. Perrez & Reicherts, 1992), which gave a signal every hour requesting information from Fred and Gina on a number of Likert scales. The seven basic items were as follows: "good–bad mood," "agitated–calm," "depressed–serene," "angry–peaceful," "hesitating–spontaneous," "lazy–active," and "lonely–cared for." Each spouse rated all items both for himself or herself and for his or her perception of the other spouse. This resulted in $k = 28$ items assessed at $n = 424$ points during the waking hours of 30 consecutive days.

The method of choice for time series analysis would be to compute an appropriate state space representation (using SAS software) of Fred and Gina's interactions (see Table 19.2). Here the first problem was encountered: If all interrelations of all 28 variables were to be assessed, a minimum of $28^2 = 784$ parameters of the model would have to be fitted; this number exceeded even the number of observations. Therefore data reduction became an obligatory first step before time series analysis could be initiated.

Data reduction was easily accomplished by means of an appropriate principal-components analysis (PCA), by which the mood items were factorized across observations (T technique; see Table 19.2). In this case

PCA showed that the seven mood items could be compressed into two factors. Factor 1 loaded on the items "good mood," "calm," "serene," "peaceful," and "cared for," and was labeled "relaxation." Factor 2 loaded on the items "spontaneous" and "active," and was labeled "spontaneity." With this two-component description, new time series of factor loadings could be generated. Then the resulting time series of these factors could be analyzed: Fred's relaxation; Fred's perception of Gina's relaxation; Fred's spontaneity; Fred's perception of Gina's spontaneity; Gina's relaxation; Gina's perception of Fred's relaxation; Gina's spontaneity; and Gina's perception of Fred's spontaneity.

Computing the state space model engendered several methodological problems. Because these were of a more technical nature, I merely list them without going into detail: The problem of missing data had to be considered; the order of the model had to be specified (lag 1 model or higher-order model?); and the stationarity of time series could become a problem.

Results. The results of the analysis of Fred and Gina's interactions are summarized by the graphs in Figure 19.1. The criterion of parsimony (holding the ratio "estimated parameters to available data" down; Akaike's information criterion) proposed a model of lag 1: This model gave all the interactions of factors at time $t - 1$ (1 hour before) with factors at time t (now). Only significant interactions are shown.

All variables were positively autocorrelated; that is, they had sequential stability. This is symbolized by the horizontal arrows in Figure 19.1. For example, if Fred's relaxation was high at time $t - 1$, it would probably be high 1 hour later (at time t). All the other arrows depicted in Figure 19.1 can be interpreted in the same manner. Gina's relaxation was related to Gina's spontaneity 1 hour later, and vice versa. The recursive temporal interactions between Gina's mood factors thus constituted a feedback subsystem in the model of the dyad. Other interactions seemed quite trivial: Gina's spontaneity enhanced Fred's perception of her spontaneity. Still other parts of the model were reminiscent of Ronald Laing's "Jack and Jill" poems (Laing, 1970). Whereas Gina's perception of Fred's spontaneity enhanced her own spontaneity, Fred's perception of Gina's relaxation tended to damp his own relaxation. Because this study is discussed here only because of the methodological paradigm used, I shall not focus on interpretations of the findings.

Discussion of Methodological Results. The method of state space representation is a linear method, because it is based on linear regressions of one (lagged) variable to another variable. Decisions for linear methods can be questionable, especially as there are theoretical reasons to assume that psychosocial systems are often intrinsically nonlinear (e.g., they may be self-organizing or chaotic; see Guastello, 1995). Unfortunately, little is known about what kind of nonlinearity has to be expected in such systems.

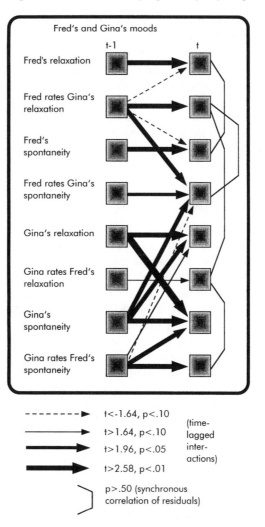

FIGURE 19.1. Graphic display of state space representation of a dyad's interactions.

Furthermore, multivariate nonlinear methods are only just being developed (Pritchard & Theiler, 1994). Therefore, it is reasonable to start from the parsimonious assumption of linearity. Our simulations with linear methods have shown that in the case of known multivariate nonlinear systems, the linear state space method correctly detects the linear interactions, whereas it misses the nonlinear ones; thus, linear methods may be trusted to give conservative results (i.e., they do not yield false positives).

The method of state space representation was applied here to model a dyadic psychosocial system. I could also have used this method as an instrument for making *predictions* about this couple's interaction. Predicting future behavior by means of time series methods has found different applications in psychology; the obvious application would be to predict individual behavior in order to intervene appropriately—the daily work of a therapist. Yet, given the tedious task of data recording, this option has scarcely been used systematically in psychology and psychopathology. Predicting is also used as a means to describe the determinism (i.e., the predictability) of a system in the context of reaching generalizations from time series models (Sugihara & May, 1990). This subject is discussed in the following section.

Single-System Approach or Multiple-Systems Approach?

The arguments and the example above have dealt with idiographic usages of the dynamic methods. In my opinion, it is one of the great advantages of this approach that single systems can be explored and modeled quantitatively. But undoubtedly we are also interested in nomothetic statements, as we wish to generalize from samples of many similar systems. To reach conclusions of this kind, the dynamic approach proceeds by combining several or many single-system studies in a systematic way. This "hybrid" approach of aggregating single-system studies is still only in its infancy (see Tschacher, 1996). Nevertheless, the prospect of "having one's cake and eating it too"—that is, of integrating the virtues of single-system modeling into the cross-sectional statistical procedures of nomothetic psychology—is very promising. I therefore outline this hybrid dynamic approach, with a special emphasis on methodological considerations.

Bootstrap Approach to Time Series Analysis

Consider the following quite common state of affairs: One has the opportunity to measure a single system extensively, but there is no available frame of reference or standard to interpret this isolated observation. It is therefore impossible to enter the cross-sectional tableau of hypothesis testing. Nonetheless, one may have found some interesting dynamic invariant in this given system (say, $\omega = 42$), but cannot interpret it (Ruelle, 1990). In other words, the ω_i of a control sample are sadly lacking.

Bootstrap testing is one possible avenue out of this impasse, because it helps to expand time series modeling by supplying cross-sectional statistics. "Bootstrapping" refers to the art of getting out of a swamp by pulling oneself up by one's bootstraps. The procedure in the context of the dynamic systems approach is to generate surrogate data based on the data of the system that is actually studied. One can consequently compute the ω_s of the surrogates and compare the actual ω of the empirical system with the distribution of these pseudocontrols (Theiler, Galdrakian, Longtin, Eubank, & Farmer, 1992; Scheier & Tschacher, 1996).

It is essential to find useful ways of generating surrogate data. One basic possibility is to randomize the sequence of the empirical time series, and perform the ω computation with a sample of randomly sequenced "time series." The results will indicate whether the sequence in the empirical time series is nonrandom with respect to measure ω. If the ω that is found empirically deviates significantly from the distribution of ω_s, we may reject the null hypothesis that the empirical system has random sequence. Additional null hypotheses can be tested (e.g., using surrogates that have the same linear autocorrelation as the empirical time series).

Several studies in the field of psychopathology have used the bootstrap method to evaluate time series (Gottschalk et al., 1995; Pezard et al., 1996; Tschacher et al., 1997). Our own study (Tschacher et al., 1997) investigated courses of schizophrenic symptomatology (consisting of daily ratings over periods of more than 200 days). The predictability of the time series was computed (the measure ω), which was then compared to predictabilities of different sets of surrogate data. We showed that 8 out of 14 empirical courses displayed the "fingerprints" of nonlinear sequences, whereas 4 courses were linear–stochastic and 2 were random sequences. This finding corroborates our assumption that schizophrenia should be viewed as a dynamic disease with nonlinear causality. Gottschalk et al. (1995) and Pezard et al. (1996) found analogous evidence in bipolar depression, using mood ratings and electroencephalographic (EEG) data, respectively.

Combining Longitudinal with Cross-Sectional Methods

The bootstrap approach is a possible way to integrate cross-sectional statistics into the longitudinal research design set forth in this chapter. In many instances, it is possible to make observations that contain dynamic as well as cross-sectional information. Such a study design provides the option of modeling/predicting each system separately, using the dynamic approach; in addition, it allows for comparisons of the single dynamic models by the further cross-sectional processing of dynamic findings. Thus the argument put forward at the beginning of this chapter—that cross-sectional analysis of dynamic state variables can be misleading—is circumvented: The values that go into statistical analysis are themselves results of a first stage of analysis.

For example, in the descriptive study of psychosocial crises mentioned earlier in this chapter (Tschacher, 1996), 34 patients used diaries to record their tension, activity, and mood throughout treatment. A control group of 20 individuals kept diaries of their daily lives. For each individual, the state space parameters were computed, yielding 9 regression values per "system" (see Figure 19.1). Then the values of the entire sample were cluster-analyzed. The clusters could be interpreted as containing individuals with similar dynamics. This method revealed that depressive patients as well as control subjects could be clearly distinguished from other patients.

When this combined method is used, several methodological considerations are necessary. The parameters that characterize the single dynamic models must be comparable, on the one hand; on the other, they should incorporate all the specific, even idiosyncratic, information of the individual dynamics. Therefore, one standard modeling technique must be found that can be meaningfully applied in each single time series analysis. Methods that filter data to account for nonstationarity (e.g., differencing techniques) cannot be used at all—or must be used in the same way in all cases of the sample. Yet the price to be paid for comparability is usually surpassed by the value of generalizability, which is supplied by the hybrid approach.

DISCUSSION

In addressing the methodological problems of family psychopathology research, I have argued in favor of a dynamic systems approach in this field. The pros and cons of the traditional cross-sectional hypothesis tests versus the longitudinal methodology of the dynamic approach have not been discussed at great length here (but see Tschacher et al., 1992; Abraham & Gilgen, 1995). In the end, both approaches may well be united in what I have termed a "hybrid" methodology. In any case, it is essential that the dimension of time be considered, either by applying time series modeling or by computing temporal invariants to be fed into a subsequent cross-sectional test. To sum up this chapter, I should like to enumerate some methodological prospects for the future of family psychopathology research, on the condition that a dynamic system approach is used.

In my view, psychology as a whole has suffered from a surplus of basic dichotomies. One such dichotomy is the mind versus body discussion: Is psychology the science of the mind, of behavior, or of brain physiology? Another, not unrelated question concerns the distinction between hermeneutic/phenomenological views and natural science views of psychology (and systemic psychology). Still another dichotomy divides psychological methodology into idiographic research on systems in the field versus experimental, laboratory-based, nomothetic research. My conclusion from watching the continuing struggle of these opposing camps is that some synthesis, Hegelian or not, is needed. I advocate a dynamic research program as a means to resolve the seemingly irreconcilable differences in psychological science.

Experiment or field study? The *raison d'être* of experimentation is detecting causality. Randomization of all potential influences except for the willfully varied independent variable cannot be achieved in the natural setting of a psychological system (e.g., a family). As is well known, co-occurrence (measured by some correlation coefficient) must not be equated with causal relation. Must we therefore resort to the laboratory and the experimental setting to differentiate causality from simple co-occurrence? I think not, for with due caution we can equate causality with time-lagged co-occurrence. The dynamic approach exploits the naturally occurring "experimentation" that results from the spontaneous fluctuations of systems' variables and their ongoing mutual reactions to one another. Thus essentially the same information about interaction is provided in repeated time series observations as in experimental settings (thereby satisfying internal validity). At the same time, the dynamic approach has the decisive advantage of greater external validity. My conclusion is that the experiment–field study dichotomy is only a superficial one, provided that a dynamic approach can be employed.

Dynamic diseases. The notion of "dynamic diseases," mentioned earlier in the chapter, was introduced by mathematical biology and applied to psychiatry early in this century (Gjessing, 1932; Cronin, 1973). In my opinion, this concept promises to yield unitary approaches to systems, regardless of what the nature of the variables may be. Of course, one must take care not to mix the levels on which measurement is performed. When, for example, schizophrenia is referred to as a dynamic disease, the dynamics of EEG measures and of behavioral ratings are not on the same time scale, nor will they show identical dynamic properties.

A *dynamic "library."* An important argument for any methodology in science is its modularity. In other words, how can the results of thousands of single studies be compared to one another? Will they lead to a synthetic view of a scientific field, or will their mere numbers discourage any attempt at developing a unifying theory? One method that is increasingly being endorsed for its relevance in this respect is statistical meta-analysis. In particular, meta-analyses have been applied to questions of clinical psychology (Grawe, Donati, & Bernauer, 1998). In the field of dynamics, Stewart (1995) has proposed using topological invariants of dynamic attractors (Abarbanel, Brown, Sidorowich, & Tsimring, 1993) as entries in a universal "library" of systems dynamics. According to this idea, research on dynamic diseases would entail the compilation of the topological properties of observed attractors in, say, schizophrenia dynamics. It might turn out that schizophrenia of the paranoid type, as documented by daily behavior ratings, is characterized best by a three-dimensional Moebius strip with a hole in the middle. I should not be surprised if the bootstrap approach of classifying single systems might eventually be the starting point for a modular library of time series in psychopathology. Effect sizes of observed time series that have been compared to several surrogate null hypotheses would be an ideal basis for such a library.

Methodology in psychopathology research should be judged not only by its potential to obtain clear results in single studies, but by its potential to organize the increment of knowledge. Methodology has a responsibility to serve theory by looking beyond isolated findings.

488   RESEARCH ISSUES

REFERENCES

Abarbanel, H. D. I., Brown, R., Sidorowich, J. J., & Tsimring, L. S. (1993). The analysis of observed chaotic data in physical systems. *Reviews of Modern Physics, 65,* 1331–1392.

Abraham, F. D., & Gilgen, A. R. (Eds.). (1995). *Chaos theory in psychology.* Westport, CT: Praeger.

Abraham, R. H., & Shaw, C. D. (1992). *Dynamics: The geometry of behavior.* Redwood City, CA: Addison-Wesley.

an der Heiden, U. (1992). Chaos in health and disease—Phenomenology and theory. In W. Tschacher, G. Schiepek, & E. J. Brunner (Eds.), *Self-organization and clinical psychology* (pp. 55–87). Berlin: Springer-Verlag.

Banerjee, S., Sibbald, P. R., & Maze, J. (1990). Quantifying the dynamics of order and organization in biological systems. *Journal of Theoretical Biology, 143,* 91–111.

Bélair, J., Glass, L., an der Heiden, U., & Milton, J. (Eds.). (1995). *Dynamical disease.* Woodbury, NY: American Institute of Physics Press.

Bloomfield, P. (1976). *Fourier analysis of time series: An introduction.* New York: Wiley.

Bortz, G. (1993). *Lehrbuch der Statistik (für Sozialwissenschaftler) [Textbook in statistics (for social scientists)].* Berlin: Springer-Verlag.

Box, G. E. P., & Jenkins, G. (1976). *Time series analysis: Forecasting and control.* San Francisco: Holden-Day.

Brunner, E. J., & Tschacher, W. (1995). Quantifizierende Inhaltsanalyse [Quantifying content analysis]. In E. König & P. Zedler (Eds.), *Bilanz qualitativer Forschung [Survey of qualitative research]* (pp. 619–632). Weinheim, Germany: Deutscher Studien Verlag.

Brunner, E. J., & Tschacher, W. (1996). Inhaltsanalyse einer Gruppensitzung: Welches Thema setzt sich in der Gruppe durch? In W. Bos & C. Tarnai (Eds.), *Computerunterstützte Inhaltsanalyse in den Empirischen Sozialwissenschaften: Theorie—Anwendung—Software [Computer-aided content analysis in the empirical social sciences: Theory—application—software]* (pp. 53–63). Münster, Germany: Waxmann.

Brunner, E. J., Tschacher, W., Ruff, A., & Quast, C. (1997). Veränderungsprozesse in Paarbeziehungen—eine empirische Studie aus der Sicht der Selbstorganisationstheorie [Process of change in a couple's relationship: An empirical study from the aspect of self-organization]. In G. Schiepek & W. Tschacher (Eds.), *Synergetik in Psychologie und Psychiatrie [Synergetics in psychology and psychiatry]* (pp. 221–234). Braunschweig, Germany: Vieweg.

Campbell, D. T., & Stanley, J. C. (1967). *Experimental and quasi-experimental designs for research.* Chicago: Rand McNally.

Cattell, R. B. (Ed.). (1966). *Handbook of multivariate experimental psychology.* Chicago: Rand McNally.

Cattell, R. B., & Warburton, F. W. (1967). *Objective personality and motivation tests.* Chicago: University of Illinois Press.

Chatfield, C. (1989). *The analysis of time series: An introduction.* London: Chapman & Hall.

Cohen, J. (1990). Things I have learned (so far). *American Psychologist, 45,* 1304–1312.

Cronin, J. (1973). The Danzinger–Elmergreen theory of periodic catatonic schizophrenia. *Bulletin Mathematical Biology, 35,* 689–707.

Crutchfield, J. P. (1994). Observing complexity and the complexity of observation. In H. Atmanspacher & G. J. Dalenoort (Eds.), *Inside versus outside* (pp. 235–272). Berlin: Springer-Verlag.

Dawis, R. V. (1987). Scale construction. *Journal of Counseling Psychology, 34,* 481–489.

Gjessing, R. (1932). Beiträge zur Kenntnis der Pathophysiologie des katatonen Stupors [Contributions to the understanding of pathophysiology in catatonic stupor]. *Archives für Psychiatrie, 96,* 319–393.

Gottman, J. M., & Roy, A. K. (1990). *Sequential analysis: A guide for behavioral researchers.* Cambridge, England: Cambridge University Press.

Gottschalk, A., Bauer, M. S., & Whybrow, P. C. (1995). Evidence of chaotic mood variation in bipolar disorder. *Archives of General Psychiatry, 52,* 947–959.

Grawe, K., Donati, R., & Bernauer, F. (1998). *Psychotherapy in transition: From speculation to science.* Seattle, WA: Hogrefe & Huber.

Green, B. F. (1981). A primer of testing. *American Psychologist, 36,* 1001–1011.

Guastello, S. J. (1995). *Chaos, catastrophe, and human affairs: Applications of nonlinear dynamics to work, organizations, and social evolution.* Hillsdale, NJ: Erlbaum.

Haken, H. (1983). *Synergetics—An introduction.* Berlin: Springer-Verlag.

Haken, H. (1996). *Principles of brain functioning: A synergetic approach to brain activity, behavior, and cognition.* Berlin: Springer-Verlag.

Hayes, A. M., & Strauss, J. L. (in press). Dynamic systems theory as a paradigm for the study of change in psychotherapy: An application to cognitive therapy for depression. *Journal of Consulting and Clinical Psychology.*

Jacobson, N. S., & Truax, P. (1991). Clinical significance: A statistical approach to defining meaningful change in psychotherapy research. *Journal of Consulting and Clinical Psychology, 59,* 12–19.

Kaplan, D., & Glass, L. (1995). *Understanding nonlinear dynamics.* New York: Springer.

Kazdin, A. E. (Ed.). (1992). *Methodological issues and strategies in clinical research.* Washington, DC: American Psychological Association.

L'Abate, L., & Baggett, M. S. (1997). *The self in the family: classification of personality, criminality, and psychopathology.* New York: Wiley.

Laing, R. D. (1970). *Knots.* London: Tavistock.

Maturana, H. R., & Varela, F. J. (1980). *Autopoiesis and cognition: The realization of the living.* Dordrecht, The Netherlands: Reidel.

Minuchin, S., Rosman, B., & Baker, L. (1978). *Psychosomatic families: Anorexia nervosa in context.* Cambridge, MA: Harvard University Press.

Nicolis, G., & Prigogine, I. (1977). *Self-organization in non-equilibrium systems.* New York: Wiley.

Perrez, M., & Reicherts, M. (1992). *Stress, coping, and health: A situation–behavior approach.* Toronto: Hogrefe & Huber.

Pezard, L., Nandrino, J.-L., Renault, B., Massioui, F. E., Allilaire, J.-F., Varela, F. J., & Martinerie, J. (1996). Depression as a dynamical disease. *Biological Psychiatry, 39,* 991–999.

Pritchard, D., & Theiler, J. (1994). Generating surrogate data for time series with several simultaneously measured variables. *Physical Review Letters, 73,* 951–954.

Rapp, P. E., Jiménez-Montano, M. A., Langs, R. J., Thomson, L., & Mees, A. I. (1991). Toward a quantitative characterization of patient–therapist communication. *Mathematical Biosciences, 105,* 207–227.

Revenstorf, D., & Vogel, B. (1989). Zur Analyse qualitativer Verlaufsdaten—ein Überblick [On the analysis of qualitative sequential data: A summary]. In F. Petermann (Ed.), *Einzelfallanalyse [Individual case analysis]* (pp. 235–256). Munich: Oldenbourg.

Rössler, O. E. (1996). *Endophysics—the world of an internal observer.* Singapore: World Scientific.

Ruelle, D. (1990). Deterministic chaos: The science and the fiction. *Proceedings of the Royal Society of London, 427A,* 241–248.

Scheier, C., & Tschacher, W. (1996). Appropriate algorithms for nonlinear time series analysis in psychology. In W. Sulis & A. Combs (Eds.), *Nonlinear dynamics in human behavior* (pp. 27–43). Singapore: World Scientific.

Sedlmeier, P., & Gigerenzer, G. (1989). Do studies of statistical power have an effect on the power of studies? *Psychological Bulletin, 105,* 309–316.

Stewart, H. B. (1995). *Recent trends in dynamical systems theory.* Lecture given at the Annual Conference of the Society for Chaos Theory in Psychology and the Life Sciences, Adelphi University, Garden City, NY.

Sugihara, G., & May, R. (1990). Nonlinear forecasting as a way of distinguishing chaos from measurement error in time series. *Nature, 344,* 734–741.

Theiler, J. (1990). Statistical precision of dimension estimators. *Physical Review A, 41,* 3038–3051.

Theiler, J., Galdrakian, B., Longtin, A., Eubank, S., & Farmer, J. D. (1992). Using surrogate data to detect nonlinearity in time series. In M. Casdagli & S. Eubank (Eds.), *Nonlinear modeling and forecasting* (pp. 163–188). Redwood City, CA: Addison-Wesley.

Tschacher, W. (1996). The dynamics of psychosocial crises—Time courses and causal models. *Journal of Nervous and Mental Disease, 184,* 172–179.

Tschacher, W. (1997). *Prozessgestalten—Theorie, Methodik und empirische Studien zur Selbstorganisation in der Psychologie [Processual Gestalt: Theory, methodology and empirical studies on self-organization in psychology].* Göttingen, Germany: Hogrefe.

Tschacher, W., & Scheier, C. (1995). Analyse komplexer psychologischer Systeme: II. Verlaufsmodelle und Komplexität einer Paartherapie [Analysis of complex psychological systems: II. Sequential models and complexity in couples therapy]. *System Familie, 8,* 160–171.

Tschacher, W., Scheier, C., & Hashimoto, Y. (1997). Dynamical analysis of schizophrenia courses. *Biological Psychiatry, 41,* 428–437.

Tschacher, W., Scheier, C., & Grawe, K. (1998). Order and pattern formation in psychotherapy. *Nonlinear Dynamics, Psychology and Life Sciences, 2,* 195–215.

Tschacher, W., Schiepek, G., & Brunner, E. J. (Eds.). (1992). *Self-organization and clinical psychology: Empirical approaches to synergetics in psychology.* Berlin: Springer-Verlag.

Tukey, J. W. (1979). Methodology and the statistician's responsibility for both accuracy and relevance. *Journal of the American Statistical Association, 74,* 786–793.

von Schlippe, A., & Schweitzer, J. (1996). *Lehrbuch der systemischen Therapie und Beratung* [*Textbook of systemic therapy and counseling*]. Göttingen, Germany: Vandenhoeck & Ruprecht.

Watzlawick, P., Beavin, J. H., & Jackson, D. D. (1967). *Pragmatics of human communication: A study of interactional patterns, pathologies, and paradoxes.* New York: Norton.

Wolf, A., Swift, J. B., Swinney, H. L., & Vastano, J. (1985). Determining Lyapounov exponents from a time series. *Physica D, 16,* 285–317.

Author Index

Page numbers in italics refer to reference list entries.

493

Subject Index